Kelly L. Stratton • Alicia K. Morgans
Editors

Urologic Oncology

Multidisciplinary Care for Patients

Springer

Editors
Kelly L. Stratton
Urology
University of Oklahoma Health
Science Center
Oklahoma City, OK, USA

Alicia K. Morgans
Medical Oncology
Dana-Farber Cancer Institute
Boston, MA, USA

ISBN 978-3-030-89890-8 ISBN 978-3-030-89891-5 (eBook)
https://doi.org/10.1007/978-3-030-89891-5

This Springer imprint is published by the registered company Springer Nature Switzerland AG
The registered company address is: Gewerbestrasse 11, 6330 Cham, Switzerland

Contents

Contributors

A. Ari Hakimi Urology Service, Department of Surgery, Memorial Sloan Kettering Cancer Center, New York, NY, USA

Mohammad Atiq National Cancer Institute, Bethesda, MD, USA

Amishi Bajaj Department of Radiation Oncology, Robert H. Lurie Comprehensive Cancer Center, Northwestern University, Feinberg School of Medicine, Chicago, IL, USA

Maria I. Carlo Department of Medicine, Memorial Sloan Kettering Cancer Center, New York, NY, USA

Heather H. Cheng Fred Hutchinson Cancer Research Center and Division of Medical Oncology, Department of Medicine, University of Washington School of Medicine, Seattle, WA, USA

Wesley H. Chou Harvard Medical School, Boston, MA, USA

Alexander P. Cole Division of Urological Surgery, Brigham and Women's Hospital, Harvard Medical School, Boston, MA, USA

Michael S. Cookson Department of Urology and Stephenson Oklahoma Cancer Center at the University of Oklahoma Health Sciences Center, Oklahoma City, OK, USA

Department of Urology, University of Oklahoma Health Sciences Center & The Stephenson Cancer Center, Oklahoma City, OK, USA

Ithaar Derweesh Department of Urology, University of California San Diego, La Jolla, CA, USA

Benjamin M. Eilender Department of Urology, Icahn School of Medicine, New York, NY, USA

Lauren A. Facchini Seattle Cancer Care Alliance, Seattle, WA, USA

Kassem S. Faraj Department of Urology, Mayo Clinic Arizona, Phoenix, AZ, USA

Yu Fujiwara Department of Medicine, Icahn School of Medicine at Mount Sinai, Mount Sinai Beth Israel, New York, NY, USA

Matthew D. Galsky Department of Medicine, Icahn School of Medicine at Mount Sinai, Mount Sinai Beth Israel, New York, NY, USA

Leonard G. Gomella The Bernard W. Godwin Jr, Department of Urology, Sidney Kimmel Cancer Center, Jefferson Health, Thomas Jefferson University, Philadelphia, PA, USA

Brendan J. Guercio Department of Medicine, Memorial Sloan Kettering Cancer Center, New York, NY, USA

Zineb Hamilou Department of Medicine, Division on Hematology Oncology, Centre Hospitalier de l'Université de Montréal, Montreal, QC, Canada

Nathan Hirshman Duke University Medical Center, Department of Medicine, Durham, NC, USA

Gopa Iyer Department of Medicine, Memorial Sloan Kettering Cancer Center, New York, NY, USA

Juan Javier-DesLoges Department of Urology, University of California San Diego, La Jolla, CA, USA

Georgia Sofia Karachaliou Duke University Hospital, Department of Medicine/ Division of Medical Oncology, Durham, NC, USA

Andrew B. Katims Department of Urology, Icahn School of Medicine, New York, NY, USA

Max F. Kelsten Department of Medicine, Feinberg School of Medicine at Northwestern University, Chicago, IL, USA

Adam S. Kibel Division of Urological Surgery, Brigham and Women's Hospital, Harvard Medical School, Boston, MA, USA

Daniel Lin Department of Urology, University of Washington, Seattle, WA, USA

Seattle Cancer Care Alliance, Seattle, WA, USA

Ravi Madan Genitourinary Malignancy Branch, National Cancer Institute, Bethesda, MD, USA

Roy Mano Department of Urology, Tel-Aviv Sourasky Medical Center, Sackler School of Medicine, Tel-Aviv University, Tel Aviv-Yafo, Israel

J. Ryan Mark Department of Urology, Sidney Kimmel Cancer Center, Thomas Jefferson University, Philadelphia, PA, USA

Viraj Master Department of Urology, Emory School of Medicine, Atlanta, GA, USA

Winship Cancer Institute, Atlanta, GA, USA

Rana R. McKay Department of Medicine/Division of Hematology-Oncology, University of California San Diego, La Jolla, CA, USA

Department of Medical Oncology, Moores UCSD Cancer Center, La Jolla, CA, USA

Hirotaka Miyashita Tisch Cancer Institute, Icahn School of Medicine at Mount Sinai, New York, NY, USA

Alicia K. Morgans Department of Medical Oncology, Dana-Farber Cancer Institute, Boston, MA, USA

Michael J. Morris Memorial Sloan Kettering Cancer Center, New York, NY, USA

Kelvin A. Moses Vanderbilt University Medical Center, Division of Urologic Oncology, Nashville, TN, USA

Kathleen M. Olson Department of Urology, Mayo Clinic Arizona, Phoenix, AZ, USA

Daniel C. Parker Department of Urology, University of Oklahoma Health Sciences Center & The Stephenson Cancer Center, Oklahoma City, OK, USA

John L. Pfail Department of Urology, Icahn School of Medicine, New York, NY, USA

Sarah P. Psutka Department of Urology, University of Washington, Seattle, WA, USA

Seattle Cancer Care Alliance, Seattle, WA, USA

Ali Aria Razmaria Memorial Sloan Kettering Cancer Center, New York, NY, USA

Soumyajit Roy Department of Radiation Oncology, Rush University Medical Center, Chicago, IL, USA

Fred Saad Department of Surgery, Division of Urology, Centre Hospitalier de l'Université de Montréal, Montreal, QC, Canada

Sean Sachdev Department of Radiation Oncology, Robert H. Lurie Comprehensive Cancer Center, Northwestern University, Feinberg School of Medicine, Chicago, IL, USA

Heiko Schoder Memorial Sloan Kettering Cancer Center, New York, NY, USA

John Sfakianos Department of Urology, Icahn School of Medicine, New York, NY, USA

Parminder Singh Department of Medicine/Division of Hematology and Oncology, Mayo Clinic Arizona, Phoenix, AZ, USA

Woodson W. Smelser Vanderbilt University Medical Center, Division of Urologic Oncology, Nashville, TN, USA

Daniel E. Spratt Department of Radiation Oncology, University Hospitals Seidman Cancer Center, Cleveland, OH, USA

Brittany M. Szymaniak Department of Urology, Feinberg School of Medicine at Northwestern University, Chicago, IL, USA

Quoc-Dien Trinh Division of Urological Surgery, Brigham and Women's Hospital, Harvard Medical School, Boston, MA, USA

Hong Truong Urology Service, Department of Surgery, Memorial Sloan Kettering Cancer Center, New York, NY, USA

Mark D. Tyson Department of Urology, Mayo Clinic Arizona, Phoenix, AZ, USA

Christopher J. D. Wallis Vanderbilt University Medical Center, Division of Urologic Oncology, Nashville, TN, USA

Elizabeth Wulff-Burchfield Internal Medicine, Divisions of Medical Oncology and Palliative Medicine, University of Kansas Medical Center, Kansas City, KS, USA

Tian Zhang Division of Hematology and Oncology, Department of Internal Medicine, University of Texas Southwestern Medical Center, Dallas, TX, USA

Chapter 1
Creating a Multidisciplinary Clinic

J. Ryan Mark and Leonard G. Gomella

Abbreviations

GU	Genitourinary
MDC	Multidisciplinary clinic
MDTB	Multidisciplinary tumor board
MIBC	Muscle-invasive bladder cancer
NAC	Neoadjuvant chemotherapy
SKCC	Sidney Kimmel Cancer Center

Introduction

Modern care of the patient with genitourinary (GU) cancer is complex. In particular, enormous controversy exists in the treatment decisions made by men diagnosed with prostate cancer. The sequence of treatments supported by international guidelines is a continuous mix of therapies delivered by highly skilled urologic, radiation, and medical oncologists. New systemic immunotherapies have toxicities outside the familiar complications of chemotherapy, often requiring input from additional specialists. The success of these and other new systemic agents has influenced the ever-evolving role of local surgical and radiation therapy for metastases, and systemic

J. R. Mark (✉)
Department of Urology, Sidney Kimmel Cancer Center, Thomas Jefferson University, Philadelphia, PA, USA
e-mail: james.r.mark@jefferson.edu

L. G. Gomella
The Bernard W. Godwin Jr, Department of Urology, Sidney Kimmel Cancer Center, Jefferson Health, Thomas Jefferson University, Philadelphia, PA, USA
e-mail: Leonard.gomella@jefferson.edu

K. L. Stratton, A. K. Morgans (eds.), *Urologic Oncology*,
https://doi.org/10.1007/978-3-030-89891-5_1

therapy is now increasingly used for localized disease – all this in an aging population with comorbidities while treating an organ system with consequential impacts on quality of life and sexual function.

How is "multidisciplinary prostate cancer care" defined? It encompasses collaborative patient care by a team of different specialists where all treatment options are discussed and individualized for each patient [1]. While this general definition exists in the field of oncology, the models of multidisciplinary clinic care can differ greatly. In its purest and arguably most effective form, a true multidisciplinary clinical setting should include real-time interaction between the various specialists and the patient. Other multidisciplinary practice models such as an agreement among specialists to follow defined care pathways or discussion of cases at tumor boards can be employed, but lack the impact of the real-time interactive model on patients, families, and trainees.

An essential element in this multidisciplinary approach to diseases such as prostate cancer is educating patients and involving them in medical decisions, a concept known as "shared decision-making." As noted by the US Institute of Medicine, shared decision-making is at the heart of patient-centered care that is "responsive to individual patient preferences, needs and values [2]." The so-called "paternalistic" approach to patient care, where physicians made the decision that they thought was best, is no longer considered to be the standard of care in medicine.

In an effort to improve the quality of care delivered by multiple specialists of different disciplines, it is unsurprising that efforts have focused on ways to streamline the patient experience and improve coordination among the care team. In our experience at our NCI-designated Sidney Kimmel Cancer Center at Thomas Jefferson University (SKCC), the multidisciplinary clinic has provided the ideal opportunity to achieve these goals and has resulted in improved satisfaction and patient outcomes [3]. We believe this is the first and longest continuously running MDC at an NCI-designated cancer center in the USA. Over the years many other centers have developed similar models of multidisciplinary clinic care. In this chapter we share our experience with this care delivery model and provide guidance to others who may be interested in developing a multidisciplinary clinic of their own.

Historical Perspective

The GU multidisciplinary clinic (MDC) at the SKCC was established in 1996 under the leadership of Dr. Leonard Gomella and radiation oncologist Dr. Richard Valicenti. While all tumor types such as bladder, kidney, and testicular are evaluated, prostate cancer diagnosis compromises up to 80% of patients seen. A major focus of our GU MDC has been to primarily help men and their families understand and face the challenging treatment decisions following a new prostate cancer diagnosis. We have been successful at using a team approach to offer men state-of-the-art oncology care by developing a clinical practice that serves as an educational resource for patients, their families, and also our residents and fellows in training. The organizational structure has changed over the years as patients' needs have evolved, but at its core the clinic has remained a place where patients with GU cancers can come to consult with urologic, radiation, and medical oncologists for education and treatment of their cancer. In 2014 we incorporated the first prostate cancer genetic testing clinic within our MDC [4].

Despite the original focus placed on prostate cancer care, the utility of the MDC extends to all our patients with genitourinary malignancies. Metastatic testicular cancer is a curable disease with combination chemotherapy and post-chemotherapy retroperitoneal lymphadenectomy. The value of a multidisciplinary approach to these typically younger men is self-evident, and the MDC at SKCC has been a convenient place to swiftly manage these men as a coordinated team. Having been operational throughout the eras of cytokine, targeted, and immunotherapies for renal cell carcinoma, our MDC has also been an invaluable location to discuss the role of cytoreductive nephrectomy, metastasectomy, and sequencing local therapy with systemic agents as well as evaluating patients for clinical trials. Small renal masses were also followed historically at the MDC where patients can discuss surveillance, partial nephrectomy, or ablative techniques together with urologists and interventional radiologists. The significant increase in the detection of small renal masses, defined as suspicious lesions less than 4 cm, resulted in us spinning off a small renal mass clinic in 1996 consisting of interventional radiologists and urologic oncologists [5]. Neoadjuvant chemotherapy prior to radical cystectomy for muscle invasive bladder cancer (MIBC) is now considered a standard of care, and we manage these patients in concert through the MDC. Specifically, for this population we have shown 70% of our patients receive neoadjuvant therapy compared to utilization rates of 20–40% reported in the literature [6]. The scenarios where patients benefit are abundant in this model across all our disease states.

Multidisciplinary clinics reflect an evolution of cancer patient care originating from multidisciplinary tumor boards (MDTBs). MDTBs have long been the mechanism to bring providers of different specialties together to discuss cancer management [7]. Patients are presented to the group for opinions on the best treatment recommendation. Alternatively, an already treated patient's case is presented as a didactic, and treatment options are discussed in retrospect. The value of MDTBs is evident as they are required for accreditation of a surgical cancer program by the American College of Surgeons Commission on Cancer Program [8].

Patients are benefitted by MDTBs as they increase adherence to national guidelines. In a study by Abraham et al., participation in a MDTB was the most significant factor contributing to guideline-based care in colorectal patients (OR 3.6, $p < 0.001$), and in another study of patients with esophageal cancer, presentation at a MDTB not only increased adherence to NCCN guidelines but also increased appropriate clinical staging (67% vs 97%, $p < 0.001$) and decreased the time to treatment (27 vs 16 days, $p < 0.001$) [9, 10]. Similar outcomes have been found when evaluating adherence to NCCN guidelines in the management of patients with prostate cancer. Hussein et al. found patients reviewed in their MDTB received treatment recommendations that were more likely to comply with NCCN guidelines than the recommendations patients received in the community (90% vs 64%, *p* not reported) [11].

Tumor boards have also been shown to influence disease management. Rao et al. describe that 26% of patients with prostate cancer presented at their MDTB had a change of the proposed treatment plan with a majority of changes made in patients with metastatic disease [12]. Scarberry et al. evaluated the impact their MDTB had in the management of patients with GU malignancies that were presented in conference. In their practice, all cancer cases are presented at MDTB, and this resulted in a management change for 18% of patients. Of particular interest is that physicians surveyed were only able to predict 10% of the cases that would have a management change illustrating, perhaps, our own bias and inability to select who should and shouldn't be presented in a multidisciplinary environment. The authors conclude that all cancer patients should be presented to a MDTB [13].

Not all studies, however, have found that MDTBs improve patient care. Lung cancer patients reviewed by Riedel et al. found no improvement in time to diagnosis or treatment following establishment of a MDTB [14]. A survey of 138 Veterans Affairs hospitals found that MDTBs did not contribute to any improvement in 20 of 27 cancer care metrics on multivariate analysis. One prostate cancer measure was noted to be improved in this study. Oral anti-androgen use before GnRH was initiated in men with metastatic disease (71% vs 82%, $p = 0.03$), though rates of adjuvant radiation therapy, concurrent ADT with EBRT, and ADT use for metastatic prostate cancer were not influenced by MDTBs [15]. The authors concluded that perhaps the structure or quality of physician involvement may have more to do with MDTB success than the format itself.

When optimized MDTBs can be an effective method of discussing complex care issues, however, Keating et al. have shown that engagement from all participating physicians is key. It has been estimated that over 50 physician hours per month are dedicated to these conferences where usually only one physician has met the patient. Therefore, the information presented regarding the patient's condition or treatment preferences is potentially biased because it was gathered viewing the problems through the prism of one specialty [7]. The MDC at SKCC was created to address these limitations by bringing the entire clinical care team to the patient and their family.

The Multidisciplinary Clinic at Sidney Kimmel Cancer Center Thomas Jefferson University

Multidisciplinary clinics vary widely in their organization as there is no universally accepted definition of this model of care. We ascribe to the principles put forth by Hong et al. that a true multidisciplinary care model fundamentally encompasses "collaborative patient care by a team of individuals where all diagnostic and treatment options are discussed and tailored for each patient." At its core, medical oncologists, radiation oncologists, and surgical oncologists are supported by pathologists, radiologists, geneticists, palliative care specialists, and representatives from nursing, nutrition, clinical trials, and social work to optimize patient care [1]. Sequential appointments in separate clinic locations coordinated by a nurse navigator as part of a cancer service line can streamline patient care; however, in developing our MDC, it was felt that true multidisciplinary care for our GU oncology patients must involve real-time interaction between the various specialists and the patient and their family. This is a necessity because treatment options and decisions can be extensive and at times controversial. The opportunity to address these issues in real time cannot be underestimated. With that philosophy in mind, we discuss the core components of our MDC at SKCC.

The basic operation of our MDC has previously been described, and our current updated 2021 organizational structure is shown in Fig. 1.1 [16]. The MDC is a weekly half-day clinic session where urologic, radiation, and medical oncologists independently evaluate and consult with a patient and their family to educate and guide their treatment decisions. Resident and fellows from their respective services participate as well as oncology trained advanced care providers. Patients are scheduled for clinic by the MDC nurse coordinator who arranges the transfer of patient records, imaging, and pathology slides. In the early days of our MDC, a post-clinic conference was held at noon to discuss the patients and their management. In the most recent iteration, all patients seen are reviewed in a MDTB conducted before the formal office hours. This conference includes participation of a pathologist and radiologist that provide second opinion reports of outside results. All available imaging and pathology are reviewed alongside the clinical history. A summary document is generated before the conference by our coordinator. Typically, the case is also reviewed and presented by a resident or fellow to the group. Possible treatment options are discussed alongside available clinical trials. A GU focused research coordinator attends the MDTB and MDC to help assess eligibility for enrollment. Additional needs are also addressed such as genetics consultation for germline testing or any anticipated additional support. Other multidisciplinary input from specialist teams like geriatric oncology or further evaluation by a dedicated molecular tumor board is considered.

Prior to arrival at the MDC, the patient is provided with educational materials by the nurse coordinator as well as relevant patient surveys such as the International Prostate Symptom Score and Sexual Activity Inventory for prostate cancer patients. Patients are then independently evaluated by each clinical service based on their clinical setting. If the situation warrants, additional consultants are added to their visit.

Separately, each physician team evaluates the patient. We encourage involvement of our trainees in this process for the interdisciplinary educational benefits this setting provides. Recommendations are discussed with the patient as in any ordinary clinic appointment before the next specialist performs their evaluation. At the conclusion of the appointment, the providers discuss their findings and, with rare exceptions, endorse the approach that was discussed at the preclinical MDTB. A representative presents the summary recommendation to the patient who then leaves the clinic with a treatment plan. Using this approach, we have been successful at

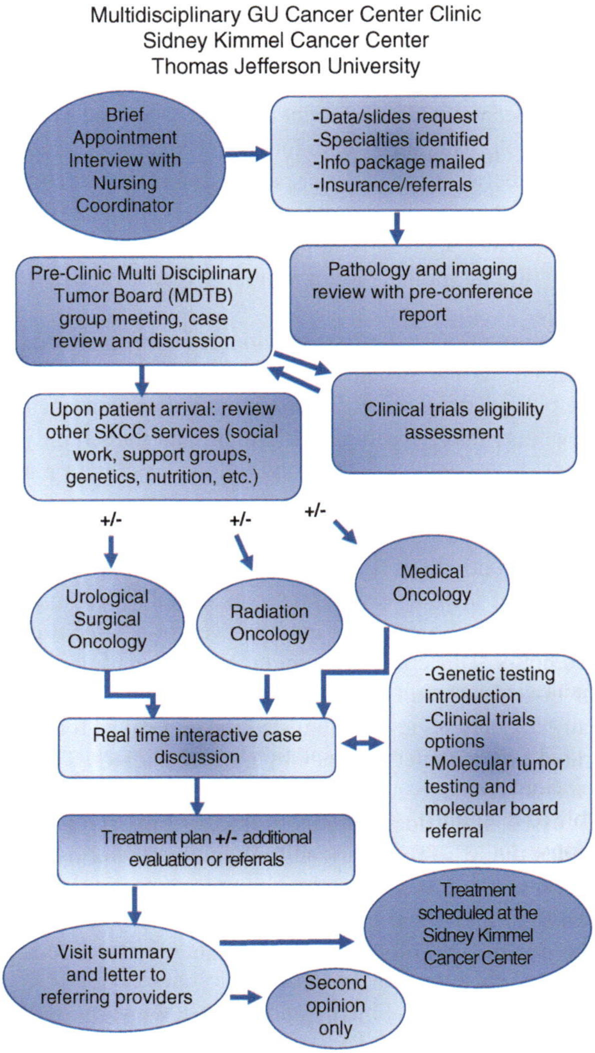

Fig. 1.1 Current 2021 organizational structure of the multidisciplinary GU cancer center clinic of the NCI-designated Sidney Kimmel Cancer Center of Thomas Jefferson University in Philadelphia. (Courtesy Dr. Leonard Gomella)

integrating the opinions of multiple specialists into a consensus recommendation. This has proven popular with patients that often receive differing recommendations from each specialist they encounter. We have reported high levels of patient satisfaction with 91% stating they were very satisfied with their care [16]. Some patients are seen for second opinions with reports returned to the consulting physicians. Retention of patients for care in our cancer center is high, and often the reason cited for remaining with our center is the seamless coordination between care teams.

There are several features of our clinic which we feel are critical to a successful MDC.

1. A dedicated nursing coordinator who is primarily responsible for scheduling patients and serves as a liaison to help patients navigate a complicated health system when arranging appointments or studies.
2. Availability of patient records, imaging, and pathology allows for true objective primary and second opinions and helps ensure accuracy of our recommendations.
3. Communication between specialists both in the preceding MDTB and during the clinic. When not in patient rooms, physicians congregate to discuss the patients. This provides additional educational exposure for our residents and fellows to learn from other disciplines.
4. Specialists express a unified therapy plan after the patient evaluation or a list of best options including clinical trial participation. The risks and benefits are discussed for all options thoroughly and by specialists with different perspectives.
5. Patient advocacy from family or close friends is encouraged. It is strongly encouraged that the patient attends the MDC with a spouse, child, relative, or close friend to support the patient during the visit.
6. A commitment to the program by the various specialists.

The organizational structure of the clinic has changed slightly through the years as noted previously. Originally the MDTB was held following the clinic. This had the advantage of all providers being familiar with the patient, but was felt to be much less efficient overall. It interfered with afternoon clinic or procedures following the MDC and created scheduling conflicts for the involved pathologist and radiologist who often have their own departmental noon conferences. Contacting the patient following the conference also led to long discussions and was felt to hinder clinical trial enrollment when trial eligibility was discussed after rather than during the visit. Patients also preferred to leave the visit with a recommendation which would otherwise be delayed in the original iteration of our clinic. Finally, the clinical space used also allows for real-time discussion among the physicians further negating the need for the post-clinic meeting.

During the 2020 pandemic, our MDC continued to be operational with approximately 60% of visits converted to virtual telehealth encounters. This was relatively easy to transform to the telehealth platform since Jefferson Health and the clinical departments have an existing long-term commitment to the expansion of telemedicine [17]. The MDC structure was largely unchanged as a virtual clinic as the MDTB was conducted as a videoconference where discussion of the clinical cases to be evaluated in the following telehealth-based MDC was possible. The nurse coordinator was also an invaluable resource for assisting patients navigating completion of staging studies in a healthcare environment that instantly became more challenging given the pressures of the novel coronavirus.

Impact of Multidisciplinary Care

Reports of our initial experience conducting prostate cancer care in the MDC at SKCC demonstrated a high level of patient satisfaction. 91% of patients were very satisfied with their care, and 96% of patients were able to make a treatment decision based on the encounter [16]. Ten years later, 97–100% of patients ranked their care as "good" or "very good" [3]. Similar results have been seen from the clinical model adapted from ours reported by Magnani where average satisfaction score was 6/7 [18]. In the case of our clinic, satisfaction levels translated into improved patient retention. In the year 2000, during an initial evaluation of our MDC, we demonstrated that 67% of patients seen only for second opinion were ultimately treated by our multidisciplinary group. By 2010, nearly all (99%) internal patients and 75% of externally referred patients elected to stay with us for their prostate cancer care [3, 16].

Patient satisfaction and retention imply that a high level of service is provided by the dedicated experts who are better able to counsel patients given the time available in the MDC. We have seen this influence our men with low-risk cancer and their understanding/acceptance of active surveillance. In our MDC, a decision counseling program was instituted to men eligible for active surveillance. Prior to their visit, 33% of men were undecided on a treatment option, and after all patients had decided on a treatment. The rate of men requesting active treatment decreased from 40% to 17%, and a preference for active surveillance increased from 27% to 83% [19]. During this same time period, only 42.1% of men in the USA with low-risk prostate cancer were treated with active surveillance identifying one quality metric of MDCs is to encourage guideline adherence for men with low-risk prostate cancer [20].

Adherence to guidelines has also been demonstrated in our MDC's utilization of neoadjuvant chemotherapy (NAC) prior to cystectomy for muscle-invasive bladder cancer. Previously published National Cancer Database rates of NAC range from 20% to 40% [21, 22]. Our cisplatin-based NAC utilization is 62.5%. In those patients who were cisplatin ineligible, our clinical trial portfolio available at the MDC expanded neoadjuvant therapies to include checkpoint inhibitors bringing total neoadjuvant therapy use to 71.8% of patients treated for muscle-invasive bladder cancer [6].

Additional improvements in care achieved by treating patients in a MDC can be observed in corrections of diagnosis. Correctly staging and assessing risk category of a patient's cancer is essential to assure the appropriate sequence of treatments is commenced. At Johns Hopkins, 13% of men with prostate cancer treated in their MDC had an upgrade in their Gleason score, while 8% were downgraded. After pathologic and radiographic review, close to 30% of men presenting to their MDC experienced a meaningful change in NCCN risk category which has considerable implications on treatment selection [23].

Colleagues working at the Prostate Cancer Programme of Milan's Istituto Nazionale dei Tumori have adapted and validated our model of multidisciplinary care at their center [18]. For those interested in establishing such a program, their conclusion that "the multidisciplinary approach needs to be adaptable to meet new needs and improve quality" must be emphasized. Since the original description of our multidisciplinary clinic established in 1996, there have been several modifications to its operational structure. As guidelines are updated and new information becomes available, these patient-centric programs must be flexible in not only their structure but in their recommendations. In the early experience of the Milan program, their data on active surveillance shows significant growth of this option in low-risk patients, from approximately 40% to over 70% between 2006 and 2010. As the concept of active surveillance became a "treatment" focus of clinical trials at their Prostate Cancer Programme, recruitment to these trials was enhanced.

Institutional benefit such as growth of one's cancer center is also gained from the MDC approach. The time invested in patient education and completeness of the evaluation from a team working in a MDC provides an excellent opportunity for discussions surrounding clinical trial enrollment. In our practice, all patients are discussed in tumor board prior to being seen, and trial eligibility is considered. Relevant trials are presented by team members along with standards of care, and a research coordinator is present on site to help with enrollment. Embedding trial coordinators within the MDC is a key strategy that has been shown to increase patient accrual. In Delaware, the ChristianaCare cancer program has reported an increase in trial enrollment from 6.4% to 13.2% from 1997 to 2002 compared to a national rate of 2.5% after starting MDCs for their breast and hepatobiliary programs [24]. The hepatobiliary MDC at Johns Hopkins increased trial enrolment from 49.2% to 77.8% after establishing their MDC, while the Hopkins prostate MDC enrolled 20% of eligible patients, and 75% of patients donated urine and/or blood for translational research [23, 25].

The theoretical benefits of a multidisciplinary clinic approach can be readily listed. Similar to our data, the Milan Prostate Programme has shown high patient satisfaction scores in the setting of a well-designed clinic. While the benefits of a multidisciplinary approach to patient care is clear, some have voiced concern to a range of over issues, including cost [26]. As described above there can be significant overhead expenditure to maintain this clinical activity. At our institution the cost of running the MDC is offset by benefits already discussed above, but also by our outcomes. We reported for the first time using our multidisciplinary clinic approach in prostate cancer that overall survival outcomes can be improved by this model. Our 5-year survival for men with localized low-risk disease approached 100% which is to be expected based on published benchmarks. However, when analyzing men with locally advanced high-risk disease, the improved outcome at our center was pronounced. For example, in men with high-risk pathologic T3 prostate cancer, 5-year survival approached 90% compared to a 78% overall survival compared to SEER (Surveillance, Epidemiology, and End Results) [3]. As others begin to care for patients in MDCs, it is essential that additional high-quality studies evaluate outcomes of this care model to further examine the cost-benefit analysis as well as report on any improvements to the model as it evolves.

Establishing a Multidisciplinary Clinic

Many US and international groups have now described their design and implementation of the multidisciplinary clinic approach to cancer care [27]. The European School of Oncology has promoted the design, implementation, and certification of prostate cancer units [28]. The MDC at SKCC has been successful over its 25 years of operations. It exists in a collegial, academic environment where the physicians are interested in not only excellent patient care but also patient satisfaction, clinical trial enrollment, and trainee education. In our healthcare delivery model, certain inefficiencies are expected and often welcomed because of our academic mission. As a consequence, our MDC structure may not be optimal for export in all situations. Local administrative and billing concerns may require an alternative organizational structure to deliver care, and each health system will have its own limitations, but also its own unique characteristics contributing to its success. Those that wish to start their own MDC will need to identify their center's capabilities during development. Following these steps may also be helpful.

The first necessary action is to secure administrative support. Improving patient care is always a priority for hospital administrators; however, this will have to be balanced against cost. A business plan can help demonstrate to hospital leadership a level of commitment to the project and should consider financial viability of the clinic and downstream benefits. How will your providers bill insurance? Will there be salary support for physician involvement? Who will staff the clinic, and will new hires be required? What is the proposed location? Knowledge of historical referral patterns and projected volume changes are key. Health systems with employed physicians should explain to administration that the decrease in billable encounters during a lower volume clinic includes an expected increase in surgical and radiation services and significant patient retention as discussed above. When private physicians will cover the clinic, administrators may be attracted to a consolidation of services to their facilities. Billing for second opinion reads by pathology and radiology is an additional opportunity for downstream revenue. It is likely that either breast, lung, gyn, colorectal, or hepatobiliary programs already have experience setting up a MDC, and their expertise navigating administrative hurdles at your institution may be an invaluable resource.

Strong physician support is paramount to a successful MDC as some physicians' business models may discourage participation. Financial incentives can favor the efficiency of one's own office. Covering a hospital location as a private physician can mean lost revenue from technical charges, loss of autonomy, and a redirection of patient referrals to the hospital's health system. Offsetting this lost revenue with guaranteed salary support for physicians in one MDC resulted in large loses for the hospital and might negatively impact administrative support [24]. Having a plan for maintaining physician engagement in a private practice environment may be more challenging than an employed or academic health system. Requiring MDC participation to remain a member of the cancer center service line is an example of how to incentivize involvement.

Another potential challenge to physician engagement is disagreement between specialists regarding appropriate treatment or turf battles which can lead to confusing and conflicting recommendations to patients. Men with localized prostate cancer are fortunate that excellent results are achieved with either surgery or radiation therapy [29]. Physicians may be biased to offer treatments they themselves deliver based on their experience or financial incentives. New technologies may be considered unproven and therefore controversial to some members of the care team while strongly endorsed by others. Large-group urology practices often have an ownership stake in a radiation center and therefore may be inclined to only discuss therapies that they are capable of providing at their facility instead of more involved regimens such as high-dose brachytherapy. If consensus is not achieved when finalizing recommendations, the MDC is unlikely to succeed in retaining patients.

We have been fortunate to practice in a collegial, patient-focused environment where the team uses our fiduciary responsibility to help patients decide on the treatment modality that offers the best results in the context of their own desired outcomes. For groups needing to align physician recommendations, it is helpful to create a consensus document of all agreed-upon evidence. Loblaw et al. have described their process in detail [30]. They first compiled a list of topics they wished to address such as who should and shouldn't be offered active surveillance or when to offer adjuvant radiation. Answers were provided by one stakeholder from each specialty, and then all members were surveyed about the extent they agreed with the answers. Consensus was achieved if >75% agreed with the wording of the answer. For items that did not reach consensus, answers were reworded and presented to the group again in a revised form for approval. The authors noted a positive shift to a more collaborative culture following this exercise.

Alongside a strong commitment from the physicians, administration needs to deliver support in terms of staffing and infrastructure. Salary support for the nurse coordinator needs to be secured at the outset. A conference room if a MDTB is not already established is needed for group discussions. A physical location for patients to be seen and the necessary staff (schedulers, medical assistants, nurses, check-in/check-out, billing) must be designated by hospital administration. Our solution was to have the MDC at SKCC in the clinical space used by the Department of Radiation Oncology at our hospital. This is a hospital-based clinic that is managed and staffed by the hospital. The urologists provide a staff member from our office who assists with surgical scheduling.

How patient encounters will be billed is dependent on clinical operations. In a true MDC where all providers are present, the patient will be charged a single technical fee either by the hospital if the office is in a designated hospital managed clinic or by the physician group that covers the office expense. Providers will then bill the appropriate E/M codes for the encounter. This will usually be HCPCS code G0463, a single new patient visit (NPV 99201-99205), or established patient visit code (EPV 99211-99215). If the clinic is designed such that all physicians see the patient at the same time, then HCPCS code G0175 can be billed if a minimum of three non-nurse specialists are present including at least one physician [31]. If HCPCS codes are not accepted by payers, then 99201-99215 can be used for the facility fee.

Physician billing is standard if patients are evaluated independently. E/M codes for new and established patients are used commensurate with documentation (99201-99215). If patients are seen simultaneously by a group of physicians, then HCPCS codes S0220 (30 min) or S0221 (60 min) may also be required. Billing on time in this scenario can be a challenge as even though a group of physicians are face to face with a patient for the entirety of the group encounter, a physician may only bill for the time they were performing the counseling. For example, a 60 min visit is divided among the providers despite all being present for the hour. Non-physician providers (psychologists, social workers) involved in multidisciplinary care can bill 99366-99368 depending on time spent in conference with the physician care team [31]. These recommendations may differ regionally and by insurance provider. It is important to discuss with your organization's billing department on how to comply with appropriate charges for your clinic's organizational structure. (It should be noted that if a MDTB is incorporated as part of the plan, it has not previously been considered billable time as the patient is not present. New Medicare rules effective January 2021 allow physicians to bill based on all time spent coordinating care that day. Whether or not time spent in MDTB will be reimbursed by payers is not known at this time.)

Finally, coordination of physician schedules and establishing a strategy for referrals will be needed. As the clinic launches, referring all newly diagnosed GU cancer patients from the participants' existing practices can help staff navigate unforeseen challenges. A marketing brochure should be distributed to physician mail lists and outreach to particular practices with a history of referrals to any members of the MDC. Hosting and advertising an event like a prostate cancer screening fair to engage community support can also increase visibility of the new clinic. As the MDC grows, it is paramount that mechanisms for data capture are instituted so that patient outcomes can be studied. Prospective studies with matched cohorts are sorely needed to improve the quality of research on the impact of MDCs [26].

Conclusion

There is a growing body of encouraging literature concerning the multidisciplinary clinic approach to prostate cancer. The complexity of modern treatment for patients with genitourinary cancer mandates coordination between urologic, radiation, and medical oncologists. Multidisciplinary clinics have emerged as a strategy to simplify the process for patients and provide a forum for clinicians of different disciplines to evaluate and discuss patient care in real time. For individuals interested in establishing a multidisciplinary prostate cancer clinic there, must be an unwavering long-term commitment from all parties, an assurance that cannot be underestimated. The institution, support staff, medical specialists, nurses, social workers, and other healthcare professionals must be partners in the vision of the center. Based on our success in GU oncology, our Sidney Kimmel Cancer Center now supports 12 other multidisciplinary clinics.

At the multidisciplinary clinic of the Sidney Kimmel Cancer Center, we have demonstrated many benefits including high levels of patient satisfaction and enhanced learning opportunities for all participants. Additional benefits of MDCs have included increased cancer program visibility, enhanced trainee education, clinical trial enrollment, and downstream institutional benefits such as patient retention. Our group has also demonstrated a defined oncologic outcome benefit to many patients with this approach.

References

1. Hong NJ, Wright FC, Gagliardi AR, Pazat LF. Examining the potential relationship between multidisciplinary cancer care and patient survival: an international literature review. J Surg Oncol. 2010;102:125–34.
2. Paget L, Han P, Nedza S, et al Patient-clinician communication: basic principles and expectations, institute of medicine discussion paper 2011. Available on line: http://www.iom.edu/Activities/Quality/~/media/Files/Activity%20Files/Quality/VSRT/Discussion%20Papers/PCCwLogos.pdf
3. Gomella LG, Lin J, Hoffman-Censits J, et al. Enhancing prostate cancer care through the multidisciplinary clinic approach: a 15-year experience. J Oncol Pract. 2010;6(6):e5–e10.
4. Giri VN, Gross L, Gomella LG, Hyatt C. How I do it: genetic counseling and genetic testing for inherited prostate cancer. Can J Urol. 2016 Apr;23(2):8247–53.
5. Lallas CD, Scotland K, Zhang M, et al. Clinical influences in the multidisciplinary management of small renal masses at a tertiary referral center. Urol Pract. 2016;3(6):468–74.
6. Smentkowski K, Glick L, Han TM, Lallas CD, Chandrasekar T, Mark JR, et al. The multidisciplinary clinic approach for bladder cancer treatment in the neoadjuvant therapy era. J Clin Oncol. 2020;38(6_suppl):475.
7. Henson DE, Frelick RW, Ford LG, et al. Results of a national survey of characteristics of hospital tumor conferences. Surg Gynecol Obstet. 1990;170:1–6.
8. Greene FL. The American joint committee on cancer: updating the strategies in cancer staging. Bull Am Coll Surg. 2002;87:13–5.
9. Abraham NS, Gossey JT, Davila JA, et al. Receipt of recommended therapy by patients with advanced colorectal cancer. Am J Gastroenterol. 2006;101:1320–8.
10. Newman EA, Guest AB, Helvie MA, et al. Changes in surgical management resulting from case review at a bresast cancer multidisciplinary tumor board. Cancer. 2006;107:2346–51.
11. Hussein A, Samoi A, Weber J, et al. Impact of a national comprehensive cancer network compliant multidisciplinary conference on treatment decisions in patients with localized prostate cancer. J Urol. 2020;203:e1198.
12. Rao K, Manya K, Azad A, et al. Uro-oncology multidisciplinary meetings at an Australian tertiary referral center – impact on clinical decision-making and implications for patient inclusion. BJU Int. 2014;114(Suppl 1):50–4.
13. Scarberry K, Ponsky L, Cherullo E, et al. Evaluating the impact of the genitourinary multidisciplinary tumour board: should every cancer patient be discussed as standard of care? Can Urol Assoc J. 2018;12(9):E403–8.
14. Riedel RF, Wang X, McCormack M, et al. Impact of a multidisciplinary thoracic oncology clinic on the timeliness of care. J Thorac Oncol. 2006;1(7):692–6.
15. Keating NL, Landrum MB, Lamont EB, et al. Tumor boards on the quality of cancer care. J Natl Cancer Inst. 2013;105(2):113–21.
16. Valicenti RK, Gomella LG, El-Gabry EA, et al. The multidisciplinary clinic approach to prostate cancer counseling and treatment. Semin Urol Oncol. 2000;18(3):188–91.

17. Glassman DT, Puri AK, Weingarten S, et al. Initial experience with telemedicine at a single institution. Urol Pract. 2018;5(5):367–71.
18. Magnani T, Valdagni R, Salvioni R, et al. The 6-year attendance of a multidisciplinary prostate cancer clinic in Italy: incidence of management changes. BJU Int. 2012;110(7):998–1003.
19. Myers RE, Leader AE, Hoffman-Censits H, et al. Decision support and shared decision making about active surveillance versus active treatment among men diagnosed with low-risk prostate cancer: a pilot study. J Canc Educ. 2018;33:180–5.
20. Mahan BA, Santino B, Franco I, et al. Use of active surveillance or watchful waiting for low-risk prostate cancer and management trends across risk groups in the United States, 2010 – 2015. JAMA. 2019;321:704–6.
21. Reardon ZD, Patel SG, Harras ZB, et al. Trends in the use of perioperative chemotherapy for localized and locally advanced muscle-invasive bladder cancer: a sign of changing tides. Eur Urol. 2015;67:165.
22. Bergerot PG, Sonpavde G, Nelson RA, et al. Trends in neoadjuvant chemotherapy (NAC) use for muscle-invasive bladder cancer (MIBC): an updated report using the National Cancer Database. J Clin Oncol. 2016;34(suppl15):4540.
23. Sundi D, Cohen JE, Cole AP, et al. Establishment of a new prostate cancer multidisciplinary clinic: format and initial experience. Prostate. 2015;75:191–9.
24. Petrelli NJ, Grusenmeyer PA. Establishing the multidisciplinary care of patients with cancer in the state of Delaware. Cancer. 2004;101:220–5.
25. Page AJ, Cosgrove D, Elnahal SM, et al. Organizing a multidisciplinary clinic. Chin Clin Oncol. 2014;3:43.
26. Osarogiagbon RU. "Like heart valve clinic, it probably saves lives, but…Who has time for that?" The challenge of disseminating multidisciplinary cancer care in the United States. Cancer. 2018;124:3656–67.
27. Gomella LG. The prostate cancer unit: a multidisciplinary approach for which the time has arrived. Eur Urol. 2011 Dec;60(6):1197–9.
28. Valdagni R, Albers P, Bangma C, et al. The requirements of a specialist Prostate Cancer Unit: a discussion paper from the European School of Oncology. Eur J Cancer. 2011 Jan;47(1):1–7.
29. Hamdy FC, Donovan JL, Lane JA, et al. 10-year outcomes after monitoring, surgery, or radiotherapy for localized prostate cancer. N Engl J Med. 2016;375(15):1415–24.
30. Loblow A, Barkin J, Buckley R, et al. Improving prostate cancer care collaboratively – a multidisciplinary, formal, consensus-based approach. Can J Urol. 2017;24(1):8646–50.
31. Parman C. Multidisciplinary clinic visits. Oncol Issues. 2018;33(5):7–10.

Chapter 2
Supportive and Palliative Care for Genitourinary Malignancies

Elizabeth Wulff-Burchfield

Abbreviations

5-HT_3RA	5-hydroxytryptamine, or serotonin, receptor antagonist
AC	Anthracycline and cyclophosphamide)
ACE	Angiotensin-converting enzyme
ADT	Androgen-deprivation therapy
ARB	Angiotensin receptor blocker
ASCO	American Society of Clinical Oncology
ASTRO	American Society for Radiation Oncology
AUA	American Urological Association
BPH	Benign prostate hyperplasia
CAPO	Canadian Association of Psychosocial Oncology
CTCAE	Common Terminology Criteria for Adverse Events
ESMO	European Society for Clinical Oncology
HoLEP	Holmium laser enucleation of the prostate
IMRT	Intensity-modulated radiotherapy
JNC	Joint National Committee
MASCC	Multinational Association for Supportive Care in Cancer
mTOR	Mammalian target of rapamycin
MUGA	Multiple-gated acquisition
NCCN	National Comprehensive Cancer Network
NK_1RA	Neurokinin-1 receptor antagonist
NSAID	Nonsteroidal anti-inflammatory drug

E. Wulff-Burchfield (✉)
Internal Medicine, Divisions of Medical Oncology and Palliative Medicine,
University of Kansas Medical Center, Kansas City, KS, USA
e-mail: ewulffburchfield@kumc.edu

K. L. Stratton, A. K. Morgans (eds.), *Urologic Oncology*,
https://doi.org/10.1007/978-3-030-89891-5_2

OIBD	Opioid-induced bowel dysfunction
ORT	Opioid Risk Tool
PDE5i	Phosphodiesterase type 5 inhibitor
PPE	Palmar-plantar erythrodysesthesia
PRN	Pro re nata, Latin for as needed
PSA	Prostate-specific antigen
RANKL	Receptor activator of nuclear factor-κB ligand
RCC	Renal cell carcinoma
SNRI	Selective norepinephrine reuptake inhibitor
SOAPP	Screener and Opioid Assessment for Patients with Pain
SSRI	Selective serotonin reuptake inhibitor
TURP	Transurethral resection of the prostate
VEGFR	Vascular endothelial growth factor receptor
VMS	Vasomotor symptoms
WHO	World Health Organization
WOCN	Wound, ostomy, and continence nurse

Despite improving cancer interventions and therapies, the experience of living with and receiving treatment for genitourinary cancers still carries significant morbidity for many patients. Substantial progress has been made toward optimizing cancer therapies from the perspective of patient-centered outcomes and quality of life; however, there is no cancer treatment or intervention that can boast total freedom from adverse side effects or outcomes. While every patient's experience is unique and our ability to predict morbidity on an individual level remains limited, the natural history of prostate, kidney, and bladder cancer, as well as their treatments, creates common themes regarding the supportive care needs for these malignancies and patient populations. These themes are readily apparent to clinicians treating these malignancies, even more so because medical providers in this position typically serve as the primary, and in some cases the only, point of contact for patients and caregivers in the setting of cancer- or treatment-related side effects. Increasing use of multimodal treatment for genitourinary malignancies can blur the line between those symptoms or issues that "belong" to medical, radiation, or urologic oncologists, palliative care, primary care, or other disciplines. Furthermore, in some cases the choice of clinician who is contacted to address a given symptom may be subject to regional, institutional or practice-related, clinician, or even patient preference. Thus, a comprehensive knowledge of supportive care needs and management strategies organized around disease type, rather than categorization "medical" or "surgical" issues, is essential to ensure that patients' needs are addressed. Therefore, some topics follow in disease-based groupings where applicable, rather than in any other configuration that would indicate a given specialty as the responsible party. Beyond these sections will follow sections dedicated to concerns common to all patients with genitourinary malignancies considerable overlap between the patient communities. Finally, the intersecting nature of supportive care needs in advanced cancer is ideally suited to involvement by specialty palliative care – specialist medical care provided by a trained multidisciplinary team of physicians, nurses, social workers, chaplains, and additional clinicians and directed toward the relief of suffering by patients and caregivers navigating a serious illness. Therefore, a section dedicated to palliative care in genitourinary malignancies will bring the chapter to a close and synthesize supportive care principles described throughout the preceding sections.

Prostate Cancer: Identity

Significant innovation in interventions and treatments for prostate cancer has led to improved disease control and survival for men with all stages of this disease. Just as men with localized or locoregionally advanced prostate cancer are experiencing improved rates of cure or long-term disease control, many men with metastatic disease are also living *with* their cancer for long periods of time. The experience of extended living *with* cancer is a recent phenomenon that remains under-recognized and poorly studied, particularly when this consists of living in a manner that is significantly and chronically altered. When coupled with the effects of prostatectomy, prostate radiation, or androgen-deprivation therapy (ADT), the experience of living with cancer or cancer chronic treatment-related effects can modify the fabric of daily life as well as self-image. Consequently, the theme of *identity* underlies some of the supportive care needs for men living on and after prostate cancer treatment.

Vasomotor Symptoms

Androgen-deprivation therapy (ADT) remains the backbone of prostate cancer therapy for many men and has a distinctive side effect profile, including vasomotor symptoms (VMS), commonly called "hot flashes" or "hot flushes." This symptom is characterized by the sensation of uncomfortable bodily warmth at ambient temperature, which may be accompanied by flushing of the skin or sweating. VMS are often spontaneous but may be prompted by physical exertion or psychosocial stress and can sometimes have a nocturnal pattern, in which circumstances they are commonly referred to as "night sweats." The relationship between VMS and androgens was first described by Huggins and Hodges in relation to surgical castration for the management of prostate cancer [1], and their work remains the backbone of the current understanding of physiology. The biological underpinnings of VMS in men on ADT are believed to be analogous to hot flashes experienced by menopausal or lactating women and can be summarized as the development of disinhibition of thermoregulatory nucleus, and therefore disinhibition of hypothalamic catecholamine signaling, that is brought about by falling levels of sex hormones [2, 3, 4]. Endogenous opioids, β-endorphins, also appear to play a role in hypothalamic catecholamine

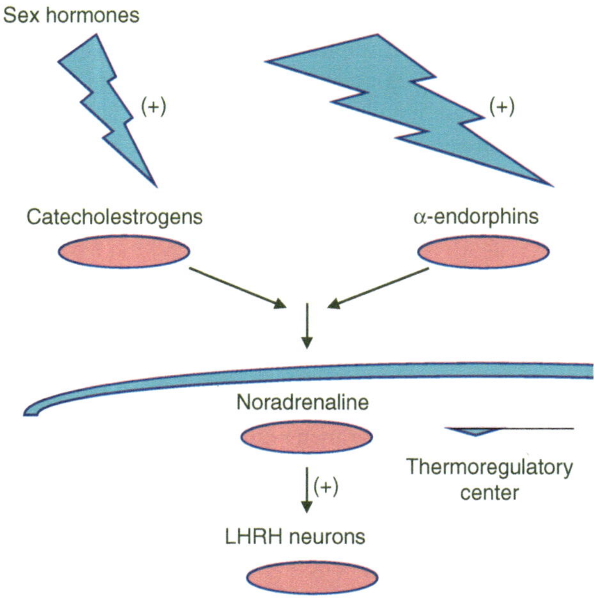

Fig. 2.1 Pathophysiology of vasomotor symptoms. (Adapted from Kouriefs et al. [280])

synthesis [5], although the interaction between peripheral levels of sex hormones, β-endorphins, and hypothalamic catecholamines is incompletely understood (Fig. 2.1). While up to 80% of men experience hot flashes [6], there is significant variability in the frequency and interference of VMS from ADT, with nearly one-third experiencing debilitating VMS [6, 7]. Evaluation of predictive factors has indicated that younger age, some genetic polymorphisms relating to neurotransmitters, vasoconstriction, and circadian rhythm may be associated with increased patient bother from hot flashes [8]; however, reports of patient weight relative to hot flash severity or interference are in conflict [8, 9]. Short of discontinuing ADT, there are no universally effective interventions for all men experiencing this symptom; however, nonpharmacologic and pharmacologic interventions have been explored and may provide relief for some men.

Nonpharmacologic interventions have been investigated, with acupuncture as the most well studied. Generally, published data indicates that acupuncture may confer an approximate 50–60% reduction in hot flashes [10–13]; however, these data are derived from small, single-arm trials and should be interpreted with caution. The issue of appropriate control in acupuncture trials is of particular relevance owing to the challenges of blinding and the uncertainty about the validity of employing sham procedures as controls [14]. Therefore, the generalizability of these data remains uncertain. To that end, a systematic review regarding acupuncture for VMS in prostate cancer failed to confirm clear evidence of benefit [15]. Other nonpharmacologic interventions for VMS lack data in patients with prostate cancer but include yoga [16] and hypnosis [17–20]. Investigation of yoga is limited to pilot data, and both interventions are currently described exclusively in women, and therefore further study is warranted before routinely integrating these into clinical practice. In conducting future trials regarding nonpharmacologic interventions for VMS, even if benefit is confirmed, the uptake may be hindered by inconsistent or unpredictable insurance coverage for these nonpharmacologic treatments [21].

Regarding pharmacologic therapies, both hormonal and nonhormonal therapies have been investigated. Among hormonal therapies, progestin treatments have the broadest foundation of data in prostate cancer. Approaches may include oral megestrol acetate [22], intramuscular administration of medroxyprogesterone acetate [23, 24], and transdermal progesterone creams [25], although there are no published, prospective, randomized data pertaining to topical progesterone interventions for *ADT-related* hot flashes. Progestin therapy is associated with a 70–90% reduction in hot flashes [22, 24], but is associated with an increased incidence of venous thromboembolic events [26], a risk that is already elevated in the setting of active malignancy and represents a leading cause of death among patients with cancer [27]. In addition to thrombotic risk, another disadvantage of progestational agents is the established side effect of weight gain [26]; given the risk of weight gain and metabolic syndrome associated with ADT [28], this is undesirable for most men. An alternative hormonal therapy is cyproterone acetate, a steroidal antiandrogen with progestational properties with similar efficacy to pure progestins [29, 30]. However, this agent is not preferred owing to its risk of hepatotoxicity [29]. Estrogens represent another class of hormonal interventions for ADT-induced VMS and include diethylstilbestrol [31–33] and transdermal estradiol [33]. Both of these therapies have been investigated for the management of VMS associated with ADT and have similar efficacy to progestational agents [31, 32]. However, estrogens have the disadvantage of higher rates of associated gynecomastia, gynecodynia, and even galactorrhea [31–33] and therefore are a less favorable pharmacologic class of agent. Consequently, among hormonal interventions for ADT-induced VMS, progestational agents have a more favorable side effect profile and should be considered the preferred hormonal agent.

Nonhormonal pharmacologic options span several classes, including anticonvulsants, antidepressants, and adrenergic blockade. Generally speaking, these classes display more variable efficacy in management of ADT-associated VMS. Among anticonvulsants, gabapentin has been evaluated at doses of 300, 600, or 900 mg per day in divided doses, and while hot flash severity was not found to be significantly improved compared to placebo, men in the highest-dosing group did report improvements in distress and quality of life as they relate to VMS, as well as satisfaction with VMS control [34]. Pregabalin has not been studied in the context of ADT-associated hot flashes, but among women on endocrine therapies for breast cancer, pregabalin reduces hot flash frequency by approximately 50–60% [35]. Both selective serotonin reuptake inhibitors (SSRIs) and serotonin-norepinephrine reuptake inhibitors (SNRIs) have also been studied as interventions for VMS. SSRIs that have been evaluated include paroxetine [36–39], citalopram [40–42], sertraline [43], and fluoxetine [42, 44], although data specific to men with ADT-related VMS is limited to pilot studies. However, among larger studies involving SSRIs for menopausal hot flashes or those associated with endocrine therapy for breast cancer, most appear to reduce hot flash frequency by 50–60%, although some data suggests that paroxetine may have a lower degree of benefit [36–39, 41–44]. Of note is that some SSRIs inhibit cytochrome P450 pathway (specifically CYP2D6) and may pose the risk of interactions with some oral cancer therapies for prostate cancer, such as abiraterone or enzalutamide [45]. SNRIs including venlafaxine and desvenlafaxine have also been evaluated for the management of VMS, including among men receiving ADT. Similarly to outcomes with SSRIs, venlafaxine [24, 46–49] and desvenlafaxine [50] are associated with a 50–60% reduction in hot flash frequency and are both safe and generally well tolerated. Finally, clonidine, an alpha adrenergic agonist, has also been evaluated for this purpose, albeit with most data again focused on menopausal hot flashes or those associated with breast cancer endocrine therapies [51–55]. However, despite achieving moderate benefit to hot flash frequency in women, randomized data has failed to show benefit among men [51] and is therefore not recommended to manage VMS in men.

Although clonidine is not recommended, anticonvulsants and antidepressants are therapies that should be considered when considering pharmacologic interventions for ADT-associated VMS. These therapies do have a lower degree of benefit than hormonal agents [24], but avoid elevating the risk of thromboembolic disease that accompanies hormonal interventions [26]. Venlafaxine and gabapentin have the highest level of evidence to support their use; however, another SSRI, SNRI, or anticonvulsant could be considered based on the need for pharmacologic intervention for other conditions (e.g., mood disorder, neuropathy). Furthermore, while these nonhormonal agents have well-described side effects, most notably xerostomia, nausea or appetite changes, or insomnia [56], the choice of agent can also be tailored in order to avoid overlapping toxicity. Finally, nonpharmacologic strategies such as acupuncture require further study before they can be widely recommended for ADT-associated VMS; however, they are unlikely to pose significant risk other than "financial toxicity" if not reimbursed by insurance.

Sexual Health and Intimacy

While occurring at a frequency similar to that of bothersome VMS for men with prostate cancer, changes to erectile function and libido represent some of the most disturbing side effects to patients facing prostate cancer and treatment. Both local and systemic therapies may impact erectile function, whereas ADT and other systemic therapies have additional impacts on libido in addition to erectile function. The impacts of local therapies on erectile function have improved with time, whereas systemic therapies have maintained near-universal impacts on libido and erectile function with prolonged exposure [57]. Prior to nerve-sparing approaches to prostatectomy, erectile dysfunction was a nearly unavoidable consequence of local therapy for prostate cancer. However, following the discovery of the cavernous nerves and evolution in the medical understanding of their role in erectile function

[58], modern surgical techniques afford many men the opportunity to pursue aggressive cancer treatment while maintaining potency. Furthermore, data have increasingly demonstrated the important temporal relationship between prostatectomy and erectile function, both in the natural history of delayed postoperative return of erectile function and in the age-related risk of permanent erectile dysfunction. Among men who undergo bilateral nerve-sparing radical prostatectomy, several prospective observational studies have demonstrated that potency rates are lowest in the immediate postoperative period and then steadily improve over a period of 18 months, ranging from 30–38% at 3 months to 59–86% at 18 months [59]. Patient age at the time of prostatectomy is an important factor in the risk of postoperative erectile dysfunction, with older men experiencing the lowest rate of erections sufficient for penetrative sexual intercourse and also the highest rate of permanent erectile dysfunction [60]. In addition to the risks of erectile dysfunction associated with prostatectomy, both external beam radiation and brachytherapy also carry the risk of this toxicity. Radiotherapy approaches for localized prostate cancer have also been transformed by data demonstrating that intensity-modulated radiotherapy (IMRT) techniques and fields that spare corporal tissues offer a meaningful improvement in the risk of post-treatment erectile dysfunction [61] analogous to what is afforded by nerve-sparing approaches to radical prostatectomy. In the modern treatment landscape, data from the Prostate Cancer Outcomes Study have indicated that 55–70% of men with adequate erectile function prior to radiation maintain erectile function following definitive radiotherapy [62]. Factors that predict for greater risk of erectile dysfunction following radiotherapy include higher pre-treatment PSA values, concurrent ADT, and pre-treatment erectile dysfunction [63]. Brachytherapy is associated with some variability in post-treatment erectile function outcomes, ranging from potency rates of 51–76% [64, 65]. As is the case with post-prostatectomy sexual outcomes, potency rates worsen with advancing patient age and pre-treatment sexual function and also appear to worsen with obese BMI [63].

For men who do experience erectile dysfunction following treatment for localized prostate cancer, both pharmacologic (oral, intraurethral, and intracavernosal agents) and nonpharmacologic interventions (vacuum-assisted devices, pelvic floor rehabilitation) can be considered as part of a program of penile rehabilitation [66, 67]. Meta-analytic data indicates that daily high-dose PDE5i therapy and pelvic floor rehabilitation are associated with significantly higher rates of recovery of erectile function following radical prostatectomy, whereas on-demand PDE5i dosing does not result in statistically better outcomes than placebo [66]. Following radiotherapy, both daily and PRN PDE5i administration is associated with significant improvement in potency, although the relative merit of daily versus on-demand PDE5i administration is unclear. Penile rehabilitation has primarily been studied in the setting of local treatment for prostate cancer, whereas the role of these strategies for men receiving ongoing ADT is less well known. Some data suggest that as many as 19% of men on ADT may maintain erectile function while on ADT [68], so for men with preserved erectile function, the aforementioned components of a penile rehabilitation program may also provide meaningful benefit to erectile function while on ADT. However, for men without erectile function while on ADT, particularly those with metastatic disease for whom a natural ADT endpoint is not recommended, it is essential for patients and their partners to assess goals for sexual activity. A high proportion of men receiving ADT for prostate cancer report a loss of sexual desire, ranging from 58 to 73% depending on the type of ADT [69], and therefore not all men receiving ADT or their partners wish to pursue sexual activity in this setting. The changed nature of sexual activity during ADT requires a higher degree of motivation [70], but for those highly motivated to maintain penetrative sexual intercourse, whether vaginal or anal, surgical implantation of a penile prosthesis may be considered [71].

Sexual activity, libido, and intimacy are interrelated, yet distinct, topics that should all be addressed in the care of men with sexual dysfunction related to prostate cancer and/or treatment. Data suggest that patients and intimate partners continue to experience notable unmet needs regarding sexuality or intimacy following prostate cancer treatment [72–74], and a number of dyadic interventions have been evaluated to improve relational intimacy. A variety of psychosocial interventions have been evaluated to improve communication and intimacy among dyads in which one partner has undergone or is undergoing treatment for prostate cancer. Interventions differ significantly in the content and aim, and results are mixed [75, 76]. Despite this lack of clear guidance from the literature, dyads affected by prostate cancer are recommended to maintain intimate physical contact with romantic partners (e.g., holding hands, spooning) and maintain open communication in order to promote relationship satisfaction.

Kidney Cancer: Variability

Among the more common GU malignancies, the management of advanced renal cell carcinoma has long been marked by a broad spectrum of clinical outcomes. Dating back to the cytokine era and continuing into the era of combination therapies with immune checkpoint inhibitors, disparate disease control and survival outcomes have been noted; a growing minority of patients experience complete responses and prolonged disease- and treatment-free survival, whereas the majority of patients do experience life expectancy limited by their kidney cancer [77]. This prognostic ambiguity for patients with advanced kidney cancer is a prominent facet of the patient and clinician experience and leaves its mark on the patient, caregiver, and clinician experience. In addition to prognostic uncertainty, medical decision-making for advanced renal cell carcinoma is more complex than over the preceding several decades due to the evolving role of cytoreductive nephrectomy. Until the availability of data from the CARMENA [78] and SURTIME [79] trials, cytoreductive nephrectomy was a mainstay treatment for all possible surgical candidates. However, the determination from these trials that up-front pharmacologic therapy may represent a non-inferior approach to up-front nephrectomy for many patients with renal cell carcinoma has led these medical decision-making discussions to include if not uncertainty, then significant nuance. The role of cytoreductive nephrectomy will likely continue to involve, but it is clear that the complexity of these medical decisions is here to stay. Due to these and other factors, the influence of *variability* represents a common thread among many of the supportive care needs specific to this population.

Unique Treatment Toxicity and Adherence

Renal cell carcinoma (RCC) has exemplified the success of targeted therapies in oncology, and while some tyrosine kinase inhibitors currently in use for the treatment of RCC have multi-kinase inhibition, the majority of targeted systemic therapies in use for the management of advanced RCC are those heavily featuring vascular endothelial growth factor receptor (VEGFR) inhibition [80]. These therapies, as well as mammalian target of rapamycin (mTOR), have a side effect profile distinct from cytotoxic chemotherapy agents, with on-target effects including hypertension, hand-foot syndrome (HFS), diarrhea, and stomatitis, among others [81]. These toxicities require directed and active management for the duration of time that patients take these therapies [82], but unfortunately patients consistently under-report toxicity while taking oral cancer agents, which can hinder efforts to effectively assess and manage these very side effects and toxicities [83]. While dose reductions and/or interruptions are considered acceptable and believed to ultimately facilitate longer-term administration of anti-cancer therapy, maintaining maximum tolerable dose density and intensity remains a priority, particularly given that a higher area under the curve (AUC) for some VEGFR TKIs is associated with superior overall survival [84]. Proactive management of common toxicities from targeted cancer therapies for RCC is possible with aggressive monitoring, implementation of prevention strategies when possible, and employing data-driven mitigation protocols.

The unique toxicity profile of VEGFR TKIs includes specific but multisystem on-target adverse effects, including dermatologic, endocrine, gastrointestinal, and cardiovascular effects. Hand-foot skin reaction or hand-foot syndrome (HFS) is a symptom associated with a number of oral cancer therapies, including all approved oral therapies for metastatic renal cell carcinoma [81], and is characterized by erythematous and/or hyperkeratotic plaques with a peripheral ring of edema on the palms and soles or other areas of significant friction while on VEGFR TKI therapy [85]. HFS associated with VEGFR TKI treatment, and to a lesser extent mTOR inhibitor therapy, is distinct from the hand-foot skin reaction that occurs in the context of cytotoxic chemotherapy, which typically results in macular erythema across the entire surface of the palms and soles, often with desquamation [86]. While not life-threatening, HFS is painful, can depress functional status, leads to dose reductions or discontinuations, creates the opportunity for superinfections, and detract from QOL [87]. Thorough pre-treatment counseling is imperative, with recommendations including prevention of significant friction, pressure, extensive heat exposure to the hands and feet, referral to podiatry for management of significant preexisting calluses, and twice-daily use of emollients that contain 10% urea. In the setting of the National Cancer Institute CTCAE grade 2 HFS, ultrapotent optical corticosteroids such as clobetasol 0.05% can be applied twice daily. Topical lidocaine can also be applied PRN for pain management with or without other oral analgesics, but if patients experience HFS refractory to the above measures, regardless of whether the severity is "intolerable grade 2" or greater, the recommendation should be to hold the agent until resolution to grade 1 or 0 and then resume at a reduced dose [85]. In addition to HFS, diffuse keratosis pilaris-like eruptions have been reported with some TKIs, characterized as widespread tiny or pinpoint hyperkeratotic papules [88]. This does not typically require treatment and resolves in conjunction with treatment discontinuation, but if patients are highly motivated to treat this, recommendations should include emollients with or without "keratolytics" such as urea or salicylic acid, as well as avoidance of hot baths and showers, which can exacerbate dry skin [89]. Finally, emergent non-melanoma skin cancers have been reported in conjunction with VEGFR TKIs, so clinicians are advised to have a low threshold for referral to dermatology for evaluation and management of skin eruptions or abnormalities.

Endocrine and gastrointestinal toxicities have been reported to variable degrees with all VEGFR TKIs used for advanced RCC. The most frequently described endocrine toxicities from VEGFR TKIs are thyroid dysfunction, typically hypothyroidism, and hypoglycemia. Hypothyroidism has been described with sunitinib, pazopanib, axitinib, and others, although the mechanism whereby these agents lead to hypothyroidism remains unknown [90]. Thyroiditis-induced thyrotoxicosis has also been described with sunitinib [91] and sorafenib [91], with eventual development of hypothyroidism. Given the high prevalence of thyroid dysfunction, clinicians are advised to monitor thyroid function at baseline and regular intervals thereafter; specific guidelines do not exist regarding this toxicity monitoring, but every 12-week intervals are generally considered acceptable, although this can and should be performed earlier in the case of symptoms suggestive of thyroid dysfunction. Hypoglycemia has been reported with multiple VEGFR TKIs, including several approved for treatment of advanced RCC [92]. Hypoglycemia may be most pronounced among patients with a diagnosis of diabetes, so in addition to routine monitoring of blood glucose levels for all patients receiving treatment with VEGFR TKIs, clinicians may consider a modest reduction in doses of medications used for treatment of diabetes [92].

Gastrointestinal and cardiovascular toxicities of VEGFR TKIs are common among patients with advanced RCC. Diarrhea is especially common and may be dose-limiting if not managed aggressively. Anti-diarrheal agents such as loperamide and diphenoxylate/atropine typically provide adequate relief, and pre-treatment counseling should include recommendations for patients to begin administering antidiarrheal agents at the first sign of loose stools [93]. Furthermore, patients should be advised to eat a bland diet when experiencing loose stools so as to avoid foods that may exacerbate this symptom. Regarding cardiovascular adverse events, hypertension is the most common, but other effects such as myocardial infarction and left ventricular dysfunction have also been reported [94]. Hypertension may develop as early as 1 week into a treatment course with VEGFR TKIs, and meta-analytic data indicates that the incidence of hypertension is approximately 23%, with a 4% incidence of high-grade hypertensive events [95], although incidence of up to 68% has been reported with some agents [96]. Oncologists should regularly screen for hypertension and manage aggressively in accordance with updated Joint National Committee guidelines [97]. ACE inhibitors and ARBs have a theoretical advantage in the management of hypertension due to VEGFR TKIs [98], so given the prominent role that these agents play in the JNC guidelines, ACE inhibitors and ARBs are a reasonable first-line agent for VEGFR TKI-induced hypertension. In addition to hypertension, myocardial infarction and heart failure have been identified as additional cardiovascular risks associated with VEGFR TKIs. Meta-analytic data has confirmed this association [95], although data is limited regarding the value of screening. However, it is generally accepted that patients with underlying cardiovascular disease or anthracycline exposure are appropriate for baseline and intermittent screening with echocardiography or MUGA scan.

Adherence and Persistence with Oral Agents

In addition to promoting a good quality of life and dignity for patients with advanced RCC, maintaining acceptable control of treatment-related side effects from TKIs is an essential component of promoting adherence, especially in light of data indicating that patient-reported bother from cancer treatment has emerged as a significant predictive factor of treatment discontinuation [99]. However, adherence, generally considered to mean patient self-administration to prescribed medications in the manner they were prescribed, is a multidimensional construct that is impacted by factors other than treatment tolerability. In addition to treatment tolerability, physical, emotional, and psychosocial factors all contribute incrementally for many patients, although these factors are weighted differently on an individual patient level. Similarly, persistence, loosely defined as consistency between the duration for which an agent is prescribed and the length of time that the patient takes it, is felt to reflect similar barriers and facilitators to adherence with regard to oral cancer therapy. With approximately 25% of anti-cancer therapy administered via the oral route [100], the proportion of oral cancer treatments for all disease is likely to increase with time, and these issues will become increasingly crucial for the practice of oncology, including across GU malignancies. Systematic review data indicates that predictors of poor adherence and persistence include adverse effects from treatment; mental health conditions, including and especially depression; inconsistent patient follow-up for scheduled visits; and compromised patient-provider relationships or mistrust or lack of belief in the prescribed treatment [101]. However, all of these barriers are themselves multifactorial, and social determinants play a prominent role in each. Clinicians can support patient adherence and persistence with oral cancer treatment by investing time in simplifying treatment schedules; encouraging patients to set reminders or use a pill box, as well as devoting time to thoroughly educate patients regarding the nature of their cancer and the risks and benefits of therapy; and assisting patients in obtaining treatment at an affordable cost [101]. Clinical pharmacists and social workers can also assist in screening for barriers to adherence and persistence and provide reinforcement for education provided to patients by clinicians.

Decisional Conflict Regarding Cytoreductive Nephrectomy

In addition to unique treatment toxicities, the patients with advanced RCC face a unique and daunting medical decision-making process regarding cytoreductive nephrectomy. Specifically, the CARMENA trial presented at the 2018 American Society of Clinical Oncology Annual Meeting has been practice-changing in the broader approach to cytoreductive nephrectomy for advanced RCC, an intervention that was previously a central tenant of RCC treatment [78]. This, as well as the SURTIME trial [79], demonstrated the non-inferiority of a surgery-sparing approach for patients receiving sunitinib for advanced renal cell carcinoma [78]. While practice-changing, the appropriate application of trial results to clinical practice has been fraught owing to the rapidly changing paradigm of first-line systemic therapy for advanced RCC. Specifically, guideline-concordant first line systemic therapy for RCC currently includes at least one immune checkpoint inhibitor agent, whereas TKI therapy was the standard of care, and therefore the control arm, at the time of the CARMENA and SURTIME trials. Therefore, the data and outcomes from the CARMENA and SURTIME trials cannot necessarily be extrapolated universally to patients diagnosed with advanced RCC in the current era. The challenges of this decision-making process ultimately rest with the treating clinicians, but surgical decision-making in other oncology patient populations indicates that decisional conflict is common [102]. Given the high stakes of the cytoreductive nephrectomy decision, support and reassurance should be offered to patients with advanced renal cell carcinoma facing decisions regarding cytoreductive nephrectomy, and whenever possible a treatment recommendation should be made by the treating clinicians rather than deferring to patients, who are unlikely to feel equipped to make this decision. Clinicians are strongly recommended to use a "best case/worst case scenario" communication and decision-making framework, adapted from Dr. Schwarze et al. [103] (Fig. 2.2). This framework begins with clinicians providing concrete descriptions of the best, worst, and most likely clinical outcomes from the two treatment paths under consideration, in this case up-front cytoreductive nephrectomy versus up-front systemic therapy, and graphical depiction drawn during the encounter and provided to the patient [103]. This communication approach shifts the focus from technical aspects of the proposed operation to a broader discussion regarding alternatives and outcomes and is feasible even in the urgent or inpatient setting [104].

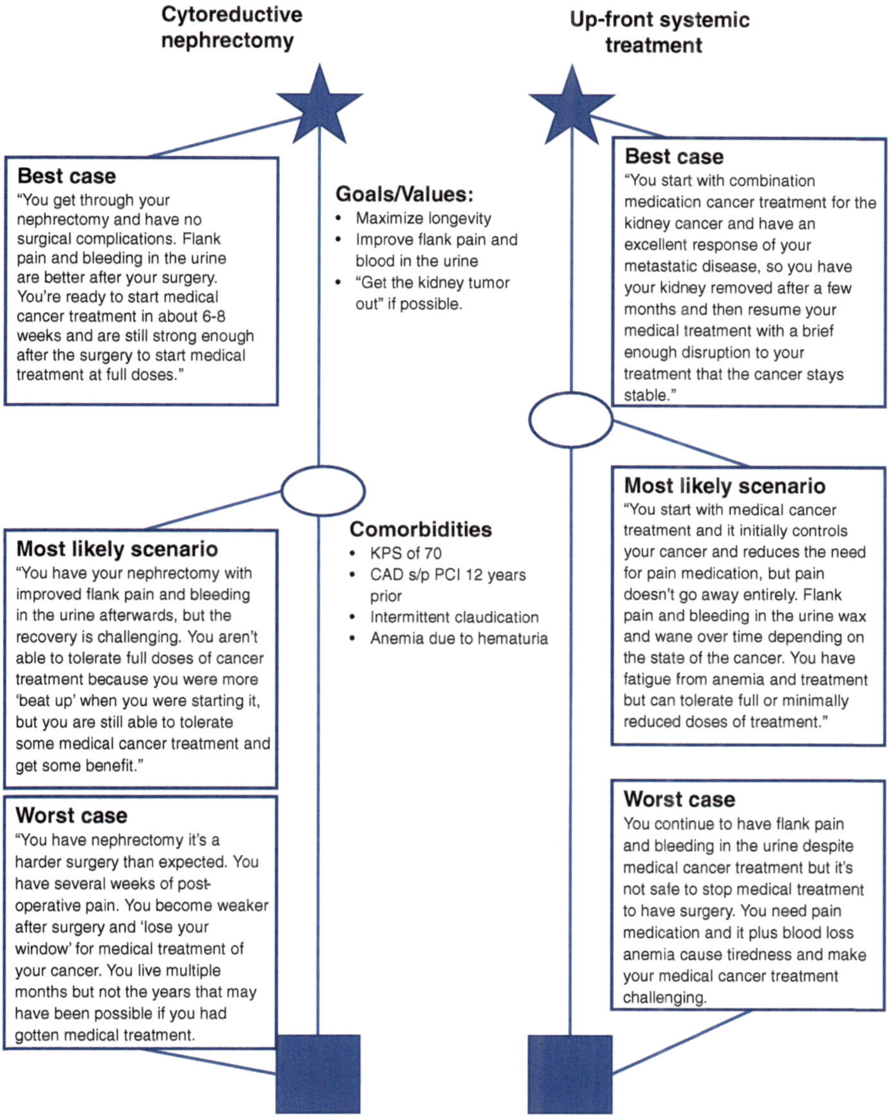

Fig. 2.2 Adaptation of "best case/worst case scenario" communication framework for discussions regarding cytoreductive nephrectomy in advanced renal cell carcinoma

Prognostic Uncertainty

The rapid innovation and evolution in treatment paradigms for advanced RCC has obscured not only surgical decision-making but also prognostication. Prognostic uncertainty is a common issue in the case of medical conditions for which there is a significant population of outliers. This is not wholly unique to renal cell carcinoma, but has been a longstanding issue in this population since the uptake of high-dose interleukin-2 and its modest rate of deep and durable responses in advanced RCC [105]. The task of cultivating prognostic awareness is a constant dilemma for oncology clinicians, and the difficulty and imprecision of this are exacerbated in settings such as RCC, as a minority of patients may achieve a complete radiographic response and long-term disease control (perhaps even treatment-free survival), whereas the majority of patients with advanced RCC have a life expectancy limited by their metastatic cancer. Availability bias is particularly relevant in advanced RCC as clinicians have extended and regular contact with patients who have experienced exceptional responses, and this can lead oncologists to experience additional cognitive dissonance with estimating survival outcomes, conveying them to patients, and integrating this into decision-making. Patient prognostic awareness may be impacted further in the era of social media, as data indicates that social media posts regarding cancer are disproportionately positive for patients both during and post-treatment, particularly in patients who self-identify as "survivors" [106]. Given these challenges, it should come as no surprise that some patients with advanced GU malignancies have poor prognostic awareness and incorrectly believe that non-curative-intent immune checkpoint inhibitor therapy is being undertaken with the intent of cure [107]. While there is no communication framework validated in the setting of immune checkpoint inhibitor therapy for advanced renal cell carcinoma, clinicians are encouraged to disclose the nature of this uncertainty and provide frequent feedback to patients as their clinical course evolves [108]. Finally, palliative care referral early in the course of metastatic cancer is associated with superior patient prognostic awareness and is appropriate for any patient with advanced cancer, including RCC [109].

Bladder Cancer: Vulnerability

Patients living with bladder cancer are often considered the more medically vulnerable subpopulation among the common GU malignancies, due to age, common comorbid conditions, and the standard use of radical cystectomy, a morbid surgery for many patients [110]. Due to these factors as well as the biology and natural history of urothelial carcinoma, outcomes have lagged behind those of other GU malignancies, both in the setting of localized and advanced disease. While novel systemic therapies and combinations are paving the way for improving clinical outcomes, the real-world experience of living with or treating bladder cancer continues to be impacted by patient comorbidity and functional impairments that influence the clinical trajectory in addition to the burdens associated with the disease itself. Furthermore, the life-changing experience of radical cystectomy results in notable alterations to body image in addition to physiology, creating the opportunity for literal and figurative exposure. Therefore, *vulnerability* is an important determinant of supportive care needs for bladder cancer patient population.

Dilemmas in Choice of Urinary Diversion

Since the adoption of radical cystectomy for the management of refractory non-muscle invasive bladder cancer and muscle-invasive bladder cancer, the question of the superior diversion technique has loomed large in the field of urology and the minds of urologists. This question has been repeatedly investigated in the broader population of patients undergoing radical cystectomy as well as distinct subpopulations, yet conflicting results indicate that this question remains unanswered. Indeed, the most appropriate metrics to define success, value, or overarching superiority in this setting remain uncertain. Survival [111], complication rates [112, 113], and health-related quality of life [114–116] have all been evaluated, with significant conflict in most domains, even in meta-analyses. Broadly, urinary and sexual symptoms may be more conspicuous in patients with orthotopic neobladder [117], yet this method may still be associated with superior quality of life [118]. However, it is essential to contextualize these findings with the data suggesting that the innate selection bias among patients offered orthotopic neobladder diversion versus ileal conduit diversion may explain a large degree of these differences in clinical and quality-of-life outcomes [119, 120]. Patients who undergo ileal conduit reconstruction have greater comorbidity, older age, and more advanced disease; thus, outcomes in morbidity, mortality, and QOL will inherently be different when patient cohorts diverge in these key criteria [119, 120]. Diversion choice may simply *not* be the primary factor in post-cystectomy quality of life, but in order to support patients in decision-making, it is appropriate for urologists to disclose that orthotopic neobladder urinary diversion may be marginally favorable among younger and/or more robust patients [121], although urinary incontinence and sexual dysfunction may be more prominent among this same cohort [117].

Ostomy Care and Management

Patients who undergo ileal conduit diversion are confronted with new anatomical and functional constraints, and it should be no surprise that the experience of living with an ostomy would create a unique profile of supportive care needs. Data indicate that patients and caregivers are often underprepared for ostomy self-management responsibilities [122], and this compounds the emotional challenges that patients face when they first encounter their ostomy postoperatively [123, 124]. Ostomy educational or training programs are generally associated with positive trends in self-care, patient empowerment, and quality of life [125, 126], and most clinicians deliver this education post-operatively [123]. However, patients and caregivers are often too overwhelmed by the medical circumstances to effectively retain a urostomy educational curriculum when delivered at this time point [127, 128], which undermines the value of the educational intervention. Caregivers play a key role in ostomy care for many patients who undergo radical cystectomy, and their involvement in urostomy training and education provides patients with meaningful support [127, 129]. Consequently, clinicians are advised to implement a standardized, preoperative urostomy educational program for patients planned for radical cystectomy and ileal conduit reconstruction and family caregivers. In addition to providing an introductory curriculum, ostomy care needs and self-management can be supported by care from an experienced wound, ostomy, and continence nurse (WOCN®), regardless of whether this is integrated into an oncology or urology clinic. The WOCN® society has interactive clinician- and patient-facing educational modules regarding peristomal skin care at no charge to users, and a number of non-profit and patient advocacy organizations provide patient-facing materials regarding urostomy function and management. Finally, several ostomy supply companies can provide patients with an ostomy "starter kit" containing a variety of pouching and skin care products, and patients report positive associations with being provided an initial bundle of pouching products [127].

Neobladder Care and Management

Even though it is not medically appropriate to offer orthotopic neobladder diversion to all patients undergoing radical cystectomy, this reconstruction approach remains valid and appropriate for many [120]. Following neobladder reconstruction, incontinence is a primary determinant of quality of life and presents challenges to adjustment [129]. However, urinary continence improves gradually over the course of 6–12 months, with daytime continence preceding nighttime continence [130]. Urinary continence does play a prominent role in health-related quality of life, and it is of note that older age appears to predict for lower quality of life in this population [131]. Given that rates of sexual dysfunction or bother may be higher in this population, both this possibility and expectations regarding incontinence are key facets of preoperative patient counseling [117]. Pelvic floor physical therapy is crucial to reestablishing continence but has an unclear role in improving symptoms of sexual dysfunction in the setting of orthotopic neobladder diversion [132].

Frailty

Age is widely accepted as a key risk factor for the development of bladder cancer [133] as well as a negative predictive factor for functional and cancer outcomes following radical cystectomy [134, 135]. Series describing older adults treated with cystectomy have indicated that carefully selected patients may still achieve operative and cancer outcomes commensurate with their younger peers, implicating factors other than chronological age contribute to cancer and operative risk in older adults [136, 137]. Frailty, a geriatric syndrome characterized as declining functional status and physical reserve as well as increased vulnerability to physiologic stressors, has been increasingly recognized as a phenotype associated with negative outcomes from cancer in many states and stages [138]. So, too, has frailty been demonstrated as a predictor of higher frequency and severity of operative complications [139, 140], mortality, and cost [141]. Newer, robotic-assisted surgical approaches to RC have proven insufficient to address all of the discrepancies in complications and outcomes experienced by older adults [142], and while chemoradiation offers an organ-sparing alternative approach, this is not appropriate or optimal for all patients [143]. Burgeoning data regarding preoperative rehabilitation ("prehab") indicate that this restorative care may be capable of overcoming some vulnerabilities associated with frailty [144], although further prospective study is necessary to determine the "dose," frequency, and duration of rehabilitation course required for benefit as well as the optimal balance between preoperative restorative care and potentially harmful delay of oncologic surgery. However, given the existing gaps in the understanding of optimal treatment choice and supportive or restorative care for frail adults with bladder cancer, the aforementioned best case scenario/worst case scenario framework [103] can enhance communication and promote goal-oriented medical care. This is highly feasible within typical preoperative workflows and high acceptability from clinicians and patients [104].

Overlapping Supportive Care

Comprehensive Pain Management

Pain management is arguably the most crucial supportive care task for clinicians to master in the management of advanced malignancies, including GU malignancies, as this is a common and distressing consequence of advanced malignancy. Valid pharmacologic and nonpharmacologic management strategies have potential to improve pain control, distress, and global quality of life for patients with neoplasm-related pain [145, 146] and often have synergistic effects when layered or combined. The two broadest categories of neural pain mechanisms are nociceptive pain, including pain directly attributable to tissue injury, and neuropathic pain, pain in a nerve distribution indirectly related to the site of tissue injury or due to nerve injury [147] (Table 2.1). A detailed pain history is crucial in order to determine the underlying neural mechanism, with the most successful pharmacologic management determined by the identified neural mechanism(s). However, even the most complete pain evaluation may not yield a single mechanism, as many patients with significant cancer pain experience a combination of both nociceptive and neuropathic pain [148].

The World Health Organization (WHO) [149], the American Society of Clinical Oncology (ASCO) [150], the National Comprehensive Cancer Network (NCCN) [151], and the European Society for Medical Oncology (ESMO) [152] have clinician guidelines for nociceptive cancer pain management, all of which recommend assessing pain regularly and initiating pharmacologic treatment based on assessed

Table 2.1 Comprehensive pain evaluation

Patient pain rating	Numerical rating scale (0–10/10) Visual analog scale Wong-Baker Faces [278]
Clinician pain interview	Location, character, intensity, and temporal pattern Triggers, aggravating factors, or alleviating factors Attempted treatments and outcome
Evaluation of neural mechanisms	Nociceptive: often aching, throbbing, or pressure-like Somatic: location easily identified (e.g., pain due to bone metastasis) Visceral: diffuse, cramping, colicky (e.g., pain due to liver capsule stretch from hepatic metastases) Neuropathic Radiculopathy: shooting or stabbing pain in a longitudinal or bandlike distribution, sometimes accompanied by paresthesias (e.g., due to spinal cord or nerve plexus injury) Neurotoxic: burning or aching, often accompanied by paresthesias (e.g., chemo-induced or diabetic neuropathy) Sympathetic (e.g., chronic regional pain syndrome following trauma to an extremity)

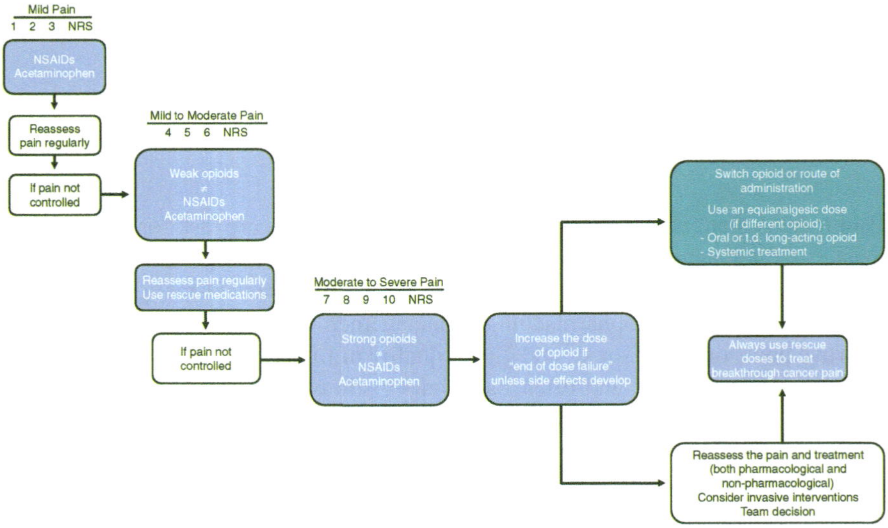

Fig. 2.3 Pharmacologic pain management algorithm. T.d. transdermal. (Adapted from Fallon et al. [152])

severity (Fig. 2.3). Over-the-counter agents including acetaminophen (paracetamol) and nonsteroidal anti-inflammatory drugs (NSAIDs) are recommended as first line for mild pain [149–152] (Table 2.1). If nociceptive pain needs exceed the analgesic capacity of acetaminophen or NSAIDs, the recommended approach in management is to consider initiation of opioid therapy. Low-potency opioids, most of which are limited to combination agents with acetaminophen in the United States, are recommended as preferred opioid for mild-to-moderate pain. These medications should be administered on a PRN basis and frequency commensurate with patients' opioid tolerance, comorbidities, and organ function, generally ranging between once every 3–4, but potentially ranging to once every 6–8 hours for patients at high risk for opioid toxicity. The choice to escalate to a higher potency opioid and/or add a long-acting agent should depend on the extent of benefit derived from low-potency therapy and the extent to which pain is intermittent or constant. Intermittent or incidental pain is generally amenable to management with short-acting opioids on a PRN basis, whereas constant pain often requires use of a scheduled long-acting agent. When starting a long-acting agent, the recommended strategy includes initiation of an agent equivalent to 50% of the total 24-hour opioid use in 1–3 divided doses, depending on the pharmacologic properties of the agent.

Opioid prescribing should also include the development of a plan for management of common opioid-related toxicities. Opioid-induced constipation, a prominent symptom that is part of the larger syndrome of opioid-induced bowel dysfunction (OIBD), affects as many as 94% of patients taking opioids for cancer pain, and its severity is often dose-related [153]. Stimulant laxatives such as bisacodyl or sennosides or osmotic agents such as magnesium citrate or lactulose have been the historic standard of care for management of opioid-induced constipation, although these are still insufficient for some patients [154]. Data regarding the efficacy of individual laxative agents is limited, but prospective, randomized data regarding docusate sodium, a commonly used surfactant agent, indicates that this agent does not improve stool consistency or frequency compared to sennosides alone [155]. Agents with novel mechanisms of action may be considered for refractory OIBD, including chloride channel activators such as lubiprostone [156] or agents targeted to peripheral μ-opioid receptors such as naloxegol [157] or methylnaltrexone [158]. Lubiprostone, naloxegol, and methylnaltrexone have not been prospectively compared, and therefore factors including route of administration (lubiprostone and naloxegol = oral, methylnaltrexone = subcutaneous), formulation of agent (lubiprostone = capsule, naloxegol = tablet), or patient preference may be used to guide decision-making. Of note is that methadone may inhibit lubiprostone-induced chloride secretion [159], thereby undermining its activity, and naloxegol and methylnaltrexone have been proposed to carry a small theoretical risk of mild central μ-opioid receptor antagonism and precipitating a pain crisis, and therefore their use should be avoided if the user's cancer pain is uncontrolled [154].

In addition to symptomatic side effects, the recent opioid epidemic makes it incumbent upon opioid prescribers to universally implement cautious and deliberate prescribing practices. Guidelines recommend risk stratification for opioid use disorder with a validated tool such as the Opioid Risk Tool (ORT) [160] or Screener and Opioid Assessment for Patients with Pain (SOAPP) [161]. Furthermore, opioid prescribers are strongly recommended to routinely query available prescription drug monitoring program (PDMP) substance monitoring databases for each patient in order to rule out any suspicious opioid-seeking behaviors [162], which have been implemented broadly in the United States. The American Society of Addiction Medicine recommends querying the available PDMP database at the time of initiation of controlled substances and then quarterly thereafter for low-risk patients [163]. However, for high-risk patients based on formal risk stratification with ORT or SOAPP, clinicians should consider monthly PDMP queries. Finally, oncology clinicians prescribing opioids for management of neoplasm-related pain are recommended to complete opioid prescribing contractual agreements with patients who will receive chronic opioid therapy, to create a framework of shared expectations with each patient regarding a single opioid prescriber policy [162].

Neuropathic pain, also called neuropathy, is a heterogeneous category of pain distinct from nociceptive pain that is best characterized as that which relates to direct nerve injury rather than that which relates to an anatomical site of tissue injury. A common but not universal facet of cancer pain [164], neuropathic pain requires careful identification and attribution, as pharmacologic and interventional strategies differ between subtypes of neuropathic pain. Criteria from the Neuropathic Pain Special Interest Group of the International Association for the Study of Pain can provide a helpful framework for identification of neuropathic pain and consider neuropathic pain that (1) follows a plausible neuroanatomical pain distribution *and* (2) has a suggestive history of a causative exposure, lesion, or condition *and* either (3) displays positive (i.e., hyperalgesia) or negative (i.e., paresthesia) sensory changes within the innervation territory of the proposed lesion *or* (4) can be confirmed by a diagnostic test (e.g., EMG) [165]. Data supports the use of anticonvulsants such as gabapentin, pregabalin, carbamazepine, oxcarbazepine, or antidepressants, particularly SNRIs and tricyclic antidepressants [166]. Many clinicians prioritize the choice of neuropathic agent based on additional medical or symptomatic needs that the agent may address (e.g., concomitant major depressive disorder); this approach has face validity and represents an appropriate decision-making process, but clinicians may also consider two systematic reviews indicating that gabapentin may have superior benefit to other adjuvant therapies for cancer-related neuropathic pain [167, 168]. Corticosteroids are an important class of adjuvant therapy for cancer pain, particularly in the setting of bone pain or visceral pain (e.g., pain related to liver capsule stretch due to malignancy) [149, 169]. However, meta-analyses have failed to uncover the ideal circumstances or dose of corticosteroids for malignant pain, although data do indicate that corticosteroids with the least mineralocorticoid activity have lower risk of adverse effects [149, 169].

Data supporting interventional approaches for chronic cancer pain are somewhat mixed, and therefore systemic pharmacologic therapy should still remain the standard of care for most cancer pain. However, specific indications such as celiac plexus neurolysis for painful pancreatic masses [170] and kyphoplasty for painful malignant compression fractures [171, 172] have been demonstrated to improve pain ratings and lower oral analgesic consumption. Just as with interventional approaches to malignant pain, nonpharmacologic treatment for cancer pain includes a broad range of approaches, spanning integrative therapies to palliative radiation. Generally, the data underlying integrative therapies are mixed, with conflicting data regarding acupuncture [173–175] and music therapy [176]. However, two meta-analyses revealed that massage therapy is associated with a significant reduction in pain for patients with cancer, although most studies were nonrandomized or randomized to no massage therapy or conventional care, rather than to enhanced usual care [177, 178]. Palliative radiation, however, has a broad evidence base to support its use in local management of painful or obstructive sites of metastatic disease, with most data indicating up to an 80% rate of improved pain control and up to a 30% rate of complete pain response [179]. Comprehensive fractionation and dosing strategies are outside the scope of this chapter, but meta-analytic data support the use of hypofractionated external beam radiation courses for palliation of symptomatic osseous metastatic disease [180], and a single-fraction or significantly hypofractionated approach to treating uncomplicated bone metastases is endorsed by ASTRO. Stereotactic radiation has a high degree of efficacy and may be considered for metastasis-directed therapy [181]. Radioisotope therapy with radium-223, while not available to all patient populations, is associated with clinically significant improvement in cancer-related bone pain and quality of life in men with metastatic, castrate-resistant prostate cancer [182]. Other radioisotope therapy (e.g., strontium-89, samarium-153) appears to have a modest degree of benefit with respect to analgesia but are associated with a higher degree of cytopenias [183].

Antiresorptive Therapy for Palliation of Bone Pain

The pharmacologic management principles, safety, and impact on fracture risk of antiresorptive therapies are thoroughly addressed in the Bone Health Management chapter, but the pain and impacts of bisphosphonates and RANKL inhibitors and other bone-targeted therapies feature heavily in supportive care for common GU malignancies. Meta-analytic data does indicate a consistent improvement in pain associated with bisphosphonates, although no clear evidence that bisphosphonates may achieve complete response of pain [149]. Based on pain response alone, there is no high-quality data available to guide choice of bisphosphonate in the management of bone metastases [149]. Monoclonal RANKL inhibitors such as denosumab demonstrate no advantage or disadvantage in pain response when compared to bisphosphonates, although differences may exist in skeletal-related events [149, 184].

Mood Disorders

The emotional and mental health consequences of a cancer diagnosis can have far-reaching impacts on quality of life [185, 186], treatment adherence [187, 188], and mortality [189]. Depression and anxiety are commonly experienced in the general population, with rates of depression approaching 15% [190], and the rate of depression in the oncology patient population is a staggering 2–3 times higher [191]. Similarly, the rate of anxiety disorders is approximately 10% in the broader population [192], but approaching twice the prevalence in the oncology patient population [193, 194]. In addition to detracting from quality of life [195], depression and anxiety negatively impact adherence to cancer treatment, which may decrease the benefit received from treatment and, therefore, survival [187, 195]. Despite the high prevalence of mood disorders among patients with cancer, recognizing and diagnosing mood disorders present unique challenges due to the frequency with which mood disorders present with physical symptoms in this population [196], which can be difficult to differentiate from other common physical symptoms associated with cancer and/or treatment [197, 198]. The American Society for Clinical Oncology (ASCO) clinical practice guideline *Screening, Assessment, and care of Anxiety and Depressive Symptoms in Adults with Cancer* [199], adapted from the Canadian Association of Psychosocial Oncology (CAPO) guideline *Screening, Assessment, and Management of Psychosocial Distress, Depression, and Anxiety in Adults with Cancer* [200], recommends universal screening for depression and anxiety multiple times throughout the cancer trajectory with validated measures. Specifically, an endorsed approach includes administration of the 2-item PHQ-9, with completion of questions 3–9 only if the patient answers "yes" to both of the first two questions [201]. When completion of the full PHQ-9 reveals moderate symptomatology, guidelines recommend pursuing expert consultation with psychiatry or psychology for diagnostic assistance, but severe symptomatology should prompt rapid treatment with a validated approach tailored to patient needs as well as available resources rather than delaying initiation of treatment to pursue ideal diagnostic evaluation [199]. Furthermore, evaluation and treatment for concurrent substance abuse are recommended in the setting of a diagnosis of major depression [199]. Distress screening is recommended as a process for evaluating symptoms of anxiety via the validated distress thermometer, and moderate to severe distress should prompt directed assessment and medical care for the identified etiology of distress, including anxiety [200]. Patients with identified distress, anxiety, and depression should be evaluated for any risk of harm to self and others [199, 200]; clinicians should be advised that assessment for suicidality does *not* increase the risk for self-harm and is considered safe, even if done repeatedly [202].

Treatment for mood disorders in patients with cancer is generally recommended to follow a risk-adapted approach, with either psychological therapy or pharmacologic therapy offered for patients with moderate depression and anxiety, and pharmacologic intervention prioritized as first-line treatment for severe mood disorders, ideally with concurrent psychological therapy [200]. There is notable variability in the prescribing patterns of SSRIs and SNRIs in the care of patients with cancer [195], and there is some controversy over the most appropriate specialty or clinician to prescribe pharmacologic therapy for severe depression and anxiety in oncology patients [191]. Psychopharmacology is growing increasingly complex with the expansion of literature exploring pharmacologic treatment of depression and anxiety in patients with cancer, but there is no one class of medication or drug within any class that has demonstrated superiority in efficacy [196]. When available, psychiatry and psychology referrals are appropriate at the time of diagnosis of moderate to severe depression and/or anxiety; however, timely consultation may not be possible in all settings, in which case primary care or the treating hematology-oncology clinician may represent the most appropriate avenue to initiate treatment. Choice of agent may be chosen based on the symptomatology of the patient's mood disorder, comorbid conditions, concurrent medications, and other symptoms that may be co-managed with the same class or drug (e.g., venlafaxine for the treatment of concomitant mood disorder and hot flashes [46], duloxetine for treatment of concurrent mood disorder and painful chemotherapy-induced neuropathy [203]).

Nausea and Vomiting

Nausea is a highly distressing complication of cancer and cancer therapy, to such an extent that the fear of these symptoms may prevent patients from pursuing cancer therapy [204–206]. When it occurs, chemotherapy-induced nausea and vomiting significantly detract from quality of life [205, 207] and may detract from functional [208] and nutritional statuses [209]. Successful prevention and management of chemotherapy-induced nausea and vomiting avoid this quality-of-life impediment and improve healthcare utilization by avoiding hospitalizations and intensive supportive care needs. Modern antiemetic regimens are associated with a rate of total nausea control, meaning no need for PRN antiemetic therapy, approaching 80%, and patients should be counseled that this is an avoidable symptom in most cases [210, 211]. Organizations including ASCO, ESMO, MASCC, and NCCN have published evidence-based guidelines to guide the choice of antiemetic regimen depending on the emetogenicity of prescribed regimens, and clinicians are encouraged to integrate them routinely into oncology practice setting for patients with genitourinary malignancies (Table 2.2).

Antiemetic therapies and interventions outside of guideline-concordant drug classes such as NK_1RA, 5-HT_3RA, corticosteroids, and dopamine receptor antagonists remain controversial and variably endorsed by guidelines. Meta-analytic data indicates that ginger supplementation improves acute chemotherapy-induced vomiting; however, the magnitude of benefit to nausea, delayed chemotherapy-induced vomiting, or quality of life remains unclear [212]. In addition, although multiple blinded, randomized controlled trials were included, all were conducted prior to adoption of four-drug antiemetic prophylaxis regimens, and therefore this is difficult to interpret in the context of current practice [212]. Despite widespread use of cannabis among patients with cancer [213], high-quality evidence regarding safety and efficacy of cannabis in the management of chemotherapy-induced nausea and vomiting is lacking, and therefore further data are required before recommendations can be made for or against its use [214], not to mention the variability in legal status of cannabis products. Finally, complementary interventions and therapies including acupuncture or acupressure, auricular therapy, hypnosis, and others have growing body of investigative literature; however, a systematic review identifies inconsistent use of randomization, appropriate controls, and blinding, leading to a high risk of bias [215]. Therefore, while many of these interventions have low risk for medical or psychological harm and therefore may be permissible even with limited efficacy data, these interventions are often costly for patients, so

Table 2.2 Comparison of antiemetic guidelines

	ASCO [211]	MASCC/ESMO [210]	NCCN [279]
High-emetic-risk regimen – non-AC	4-drug regimen including NK_1RA + 5-HT_3RA + dexamethasone + olanzapine	3–4 drug regimen including NK_1RA + 5-HT_3RA + dexamethasone ± olanzapine	Three regimen options: 1) 4-drug regimen (preferred) including NK_1RA + 5-HT_3RA + dexamethasone + olanzapine 2) 3-drug regimen including palonosetron + dexamethasone + olanzapine 3) 3-drug regimen including NK_1RA + 5-HT_3RA + dexamethasone
High-emetic-risk regimen – AC (anthracycline and cyclophosphamide)	4-drug regimen including NK_1RA + 5-HT_3RA + dexamethasone + olanzapine	3–4 drug regimen including NK_1RA + 5-HT_3RA + dexamethasone ± olanzapine	Three regimen options: 1) 4-drug regimen (preferred) including NK_1RA + 5-HT_3RA + dexamethasone + olanzapine 2) 3-drug regimen including palonosetron + dexamethasone + olanzapine 3) 3-drug regimen including NK_1RA + 5-HT_3RA + dexamethasone
Moderate-emetic-risk regimen – non-carboplatin	2-drug regimen including 5-HT_3RA + dexamethasone	2-drug regimen including NK_1RA + 5-HT_3RA + dexamethasone ± olanzapine	Three regimen options: 1) 2-drug regimen including 5-HT_3RA + dexamethasone 2) 3-drug regimen including palonosetron + dexamethasone + olanzapine 3) 3-drug regimen including NK_1RA + 5-HT_3RA + dexamethasone

Moderate-emetic-risk regimen – carboplatin AUC ≥ 4	3-drug regimen including $NK_1RA + 5\text{-}HT_3RA$ + dexamethasone	3-drug regimen including $NK_1RA + 5\text{-}HT_3RA$ + dexamethasone	Three regimen options: 1) 2-drug regimen including $5\text{-}HT_3RA$ + dexamethasone 2) 3-drug regimen including palonosetron + dexamethasone + olanzapine 3) 3-drug regimen including $NK_1RA + 5\text{-}HT_3RA$ + dexamethasone
Low-emetic-risk regimen	2-drug regimen including $5\text{-}HT_3RA$ + dexamethasone	Three 1-drug regimen options: 1) $5\text{-}HT_3RA$ 2) Dexamethasone 3) Dopamine receptor antagonist (metoclopramide or prochlorperazine)	Three 1-drug regimen options: 1) Dexamethasone 2) Dopamine receptor antagonist (metoclopramide or prochlorperazine) 3) $5\text{-}HT_3RA$
Minimal-emetic-risk regimen	No routine prophylaxis		

the "financial toxicity" of these interventions must be weighed against the potential for benefit [216].

Chronic Lower Urinary Tract Symptoms

Chronic urinary symptoms are commonly experienced by patients living with or treated for GU malignancies, ranging from obstructive symptoms to urinary frequency to incontinence. These can significantly impact patient quality of life and may have far-reaching impacts on employment, relationships, and psychosocial functioning, in addition to physical health. Voiding dysfunction is itself a common presenting symptom among patients with prostate and bladder cancer, and this can persist or develop following definitive treatment or in the setting of advanced disease with intact primary tumors or recurrence. When evaluating obstructive symptoms, a thorough history is key to determining the likely etiology for all patients, but more cystoscopic or urodynamic assessment may be required in patients with prior prostate, bladder, or pelvic surgery or radiation in order to evaluate for disease recurrence or etiologies that may require operative management (e.g., urethral stricture). Pharmacologic treatment with alpha-1-adrenoceptor agents such as alfuzosin, doxazosin, silodosin, tamsulosin, and terazosin or 5-alpha reductase inhibitors such has dutasteride or finasteride has an important role in the management of benign prostatic hyperplasia [217], but the defined role in the setting of malignancy remains unclear. These classes of agents, preferably administered in combination, may be considered in the setting of malignancy if the prescriber suspects a component of BPH. In addition to BPH, alpha-1-adrenoceptor agents have a high degree of efficacy in palliating acute radiation-induced urethritis and should also be considered first-line treatment in this setting [218]. However, if malignant bladder outlet obstruction is suspected, treatment of malignancy, either with pharmacologic management, radiation, or surgical management, should be pursued whenever possible [219]. Palliative radiotherapy for refractory bladder outlet obstruction is highly effective in the setting of bladder outlet obstruction from prostate cancer [220] and should be considered early in these settings for patients whose symptoms do not respond to pharmacologic management. However, in refractory cases, surgical or interventional management may represent the most effective strategy.

In the setting of ineffective or unavailable pharmacologic or noninvasive interventions, operative transurethral resection of the prostate (TURP) [221–224] or bladder tumors (TURBT) [225] and holmium laser enucleation of the prostate (HoLEP) [222, 226] have demonstrated safety and at least short-term efficacy for bladder outlet obstruction in the setting of refractory genitourinary malignancies, whereas water vapor thermal therapy and prostatic urethral lift are less established in the setting of bladder outlet obstruction due to malignancy. Palliative cystoprostatectomy may be considered for select cases of incurable prostate [227] and bladder [228] cancer, although clinicians should be advised to clearly communicate the palliative intent, as there is a high risk of patients misperceiving the intent of the surgical intervention, particularly when urgent [229]. As with urethral obstruction, ureteral obstruction is a common consequence of advanced genitourinary malignancies. Percutaneous nephrostomy tube placement and ureteral stent placement have an important role in the palliation of ureteric obstruction, each with advantages and disadvantages [230, 231]. Percutaneous nephrostomy tube placement should be considered the standard of care for patients with extrinsic compression of the ureters given the notably higher rate of stent failure in the setting of nephrostomy tube placement [231, 232]; however, for intrinsic ureteric obstruction, the decision-making regarding ureteral stent versus percutaneous nephrostomy tube placement should incorporate feasibility of stenting in addition to patient preference [231].

Overactive bladder and incontinence can represent other consequences of tumor or treatment, both acutely and later in the disease or treatment course. These symptoms can be disruptive to daily activities and sleep, both of which detract from quality of life. Pharmacologic management is possible in many cases with antispasmodic agents, although the potential for benefit with these medications should be balanced with the risk of urinary retention [233, 234]. Procedural intervention may also be appropriate for some cases of bladder spasticity, including injection of botulinum toxin A which may offer relief from refractory symptoms [235]. While rates and severity of postoperative incontinence have improved in conjunction with advancing surgical and radiation techniques [236, 237], this distressing consequence of GU malignancies and their treatment remains a common symptom for patients with such malignancies. Pelvic floor rehabilitation [238–240] and biofeedback [241] are recommended early in the postoperative or post-radiation course for patients who receive local treatment for GU malignancies, but surgical approaches to management should be delayed by at least 1 year postoperative given that incontinence may improve over a period of months [242]. At any point, consultation with a urologist specializing in men's health can help create a comprehensive plan and help set expectations and benchmarks for recovery.

Hematuria

Similar to voiding dysfunction, hematuria represents both a frequent presenting symptom for GU malignancies but can also be a late consequence of malignancy or treatment. This symptom can be frightening to patients and caregivers and also increases the risk for anemia and associated consequences [243], pain, and clot retention. While the underlying cause of gross hematuria is often apparent for patients with a known malignancy, if the etiology is in question, urinalysis and urine culture, CT imaging, and flexible cystoscopy should be considered essential tools in the workup [244]. Flexible cystoscopy is safe even among frail patients or those with advanced cancer and is of supreme value when evaluating for a lower urinary tract cause of gross hematuria [244]. In the setting of malignant etiologies of hematuria, catheter placement and irrigation remain the first-line intervention in most cases. However, for refractory hematuria of malignant etiologies, "hemostatic" radiotherapy is an effective and noninvasive treatment [245–247]. Hemostatic doses of radiotherapy in the palliative setting typically range from 30 to 36 Gy, although the literature demonstrates some variability in recommended dose, and the rate of response is high, ranging from 80% to 100% [220, 246, 248]. Intravesical aminocaproic acid, alum, silver nitrate, or prostaglandin administration may be considered in the management of bladder hemorrhage refractory to radiotherapy or if radiotherapy or palliative urinary diversion is not possible or medically appropriate; of note is that aminocaproic acid, alum, and prostaglandin administration are considered preferable to formalin if an intravesical approach to palliative management of refractory hematuria is deemed necessary [249]. Interventional radiology approaches such as vesical artery embolization [250] or prostatic artery embolization [251, 252] are not available in all settings, but may be considered for refractory bladder or prostatic hemorrhage, respectively. Finally, late effects of radiotherapy may also result in clinically significant bladder hemorrhage from radiation cystitis [253]. Hyperbaric oxygen therapy [254], which is believed to promote healing by elevating tissue oxygenation and promoting angiogenesis, is a preferred noninvasive intervention for late or chronic radiation cystitis, with success rates as high as 85% [255, 256]. However, in cases where hyperbaric oxygen is unavailable or a patient is not stable enough to undergo this therapy, the aforementioned intravesical therapies or urinary diversion may be considered, depending on the clinical circumstances and available resources.

While noninvasive interventions are preferred whenever possible for refractory hematuria derived from the bladder, interventional approaches remain the current standard for refractory hematuria due to renal hemorrhage. Palliative nephrectomy remains an important consideration for patients with symptomatic renal masses and has been demonstrated to reduce flank pain and the need for blood transfusions [257]. However, renal artery embolization was described several decades ago as an intervention for refractory renal hemorrhage in patients unfit for operative management and may be considered an alternative to operative management if surgery is medically inappropriate [258, 259]. Post-embolization syndrome, a syndrome comprised of a flulike illness with pain, fever, and sometime nausea, is, however, an expected consequence of renal artery embolization but responds well to antipyretic and antiemetic therapy [260]. Radiofrequency ablation [261] and stereotactic radiotherapy [262, 263] are minimally noninvasive interventions increasing in use and prominence for the management of refractory renal hemorrhage due to inoperable renal cell carcinoma, although prospective, randomized data is lacking for these interventions.

Palliative Care

Even in the current era of rapidly improving technology in many fields, some patients will still ultimately die of their cancer or will experience their cancer in the setting of significant other medical complexity. Patients in circumstances such as

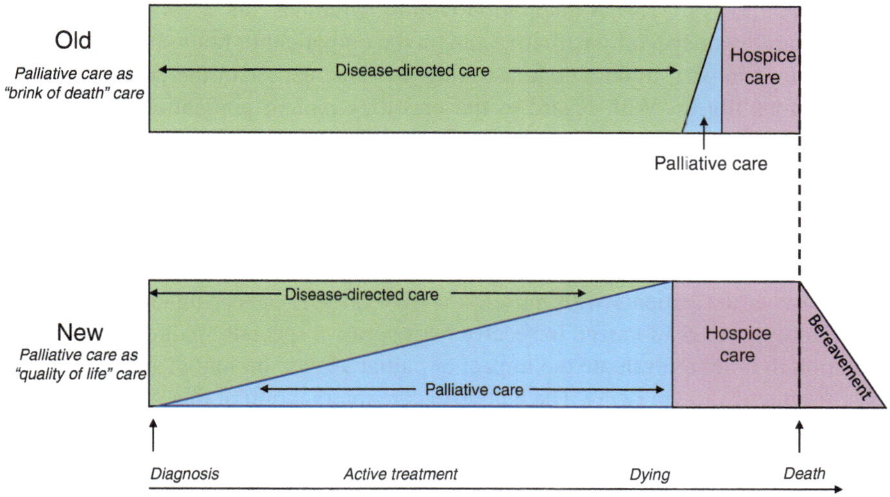

Fig. 2.4 Depiction of concurrent palliative care. (Adapted from Buss et al. [281])

these typically experience escalating symptom burden as they approach the end of their life [264], and thus it is the moral imperative of clinicians who treat and support patients with advanced malignancy to understand the unique global needs in order to anticipate and successfully address them. The field of palliative care is a discipline focused on the relief of suffering for patients with serious illnesses and their families/caregivers [265] and is well suited to address these symptoms and quality of life needs. This field exists on a spectrum with hospice care, and while it is frequently conflated with hospice, it is intended to provide supportive care concurrent with, rather than as an alternative to, conventional cancer care [265] (Fig. 2.4). There exist two general forms of palliative care: primary palliative care and secondary palliative care [266]. Primary palliative care includes basic supportive care that can be carried out by providers of any training or specialty. This includes uncomplicated pain or symptom management, assessment for depression or anxiety, evaluation of general goal concordance with treatments being offered. Specialty palliative care is typically carried out by clinicians who have completed subspecialty training (e.g., fellowship training in Hospice and Palliative Medicine, End-of-Life Nursing Education Consortium [ELNEC] training for nurses or advance practice nurses) and conducted this in a consultative capacity via a multidisciplinary team. Specialty palliative care is ideally suited for complex pain and symptom management, challenging communication needs, nuanced goals of care and medical decision-making discussions, and for the support of patient, caregiver, or medical team distress.

Palliative care is most commonly available in the inpatient setting, with up to 72% of hospitals with 50 or more beds reporting availability of a palliative care program [267]. However, specialty palliative care has an increasing presence in ambulatory, long-term care, and home health settings [268]. Improving accessibility to palliative care services naturally facilitates care beyond acute and end-of-life needs and allows for earlier integration with longitudinal cancer care. The increasing availability of specialty palliative care in the outpatient or home-based setting is due, at least in part, to data demonstrating its value earlier in the care of patients with serious illness. With regard to the oncology patient population, a landmark 2010 study by Temel et al. demonstrated improvement in depression, symptom control, and avoidance of aggressive care at the end of life, all of which were accomplished without shortening life expectancy [269]. Further data followed in other cancer populations, including patients with small-cell lung cancer [270], metastatic GI cancers [270], and muscle-invasive bladder cancer [271]. In an innovative study by Rabow et al., patients with muscle-invasive bladder cancer undergoing radical cystectomy were randomized to receive perioperative specialty palliative care consultation in order to evaluate the impact of palliative care on mood, symptoms, and post-traumatic growth [271]. The palliative care intervention of this study was associated with improved depression, fatigue, quality of life, and post-traumatic growth [271]. Despite this data reinforcing the value of palliative care in bladder cancer, recent data demonstrates that uptake of palliative care services is disproportionately low, only 3.6%, among patients diagnosed with bladder cancer [272]. Barriers to palliative care use in this population are unclear but given the high morbidity and mortality of muscle-invasive bladder cancer, research efforts directed toward ameliorating this discrepancy are sorely needed.

Patients diagnosed with advanced renal cell carcinoma [273], and prostate cancer [274], however, appear to be accessing palliative care at rates more commensurate with the broader advanced cancer population, and these rates are rising [273, 274]. Despite variability in palliative care uptake among patients with GU malignancies, there is a strong evidence base to support integration of palliative care into urology clinic workflows. Feedback from patients and urology clinic physicians and providers reinforces the feasibility of such an approach, and patient care is positively impacted by specialty expertise in supportive care and symptom management. Furthermore, clinicians participating in this model benefit from increased knowledge about patient values and needs, which can be incorporated into medical decision-making [275, 276]. Due to the existing and worsening palliative care workforce shortage [277], it is unlikely that the integrated palliative care model will form the new standard of care; however, it reinforces the value of this modality of care among patients with GU malignancies and serves as a call for all clinicians treating patients with these conditions to consult with specialty palliative care when indicated in order to improve patient quality of life and quality of care.

References

1. Huggins C, Hodges CV. Studies on prostatic cancer – I. The effect of castration, of estrogen and of androgen injection on serum phosphatases in metastatic carcinoma of the prostate. Cancer Res. 1941;1(4):293–7.
2. Shanafelt TD, Barton DL, Adjei AA, Loprinzi CL. Pathophysiology and treatment of hot flashes. Mayo Clin Proc. 2002;77(11):1207–18. https://doi.org/10.4065/77.11.1207.

3. Beckman AL. Effect of intrahypothalamic norepinephrine on thermoregulatory responses in the rat. Am J Phys. 1970;218(6):1596–604. https://doi.org/10.1152/ajplegacy.1970.218.6.1596.
4. Paul SM, Axelrod J. Catechol estrogens: presence in brain and endocrine tissues. Science. 1977;197(4304):657–9. https://doi.org/10.1126/science.877577.
5. Dyer RG, Grossmann R. Opioid modulation of the response of preoptic neurons to stimulation of the ventral noradrenergic tract in female rats. J Physiol Lond. 1988;400:631–44. https://doi.org/10.1113/jphysiol.1988.sp017140.
6. Sharifi N, Gulley JL, Dahut WL. Androgen deprivation therapy for prostate cancer. JAMA: J Am Med Assoc. 2005;294(2):238–44. https://doi.org/10.1001/jama.294.2.238.
7. Holzbeierlein JM, McLaughlin MD, Thrasher JB. Complications of androgen deprivation therapy for prostate cancer. Curr Opin Urol. 2004;14(3):177–83. https://doi.org/10.1097/00042307-200405000-00007.
8. Gonzalez BD, Jim HSL, Donovan KA, Small BJ, Sutton SK, Park J, et al. Course and moderators of hot flash interference during androgen deprivation therapy for prostate cancer: a matched comparison. J Urol. 2015;194(3):690–5. https://doi.org/10.1016/j.juro.2015.03.026.
9. Iversen P, Karup C, van der Meulen E, Tanko LB, Huhtaniemi I. Hot flushes in prostatic cancer patients during androgen-deprivation therapy with monthly dose of degarelix or leuprolide. Prostate Cancer Prostatic Dis. 2011;14(2):184–90. https://doi.org/10.1038/pcan.2011.11.
10. Ashamalla H, Jiang ML, Guirguis A, Peluso F, Ashamalla M. Acupuncture for the alleviation of hot flashes in men treated with androgen ablation therapy. Int J Radiat Oncol Biol Phys. 2011;79(5):1358–63. https://doi.org/10.1016/j.ijrobp.2010.01.025.
11. Beer TM, Benavides M, Emmons SL, Hayes M, Liu G, Garzotto M, et al. Acupuncture for hot flashes in patients with prostate cancer. Urology. 2010;76(5):1182–8. https://doi.org/10.1016/j.urology.2010.03.033.
12. Hammar M, Frisk J, Grimas O, Hook M, Spetz AC, Wyon Y. Acupuncture treatment of vasomotor symptoms in men with prostatic carcinoma: a pilot study. J Urol. 1999;161(3):853–6.
13. Frisk J, Spetz AC, Hjertberg H, Petersson B, Hammar M. Two modes of acupuncture as a treatment for hot flushes in men with prostate cancer--a prospective multicenter study with long-term follow-up. Eur Urol. 2009;55(1):156–63. https://doi.org/10.1016/j.eururo.2008.02.002.
14. Kaptchuk TJ. Placebo effects in acupuncture. Med Acupunct. 2020;32(6):352–6. https://doi.org/10.1089/acu.2020.1483.
15. Lee MS, Kim KH, Shin BC, Choi SM, Ernst E. Acupuncture for treating hot flushes in men with prostate cancer: a systematic review. Support Care Cancer. 2009;17(7):763–70. https://doi.org/10.1007/s00520-009-0589-3.
16. Avis NE, Legault C, Russell G, Weaver K, Danhauer SC. Pilot study of integral yoga for menopausal hot flashes. Menopause. 2014;21(8):846–54. https://doi.org/10.1097/GME.0000000000000191.
17. Elkins G, Johnson A, Fisher W, Sliwinski J, Keith T. A pilot investigation of guided self-hypnosis in the treatment of hot flashes among postmenopausal women. Int J Clin Exp Hypn. 2013;61(3):342–50. https://doi.org/10.1080/00207144.2013.784112.
18. Elkins GR, Fisher WI, Johnson AK, Carpenter JS, Keith TZ. Clinical hypnosis in the treatment of postmenopausal hot flashes: a randomized controlled trial. Menopause. 2013;20(3):291–8. https://doi.org/10.1097/GME.0b013e31826ce3ed.
19. Elkins G, Marcus J, Stearns V, Perfect M, Rajab MH, Ruud C, et al. Randomized trial of a hypnosis intervention for treatment of hot flashes among breast cancer survivors. J Clin Oncol. 2008;26(31):5022–6. https://doi.org/10.1200/JCO.2008.16.6389.
20. Elkins G, Marcus J, Stearns V, Hasan Rajab M. Pilot evaluation of hypnosis for the treatment of hot flashes in breast cancer survivors. Psychooncology. 2007;16(5):487–92. https://doi.org/10.1002/pon.1096.
21. Bleck R, Marquez E, Gold MA, Westhoff CL. A scoping review of acupuncture insurance coverage in the United States. Acupunct Med. 2020:964528420964214. https://doi.org/10.1177/0964528420964214.

22. Loprinzi CL, Michalak JC, Quella SK, Ofallon JR, Hatfield AK, Nelimark RA, et al. Megestrol-acetate for the prevention of hot flashes. N Engl J Med. 1994;331(6):347–52. https://doi.org/10.1056/Nejm199408113310602.
23. Bertelli G, Venturini M, Del Mastro L, Bergaglio M, Sismondi P, Biglia N, et al. Intramuscular depot medroxyprogesterone versus oral megestrol for the control of postmenopausal hot flashes in breast cancer patients: a randomized study. Ann Oncol. 2002;13(6):883–8. https://doi.org/10.1093/annonc/mdf151.
24. Irani J, Salomon L, Oba R, Bouchard P, Mottet N. Efficacy of venlafaxine, medroxyprogesterone acetate, and cyproterone acetate for the treatment of vasomotor hot flushes in men taking gonadotropin-releasing hormone analogues for prostate cancer: a double-blind, randomised trial. Lancet Oncol. 2010;11(2):147–54. https://doi.org/10.1016/S1470-2045(09)70338-9.
25. Leonetti HB, Longo S, Anasti JN. Transdermal progesterone cream for vasomotor symptoms and postmenopausal bone loss. Obstet Gynecol. 1999;94(2):225–8. https://doi.org/10.1016/S0029-7844(99)00266-5.
26. Ruiz Garcia V, Lopez-Briz E, Carbonell Sanchis R, Gonzalvez Perales JL, Bort-Marti S. Megestrol acetate for treatment of anorexia-cachexia syndrome. Cochrane Database Syst Rev. 2013;(3):CD004310. https://doi.org/10.1002/14651858.CD004310.pub3.
27. Khorana AA, Francis CW, Culakova E, Kuderer NM, Lyman GH. Thromboembolism is a leading cause of death in cancer patients receiving outpatient chemotherapy. J Thromb Haemost. 2007;5(3):632–4. https://doi.org/10.1111/j.1538-7836.2007.02374.x.
28. Braga-Basaria M, Muller D, Carducci M, Egan J, John M, Dobs A, et al. Metabolic syndrome in men with prostate cancer undergoing long-term androgen deprivation therapy. J Androl. 2006:92.
29. Eaton AC, McGuire N. Cyproterone acetate in treatment of post-orchidectomy hot flushes. Double-blind cross-over trial. Lancet. 1983;2(8363):1336–7. https://doi.org/10.1016/s0140-6736(83)91092-9.
30. Ronzoni G, De Giovanni L, Menchinelli P, Meneschincheri M. Therapy of vasomotor syndrome in the treatment of advanced prostatic cancer: apropos of 37 cases. Arch Ital Urol Androl. 1998;70(1):37–40.
31. Atala A, Amin M, Harty JI. Diethylstilbestrol in treatment of postorchiectomy vasomotor symptoms and its relationship with serum follicle-stimulating-hormone, luteinizing-hormone, and testosterone. Urology. 1992;39(2):108–10. https://doi.org/10.1016/0090-4295(92)90264-W.
32. Miller JI, Ahmann FR. Treatment of castration-induced menopausal symptoms with low-dose diethylstilbestrol in men with advanced prostate-cancer. Urology. 1992;40(6):499–502. https://doi.org/10.1016/0090-4295(92)90401-H.
33. Gerber GS, Zagaja GP, Ray PS, Rukstalis DB. Transdermal estrogen in the treatment of hot flushes in men with prostate cancer. Urology. 2000;55(1):97–101. https://doi.org/10.1016/S0090-4295(99)00370-2.
34. Loprinzi CL, Dueck AC, Khoyratty BS, Barton DL, Jafar S, Rowland KM Jr, et al. A phase III randomized, double-blind, placebo-controlled trial of gabapentin in the management of hot flashes in men (N00CB). Ann Oncol. 2009;20(3):542–9. https://doi.org/10.1093/annonc/mdn644.
35. Loprinzi CL, Qin R, Balcueva EP, Flynn KA, Rowland KM Jr, Graham DL, et al. Phase III, randomized, double-blind, placebo-controlled evaluation of pregabalin for alleviating hot flashes, N07C1. J Clin Oncol. 2010;28(4):641–7. https://doi.org/10.1200/JCO.2009.24.5647.
36. Loprinzi CL, Barton DL, Carpenter LA, Sloan JA, Novotny PJ, Gettman MT, et al. Pilot evaluation of paroxetine for treating hot flashes in men. Mayo Clin Proc. 2004;79(10):1247–51. https://doi.org/10.4065/79.10.1247.
37. Stearns V, Isaacs C, Rowland J, Crawford J, Ellis MJ, Kramer R, et al. A pilot trial assessing the efficacy of paroxetine hydrochloride (Paxil (R)) in controlling hot flashes in breast cancer survivors. Ann Oncol. 2000;11(1):17–22. https://doi.org/10.1023/A:1008382706068.
38. Stearns V, Slack R, Greep N, Henry-Tilman R, Osborne M, Bunnell C, et al. Paroxetine is an effective treatment for hot flashes: results from a prospective randomized clinical trial. J Clin Oncol. 2005;23(28):6919–30. https://doi.org/10.1200/Jco.2005.10.081.

39. Stearns V, Beebe KL, Iyengar M, Dube E. Paroxetine controlled release in the treatment of menopausal hot flashes – a randomized controlled trial. JAMA: J Am Med Assoc. 2003;289(21):2827–34. https://doi.org/10.1001/jama.289.21.2827.
40. Loprinzi CL, Flynn PJ, Carpenter LA, Atherton P, Barton DL, Shanafelt TD, et al. Pilot evaluation of citalopram for the treatment of hot flashes in women with inadequate benefit from venlafaxine. J Palliat Med. 2005;8(5):924–30. https://doi.org/10.1089/jpm.2005.8.924.
41. Barton DL, LaVasseur BI, Sloan JA, Stawis AN, Flynn KA, Dyar M, et al. Phase III, placebo-controlled trial of three doses of citalopram for the treatment of hot flashes: NCCTG trial N05C9. J Clin Oncol. 2010;28(20):3278–83. https://doi.org/10.1200/Jco.2009.26.6379.
42. Suvanto-Luukkonen E, Koivunen R, Sundstrom H, Bloigu R, Kaljalainen E, Haiva-Mallinen L, et al. Citalopram and fluoxetine in the treatment of postmenopausal symptoms: a prospective, randomized, 9-month, placebo-controlled, double-blind study. Menopause: J N Am Menopause Soc. 2005;12(1):18–26. https://doi.org/10.1097/00042192-200512010-00006.
43. Roth AJ, Scher HI. Sertraline relieves hot flashes secondary to medical castration as treatment of advanced prostate cancer. Psychooncology. 1998;7(2):129–32. https://doi.org/10.1002/(SICI)1099-1611(199803/04)7:2<129::AID-PON294>3.0.CO;2-T.
44. Loprinzi CL, Sloan JA, Perez EA, Quella SK, Stella PJ, Mailliard JA, et al. Phase III evaluation of fluoxetine for treatment of hot flashes. J Clin Oncol. 2002;20(6):1578–83. https://doi.org/10.1200/JCO.2002.20.6.1578.
45. Benoist GE, Hendriks RJ, Mulders PFA, Gerritsen WR, Somford DM, Schalken JA, et al. Pharmacokinetic aspects of the two novel oral drugs used for metastatic castration-resistant prostate cancer: abiraterone acetate and enzalutamide. Clin Pharmacokinet. 2016;55(11):1369–80. https://doi.org/10.1007/s40262-016-0403-6.
46. Barton D, La Vasseur B, Loprinzi C, Novotny P, Wilwerding MB, Sloan J. Venlafaxine for the control of hot flashes: results of a longitudinal continuation study. Oncol Nurs Forum. 2002;29(1):33–40. https://doi.org/10.1188/02.ONF.33-40.
47. Bordeleau L, Pritchard KI, Loprinzi CL, Ennis M, Jugovic O, Warr D, et al. Multicenter, randomized, cross-over clinical trial of venlafaxine versus gabapentin for the management of hot flashes in breast cancer survivors. J Clin Oncol. 2010;28(35):5147–52. https://doi.org/10.1200/JCO.2010.29.9230.
48. Loprinzi CL, Levitt R, Barton D, Sloan JA, Dakhil SR, Nikcevich DA, et al. Phase III comparison of depomedroxyprogesterone acetate to venlafaxine for managing hot flashes: North Central Cancer Treatment Group Trial N99C7. J Clin Oncol. 2006;24(9):1409–14. https://doi.org/10.1200/JCO.2005.04.7324.
49. Quella SK, Loprinzi CL, Sloan J, Novotny P, Perez EA, Burch PA, et al. Pilot evaluation of venlafaxine for the treatment of hot flashes in men undergoing androgen ablation therapy for prostate cancer. J Urol. 1999;162(1):98–102. https://doi.org/10.1097/00005392-199907000-00024.
50. Speroff L, Gass M, Constantine G, Olivier S, Investigators S. Efficacy and tolerability of desvenlafaxine succinate treatment for menopausal vasomotor symptoms – a randomized controlled trial. Obstet Gynecol. 2008;111(1):77–87. https://doi.org/10.1097/01.AOG.0000297371.89129.b3.
51. Loprinzi CL, Goldberg RM, Ofallon JR, Quella SK, Miser AW, Mynderse LA, et al. Transdermal clonidine for ameliorating postorchiectomy hot flashes. J Urol. 1994;151(3):634–6. https://doi.org/10.1016/S0022-5347(17)35034-6.
52. Goldberg RM, Loprinzi CL, Ofallon JR, Veeder MH, Miser AW, Mailliard JA, et al. Transdermal clonidine for ameliorating tamoxifen-induced hot flashes. J Clin Oncol. 1994;12(1):155–8. https://doi.org/10.1200/Jco.1994.12.1.155.
53. Laufer LR, Erlik Y, Meldrum DR, Judd HL. Effect of clonidine on hot flashes in postmenopausal women. Obstet Gynecol. 1982;60(5):583–6.
54. Clayden JR, Bell JW, Pollard P. Menopausal flushing – double-blind trial of a non-hormonal medication. Br Med J. 1974;1(5905):409–12. https://doi.org/10.1136/bmj.1.5905.409.
55. Schindler AE, Muller D, Keller E, Goser R, Runkel F. Studies with clonidine (Dixarit) in menopausal women. Arch Gynecol. 1979;227(4):341–7. https://doi.org/10.1007/Bf02109923.

56. Jones JM, Kohli M, Loprinzi CL. Androgen deprivation therapy-associated vasomotor symptoms. Asian J Androl. 2012;14(2):193–7. https://doi.org/10.1038/aja.2011.101.
57. Corona G, Filippi S, Comelio P, Bianchi N, Frizza F, Dicuio M, et al. Sexual function in men undergoing androgen deprivation therapy. Int J Impot Res. 2021. https://doi.org/10.1038/s41443-021-00418-7.
58. Walsh PC. The discovery of the cavernous nerves and development of nerve sparing radical retropubic prostatectomy. J Urol. 2007;177(5):1632–5. https://doi.org/10.1016/j.juro.2007.01.012.
59. Walsh PC, Marschke P, Ricker D, Burnett AL. Patient-reported urinary continence and sexual function after anatomic radical prostatectomy. Urology. 2000;55(1):58–61. https://doi.org/10.1016/S0090-4295(99)00397-0.
60. Kundu SD, Roehl KA, Eggener SE, Antenor JAV, Han M, Catalona WJ. Potency, continence and complications in 3,477 consecutive radical retropubic prostatectomies. J Urol. 2004;172(6):2227–31. https://doi.org/10.1097/01.ju.0000145222.94455.73.
61. Buyyounouski MK, Horwitz EM, Price RA, Hanlon AL, Uzzo RG, Pollack A. Intensity-modulated radiotherapy with MRI simulation to reduce doses received by erectile tissue during prostate cancer treatment. Int J Radiat Oncol. 2004;58(3):743–9. https://doi.org/10.1016/S0360-3016(03)01617-1.
62. Hamilton AS, Stanford JL, Gilliland FD, Albertsen PC, Stephenson RA, Hoffman RM, et al. Health outcomes after external-beam radiation therapy for clinically localized prostate cancer: results from the prostate cancer outcomes study. J Clin Oncol. 2001;19(9):2517–26. https://doi.org/10.1200/Jco.2001.19.9.2517.
63. Alemozaffar M, Regan MM, Cooperberg MR, Wei JT, Michalski JM, Sandler HM, et al. Prediction of erectile function following treatment for prostate cancer. JAMA: J Am Med Assoc. 2011;306(11):1205–14. https://doi.org/10.1001/jama.2011.1333.
64. Potters L, Torre T, Fearn PA, Leibel SA, Kattan MW. Potency after permanent prostate brachytherapy for localized prostate cancer. Int J Radiat Oncol Biol Phys. 2001;50(5):1235–42. https://doi.org/10.1016/S0360-3016(01)01578-4.
65. Merrick GS, Butler WM, Wallner KE, Galbreath RW, Anderson RL, Kurko BS, et al. Erectile function after prostate brachytherapy. Int J Radiat Oncol Biol Phys. 2005;62(2):437–47. https://doi.org/10.1016/j.ijrobp.2004.10.001.
66. Sari Motlagh R, Abufaraj M, Yang L, Mori K, Pradere B, Laukhtina E, et al. Penile rehabilitation strategy after nerve sparing radical prostatectomy: a systematic review and network meta-analysis of randomized trials. J Urol. 2021;205(4):1018–30. https://doi.org/10.1097/JU.0000000000001584.
67. Nicolai M, Urkmez A, Sarikaya S, Fode M, Falcone M, Albersen M, et al. Penile rehabilitation and treatment options for erectile dysfunction following radical prostatectomy and radiotherapy: a systematic review. Front Surg. 2021;8:636974. https://doi.org/10.3389/fsurg.2021.636974.
68. Rousseau L, Dupont A, Labrie F, Couture M. Sexuality changes in prostate cancer patients receiving antihormonal therapy combining the antiandrogen flutamide with medical (LHRH agonist) or surgical castration. Arch Sex Behav. 1988;17(1):87–98. https://doi.org/10.1007/BF01542054.
69. Potosky AL, Knopf K, Clegg LX, Albertsen PC, Stanford JL, Hamilton AS, et al. Quality-of-life outcomes after primary androgen deprivation therapy: results from the Prostate Cancer Outcomes Study. J Clin Oncol. 2001;19(17):3750–7. https://doi.org/10.1200/JCO.2001.19.17.3750.
70. Schover LR. Sexual healing in patients with prostate cancer on hormone therapy. Am Soc Clin Oncol Educ Book. 2015:e562–6. https://doi.org/10.14694/EdBook_AM.2015.35.e562.
71. Levine LA, Estrada CR, Morgentaler A. Mechanical reliability and safety of, and patient satisfaction with the Ambicor inflatable penile prosthesis: results of a 2 center study. J Urol. 2001;166(3):932–7. https://doi.org/10.1016/S0022-5347(05)65867-3.
72. Alexis O, Worsley AJ. The experiences of gay and bisexual men post-prostate cancer treatment: a meta-synthesis of qualitative studies. Am J Mens Health. 2018;12(6):2076–88. https://doi.org/10.1177/1557988318793785.

73. Watson E, Shinkins B, Frith E, Neal D, Hamdy F, Walter F, et al. Symptoms, unmet needs, psychological well-being and health status in survivors of prostate cancer: implications for redesigning follow-up. BJU Int. 2016;117(6B):E10–9. https://doi.org/10.1111/bju.13122.
74. Goonewardene SS, Persad R. Psychosexual care in prostate cancer survivorship: a systematic review. Translat Androl Urol. 2015;4(4):413–20. https://doi.org/10.3978/j.issn.2223-4683.2015.08.04.
75. Manne SL, Kashy DA, Zaider T, Kissane D, Lee D, Kim IY, et al. Couple-focused interventions for men with localized prostate cancer and their spouses: a randomized clinical trial. Br J Health Psychol. 2019;24(2):396–418. https://doi.org/10.1111/bjhp.12359.
76. Wootten AC, Abbott JM, Farrell A, Austin DW, Klein B. Psychosocial interventions to support partners of men with prostate cancer: a systematic and critical review of the literature. J Cancer Surviv. 2014;8(3):472–84. https://doi.org/10.1007/s11764-014-0361-7.
77. Albiges L, Tannir NM, Burotto M, McDermott D, Plimack ER, Barthelemy P, et al. Nivolumab plus ipilimumab versus sunitinib for first-line treatment of advanced renal cell carcinoma: extended 4-year follow-up of the phase III CheckMate 214 trial. Esmo Open. 2020;5(6):ARTN e001079. https://doi.org/10.1136/esmoopen-2020-001079.
78. Mejean A, Ravaud A, Thezenas S, Colas S, Beauval JB, Bensalah K, et al. Sunitinib alone or after nephrectomy in metastatic renal-cell carcinoma. N Engl J Med. 2018;379(5):417–27. https://doi.org/10.1056/NEJMoa1803675.
79. Bex A, Mulders P, Jewett M, Wagstaff J, van Thienen JV, Blank CU, et al. Comparison of immediate vs deferred cytoreductive nephrectomy in patients with synchronous metastatic renal cell carcinoma receiving sunitinib: the SURTIME randomized clinical trial (vol 5, pg 164, 2018). Jama Oncol. 2019;5(2):271. https://doi.org/10.1001/jamaoncol.2019.0117.
80. Hofmann F, Hwang EC, Lam TBL, Bex A, Yuan YH, Marconi LSO, et al. Targeted therapy for metastatic renal cell carcinoma. Cochrane Database Syst Rev. 2020(10):ARTN CD012796. https://doi.org/10.1002/14651858.CD012796.pub2.
81. Hutson TE, Figlin RA, Kuhn JG, Motzer RJ. Targeted therapies for metastatic renal cell carcinoma: an overview of toxicity and dosing strategies. Oncologist. 2008;13(10):1084–96. https://doi.org/10.1634/theoncologist.2008-0120.
82. Jonasch E, Pagliaro LC, Tannir NM. Long-term management of patients with metastatic renal cell carcinoma on targeted agents. Expert Rev Anticancer Ther. 2010;10(12):1883–9. https://doi.org/10.1586/Era.10.195.
83. Gandhi S, Day L, Paramsothy T, Giotis A, Ford M, Boudreau A, et al. Oral anticancer medication adherence, toxicity reporting, and counseling: a study comparing health care providers and patients J Oncol Pract. 2015;11(6):498-+. https://doi.org/10.1200/Jop.2015.004572.
84. Houk BE, Bello CL, Poland B, Rosen LS, Demetri GD, Motzer RJ. Relationship between exposure to sunitinib and efficacy and tolerability endpoints in patients with cancer: results of a pharmacokinetic/pharmacodynamic meta-analysis. Cancer Chemother Pharmacol. 2010;66(2):357–71. https://doi.org/10.1007/s00280-009-1170-y.
85. McLellan B, Kerr H. Cutaneous toxicities of the multikinase inhibitors sorafenib and sunitinib. Dermatol Ther. 2011;24(4):396–400. https://doi.org/10.1111/j.1529-8019.2011.01435.x.
86. Kwakman JJM, Elshot YS, Punt CJA, Koopman M. Management of cytotoxic chemotherapy-induced hand-foot syndrome. Oncol Rev. 2020;14(1):57–63. https://doi.org/10.4081/oncol.2020.442.
87. Nardone B, Hensley JR, Kulik L, West DP, Mulcahy M, Rademaker A, et al. The effect of hand-foot skin reaction associated with the multikinase inhibitors sorafenib and sunitinib on health-related quality of life. J Drugs Dermatol. 2012;11(11):e61–5.
88. Franck N, Barete S, Moguelet P, Blanchet B, Carlotti A, Ropert S, et al. Spiny follicular hyperkeratosis eruption: a new cutaneous adverse effect of sorafenib. J Clin Oncol. 2010;28(31):E640–E2. https://doi.org/10.1200/Jco.2010.31.3783.
89. James WD, Elston DM, Berger TG. Andrews' diseases of the skin: clinical dermatology. 12th ed. Philadelphia: Elsevier; 2016.
90. Torino F, Corsello SM, Longo R, Barnabei A, Gasparini G. Hypothyroidism related to tyrosine kinase inhibitors: an emerging toxic effect of targeted therapy. Nat Rev Clin Oncol. 2009;6(4):219–28. https://doi.org/10.1038/nrclinonc.2009.4.

91. Grossmann M, Premaratne E, Desai J, Davis ID. Thyrotoxicosis during sunitinib treatment for renal cell carcinoma. Clin Endocrinol. 2008;69(4):669–72. https://doi.org/10.1111/j.1365-2265.2008.03253.x.
92. Agostino NM, Chinchilli VM, Lynch CJ, Koszyk-Szewczyk A, Gingrich R, Sivik J, et al. Effect of the tyrosine kinase inhibitors (sunitinib, sorafenib, dasatinib, and imatinib) on blood glucose levels in diabetic and nondiabetic patients in general clinical practice. J Oncol Pharm Pract. 2011;17(3):197–202. https://doi.org/10.1177/1078155210378913.
93. Appleby L, Morrissey S, Bellmunt J, Rosenberg J. Management of treatment-related toxicity with targeted therapies for renal cell carcinoma: evidence-based practice and best practices. Hematol Oncol Clin N. 2011;25(4):893-+. https://doi.org/10.1016/j.hoc.2011.05.004.
94. Hall PS, Harshman LC, Srinivas S, Witteles RM. The frequency and severity of cardiovascular toxicity from targeted therapy in advanced renal cell carcinoma patients. JACC Heart Fail. 2013;1(1):72–8. https://doi.org/10.1016/j.jchf.2012.09.001.
95. Totzeck M, Mincu RI, Mrotzek S, Schadendorf D, Rassaf T. Cardiovascular diseases in patients receiving small molecules with anti-vascular endothelial growth factor activity: a meta-analysis of approximately 29,000 cancer patients. Eur J Prev Cardiol. 2018;25(5):482–94. https://doi.org/10.1177/2047487318755193.
96. Schlumberger M, Tahara M, Wirth LJ, Robinson B, Brose MS, Elisei R, et al. Lenvatinib versus placebo in radioiodine-refractory thyroid cancer. N Engl J Med. 2015;372(7):621–30. https://doi.org/10.1056/NEJMoa1406470.
97. Cifu AS, Davis AM. Prevention, detection, evaluation, and management of high blood pressure in adults. JAMA: J Am Med Assoc. 2017;318(21):2132–4. https://doi.org/10.1001/jama.2017.18706.
98. Izzedine H, Derosa L, Le Teuff G, Albiges L, Escudier B. Hypertension and angiotensin system inhibitors: impact on outcome in sunitinib-treated patients for metastatic renal cell carcinoma. Ann Oncol. 2015;26(6):1128–33. https://doi.org/10.1093/annonc/mdv147.
99. Pearman TP, Beaumont JL, Mroczek D, O'Connor M, Cella D. Validity and usefulness of a single-item measure of patient-reported bother from side effects of cancer therapy. Cancer-Am Cancer Soc. 2018;124(5):991–7. https://doi.org/10.1002/cncr.31133.
100. Banna GL, Collova E, Gebbia V, Lipari H, Giuffrida P, Cavallaro S, et al. Anticancer oral therapy: emerging related issues. Cancer Treat Rev. 2010;36(8):595–605. https://doi.org/10.1016/j.ctrv.2010.04.005.
101. Ruddy K, Mayer E, Partridge A. Patient adherence and persistence with oral anticancer treatment. CA: Cancer J Clin. 2009;59(1):56–66. https://doi.org/10.3322/caac.20004.
102. ter Stege JA, Oldenburg HSA, Woerdeman LAE, Witkamp AJ, Kieffer JM, van Huizum MA, et al. Decisional conflict in breast cancer patients considering immediate breast reconstruction. Breast. 2021;55:91–7. https://doi.org/10.1016/j.breast.2020.12.001.
103. Schwarze ML, Kehler JM, Campbell TC. Navigating high risk procedures with more than just a street map. J Palliat Med. 2013;16(10):1169–71. https://doi.org/10.1089/jpm.2013.0221.
104. Taylor LJ, Nabozny MJ, Steffens NM, Tucholka JL, Brasel KJ, Johnson SK, et al. A framework to improve surgeon communication in high-stakes surgical decisions best case/worst case. JAMA Surg. 2017;152(6):531–8. https://doi.org/10.1001/jamasurg.2016.5674.
105. Rosenberg SA, Yang JC, Topalian SL, Schwartzentruber DJ, Weber JS, Parkinson DR, et al. Treatment of 283 consecutive patients with metastatic melanoma or renal-cell cancer using high-dose bolus interleukin-2. JAMA: J Am Med Assoc. 1994;271(12):907–13. https://doi.org/10.1001/jama.271.12.907.
106. Warner EL, Ellington L, Kirchhoff AC, Cloyes KG. Acquisition of social support and linguistic characteristics of social media posts about young adult cancer. J Adolesc Young Adult Oncol. 2018;7(2):196–203. https://doi.org/10.1089/jayao.2017.0076.
107. Bergerot CD, Bergerot PG, Philip EJ, Hsu JA, Dizman N, Vaishampayan U, et al. Perception of cure among patients with metastatic genitourinary cancer initiating immunotherapy. J Immunother Cancer. 2019;7(1):71. https://doi.org/10.1186/s40425-019-0557-5.
108. Temel JS, Shaw AT, Greer JA. Challenge of prognostic uncertainty in the modern era of cancer therapeutics. J Clin Oncol. 2016;34(30):3605–8. https://doi.org/10.1200/jco.2016.67.8573.

109. Temel JS, Greer JA, Admane S, Gallagher ER, Jackson VA, Lynch TJ, et al. Longitudinal perceptions of prognosis and goals of therapy in patients with metastatic non-small-cell lung cancer: results of a randomized study of early palliative care. J Clin Oncol. 2011;29(17):2319–26. https://doi.org/10.1200/JCO.2010.32.4459.
110. Witjes JA, Bruins HM, Cathomas R, Comperat EM, Cowan NC, Gakis G, et al. European Association of Urology guidelines on muscle-invasive and metastatic bladder cancer: summary of the 2020 guidelines. Eur Urol. 2021;79(1):82–104. https://doi.org/10.1016/j.eururo.2020.03.055.
111. Su XH, Wu KH, Wang S, Su W, Li CY, Li BK, et al. The impact of orthotopic neobladder vs ileal conduit urinary diversion after cystectomy on the survival outcomes in patients with bladder cancer: a propensity score matched analysis. Cancer Med-US. 2020;9(20):7590–600. https://doi.org/10.1002/cam4.3404.
112. Browne E, Lawrentschuk N, Jack GS, Davis NF. A systematic review and meta-analysis of the long-term outcomes of ileal conduit and orthotopic neobladder urinary diversion. CUAJ-Can Urol Assoc J. 2021;15(1):E48–57. https://doi.org/10.5489/cuaj.6466.
113. Demaegd L, Albersen M, Muilwijk T, Milenkovic U, Moris L, Everaerts W, et al. Comparison of postoperative complications of ileal conduits versus orthotopic neobladders. Transl Androl Urol. 2020;9(6):2541–54. https://doi.org/10.21037/tau-20-713.
114. Ziouziou I, Irani J, Wei JT, Karmouni T, El Khader K, Koutani A, et al. Ileal conduit vs orthotopic neobladder: which one offers the best health-related quality of life in patients undergoing radical cystectomy? A systematic review of literature and meta-analysis. Progres En Urologie. 2018;28(5):241–50. https://doi.org/10.1016/j.purol.2018.02.001.
115. Shi HC, Yu H, Bellmunt J, Leow JJ, Chen XY, Guo CC, et al. Comparison of health-related quality of life (HRQoL) between ileal conduit diversion and orthotopic neobladder based on validated questionnaires: a systematic review and meta-analysis. Qual Life Res. 2018;27(11):2759–75. https://doi.org/10.1007/s11136-018-1902-8.
116. Cerruto MA, D'Elia C, Siracusano S, Saleh O, Gacci M, Cacciamani G, et al. Health-related quality of life after radical cystectomy for bladder cancer in elderly patients with ileal orthotopic neobladder or ileal conduit: results from a multicentre cross-sectional study using validated questionnaires. Urol Int. 2018;100(3):346–52. https://doi.org/10.1159/000487644.
117. Goldberg H, Baniel J, Mano R, Rotlevy G, Kedar D, Yossepowitch O. Orthotopic neobladder vs. ileal conduit urinary diversion: a long-term quality-of -life comparison. Urol Oncol-Semin Ori. 2016;34(3):ARTN 121.e1. https://doi.org/10.1016/j.urolonc.2015.10.006.
118. Singh V, Yadav R, Sinha RJ, Gupta DK. Prospective comparison of quality-of-life outcomes between ileal conduit urinary diversion and orthotopic neobladder reconstruction after radical cystectomy: a statistical model. BJU Int. 2014;113(5):726–32. https://doi.org/10.1111/bju.12440.
119. Crozier J, Hennessey D, Sengupta S, Bolton D, Lawrentschuk N. A systematic review of ileal conduit and neobladder outcomes in primary bladder cancer. Urology. 2016;96:74–9. https://doi.org/10.1016/j.urology.2016.06.034.
120. Almassi N, Bochner BH. Ileal conduit or orthotopic neobladder: selection and contemporary patterns of use. Curr Opin Urol. 2020;30(3):415–20. https://doi.org/10.1097/Mou.0000000000000738.
121. Ali AS, Hayes MC, Birch B, Dudderidge T, Somani BK. Health related quality of life (HRQoL) after cystectomy: comparison between orthotopic neobladder and ileal conduit diversion. Eur J Surg Oncol: EJSO. 2015;41(3):295–9. https://doi.org/10.1016/j.ejso.2014.05.006.
122. Werth SL, Schutte DL, Stommel M. Bridging the gap perceived educational needs in the inpatient to home care setting for the person with a new ostomy. J Wound Ostomy Cont Nurs. 2014;41(6):566–72. https://doi.org/10.1097/Won.0000000000000081.
123. Metcalf C. Stoma care: empowering patients through teaching practical skills. Br J Nurs. 1999;8(9):593–600. https://doi.org/10.12968/bjon.1999.8.9.6621.
124. Vujnovich A. Pre and post-operative assessment of patients with a stoma. Nurs Stand. 2008;22(19):50–6; quiz 8. https://doi.org/10.7748/ns2008.01.22.19.50.c6315.

125. Quirk H, Rosario DJ, Bourke L. Supportive interventions to improve physiological and psychological health outcomes among patients undergoing cystectomy: a systematic review. BMC Urol. 2018;18(1):71. https://doi.org/10.1186/s12894-018-0382-z.
126. Danielsen AK, Burcharth J, Rosenberg J. Patient education has a positive effect in patients with a stoma: a systematic review. Colorectal Dis. 2013;15(6):e276–e83. https://doi.org/10.1111/codi.12197.
127. Wulff-Burchfield EM, Potts M, Glavin K, Mirza M. A qualitative evaluation of a nurse-led pre-operative stoma education program for bladder cancer patients. Support Care Cancer. 2021. https://doi.org/10.1007/s00520-021-06093-0.
128. Mohamed NE, Pisipati S, Lee CT, Goltz HH, Latini DM, Gilbert FS, et al. Unmet informational and supportive care needs of patients following cystectomy for bladder cancer based on age, sex, and treatment choices. Urol Oncol Semin Ori Investig. 2016;34(12):531-e7. https://doi.org/10.1016/j.urolonc.2016.06.010.
129. Paterson C, Jensen BT, Jensen JB, Nabi G. Unmet informational and supportive care needs of patients with muscle invasive bladder cancer: a systematic review of the evidence. Eur J Oncol Nurs. 2018;35:92–101. https://doi.org/10.1016/j.ejon.2018.05.006.
130. Beduk Y, Turkolmez K, Baltaci S, Gogus C. Comparison of clinical and urodynamic outcome in orthotopic ileocaecal and ileal neobladder. Eur Urol. 2003;43(3):258–62. https://doi.org/10.1016/s0302-2838(03)00042-3.
131. Imbimbo C, Mirone V, Siracusano S, Niero M, Cerruto MA, Lonardi C, et al. Quality of life assessment with orthotopic ileal neobladder reconstruction after radical cystectomy: results from a prospective Italian Multicenter Observational Study. Urology. 2015;86(5):974–80. https://doi.org/10.1016/j.urology.2015.06.058.
132. Haisfield-Wolfe ME, Schoenberg M, Welch J, Huang Y. Improving the quality of continence for bladder cancer patients recovering after a cystectomy with neobladder reconstruction. Oncol Nurs Forum. 2004;31(2):412.
133. Messing EM. Urothelial tumors of the bladder. In: Wein AJ, editor. Campbell-Walsh urology. Philadelphia: Saunders Elsevier; 2008. p. 2407–46.
134. Figueroa AJ, Stein JP, Dickinson M, Skinner EC, Thangathurai D, Mikhail MS, et al. Radical cystectomy for elderly patients with bladder carcinoma – an updated experience with 404 patients. Cancer-Am Cancer Soc. 1998;83(1):141–7. https://doi.org/10.1002/(Sici)1097-0142(19980701)83:1<141::Aid-Cncr19>3.0.Co;2-X.
135. Nielsen ME, Shariat SF, Karakiewicz PI, Lotan Y, Rogers CG, Amiel GE, et al. Advanced age is associated with poorer bladder cancer-specific survival in patients treated with radical cystectomy. Eur Urol. 2007;51(3):699–708. https://doi.org/10.1016/j.eururo.2006.11.004.
136. Tyritzis SI, Anastasiou I, Stravodimos KG, Alevizopoulos A, Kollias A, Balangas A, et al. Radical cystectomy over the age of 75 is safe and increases survival. BMC Geriatr. 2012;12:Artn 18. https://doi.org/10.1186/1471-2318-12-18.
137. Chang SS, Alberts G, Cookson MS, Smith JA. Radical cystectomy is safe in elderly patients at high risk. J Urol. 2001;166(3):938–40. https://doi.org/10.1016/S0022-5347(05)65868-5.
138. Ethun CG, Bilen MA, Jani AB, Maithel SK, Ogan K, Master VA. Frailty and cancer: implications for oncology surgery, medical oncology, and radiation oncology. CA-Cancer J Clin. 2017;67(5):363–77. https://doi.org/10.3322/caac.21406.
139. Chappidi MR, Kates M, Patel HD, Tosoian JJ, Kaye DR, Sopko NA, et al. Frailty as a marker of adverse outcomes in patients with bladder cancer undergoing radical cystectomy. Urol Oncol Semin Ori. 2016;34(6):256-e1. https://doi.org/10.1016/j.urolonc.2015.12.010.
140. Burg ML, Clifford TG, Bazargani ST, Lin-Brande M, Miranda G, Cai J, et al. Frailty as a predictor of complications after radical cystectomy: a prospective study of various preoperative assessments. Urol Oncol-Semin Ori. 2019;37(1):40–7. https://doi.org/10.1016/j.urolonc.2018.10.002.
141. Palumbo C, Knipper S, Pecoraro A, Rosiello G, Luzzago S, Deuker M, et al. Patient frailty predicts worse perioperative outcomes and higher cost after radical cystectomy. Surg Oncol-Oxford. 2020;32:8–13. https://doi.org/10.1016/j.suronc.2019.10.014.

142. Bochner BH, Dalbagni G, Sjoberg DD, Silberstein J, Paz GEK, Donat SM, et al. Comparing open radical cystectomy and robot-assisted laparoscopic radical cystectomy: a randomized clinical trial. Eur Urol. 2015;67(6):1042–50. https://doi.org/10.1016/j.eururo.2014.11.043.
143. Ritch CR, Balise R, Prakash NS, Alonzo D, Almengo K, Alameddine M, et al. Propensity matched comparative analysis of survival following chemoradiation or radical cystectomy for muscle-invasive bladder cancer. BJU Int. 2018;121(5):745–51. https://doi.org/10.1111/bju.14109.
144. Jensen BT, Lauridsen SV, Jensen JB. Prehabilitation for major abdominal urologic oncology surgery. Curr Opin Urol. 2018;28(3):243–50. https://doi.org/10.1097/Mou.0000000000000487.
145. Wiffen PJ, Wee B, Derry S, Bell RF, Moore RA. Opioids for cancer pain – an overview of Cochrane reviews. Cochrane Database Syst Rev. 2017;7:CD012592. https://doi.org/10.1002/14651858.CD012592.pub2.
146. Wiffen PJ, Wee B, Moore RA. Oral morphine for cancer pain. Cochrane Database Syst Rev. 2016;4:CD003868. https://doi.org/10.1002/14651858.CD003868.pub4.
147. Casey KL. Neural mechanisms of pain: an overview. Acta Anaesthesiol Scand Suppl. 1982;74:13–20. https://doi.org/10.1111/j.1399-6576.1982.tb01838.x.
148. Portenoy RK, Ahmed E. Cancer pain syndromes. Hematol Oncol Clin North Am. 2018;32(3):371–86. https://doi.org/10.1016/j.hoc.2018.01.002.
149. WHO guidelines for the pharmacological and radiotherapeutic management of cancer pain in adults and adolescents. WHO guidelines approved by the Guidelines Review Committee. Geneva; 2018.
150. Paice JA, Portenoy R, Lacchetti C, Campbell T, Cheville A, Citron M, et al. Management of chronic pain in survivors of adult cancers: American Society of Clinical Oncology clinical practice guideline. J Clin Oncol. 2016;34(27):3325–45. https://doi.org/10.1200/JCO.2016.68.5206.
151. Swarm RA, Paice JA, Anghelescu DL, Are M, Bruce JY, Buga S, et al. Adult cancer pain, version 3.2019, NCCN clinical practice guidelines in oncology. J Natl Compr Cancer Netw. 2019;17(8):977–1007. https://doi.org/10.6004/jnccn.2019.0038.
152. Fallon M, Giusti R, Aielli F, Hoskin P, Rolke R, Sharma M, et al. Management of cancer pain in adult patients: ESMO clinical practice guidelines. Ann Oncol. 2018;29(Suppl 4):iv166–iv91. https://doi.org/10.1093/annonc/mdy152.
153. Sykes NP. The relationship between opioid use and laxative use in terminally ill cancer patients. Palliat Med. 1998;12(5):375–82. https://doi.org/10.1191/026921698674125048.
154. Poulsen JL, Brock C, Olesen AE, Nilsson M, Drewes AM. Evolving paradigms in the treatment of opioid-induced bowel dysfunction. Ther Adv Gastroenterol. 2015;8(6):360–72. https://doi.org/10.1177/1756283X15589526.
155. Tarumi Y, Wilson MP, Szafran O, Spooner GR. Randomized, double-blind, placebo-controlled trial of oral docusate in the management of constipation in hospice patients. J Pain Symptom Manag. 2013;45(1):2–13. https://doi.org/10.1016/j.jpainsymman.2012.02.008.
156. Camilleri M, Drossman DA, Becker G, Webster LR, Davies AN, Mawe GM. Emerging treatments in neurogastroenterology: a multidisciplinary working group consensus statement on opioid-induced constipation. Neurogastroenterol Motil. 2014;26(10):1386–95. https://doi.org/10.1111/nmo.12417.
157. Chey WD, Webster L, Sostek M, Lappalainen J, Barker PN, Tack J. Naloxegol for opioid-induced constipation in patients with noncancer pain. N Engl J Med. 2014;370(25):2387–96. https://doi.org/10.1056/NEJMoa1310246.
158. Thomas J, Karver S, Cooney GA, Chamberlain BH, Watt CK, Slatkin NE, et al. Methylnaltrexone for opioid-induced constipation in advanced illness. N Engl J Med. 2008;358(22):2332–43. https://doi.org/10.1056/NEJMoa0707377.
159. Cuppoletti J, Chakrabarti J, Tewari K, Malinowska DH. Methadone but not morphine inhibits lubiprostone-stimulated Cl- currents in T84 intestinal cells and recombinant human

ClC-2, but not CFTR Cl- currents. Cell Biochem Biophys. 2013;66(1):53–63. https://doi.org/10.1007/s12013-012-9406-6.
160. Webster LR, Webster RM. Predicting aberrant behaviors in opioid-treated patients: preliminary validation of the opioid risk tool. Pain Med. 2005;6(6):432–42. https://doi.org/10.1111/j.1526-4637.2005.00072.x.
161. Butler SF, Budman SH, Fernandez KC, Fanciullo GJ, Jamison RN. Cross-validation of a screener to predict opioid misuse in chronic pain patients (SOAPP-R). J Addict Med. 2009;3(2):66–73. https://doi.org/10.1097/ADM.0b013e31818e41da.
162. Dalal S, Bruera E. Pain management for patients with advanced cancer in the opioid epidemic era. Am Soc Clin Oncol Educ Book. 2019;39:24–35. https://doi.org/10.1200/EDBK_100020.
163. Directors ABo. Prescription drug monitoring programs (PDMPs). 2018. Accessed.
164. Bennett MI, Rayment C, Hjermstad M, Aass N, Caraceni A, Kaasa S. Prevalence and aetiology of neuropathic pain in cancer patients: a systematic review. Pain. 2012;153(2):359–65. https://doi.org/10.1016/j.pain.2011.10.028.
165. Ochoa JL. Neuropathic pain: redefinition and a grading system for clinical and research purposes. Neurology. 2009;72(14):1282–3. https://doi.org/10.1212/01.wnl.0000346325.50431.5f.
166. Finnerup NB, Attal N, Haroutounian S, McNicol E, Baron R, Dworkin RH, et al. Pharmacotherapy for neuropathic pain in adults: a systematic review and meta-analysis. Lancet Neurol. 2015;14(2):162–73. https://doi.org/10.1016/S1474-4422(14)70251-0.
167. van den Beuken-van Everdingen MHJ, de Graeff A, Jongen JLM, Dijkstra D, Mostovaya I, Vissers KC, et al. Pharmacological treatment of pain in cancer patients: the role of adjuvant analgesics, a systematic review. Pain Pract. 2017;17(3):409–19. https://doi.org/10.1111/papr.12459.
168. Bennett MI. Effectiveness of antiepileptic or antidepressant drugs when added to opioids for cancer pain: systematic review. Palliat Med. 2011;25(5):553–9. https://doi.org/10.1177/0269216310378546.
169. Haywood A, Good P, Khan S, Leupp A, Jenkins-Marsh S, Rickett K, et al. Corticosteroids for the management of cancer-related pain in adults. Cochrane Database Syst Rev. 2015(4):ARTN CD010756. https://doi.org/10.1002/14651858.CD010756.pub2.
170. Arcidiacono PG, Calori G, Carrara S, McNicol ED, Testoni PA. Celiac plexus block for pancreatic cancer pain in adults. Cochrane Database Syst Rev. 2011;(3):CD007519. https://doi.org/10.1002/14651858.CD007519.pub2.
171. Fourney DR, Schomer DF, Nader R, Chlan-Fourney J, Suki D, Ahrar K, et al. Percutaneous vertebroplasty and kyphoplasty for painful vertebral body fractures in cancer patients. J Neurosurg. 2003;98(1 Suppl):21–30. https://doi.org/10.3171/spi.2003.98.1.0021.
172. Berenson J, Pflugmacher R, Jarzem P, Zonder J, Schechtman K, Tillman JB, et al. Balloon kyphoplasty versus non-surgical fracture management for treatment of painful vertebral body compression fractures in patients with cancer: a multicentre, randomised controlled trial. Lancet Oncol. 2011;12(3):225–35. https://doi.org/10.1016/S1470-2045(11)70008-0.
173. Paley CA, Johnson MI, Tashani OA, Bagnall AM. Acupuncture for cancer pain in adults. Cochrane Database Syst Rev. 2015(10): ARTN CD007753. https://doi.org/10.1002/14651858.CD007753.pub3.
174. Garcia MK, McQuade J, Haddad R, Patel S, Lee R, Yang PY, et al. Systematic review of acupuncture in cancer care: a synthesis of the evidence. J Clin Oncol. 2013;31(7):952–60. https://doi.org/10.1200/Jco.2012.43.5818.
175. Choi TY, Lee MS, Kim TH, Zaslawski C, Ernst E. Acupuncture for the treatment of cancer pain: a systematic review of randomised clinical trials. Support Care Cancer. 2012;20(6):1147–58. https://doi.org/10.1007/s00520-012-1432-9.
176. Kwekkeboom KL, Cherwin CH, Lee JW, Wanta B. Mind-body treatments for the pain-fatigue-sleep disturbance symptom cluster in persons with cancer. J Pain Symptom Manag. 2010;39(1):126–38. https://doi.org/10.1016/j.jpainsymman.2009.05.022.

177. Boyd C, Crawford C, Paat CF, Price A, Xenakis L, Zhang W, et al. The impact of massage therapy on function in pain populations-a systematic review and meta-analysis of randomized controlled trials: part II, cancer pain populations. Pain Med. 2016;17(8):1553–68. https://doi.org/10.1093/pm/pnw100.
178. Lee SH, Kim JY, Yeo S, Kim SH, Lim S. Meta-analysis of massage therapy on cancer pain. Integr Cancer Ther. 2015;14(4):297–304. https://doi.org/10.1177/1534735415572885.
179. Lutz S, Balboni T, Jones J, Lo S, Petit J, Rich SE, et al. Palliative radiation therapy for bone metastases: update of an ASTRO evidence-based guideline. Pract Radiat Oncol. 2017;7(1):4–12. https://doi.org/10.1016/j.prro.2016.08.001.
180. Chow R, Hoskin P, Hollenberg D, Lam M, Dennis K, Lutz S, et al. Efficacy of single fraction conventional radiation therapy for painful uncomplicated bone metastases: a systematic review and meta-analysis. Ann Palliat Med. 2017;6(2):125–42. https://doi.org/10.21037/apm.2016.12.04.
181. Bhattacharya IS, Hoskin PJ. Stereotactic body radiotherapy for spinal and bone metastases. Clin Oncol. 2015;27(5):298–306. https://doi.org/10.1016/j.clon.2015.01.030.
182. Sartor O, Coleman R, Nilsson S, Heinrich D, Helle SI, O'Sullivan JM, et al. Effect of radium-223 dichloride on symptomatic skeletal events in patients with castration-resistant prostate cancer and bone metastases: results from a phase 3, double-blind, randomised trial. Lancet Oncol. 2014;15(7):738–46. https://doi.org/10.1016/S1470-2045(14)70183-4.
183. Roque IFM, Martinez-Zapata MJ, Scott-Brown M, Alonso-Coello P. Radioisotopes for metastatic bone pain. Cochrane Database Syst Rev. 2011;(7):CD003347. https://doi.org/10.1002/14651858.CD003347.pub2.
184. Porta-Sales J, Garzon-Rodriguez C, Llorens-Torrome S, Brunelli C, Pigni A, Caraceni A. Evidence on the analgesic role of bisphosphonates and denosumab in the treatment of pain due to bone metastases: a systematic review within the European Association for Palliative Care guidelines project. Palliat Med. 2017;31(1):5–25. https://doi.org/10.1177/0269216316639793.
185. Saini A, Berruti A, Cracco C, Sguazzotti E, Porpiglia F, Russo L, et al. Psychological distress in men with prostate cancer receiving adjuvant androgen-deprivation therapy. Urol Oncol. 2013;31(3):352–8. https://doi.org/10.1016/j.urolonc.2011.02.005.
186. Smith EM, Gomm SA, Dickens CM. Assessing the independent contribution to quality of life from anxiety and depression in patients with advanced cancer. Palliat Med. 2003;17(6):509–13. https://doi.org/10.1191/0269216303pm781oa.
187. DiMatteo MR, Haskard-Zolnierek KB. Impact of depression on treatment adherence and survival from cancer. In: Kissane DW, Maj M, Sartorius N, editors. World psychiatric association titles on depression depression and cancer. Wiley-Blackwell; 2011. p. 101–24.
188. DiMatteo MR, Lepper HS, Croghan TW. Depression is a risk factor for noncompliance with medical treatment – meta-analysis of the effects of anxiety and depression on patient adherence. Arch Intern Med. 2000;160(14):2101–7. https://doi.org/10.1001/archinte.160.14.2101.
189. Weis J, Heckl U. Influence of psychological response on survival in breast cancer: a population-based cohort study. Strahlenther Onkol. 2000;176(5):241–2.
190. Hirschfeld RM, Keller MB, Panico S, Arons BS, Barlow D, Davidoff F, et al. The National Depressive and Manic-Depressive Association consensus statement on the undertreatment of depression. JAMA. 1997;277(4):333–40.
191. Pasquini M, Biondi M. Depression in cancer patients: a critical review. Clin Pract Epidemiol Ment Health. 2007;3:2. https://doi.org/10.1186/1745-0179-3-2.
192. Baxter AJ, Scott KM, Vos T, Whiteford HA. Global prevalence of anxiety disorders: a systematic review and meta-regression. Psychol Med. 2013;43(5):897–910. https://doi.org/10.1017/S003329171200147x.
193. Mitchell AJ, Chan M, Bhatti H, Halton M, Grassi L, Johansen C, et al. Prevalence of depression, anxiety, and adjustment disorder in oncological, haematological, and palliative-care settings: a meta-analysis of 94 interview-based studies. Lancet Oncol. 2011;12(2):160–74. https://doi.org/10.1016/S1470-2045(11)70002-X.

194. Linden W, Vodermaier A, MacKenzie R, Greig D. Anxiety and depression after cancer diagnosis: prevalence rates by cancer type, gender, and age. J Affect Disord. 2012;141(2–3):343–51. https://doi.org/10.1016/j.jad.2012.03.025.
195. Ashbury FD, Madlensky L, Raich P, Thompson M, Whitney G, Hotz K, et al. Antidepressant prescribing in community cancer care. Support Care Cancer. 2003;11(5):278–85. https://doi.org/10.1007/s00520-003-0446-8.
196. Fisch M. Treatment of depression in cancer. J Natl Cancer Inst Monogr. 2004;32:105–11. https://doi.org/10.1093/jncimonographs/lgh011.
197. Walsh D, Donnelly S, Rybicki L. The symptoms of advanced cancer: relationship to age, gender, and performance status in 1,000 patients. Support Care Cancer. 2000;8(3):175–9. https://doi.org/10.1007/s005200050281.
198. Portenoy RK, Thaler HT, Kornblith AB, Lepore JM, Friedlanderklar H, Coyle N, et al. Symptom prevalence, characteristics and distress in a cancer population. Qual Life Res. 1994;3(3):183–9. https://doi.org/10.1007/Bf00435383.
199. Andersen BL, Rowland JH, Somerfield MR. Screening, assessment, and care of anxiety and depressive symptoms in adults with cancer: an American Society of Clinical Oncology guideline adaptation. J Oncol Pract. 2015;11(2):133–U499. https://doi.org/10.1200/Jop.2014.002311.
200. Howell D, Heshavarz H, Esplen MJ, Hack T, Hamel M, Howes J, et al. Pan-Canadian practice guideline: screening, assessment and management of psychosocial distress, depression and anxiety in adults with cancer, Version 2. 2015. https://www.capo.ca/resources/Documents/Guidelines/3APAN--~1.PDF. Accessed.
201. Arroll B, Goodyear-Smith F, Crengle S, Gunn J, Kerse N, Fishman T, et al. Validation of PHQ-2 and PHQ-9 to screen for major depression in the primary care population. Ann Fam Med. 2010;8(4):348–53. https://doi.org/10.1370/afm.1139.
202. Law MK, Furr RM, Arnold EM, Mneimne M, Jaquett C, Fleeson W. Does assessing suicidality frequently and repeatedly cause harm? A randomized control study. Psychol Assess. 2015;27(4):1171–81. https://doi.org/10.1037/pas0000118.
203. Smith EML, Pang H, Cirrincione C, Fleishman S, Paskett ED, Ahles T, et al. Effect of duloxetine on pain, function, and quality of life among patients with chemotherapy-induced painful peripheral neuropathy a randomized clinical trial. JAMA: J Am Med Assoc. 2013;309(13):1359–67. https://doi.org/10.1001/jama.2013.2813.
204. Hickok JT. Prevalence and severity of acute and delayed NV association with 3 highly emetogenic chemotherapies. Support Care Cancer. 2001;9:289.
205. Ballatori E, Roila F, Ruggeri B, Betti M, Sarti S, Soru G, et al. The impact of chemotherapy-induced nausea and vomiting on health-related quality of life. Support Care Cancer. 2007;15(2):179–85. https://doi.org/10.1007/s00520-006-0109-7.
206. Passik SD, Kirsh KL, Rosenfeld B, McDonald MV, Theobald DE. The changeable nature of patients' fears regarding chemotherapy: implications for palliative care. J Pain Symptom Manag. 2001;21(2):113–20. https://doi.org/10.1016/S0885-3924(00)00249-9.
207. Chasen M, Urban L, Schnadig I, Rapoport B, Powers D, Arora S, et al. Rolapitant improves quality of life of patients receiving highly or moderately emetogenic chemotherapy. Support Care Cancer. 2017;25(1):85–92. https://doi.org/10.1007/s00520-016-3388-7.
208. Lee J, Dibble SL, Pickett M, Luce J. Chemotherapy-induced nausea/vomiting and functional status in women treated for breast cancer. Cancer Nurs. 2005;28(4):249–55.
209. Davidson W, Teleni L, Muller J, Ferguson M, McCarthy AL, Vick J, et al. Malnutrition and chemotherapy-induced nausea and vomiting: implications for practice. Oncol Nurs Forum. 2012;39(4):398. https://doi.org/10.1188/12.Onf.E340-E345.
210. Aapro M, Gralla RJ, Herrstedt J, Molassiotis A, Roila F. MASCC/ESMO antiemetic guideline 2016 with updates in 2019. 2019. Accessed.
211. Hesketh PJ, Kris MG, Basch E, Bohlke K, Barbour SY, Clark-Snow RA, et al. Antiemetics: ASCO guideline update. J Clin Oncol. 2020;38(24):2782–97. https://doi.org/10.1200/JCO.20.01296.

212. Crichton M, Marshall S, Marx W, McCarthy AL, Isenring E. Efficacy of ginger (Zingiber officinale) in ameliorating chemotherapy-induced nausea and vomiting and chemotherapy-related outcomes: a systematic review update and meta-analysis. J Acad Nutr Diet. 2019;119(12):2055–68. https://doi.org/10.1016/j.jand.2019.06.009.
213. Pergam SA, Woodfield MC, Lee CM, Cheng GS, Baker KK, Marquis SR, et al. Cannabis use among patients at a comprehensive cancer center in a state with legalized medicinal and recreational use. Cancer. 2017;123(22):4488–97. https://doi.org/10.1002/cncr.30879.
214. Smith LA, Azariah F, Lavender VTC, Stoner NS, Bettiol S. Cannabinoids for nausea and vomiting in adults with cancer receiving chemotherapy. Cochrane Database Syst Rev. 2015(11): ARTN CD009464. https://doi.org/10.1002/14651858.CD009464.pub2.
215. Cherwin C, Nakad L, Albashayreh A. Systematic review of nonpharmacologic approaches for the management of gastrointestinal symptoms. Oncol Nurs Forum. 2019;46(1):E1–E21. https://doi.org/10.1188/19.Onf.E1-E21.
216. Han S, Jang BH, Suh HS, Hwang DS. Complementary medicine use and costs in patients with breast cancer who experienced treatment-related side effects: a cross-sectional survey in Korea. Complement Ther Med. 2019;44:210–7. https://doi.org/10.1016/j.ctim.2019.04.013.
217. McConnell JD, Roehrborn CG, Bautista OM, Andriole GL Jr, Dixon CM, Kusek JW, et al. The long-term effect of doxazosin, finasteride, and combination therapy on the clinical progression of benign prostatic hyperplasia. N Engl J Med. 2003;349(25):2387–98. https://doi.org/10.1056/NEJMoa030656.
218. Prosnitz RG, Schneider L, Manola J, Rocha S, Loffredo M, Lopes L, et al. Tamsulosin palliates radiation-induced urethritis in patients with prostate cancer: results of a pilot study. Int J Radiat Oncol Biol Phys. 1999;45(3):563–6. https://doi.org/10.1016/S0360-3016(99)00246-1.
219. Ok JH, Meyers FJ, Evans CP. Medical and surgical palliative care of patients with urological malignancies. J Urol. 2005;174(4 Pt 1):1177–82. https://doi.org/10.1097/01.ju.0000173077.84274.01.
220. Cameron MG, Kersten C, Guren MG, Fossa SD, Vistad I. Palliative pelvic radiotherapy of symptomatic incurable prostate cancer – a systematic review. Radiother Oncol. 2014;110(1):55–60. https://doi.org/10.1016/j.radonc.2013.08.008.
221. Qu M, Zhu F, Chen H, Lian BJ, Jia ZP, Shi ZK, et al. Palliative transurethral resection of the prostate in patients with metastatic prostate cancer: a prospective study of 188 patients. J Endourol. 2019;33(7):570–5. https://doi.org/10.1089/end.2019.0108.
222. Javanmard B, Hadad AH, Yaghoobi M, Lotfi B. Diode laser ablation of prostate and channel transurethral resection of prostate in patients with prostate cancer and bladder outlet obstruction symptoms. Urol J. 2014;11(4):1788–91.
223. Marszalek M, Ponholzer A, Rauchenwald M, Madersbacher S. Palliative transurethral resection of the prostate: functional outcome and impact on survival. BJU Int. 2007;99(1):56–9. https://doi.org/10.1111/j.1464-410X.2006.06529.x.
224. Crain DS, Amling CL, Kane CJ. Palliative transurethral prostate resection for bladder outlet obstruction in patients with locally advanced prostate cancer. J Urol. 2004;171(2):668–71. https://doi.org/10.1097/01.ju.0000104845.24632.92.
225. Sagalowsky AI. Feasibility of radical transurethral resection as monotherapy for selected patients with muscle invasive bladder cancer. J Urol. 2010;184(2):480–1. https://doi.org/10.1016/j.juro.2010.04.085.
226. Becker A, Placke A, Kluth L, Schwarz R, Isbarn H, Chun F, et al. Holmium laser enucleation of the prostate is safe in patients with prostate cancer and lower urinary tract symptoms-a retrospective feasibility study. J Endourol. 2014;28(3):335–41. https://doi.org/10.1089/end.2013.0432.
227. Leibovici D, Kamat AM, Pettaway CA, Pagliaro L, Rosser CJ, Logothetis C, et al. Cystoprostatectomy for effective palliation of symptomatic bladder invasion by prostate cancer. J Urol. 2005;174(6):2186–90. https://doi.org/10.1097/01.ju.0000181826.65272.7b.
228. Goonewardene SS, Venti K, Bahl A, Persad R, Motiwala H, Abdala D. The role of palliative cystectomy in bladder cancer. In: Management of muscle invasive bladder cancer. management of urology. Cham: Springer; 2021.

229. Hamilton TD, Selby D, Tsang ME, Kim A, Wright FC. Patients' perceptions of palliative surgical procedures: a qualitative analysis. Ann Palliat Med. 2017;6:S77–84. https://doi.org/10.21037/apm.2017.01.04.
230. Allen DJ, Longhorn SE, Philp T, Smith RD, Choong S. Percutaneous urinary drainage and ureteric stenting in malignant disease. Clin Oncol-UK. 2010;22(9):733–9. https://doi.org/10.1016/j.clon.2010.07.004.
231. Kouba E, Wallen EM, Pruthi RS. Management of ureteral obstruction due to advanced malignancy: optimizing therapeutic and palliative outcomes. J Urol. 2008;180(2):444–50. https://doi.org/10.1016/j.juro.2008.04.008.
232. Yossepowitch O, Lifshitz DA, Dekel Y, Gross M, Keidar DM, Neuman M, et al. Predicting the success of retrograde stenting for managing ureteral obstruction. J Urol. 2001;166(5):1746–9. https://doi.org/10.1016/S0022-5347(05)65666-2.
233. Parsons JK, Dahm P, Kohler TS, Lerner LB, Wilt TJ. Surgical management of lower urinary tract symptoms attributed to benign prostatic hyperplasia: AUA guideline amendment 2020. J Urol. 2020;204(4):799–804. https://doi.org/10.1097/JU.0000000000001298.
234. Walton A. Managing overactive bladder symptoms in a palliative care setting. J Palliat Med. 2014;17(1):118–21. https://doi.org/10.1089/jpm.2012.0116.
235. Lightner DJ, Gomelsky A, Souter L, Vasavada SP. Diagnosis and treatment of overactive bladder (non-neurogenic) in adults: AUA/SUFU guideline amendment 2019. J Urol. 2019;202(3):558–63. https://doi.org/10.1097/JU.0000000000000309.
236. Michaelson MD, Cotter SE, Gargollo PC, Zietman AL, Dahl DM, Smith MR. Management of complications of prostate cancer treatment. CA-Cancer J Clin. 2008;58(4):196–213. https://doi.org/10.3322/Ca.2008.0002.
237. Konety BR, Sadetsky N, Carroll PR. Recovery of urinary continence following radical prostatectomy: the impact of prostate volume – analysis of data from the CaPSURE (TM) database. J Urol. 2007;177(4):1423–5. https://doi.org/10.1016/j.juro.2006.11.089.
238. Bailey GC, Blackburne A, Ziegelmann MJ, Lightner DJ. Outcomes of surgical management in patients with stress urinary incontinence and/or neovesicovaginal fistula after orthotopic neobladder diversion. J Urol. 2016;196(5):1478–83. https://doi.org/10.1016/j.juro.2016.06.009.
239. Milios JE, Ackland TR, Green DJ. Pelvic floor muscle training in radical prostatectomy: a randomized controlled trial of the impacts on pelvic floor muscle function and urinary incontinence. BMC Urol. 2019;19(1):ARTN 116. https://doi.org/10.1186/s12894-019-0546-5.
240. Wang W, Huang QM, Liu FP, Mao QQ. Effectiveness of preoperative pelvic floor muscle training for urinary incontinence after radical prostatectomy: a meta-analysis. BMC Urol. 2014;14:Artn 99. https://doi.org/10.1186/1471-2490-14-99.
241. Sciarra A, Mariotti G. Recovery of urinary continence after radical prostatectomy using early vs late pelvic floor electrical stimulation and biofeedback-associated treatment. Urology. 2015;86(1):121. https://doi.org/10.1016/j.urology.2015.02.066.
242. Eastham JA, Kattan MW, Rogers E, Goad JR, Ohori M, Boone TB, et al. Risk factors for urinary incontinence after radical prostatectomy. J Urol. 1996;156(5):1707–13. https://doi.org/10.1016/S0022-5347(01)65488-0.
243. Nalesnik JG, Mysliwiec AG, Canby-Hagino E. Anemia in men with advanced prostate cancer: incidence, etiology, and treatment. Rev Urol. 2004;6(1):1–4.
244. Avellino GJ, Bose S, Wang DS. Diagnosis and Management of Hematuria. Surg Clin North Am. 2016;96(3):503–15. https://doi.org/10.1016/j.suc.2016.02.007.
245. Cameron MG, Kersten C, Vistad I, van Helvoirt R, Weyde K, Undseth C, et al. Palliative pelvic radiotherapy for symptomatic incurable prostate cancer – a prospective multicenter study. Radiother Oncol. 2015;115(3):314–20. https://doi.org/10.1016/j.radonc.2015.05.021.
246. Tey J, Ho F, Koh WY, Chia D, Ooi KH, Tuan JKL, et al. Palliative radiotherapy for bladder cancer: a systematic review and meta-analysis. Acta Oncol. 2021. https://doi.org/10.1080/0284186x.2021.1880025.
247. Boyer MJ, Salama JK, Lee WR. Palliative radiotherapy for prostate cancer. Oncology-New York. 2014;28(4):306–12.

248. Tey J, Soon YY, Cheo T, Ooi KH, Ho F, Vellayappan B, et al. Efficacy of palliative bladder radiotherapy for hematuria in advanced bladder cancer using contemporary radiotherapy techniques. In Vivo. 2019;33(6):2161–7. https://doi.org/10.21873/invivo.11718.
249. Abt D, Bywater M, Engeler DS, Schmid HP. Therapeutic options for intractable hematuria in advanced bladder cancer. Int J Urol. 2013;20(7):651–60. https://doi.org/10.1111/iju.12113.
250. Mohan S, Kumar S, Dubey D, Phadke RV, Baijal SS, Kathuria M. Superselective vesical artery embolization in the management of intractable hematuria secondary to hemorrhagic cystitis. World J Urol. 2019;37(10):2175–82. https://doi.org/10.1007/s00345-018-2604-0.
251. Kably I, Acharya V, Richardson AJ, Bhatia S. Prostatic artery embolization in refractory hematuria of prostatic origin. Tech Vasc Interv Radiol. 2020;23(3):ARTN 100694. https://doi.org/10.1016/j.tvir.2020.100694.
252. Kably I, Pereira K, Chong W, Bhatia S. Prostate artery embolization (PAE) in the management of refractory hematuria of prostatic origin secondary to iatrogenic urological trauma: a safe and effective technique. Urology. 2016;88:218–21. https://doi.org/10.1016/j.urology.2015.10.025.
253. Moreno JG, Ahlering TE. Late local complications after definitive radiotherapy for prostatic adenocarcinoma. J Urol. 1992;147(3):926–8. https://doi.org/10.1016/S0022-5347(17)37424-4.
254. Del Pizzo JJ, Chew BH, Jacobs SC, Sklar GN. Treatment of radiation induced hemorrhagic cystitis with hyperbaric oxygen: long-term followup. J Urol. 1998;160(3):731–3. https://doi.org/10.1016/S0022-5347(01)62770-8.
255. Mougin J, Souday V, Martin F, Azzouzi AR, Bigot P. Evaluation of hyperbaric oxygen therapy in the treatment of radiation-induced hemorrhagic cystitis. Urology. 2016;94:42–6. https://doi.org/10.1016/j.urology.2016.04.015.
256. Oscarsson N, Arnell P, Lodding P, Ricksten SE, Seeman-Lodding H. Hyperbaric oxygen treatment in radiation-induced cystitis and proctitis: a prospective cohort study on patient-perceived quality of recovery. Int J Radiat Oncol Biol Phys. 2013;87(4):670–5. https://doi.org/10.1016/j.ijrobp.2013.07.039.
257. Middleton AW. Indications for and results of nephrectomy for metastatic renal-cell carcinoma. Urol Clin N Am. 1980;7(3):711–7.
258. Ekelund L, Karp W, Mansson W, Olsson AM. Palliative embolization of renal tumors – follow-up of 19 cases. Urol Radiol. 1981;3(1):13–8. https://doi.org/10.1007/Bf02938624.
259. Ekelund L, Mansson W, Olsson AM, Stigsson L. Palliative embolization of arterial renal tumor supply – results in 10 cases. Acta Radiol Diagn. 1979;20(2):323–36. https://doi.org/10.1177/028418517902000205.
260. Munro NP, Woodhams S, Nawrocki JD, Fletcher MS, Thomas PJ. The role of transarterial embolization in the treatment of renal cell carcinoma. BJU Int. 2003;92(3):240–4. https://doi.org/10.1046/j.1464-410X.2003.04314.x.
261. Matuszewski M, Krajka K. Radio-frequency ablation: new technology for palliative treatment of hematuria in disseminated renal cell carcinoma. Scand J Urol Nephrol. 2007;41(6):563–4. https://doi.org/10.1080/00365590701308495.
262. Nikolaev A, Benda R. Palliative radiation therapy for symptomatic control of inoperable renal cell carcinoma. Urol Case Rep. 2016;4:51–2. https://doi.org/10.1016/j.eucr.2015.09.006.
263. Francolini G, Detti B, Ingrosso G, Desideri I, Becherini C, Carta G, et al. Stereotactic body radiation therapy (SBRT) on renal cell carcinoma, an overview of technical aspects, biological rationale and current literature. Crit Rev Oncol Hematol. 2018;131:24–9. https://doi.org/10.1016/j.critrevonc.2018.08.010.
264. Verkissen MN, Hjermstad MJ, Van Belle S, Kaasa S, Deliens L, Pardon K. Quality of life and symptom intensity over time in people with cancer receiving palliative care: results from the international European Palliative Care Cancer Symptom study. Plos One. 2019;14(10):ARTN e0222988. https://doi.org/10.1371/journal.pone.0222988.

265. About Palliative Care. https://www.capc.org/about/palliative-care/. Accessed 27 Mar 2019.
266. von Gunten CF. Secondary and tertiary palliative care in US hospitals. JAMA: J Am Med Assoc. 2002;287(7):875–81. https://doi.org/10.1001/jama.287.7.875.
267. Morrison SM, Meier DE: America's care of serious illness: a state-by-state report card on access to palliative care in our nation's hospitals. 2019. https://reportcard.capc.org/wp--content/uploads/2020/05/CAPC_State-by-State-Report-Card_051120.pdf. Accessed.
268. Calton BA, Alvarez-Perez A, Portman DG, Ramchandran KJ, Sugalski J, Rabow MW. The current state of palliative care for patients cared for at leading US cancer centers: the 2015 NCCN Palliative Care Survey. J Natl Compr Cancer Netw. 2016;14(7):859–66. https://doi.org/10.6004/jnccn.2016.0090.
269. Temel JS, Greer JA, Muzikansky A, Gallagher ER, Admane S, Jackson VA, et al. Early palliative care for patients with metastatic non-small-cell lung cancer. N Engl J Med. 2010;363(8):733–42. https://doi.org/10.1056/NEJMoa1000678.
270. El-Jawahri A, Greer JA, Pirl WF, Park ER, Jackson VA, Back AL, et al. Effects of early integrated palliative care on caregivers of patients with lung and gastrointestinal cancer: a randomized clinical trial. Oncologist. 2017. https://doi.org/10.1634/theoncologist.2017-0227.
271. Rabow MW, Benner C, Shepard N, Meng MV. Concurrent urologic and palliative care after cystectomy for treatment of muscle-invasive bladder cancer. Urol Oncol. 2015;33(6):267 e23–9. https://doi.org/10.1016/j.urolonc.2015.02.012.
272. Hugar LA, Lopa SH, Yabes JG, Yu JA, Turner RM 2nd, Fam MM, et al. Palliative care use amongst patients with bladder cancer. BJU Int. 2019;123(6):968–75. https://doi.org/10.1111/bju.14708.
273. Patel HV, Sterling J, Srivastava A, Kim S, Saraiya B, Mayer TM, et al. Factors associated with palliative care utilization in advanced and metastatic renal cell carcinom. In: 19th annual meeting of the International Kidney Cancer Symposium (IKCS 2020); 2020.
274. Roeland EJ, Triplett DP, Matsuno RK, Boero IJ, Hwang L, Yeung HN, et al. Patterns of palliative care consultation among elderly patients with cancer. J Natl Compr Canc Ne. 2016;14(4):439–45. https://doi.org/10.6004/jnccn.2016.0050.
275. Huen K, Huang C, Liu H, Kwan L, Pannell S, Laviana A, et al. Outcomes of an integrated urology-palliative care clinic for patients with advanced urological cancers: maintenance of quality of life and satisfaction and high rate of hospice utilization through end of life. Am J Hosp Palliat Care. 2019;36(9):801–6. https://doi.org/10.1177/1049909119833663.
276. Bergman J. Community-partnered collaboration to build an integrated palliative care clinic: the view from urology. Am J Hosp Palliat Med. 33(2):164–70. https://doi.org/10.1177/1049909114555156.
277. Kamal AH, Bull JH, Swetz KM, Wolf SP, Shanafelt TD, Myers ER. Future of the palliative care workforce: preview to an impending crisis. Am J Med. 2017;130(2):113–4. https://doi.org/10.1016/j.amjmed.2016.08.046.
278. Wong DL, Baker CM. Pain in children: comparison of assessment scales. Pediatr Nurs. 1988;14(1):9–17.
279. Antiemesis (Version 1.2021). 2021. https://www.nccn.org/professionals/physician_gls/pdf/antiemesis.pdf. Accessed 12 Mar 2021.
280. Kouriefs C, Georgiou M, Ravi R, et al. Hot flushes and prostate cancer: pathogenesis and treatment. BJU Int. 2002;89:379–83.
281. Buss MK, Rock LK, McCarthy EP. Understanding palliative care and hospice: a review for primary care providers. Mayo Clin Proc. 2017;92(2):280–6.

Chapter 3
Operationalizing Genetic Testing in the Care of Patients with Prostate Cancer

Brittany M. Szymaniak, Lauren A. Facchini, Max F. Kelsten, Heather H. Cheng, and Alicia K. Morgans

Abbreviations

DTC	Direct to consumer
GINA	Genetic Information Nondiscrimination Act
NCCN	National Comprehensive Cancer Network
NSGC	National Society of Genetic Counselors
VUS	Variant of uncertain significance

Brittany M. Szymaniak and Lauren A. Facchini contributed equally with all other contributors.

B. M. Szymaniak
Department of Urology, Feinberg School of Medicine at Northwestern University, Chicago, IL, USA
e-mail: brittany.szymaniak@nm.org

L. A. Facchini
Seattle Cancer Care Alliance, Seattle, WA, USA
e-mail: lfacchini@seattlecca.org

M. F. Kelsten
Department of Medicine, Feinberg School of Medicine at Northwestern University, Chicago, IL, USA
e-mail: max.kelsten@northwestern.edu

H. H. Cheng
Fred Hutchinson Cancer Research Center and Division of Medical Oncology, Department of Medicine, University of Washington School of Medicine, Seattle, WA, USA
e-mail: hhcheng@uw.edu

A. K. Morgans (✉)
Department of Medical Oncology, Dana-Farber Cancer Institute, Boston, MA, USA
e-mail: aliciak_morgans@dfci.harvard.edu

K. L. Stratton, A. K. Morgans (eds.), *Urologic Oncology*,
https://doi.org/10.1007/978-3-030-89891-5_3

Introduction

Germline genetic testing for prostate cancer was formally included into the National Comprehensive Cancer Network (NCCN) testing criteria in 2018 due to data that associated hereditary prostate cancer with the *BRCA1* and *BRCA2* genes [1, 2]. This expanded the indications for genetic testing and allowed for a more comprehensive genetic risk assessment for patients and their families. With the added emphasis of genetic testing to determine eligibility for targeted prostate cancer therapies, such as PARP inhibitors, there is now an increased demand for access to genetic counseling services. This chapter aims to address the various components of the genetic counseling and testing process to provide a framework of care that includes urologists, GU oncologists, and genetics providers in an effort to support optimal multidisciplinary collaboration.

Germline Genetic Testing

Prostate Cancer Genetics

Germline variants in patients with prostate cancer have been well documented in recent years. It is estimated that ~5–10% of patients with prostate cancer and ~10–15% of men with metastatic prostate cancer have an identifiable germline variant, which is in line with the prevalence of germline variants in other hereditary types of cancer [2–5]. Approximately 20–30% of prostate cancer cases can be classified as "familial," meaning there are more incidences of prostate cancer in the family than expected by sporadic chance, but an underlying cause is unknown [6]. Familial prostate cancer may be caused by multiple unidentified genetic risk factors, environmental risk factors, or a combination of both.

Genes associated with hereditary cancer can be categorized in three ways: high-risk, moderate-/low-risk, or preliminary-evidence [7]. High-risk genes have established cancer risks that are significantly elevated above the general population and have well-established screening guidelines. Moderate-/low-risk genes have cancer risks that are only moderately elevated compared to the general population and may have screening recommendations. Preliminary-evidence genes do not have clearly defined cancer risks and do not have established screening recommendations. It is important to recognize the overlap between these categories in regard to their various associated cancer risks, which can make navigating prostate cancer genetics more complex. For example, while *ATM* and *CHEK2* are considered moderate-risk breast cancer genes and have corresponding screening recommendations, their association with prostate cancer is still relatively new, and there are no established screening guidelines. Furthermore, *PALB2* is considered a high-risk gene for breast cancer, but preliminary evidence for prostate cancer. Thus, while there may be limited clinical impact for these men outside of possible qualifications for genetically targeted therapies, there may still be important risks to consider for other relatives.

Provider and patient expectations must be aligned to recognize that the majority of germline tests will be negative, and of the positive results, not all will not have treatment or screening implications. *BRCA2* variants contribute to the majority of germline pathogenic variants in the metastatic disease setting, accounting for >40% of results [2]. In general, moderate-risk genes are more common in the population (1 in 100 people), while high-risk genes are rarer (1 in 300–500 people), so an individual is more likely to have a positive result in a moderate−/low-risk gene [7]. However, this risk may vary by heritage. For example, for individuals of Ashkenazi Jewish ancestry, the carrier rate of a *BRCA1/2* pathogenic variant is ~1/40 due to the presence of three founder variants, a rate significantly higher than average [8]. Nonetheless, the overall chance to detect a positive result is quite low, since only ~5–10% of men with prostate cancer will test positive.

Genetic Testing Models

Given the integral role of genetic testing in the care of patients with prostate cancer, germline testing is quickly becoming a new standard of care. However, there are multiple time-points during a patient's care to consider discussing genetic testing, such as at the time of diagnosis, upon disease progression, or in parallel with somatic tumor testing.

The first step in incorporating genetics into the workflow is establishing the approach the clinic will take for germline genetic testing. This will allow for the most optimal method to operationalize the process of genetic testing in a streamlined fashion that will fit best for the specific clinic. The following models were outlined by Giri et al. and Szymaniak-Facchini et al. and are briefly summarized below [9, 10]:

1. A patient is referred to a genetic counselor for an assessment and discussion of genetic testing if indicated.
2. The entirety of the genetic testing process, pre- and post-test, is completed by the urologist or GU oncology team.
3. The genetic testing is initiated within the clinic, and the patient is referred to a genetic counselor for post-test counseling.

Both Giri et al. and Szymaniak-Facchini et al. provide an in-depth review of the components of the genetic testing process that details the responsibilities and knowledge required of providers [9, 10].

Although genetic testing for patients with prostate cancer is expanding into new standards of care, the implications may be different depending on the disease state. Testing at the time of diagnosis may have different management discussions compared to at metastatic disease recurrence or when done in parallel with somatic tumor testing for treatment decision-making.

Identifying Patients Appropriate for Genetic Counseling and Testing

Germline genetic testing is now routinely recommended for men with high-risk or very-high-risk localized prostate cancer, intraductal/cribriform histology, and metastatic prostate cancer [1]. Men with prostate cancer who are of Ashkenazi Jewish ancestry or with family histories of early-onset breast cancer (under age 50), ovarian cancer, pancreatic cancer, or metastatic or intraductal/cribriform prostate cancer or with multiple relatives with breast or prostate cancer (any grade) should also be offered testing [1]. Because these recommendations are frequently changing, care teams must both remain up to date with the most recent guidelines and have a plan to consistently screen and identify patients who meet criteria.

A thorough family history can help determine which patients should be offered genetic testing, identify the most appropriate test to offer, and inform next steps if germline testing is negative or inconclusive. Genetic counselors typically complete three- to four-generation pedigrees prior to ordering testing, which include information on ages, cause of death, cancer histories (types of cancer and age of onset), prior genetic testing, and ancestry of both maternal and paternal relatives. Collecting this detailed history may not be feasible for all GU providers during routine visits, but family history questionnaires and online pedigree tools can help collect this information in a fast and systematic way. If there are other types of cancers observed in the family, GU providers may want to consider expanding testing to include genes related to the other cancer types or referring the patient to genetics before ordering testing. Additionally, if there is a known pathogenic variant in the family, it is important to confirm that the genetic test will include evaluation of the familial variant. GU providers should be cautious when ordering single site testing, especially in families of Ashkenazi Jewish ancestry or families with unexplained cancer histories.

Pre-test Education and Informed Consent

Prior to ordering genetic testing, each patient should have a basic understanding of the purpose of genetic testing and the potential benefits and limitations of the test. They should also have an opportunity to ask questions and have concerns addressed. Several major medical societies, such as the National Society of Genetic Counselors and the American Society of Clinical Oncology, have published guidelines reviewing the components of pre-test counseling and informed consent, which can serve as a guide for GU providers [11, 12]. Educational handouts, videos, or group counseling sessions can be an alternative or supplement to traditional in-person pre-test education. Development of these resources is another opportunity for GU and genetics providers to collaborate.

Genetic privacy and discrimination are often common concerns for patients, especially in the era of patient-directed and direct-to-consumer (DTC) testing. GU providers should be versed in the differences between patient-directed or DTC and clinical testing [10]. They should also be familiar with the Genetic Information Nondiscrimination Act (GINA), which applies to places of employment and health insurance, but does not apply to life, disability, or long-term care insurance. Patients with significant hesitations, questions, or a poor understanding of genetic testing may benefit from a pre-test counseling session with a genetics provider.

It is important to keep in mind that not every patient will be interested in pursuing germline genetic testing and that the testing process is voluntary. Patients may be overwhelmed with a new diagnosis and/or the complex decisions that need to be made surrounding treatment and, therefore, may not be in the right mental or emotional place to consider adding on this type of testing [13, 14]. Additionally, some patients may prefer not to learn this type of information since it may lead to feelings of guilt or distress [15, 16]. Each patient will be unique in their preferences, which underscores the need for appropriate pre-test education and informed consent. Providers can consider raising this topic with their patients across multiple appointments, laying the groundwork for when a patient may be ready to discuss in more detail.

Test Selection

As part of a typical pre-test genetic counseling session, there is discussion of the specific genes or panels that are indicated based on the personal and family history of cancer (i.e., hereditary pancreas cancer panel based on a history of pancreas cancer). There is also a shared decision-making discussion about the scope of the testing (targeted vs comprehensive) based on the patient's preferences and goals. However, this type of nuanced discussion of family history and delineation of specific genes to be tested is not always realistically feasible if genetic testing is being initiated with a GU provider. Thus, it is critical that clinics develop a strategy for test selection that will encompass the most appropriate genes for their prostate cancer patients.

Many genetic testing laboratories now offer prostate cancer-specific panels, which evaluate known genes associated with prostate cancer. These pre-selected panels may be more easily implemented in a GU provider's practice. However, based on an individual patient's risk and family history, there may be additional genes for which testing is indicated. This type of testing approach might be more appropriate for testing models that involve a post-test referral to a genetic counselor. Depending on the testing laboratory, there are options to reflex to a larger panel at no additional cost within a set time-window (usually 90 days) from the release of the initial test report, which can allow a genetic counselor to include testing for other appropriate genes based on the full assessment of the family history.

In contrast, guidelines-based, comprehensive panels cover a wide range of hereditary cancer genes. The genes included in these panels often have well-defined cancer risks and management recommendations. This type of comprehensive panel may be an appropriate option for clinics ordering testing up front in order to capture more genes that might be relevant to the wider family history. However, this should not be a substitute for collecting a thorough family history, since this can still influence screening recommendations. Furthermore, some patients may be less receptive to comprehensive testing, which highlights the critical importance of informed consent.

Insurance coverage for genetic testing can be variable and is often dependent on the specifics of the plan. Payers have historically based their criteria on the NCCN High Risk: Breast, Ovarian, and Pancreas guidelines, but coverage is not always aligned with the most update-to-date NCCN recommendations, and insurers may develop their own stricter criteria [1]. To minimize unanticipated expenses, many testing laboratories will contract with various payers and perform a benefits investigation to estimate the out-of-pocket cost for the patient. In addition, many testing laboratories offer fixed patient-pay prices of $250 or less. Laboratories may also offer financial assistance or sponsored (no cost) testing. During a genetic counseling appointment, the logistics of testing and cost are discussed. However, if testing is being ordered in the clinic, it is important to have the specifics of the testing laboratory's billing available so patients can make an informed decision about whether testing is within their budget.

Results Delivery

Post-test counseling and result delivery will depend on the genetic testing model determined by each clinic. As outlined by Giri et al. and Szymaniak-Facchini et al., GU providers have the option to [9, 10]:

1. Refer all patients to genetics for post-test counseling regardless of results.
2. Deliver all results, provide post-test counseling, and refer to genetics only in complex cases or by patient request.
3. Deliver negative results and refer patients with a positive result or a concerning variant of uncertain significance (VUS) to genetics for post-test counseling.

Regardless of the model utilized, a clear strategy should be in place to ensure results are returned in a timely and organized manner. A copy of the test report should be in the patient's medical record and offered to the patient, especially in the event of a positive test result.

When discussing results with patients, providers should be conscious of these key points:

- *Negative results.* A negative result lowers but does not eliminate the risk for a hereditary cancer predisposition. Cancer screening for the patient and their family should be based on their personal risk factors and family history. If a patient's personal or family history changes, or new options arise for testing, it may be worthwhile to review with genetics if updated testing or additional screening is recommended.

- *Positive results*. If a pathogenic or likely pathogenic variant is identified, providers should review the cancer risks associated with the variant in order to recommend further cancer screening and specialist referrals as indicated. Possible treatment implications and research opportunities should also be discussed, particularly for patients with metastatic disease and variants in DNA repair genes or mismatch repair genes. Patients should be strongly encouraged to discuss the results with their at-risk relatives for cascade testing, including both male and female relatives, and to meet with genetic counselor if one has not been involved to this point – to provide support for patients, some of whom may find this process stressful, and to ensure medically accurate information and cascade testing discussions.
- *VUS results*. Variants of uncertain significance are the second most common result, and the likelihood of detecting a VUS increases with larger panels [7]. Given that the overwhelming majority of VUS results are later reclassified as benign, providers should be careful when reviewing VUS results with patients and stress the uncertainty of whether the genetic variant is disease-causing or benign [17]. Until reclassified as pathogenic or expertly reviewed by a genetics provider, VUS results should be treated as negative results, and any screening and/or treatment recommendations should be based on a patient's personal and family history. Testing family members for VUS results is not recommended unless in the context of research or a VUS resolution program. Patients should be encouraged to check in with providers every few years to see if there are updates to the VUS classification. If a laboratory reclassifies a variant, they will issue an amended report to the ordering provider. It is therefore the ordering provider's responsibility to follow up with patients over time regarding any classification changes.

Variants of uncertain significance can be challenging results both for patients and providers. Incorrect interpretation of VUS results can lead to mismanagement of patient care, unnecessary screening, and inappropriate testing [18]. For providers, lack of genetic training and confirmation biases can lead to an over suspicion of the pathogenicity of a VUS [18]. While a VUS result may seem consistent with the patient's clinical presentation, providers should remember that >90% of VUS are later reclassified as benign and be hesitant to conclude that a VUS had any role in the patient's personal or family history without significant supporting data [17]. To help gather this data, providers can consider enrolling patients in VUS resolution programs through genetic testing laboratories or academic centers. These programs may offer family segregation studies, RNA analysis, or somatic/tumor testing, all of which can aid in the classification of variants. Genetic counselors are also widely available at most laboratories to assist providers in the interpretation of VUS results and discuss resolution study options.

Somatic Testing

Germline genetic testing assesses for pathogenic variants in genes inherited from parents that can predispose an individual to cancer. Alternatively, somatic genetic testing assesses for acquired, tissue-specific genetic alterations within an individual's tumor. The purposes of somatic testing in prostate cancer are to determine clinical risk (i.e., death or metastatic disease within a certain time frame) in order to aid with treatment planning, targeted therapies based on the genetic composition of the tumor, and eligibility for clinical trials.

There is the possibility of identifying a somatic variant that may be suspicious for germline origin, such as a *BRCA2* variant. This becomes particularly relevant in the setting of paired somatic and germline testing. Typically, the germline (blood) sample is used to "subtract out" the background genetic information to identify the genetic data specific to the tumor. However, since the germline is being analyzed, the laboratory may also report germline variants. Germline testing in this context may not be clinically validated, so additional germline or confirmatory testing may be needed.

Though somatic and germline testing each has unique indications, their synergistic effect can provide great clinical benefit since both tests may identify eligibility for genetically targeted therapies, such as PARP inhibitors and checkpoint inhibitors. Furthermore, if a patient undergoes germline genetic testing and does not have a pathogenic or likely pathogenic variant identified, this does not eliminate the possibility of a relevant somatic variant. Conversely, if a suspicious somatic variant is identified, germline genetic testing may be needed to determine the clinical relevance of this finding. Therefore, conducting germline testing at the time of somatic testing is a reasonable and potentially beneficial clinical approach.

Cascade Testing

Cascade testing, the clinical investigations of a proband's family members following the identification of a positive test result, is an important concept that should be discussed with patients. Targeted familial testing for relatives can clarify cancer risks and determine the most appropriate screening and risk-reducing strategies. Additionally, several cancer genes have risks for autosomal recessive conditions, and knowledge of carrier status can inform reproductive decisions [7]. Despite potential benefits, studies have shown that uptake for cascade testing is low [19, 20]. One contributing reason is that cascade testing relies on the affected proband sharing the information with the at-risk family members. This responsibility can be difficult when a patient may be in the midst of cancer treatment [21]. For this reason, it can be helpful to provide patients with resources, such as family letters and support groups, and stress the importance of sharing this information with family not just at the results disclosure, but in follow-up visits as well. Several laboratories also offer free familial testing within a set number of days (i.e., 90 days) after the proband's testing, which can be another incentive for the patient to share the results with the relatives.

Unaffected relatives who test positive, particularly for a high-risk variant, can be followed in high-risk surveillance and prevention programs. There may also be long-term follow-up studies that these individuals can enroll in to help improve our understanding of the natural history of these syndromes. Relatives who test positive for preliminary evidence or moderate-/low-risk prostate variants may want to consider checking in every few years with genetics to see if there are updates to the risk assessment or screening recommendations. Enrolling in variant registries, such as PROMPT, should also be encouraged.

Identifying and Overcoming Barriers

Cementing the Genetic and GU Clinical Team Partnership

Due to the relatively recent incorporation of germline testing for men with prostate cancer into guidelines, the importance of testing continues to be under-recognized among prostate cancer clinical care teams. Additionally, important working relationships between genetic counselors and members of the urology and GU oncology communities are still being established. The evolution of optimal care standards for germline genetic testing in prostate cancer creates an opportunity and need to establish partnerships between genetic counselors and GU clinical teams to meet the challenge. However, before developing this infrastructure, it is critical to first understand the notable barriers to implementation.

1. *There are a limited number of genetic counselors.* Despite a workforce supply and demand assessment from the Genetic Counselor Workforce Working Group in 2016 that raised concerns about an impending shortage of genetic counselors, the expansion of the workforce has significantly outpaced their predictions [22, 23]. This success is largely due to the creation of additional training programs and the expansion of existing programs. Within the next 5 years, it is predicted that there will be close to 7500 practicing genetic counselors compared to ~5100 in 2019 [23].
2. *There is limited access to genetic counselors.* There is an overarching challenge of providers being able to effectively access genetic counselors, especially if none are located at their institution or within their practice. While historically genetic counselors have been located at academic centers and hospitals in urban areas, genetic counselors are available at genetic testing companies and private, stand-alone genetic counseling services that offer telemedicine consultations [24, 25]. Moreover, there has been a recent expansion of telemedicine services in response to the COVID-19 pandemic, which opens up additional options for patients. The National Society of Genetic Counselors (NSGC) has a "Find a Genetic Counselor" directory of both US and Canadian genetic counselors who offer in-person and telemedicine services.
3. *There is a lack of comfort regarding genetics knowledge among urology and oncology clinicians.* Despite limited genetics training for medical professionals, there is a significant demand on providers to interpret and incorporate various genetic information into their everyday practice. This increased complexity may

lead to under-recognition of the need for a genetics evaluation, inappropriate testing, and misinformation regarding results [26, 27, 28].

Despite these challenges, there are multiple ways to overcome these barriers to provide multidisciplinary care incorporating the expertise of both genetic counselors and GU providers.

- *Alternative delivery models.* A blended clinical approach that allows for initiation of genetic testing in the clinic with a subsequent referral to a genetic counselor for post-test discussion. This particular model has received a high degree of consensus among multiple disciplines [29]. The utilization of telehealth (telephone, video) can improve access to consults for genetic counseling.
- *Multidisciplinary clinics.* Providers can take advantage of genetic counselors within their institutions and/or advocate for hiring new genetic counselors.
- *Tumor boards.* The inclusion of genetics experts during institutional GU tumor boards can aid in the identification of appropriate patients for genetic testing, as well as reviewing results.
- *Educational opportunities.* The City of Hope Comprehensive Cancer Center offers an intensive, 12-week-long cancer genetics course for physicians, physician assistants, nurses, genetic counselors, and other healthcare professionals to gain comfort with and knowledge of the integration of genetic information into oncology practice. Clinical teams can limit the need to hire additional staff by sponsoring a designated person among their existing group to take advantage of such educational opportunities and bring the needed expertise back to the practice. In addition, urologists and GU oncologists could invite a genetic counselor for a grand-rounds presentation, partner with a genetic counselor to participate in a lecture for residents or other learners, or utilize resources available through AUA and ASCO to supplement team member knowledge in the area of cancer genetics.

Patient Disparities

Like many areas of medicine, disparities within access and uptake of genetic services are well documented, and solutions to provide equitable care are urgently needed. Patients of disadvantaged socioeconomic backgrounds and racial/ethnic minorities are less likely to be referred to genetics and less likely to consent to testing [30–32]. Additionally, men are significantly less likely to pursue testing for *BRCA1/2* compared to women, despite the known cancer risks for men [33]. These issues affect not only patients and their family members but also the genetic community as a whole. Variant classification, risk stratification, and gene discovery rely on comprehensive genomic data from individuals of all backgrounds and ancestries. Since the majority of genomic data has been historically collected from individuals of European ancestry, data for minority groups lags behind, which can lead to increased VUS detection and decreased utility of testing overall [30]. As GU providers implement genetic testing into their clinical practice, it will be essential to understand these disparities and recognize existing biases so that we can actively work together to provide equal access to care.

There is still limited data available about prostate cancer patients' perceptions, expectations, and needs related to genetic testing. More research is needed to better define the barriers to testing on the patient-facing side, especially since the concept of genetic testing is not as highly publicized for this patient population. However, Greenberg et al. recently published results from a focus group study of men with prostate cancer that concluded that referring providers can utilize their relationships with these patients to personalize the discussion of genetic testing and help determine the most appropriate timing during the treatment process [34]. This emphasizes that GU and genetics providers are in a unique position to help address these barriers and improve care for patients with prostate cancer.

Key Takeaway

As GU clinics either begin to incorporate germline genetic testing into their practices or expand their existing efforts, a partnership with genetics is highly encouraged to provide the most optimal care for patients. While the genetic testing process can be complex and nuanced, there are both laboratory and clinical genetic counselors available to help.

References

1. Daly MB, Pilarski R, Yurgelun MB, Berry MP, Buys SS, Dickson P, et al. NCCN guidelines insights: genetic/familial high-risk assessment: breast, ovarian, and pancreatic, version 1.2020. J Natl Compr Cancer Netw. 2020;18(4):380–91.
2. Pritchard CC, Mateo J, Walsh MF, De Sarkar N, Abida W, Beltran H, et al. Inherited DNA-repair gene mutations in men with metastatic prostate cancer. N Engl J Med. 2016;375(5):443–53.
3. Leongamornlert D, Saunders E, Dadaev T, Tymrakiewicz M, Goh C, Jugurnauth-Little S, et al. Frequent germline deleterious mutations in DNA repair genes in familial prostate cancer cases are associated with advanced disease. Br J Cancer. 2014;110(6):1663–72.
4. Isaacsson Velho P, Silberstein JL, Markowski MC, Luo J, Lotan TL, Isaacs WB, Antonarakis ES. Intraductal/ductal histology and lymphovascular invasion are associated with germline DNA-repair gene mutations in prostate cancer. Prostate. 2018;78(5):401–7.
5. Abida W, Armenia J, Gopalan A, Brennan R, Walsh M, Barron D, et al. Prospective genomic profiling of prostate cancer across disease states reveals germline and somatic alterations that may affect clinical decision making. JCO Precis Oncol. 2017;2017:PO.17.00029.
6. Giri VN, Beebe-Dimmer JL. Familial prostate cancer. Semin Oncol. 2016;43(5):560–5.
7. Price KS, Svenson A, King E, Ready K, Lazarin GA. Inherited cancer in the age of next-generation sequencing. Biol Res Nurs. 2018;20(2):192–204.
8. Roa BB, Boyd AA, Volcik K, Richards CS. Ashkenazi Jewish population frequencies for common mutations in BRCA1 and BRCA2. Nat Genet. 1996;14(2):185–7.

9. Giri VN, Hyatt C, Gomella LG. Germline testing for men with prostate cancer: navigating an expanding new world of genetic evaluation for precision therapy and precision management. J Clin Oncol. 2019;37(17):1455–9.
10. Szymaniak BM, Facchini LA, Giri VN, Antonarakis ES, Beer TM, Carlo MI, et al. Practical considerations and challenges for germline genetic testing in patients with prostate cancer: recommendations from the germline genetics working group of the PCCTC. JCO Oncol Pract. 2020;16(12):811–9.
11. Riley BD, Culver JO, Skrzynia C, Senter LA, Peters JA, Costalas JW, et al. Essential elements of genetic cancer risk assessment, counseling, and testing: updated recommendations of the National Society of Genetic Counselors. J Genet Couns. 2012;21(2):151–61.
12. Robson ME, Bradbury AR, Arun B, Domchek SM, Ford JM, Hampel HL, et al. American Society of Clinical Oncology policy statement update: genetic and genomic testing for cancer susceptibility. J Clin Oncol. 2015;33(31):3660–7.
13. Halverson CME, Wessinger BC, Clayton EW, Wiesner GL. Patients' willingness to reconsider cancer genetic testing after initially declining: mention it again. J Genet Couns. 2020;29(1):18–24.
14. Ardern-Jones A, Kenen R, Eeles R. Too much, too soon? Patients and health professionals' views concerning the impact of genetic testing at the time of breast cancer diagnosis in women under the age of 40. Eur J Cancer Care (Engl). 2005;14(3):272–81.
15. Culver JO, Ricker CN, Bonner J, Kidd J, Sturgeon D, Hodan R, et al. Psychosocial outcomes following germline multigene panel testing in an ethnically and economically diverse cohort of patients. Cancer. 2021;127(8):1275–85. Epub 2020 Dec 15.
16. Graves KD, Gatammah R, Peshkin BN, Krieger A, Gell C, Valdimarsdottir HB, Schwartz MD. BRCA1/2 genetic testing uptake and psychosocial outcomes in men. Familial Cancer. 2011;10(2):213–23.
17. Mersch J, Brown N, Pirzadeh-Miller S, Mundt E, Cox HC, Brown K, et al. Prevalence of variant reclassification following hereditary cancer genetic testing. JAMA. 2018;320(12):1266–74.
18. Macklin SK, Jackson JL, Atwal PS, Hines SL. Physician interpretation of variants of uncertain significance. Familial Cancer. 2019;18(1):121–6.
19. Seven M, Shah LL, Yazici H, Daack-Hirsch S. From Probands to relatives: communication of genetic risk for hereditary breast-ovarian cancer and its influence on subsequent testing. Cancer Nurs. Epub 2020 Aug 13
20. Menko FH, Ter Stege JA, van der Kolk LE, Jeanson KN, Schats W, Moha DA, et al. The uptake of presymptomatic genetic testing in hereditary breast-ovarian cancer and Lynch syndrome: a systematic review of the literature and implications for clinical practice. Familial Cancer. 2019;18(1):127–35.
21. Katz SJ, Kurian AW, Morrow M. Treatment decision making and genetic testing for breast cancer: mainstreaming mutations. JAMA. 2015;314(10):997–8.
22. Hoskovec JM, Bennett RL, Carey ME, DaVanzo JE, Dougherty M, Hahn SE, et al. Projecting the supply and demand for certified genetic counselors: a workforce study. J Genet Couns. 2018;27(1):16–20.
23. National Society of Genetic Counselors [Internet]. Genetic Counselor Workforce Initiatives; [cited 2021 Feb 28]. Available from: https://www.nsgc.org/page/genetic-counselor-workforce-initiatives-532.
24. US Bureau of Labor Statistics [Internet]. Occupational Outlook Handbook: Genetic Counselors; [cited 2021 Feb 28]. Available from: https://www.bls.gov/ooh/healthcare/genetic-counselors.htm.
25. Maiese DR, Keehn A, Lyon M, Flannery D, Watson M, Working Groups of the National Coordinating Center for Seven Regional Genetics Service Collaboratives. Current conditions in medical genetics practice. Genet Med. 2019;21(8):1874–7.
26. Bellcross CA, Kolor K, Goddard KA, Coates RJ, Reyes M, Khoury MJ. Awareness and utilization of BRCA1/2 testing among U.S. primary care physicians. Am J Prev Med. 2011;40(1):61–6.

27. Plon SE, Cooper HP, Parks B, Dhar SU, Kelly PA, Weinberg AD, et al. Genetic testing and cancer risk management recommendations by physicians for at-risk relatives. Genet Med. 2011;13(2):148–54.
28. Mahon SM. Errors in genetic testing: common causes and strategies for prevention. Clin J Oncol Nurs. 2017;21(6):673–6.
29. Giri VN, Knudsen KE, Kelly WK, Cheng HH, Cooney KA, Cookson MS, et al. Implementation of germline testing for prostate cancer: Philadelphia prostate cancer consensus conference 2019. J Clin Oncol. 2020;38(24):2798–811.
30. Saulsberry K, Terry SF. The need to build trust: a perspective on disparities in genetic testing. Genet Test Mol Biomarkers. 2013;17(9):647–8.
31. Hann KEJ, Freeman M, Fraser L, Waller J, Sanderson SC, Rahman B, et al. PROMISE study team. Awareness, knowledge, perceptions, and attitudes towards genetic testing for cancer risk among ethnic minority groups: a systematic review. BMC Public Health. 2017;17(1):503.
32. Paller CJ, Wang L, Brawley OW. Racial inequality in prostate cancer outcomes-socioeconomics, not biology. JAMA Oncol. 2019;5(7):983–4.
33. Childers KK, Maggard-Gibbons M, Macinko J, Childers CP. National Distribution of cancer genetic testing in the United States: evidence for a gender disparity in hereditary breast and ovarian cancer. JAMA Oncol. 2018;4(6):876–9.
34. Greenberg S, Slager S, Neil BO, Cooney K, Maughan B, Stopa N, et al. What men want: qualitative analysis of what men with prostate cancer (PCa) want to learn regarding genetic referral, counseling, and testing. Prostate. 2020;80(5):441–50.

Chapter 4
High-Risk Localized Prostate Cancer

Alexander P. Cole, Quoc-Dien Trinh, and Adam S. Kibel

High-risk prostate cancer comprises approximately one fifth of cases of localized disease [1]. These men often are curable, but also are at high risk for occult metastatic disease. Appropriate treatment is therefore paramount. The proportion of men with high-risk localized prostate cancer has increased in recent years – this has been attributed to recent decrease in the diagnosis of low-risk disease with lower utilization of PSA (prostate-specific antigen) screening [2–4]. Other factors such as diet and behavioral changes, demographic shifts, and less use of surgery for benign prostatic disease may also be at play [5].

In contrast to low-risk prostate cancer, mature long-term survival data during the PSA screening era has underscored the high probability of high-risk patients developing metastases and dying from their disease [6–8]. While some men "progress" to metastatic disease, it is likely that many of these men in fact have undetectable micro metastatic disease at the time of diagnosis. A cancer of 1 mm diameter – well below detection level for cross-sectional imaging – will typically be made up of about 100,000 cells, and therefore these micro-focal metastatic cancers may go undetected at the time of diagnosis. Treatment has evolved to address this, often combining local therapy with systemic treatments – making multimodality treatment a hallmark of high-risk prostate cancer management.

This increased complexity of high-risk disease means that treatment is challenging and time-consuming and involves multiple specialties. This complexity is reflected in the large proportion of men with high-risk prostate cancer who do not receive guideline-concordant treatment. In their study of 8229 men in 7 state cancer registries, Hamilton et al. showed that only 52.7% men in the National Comprehensive Cancer Network (NCCN) high-risk disease group received guideline-concordant

A. P. Cole · Q.-D. Trinh · A. S. Kibel (✉)
Division of Urological Surgery, Brigham and Women's Hospital, Harvard Medical School, Boston, MA, USA
e-mail: apcole@bwh.harvard.edu; akibel@bwh.harvard.edu

K. L. Stratton, A. K. Morgans (eds.), *Urologic Oncology*,
https://doi.org/10.1007/978-3-030-89891-5_4

care with the majority of the remainder (32.6% of the total) receiving less aggressive therapy than recommended [9]. Factors associated with non-guideline-concordant care include African American race and lack of insurance [10, 11]. Undertreatment has also been noted among healthy older men – perhaps due to physicians' tendency to underestimate life expectancies [12].

In this chapter we will outline the diagnosis and management of high-risk prostate cancer, emphasizing core management concepts as well as recent advances.

Defining High-Risk Prostate Cancer

Since the original risk group definitions described by D'Amico et al. in the late 1990s, the stratification of localized prostate cancer into risk groups based on PSA, Gleason grade, and clinical stage has been a key tool for informing treatment decisions [13]. While prostate cancer risk exists on a clinical spectrum, historical practice has been to categorize men into low-, intermediate-, and high-risk categories.

The original D'Amico high-risk group was comprised of men with T2c or PSA level ≥20 ng/mL or Gleason score ≥8. These categories were generated using risk of biochemical recurrence after surgery or radiation. Over the intervening years, the definition of high-risk disease has undergone gradual shifts, and there are now a number of definitions in use (Table 4.1). The degree of uncertainty regarding the definition of locally advanced prostate cancer was underscored in a 2007 survey of more than 150 UK oncologists and urologists: 95 different answers were given when respondents were asked about the definition of high-risk prostate cancer [14]. In a similar vein, a study of nearly 5000 men treated with radical prostatectomy at Memorial Sloan Kettering Cancer Center in New York found that the proportion of men defined as high risk ranged from 3% to 38% depending on the definition used; outcomes also varied between them, with 5-year biochemical recurrence rates between 49% and 80% depending on which definition was used [15].

Alongside the risk groups which classically utilized PSA, Gleason score, and stage, there are approaches which seek to improve upon risk stratification by adding other readily available clinical variables. The Cancer of the Prostate Risk Assessment (CAPRA) score utilizes age, PSA, clinical stage, Gleason grade, and percentage of positive systematic biopsy cores to predict risk of recurrence for localized disease [16]. In the targeted biopsy era, the relevance of the number of positive cores from

Table 4.1 Definitions of high-risk prostate cancer

Professional organization	Definition(s)
American Urological Association [13, 109]	PSA ≥20 ng/ml or GS ≥8 or c ≥T2c
European Association of Urology [110]	PSA ≥20 ng/ml or GS ≥8 or c ≥T3a
National Comprehensive Cancer Network [111]	PSA ≥20 ng/ml or GS ≥8 or c ≥T3a
Radiation Therapy Oncology Group [112]	GS = 7 with cT3 or N1 GS ≥8 and cT1–2

the lesion is of unclear relevance. A more integrated risk stratification approach, such as the well-known Kattan and Briganti nomograms, uses regression models to provide a continuous estimate of risk [17, 18].

It should be noted that all of the components of historical risk stratification score (PSA, grade, and stage) have important limitations. First, serum PSA levels have numerous benign sources of elevation and may be impacted by patient age, race, and genetics as well as prostate size, recent instrumentation, and inflammation. Second, Gleason grading has evolved over the past few decades with a noticeable grade inflation occurring. Albertsen et al. found an upward shift in Gleason grading when experienced pathologists re-reviewed slides from the early 1990s, with 55% of the needle cores upgraded [19]. Further emphasizing the potential impact of grade inflation, a group of Swedish researchers recently compared a contemporary cohort of surgically treated men in their national cancer registry using the same stage and grade criteria as one of the major Scandinavian trials in the 1990s. They found that men diagnosed and treated in the 1990s had similar prostate cancer-specific mortality as men in a contemporary time period with *one-unit higher* Gleason grade group [20]. Finally, stage migration has occurred: The widespread adoption of cross-sectional imaging of the prostate for local staging, mainly multi-parametric MRI (mpMRI), has increased the ability to identify extra prostatic extension. It is likely that large numbers of men now staged as cT3a or cT3b on the basis of MRI would have been staged as cT2 or even cT1c in the pre-MRI era.

Further increasing the complexity of risk stratification, biomarkers have been developed to assist with determining which patients have potentially lethal disease despite lower Gleason score. The Genomic Prostate Score (Oncotype Dx) is a 17-gene assay which predicts pathologic outcomes after prostatectomy [21, 22]. The Decipher score is an RNA-based assay which predicts metastasis after radical prostatectomy [23]. The Prolaris test is a measure of cell cycle progression associated with prostate cancer-specific mortality for several treatments in low-risk men [24]. While none of these tests is specifically designed as a predictive biomarker (e.g., for the effectiveness of any *specific therapies*), the presence of a higher or lower than expected score may spur more or less aggressive therapies for men in borderline risk categories.

In addition to the increased ability to identify local invasion, mpMRI may also provide insight into disease biology. These protocols combine T2 sequences with dynamic contrast enhancement and diffusion weighted imaging. It therefore identifies changes which closely track three of the six hallmarks of cancer including angiogenesis, cellularity, and invasiveness [25]. The use of mpMRI visibility to identify high-risk prostate cancers is supported by molecular data. Visible tumors are enriched with molecular features of tumor development and aggressivity, including activation of proliferative signaling, DNA damage, and inflammation [26]. Indeed, MRI-visible tumors are significantly enriched with molecular features of progression, including, *PTEN* loss, biochemical recurrence-associated genes (e.g., *CENPF*), and raised genomic scores (e.g., Oncotype Dx, Decipher, and Prolaris) compared to non-visible disease [26]. Visible tumors nearly always have some component of Gleason pattern 4 cancer. Emerging data suggest there are distinct clinical phenotypes of mpMRI visible versus non-visible tumors, which closely mirrors the distinction in clinical aggressiveness between Gleason grade groups [8, 27].

Ultimately, these details can be distilled into a conceptual definition of high-risk disease – it is prostate cancer – which is clinically localized but where a relatively high probability exists of occult, subclinical metastases. As a result, multimodality treatment is the guiding concept behind most high-risk prostate cancer treatment and will be the topic of the remainder of this chapter.

Treatment

Observation

Unlike the case with low- and intermediate-risk prostate cancer, there is relatively little controversy that men with high-risk prostate cancer have a high chance of dying from their disease if untreated. In the 20-year follow-up of the landmark Prostate Cancer Outcomes Study, Albertson et al. demonstrated that men with low-risk disease treated with either surgery or hormone therapy are unlikely to die from prostate cancer. The same is not true in men with high-risk disease (defined in his study as Gleason score 8–10) who received either observation or hormones. In this group, 66 out of 100 men died of prostate cancer at 20-year follow-up [28]. The risk of dying from prostate cancer was even present in the subgroup of relatively older men. Even among the oldest subgroup of men over 70 years of age with high-risk disease, nearly two thirds of men died of prostate cancer. While appropriate for men in lower risk categories, observation is rarely appropriate for men with high-risk disease, even for those in advanced age ranges [12].

Radiation and ADT

The use of radiation for prostate cancer dates to the first decade of the twentieth century [29, 30], and androgen deprivation therapy (ADT) has been a backbone of systemic therapy for prostate cancer since the 1940s [31]. The approach of combining these two modalities for high-risk disease was first investigated the 1960s [32]. These early studies were based on the belief that smaller tumors could be more effectively treated with radiation and the clinical observation that hormone therapy could effectively reduce the size of tumors. Unfortunately these early trials faced hurdles related to substantial toxicities of hormonal therapies available at that time, which was largely diethylstilbestrol, a medication with substantial cardiac and thrombogenic risks [33, 34]. As new hormonal agents were developed, toxicities were lessened. Reanalysis of prior trial data and two small Radiation Therapy Oncology Group (RTOG) phase II trials in the 1980s suggested that concomitant radiation and androgen suppression could reduce tumor burden and improve clinical response with acceptable toxicities [35–37].

On the basis of these results, RTOG 8610 evaluated the benefit of neoadjuvant ADT plus radiation therapy versus radiation therapy alone. The initial results from this trial, published in 1995, demonstrated that men with locally advanced disease had increased local control and disease-free survival when pelvic radiation was combined with short-term ADT [38].

Duration of ADT

In the 1990s, a series of trials provided definitive evidence supporting the combination of radiation and ADT. The first trial to prospectively demonstrate a survival benefit for ADT plus radiation in *high-risk* disease was EORTC 22863, published in 1997 by Bolla et al. which demonstrated an improvement in survival from 39.8% to 58.1% at 10-year follow-up. Unlike the shorter-duration ADT employed in the RTOG trials, this study used radiotherapy with or without 3 years of ADT [39–41].

Further evidence of the importance of longer-duration ADT was provided by EORTC 22961, a follow-up study that examined the duration of ADT. In EORTC 22961, men were recruited with locally advanced prostate cancer (cT2c to cT4, clinical nodal stages N0 to N2). All subjects received EBRT and 6 months of ADT, and those in the extended arm received an additional 30 months of ADT (3 years total). The 6-month ADT group had worse cancer-specific mortality compared to the 36-month ADT group (4.7% versus 3.2% at 5 years, hazard ratio 1.71, 95% CI 1.14–2.57). Overall mortality was also worse in the short-term group (19.0% versus 15.2% at 5 years, hazard ratio of 1.42, 95% CI 1.09–1.85) [42].

The RTOG 9202 trial further refined the question of ADT duration. This trial randomized men with cT2 or cT4 disease to 28 months vs. 4 months ADT and radiotherapy. Horwitz et al. report their 10-year follow-up which revealed superior disease-free survival, local progression, metastasis, and biochemical-free survival in the long-term ADT group. Disease-free survival improved from 83.9% to 88.7% at 10 years ($p = 0.0042$) although overall survival was no different – 51.6% versus 53.9% ($p = 0.36$) [43]. Lastly, in RTOG 8531, a total of 977 men with palpable extraprostatic extension were randomized to radiation alone or radiation with lifelong ADT. The men who received combination therapy with lifelong ADT had lower 10-year cancer-specific mortality 16% vs. 22% ($p = 0.005$) and improved survival 49% vs. 39% ($p = 0.002$) [44]. A systematic review examining pooled data from six studies of varying duration of ADT confirmed that longer duration improves overall and disease-specific survival in intermediate- and high-risk prostate cancer patients [45]. Current guidelines for men with high-risk disease thus support the use of ADT for 2 or 3 years [46].

The finding of improved survival in combination ADT plus RT led some to question whether it was simply the case that ADT itself was responsible for the survival benefit. The relative contribution of RT was evaluated in two trials. In the

Scandinavian Prostate Cancer Group-7 trial, Widmark et al. randomized 875 men with locally advanced cancer to receive 3 months of androgen deprivation therapy and RT followed by lifelong flutamide versus ADT alone. After a median follow-up of 7.6 years, they report that the addition of local radiotherapy to ADT halved the 10-year prostate cancer-specific mortality and resulted in a 10-year overall survival rate of 70% compared to 61% in the ADT monotherapy group [47]. Warde et al. reported a similar multi-institutional trial which recruited men with locally advanced prostate cancer (broadened to include localized disease with a PSA >40 ng/dl or PSA >20 ng/dl and Gleason score 8) [29]. Men were randomized to lifelong ADT with or without external beam radiation to the prostate, seminal vesicles, and pelvic nodes. The authors report a prolonged 7-year OS of 74% compared to 66% in the ADT monotherapy group. Taken together, these results support the synergistic effect of radiation plus ADT.

Combination Radiotherapy

Given the importance of local therapy, the question arose whether increasing the intensity of local therapy for high-risk prostate cancer could further improve disease control and survival. It had been shown that adding brachytherapy to external beam radiation increases the radiation dose by approximately 50% [48, 49]. The ASCENDE-RT trial addressed the clinical benefit of brachytherapy boost. This study enrolled men with intermediate- and high-risk localized prostate cancer. All men received 12 months of ADT and 23 fractions of pelvic radiation to the prostate, seminal vesicles, and regional lymph nodes. The EBRT boost arm then received an additional 16 fractions of radiation to the prostate, whereas the experimental brachytherapy boost arm received brachytherapy implants to the prostate. Over a median follow-up of 6.7 years, Morris et al. reported a substantial improvement in progression-free survival in the brachytherapy boost group (83% versus 63%) [50]. The survival benefit of this approach was also investigated in two retrospective studies. One utilized institutional results, and the second employed high-quality national cancer registry data. Both showed improved survival with EBRT plus brachytherapy with ADT versus EBRT with ADT alone [51, 52]. The limitations retrospective analysis notwithstanding [53], these two studies support the effectiveness of brachytherapy boost in a real-world setting. Importantly, the benefit must be balanced against the significantly higher toxicities in the combined EBRT plus brachytherapy group. This improved progression-free survival came at the cost of a higher rate of high-grade GU toxicity in the combined EBRT+ brachytherapy group. In the brachytherapy boost group, the proportion of men with grade 3 or higher GU toxicity was 7.0% at 2 years and 8.6% at 5 years versus 1.1% at 2 years and 2.2% at 5 years (*P* 0.005 and 0.058, respectively) [54].

The toxicities of radiohormonal therapy are not simply radiation-related. ADT causes metabolic, GI, cardiovascular, and cognitive side effects [55–58]. In 2008, D'Amico et al. reported results of a single institution trial which randomized men with high-risk disease to 6 months of ADT plus RT versus RT alone. They also performed an analysis stratified by comorbidity. In their initial results, the authors report a greater hazard of all-cause mortality in the radiation therapy monotherapy group versus the combined ADT + RT group (HR 1.8, 95% CI 1.1–2.9) with a 5-yr OS of 88% vs. 78%. Importantly, they determined that ADT only conferred a benefit in low-comorbidity group which suggests a potential interaction between ADT and comorbidity status [59]. Further supporting this, in their long-term follow, D'Amico et al. report that the high-comorbidity group actually had worse overall, cardiac, and all-cause mortality in men who received combined therapy with both ADT and RT. This supports the conclusion that ADT only improved outcomes in men with few comorbidities and the toxicity in high-comorbidity patients may result in greater net harm [60]. These results underscore that ADT can yield dramatic benefits in terms of cancer outcomes, but the metabolic and cardiac implications should be weighed against the improved cure rates.

Surgery for High-Risk Prostate Cancer

With the risks of ADT and radiation therapy in mind, some have emphasized surgical treatment of high-risk prostate cancer. Landmark trials from Sweden and the United States evaluating surgery versus watchful waiting support the conclusion that surgery is appropriate for many men with high-risk prostate cancer.

In the Scandinavian Prostate Cancer Group-4 (SPCG-4) trial 18-year follow-up, there was a significant reduction in mortality and metastatic disease among men who received prostatectomy for localized prostate cancer [8]. Curiously there was no significant benefit of surgery for men with highest-risk disease. The authors of the SPCG-4 acknowledge this surprising finding and suggest that many men in the high-risk group may in fact have been diverted to non-surgical treatments regardless of being randomized to surgery or watchful waiting. In addition, they may have been such high risk that they had occult metastatic disease and therefore unlikely to benefit. The US-based Prostate Cancer Intervention Versus Observation Trial (PIVOT) did not demonstrate a survival benefit for surgical treatment versus observation among the entire cohort but did show that cancer mortality was lower in the surgically treated men with D'Amico high-risk prostate disease [61, 62]. While the ProtecT trial is often cited in the debate on surgical treatment, it has limited information for the management of high-risk disease. Hamdy et al. randomized 1643 men to surgery, radiation, and active management. They report no difference in prostate cancer-specific mortality between groups [63]. However, the study comprised nearly all low- and intermediate-risk cases, and therefore its results should not be used to guide treatment of high-risk disease [64].

There is a body of retrospective data supporting surgery for localized high-risk disease as well as clear potential benefits to this approach [65, 66]. The most obvious of these is the potential for cure with a single procedure. Nomograms for men with localized disease suggest durable cure rate of >50% for some men with high-risk localized disease fully resected at the time of prostatectomy and an overall survival approaching 100% at 10 years [17].

Radical prostatectomy provides highly accurate staging information which improves risk stratification and subsequent treatment. A recent study from Duke showed that among men whose *only* high-risk feature was Gleason 8 disease, 60% were downgraded at the time of radical prostatectomy (e.g., from Gleason 8 to Gleason 7) [67]. Given that intensity of treatment, particularly use of ADT, is in large part driven by grade, a large portion of men with biopsy Gleason 4 + 4 disease may well be getting overtreated or paradoxically have curative treatment withheld by the false belief that their cancer is incurable.

Salvage Therapies for High-Risk Disease

Treatment of Adverse Pathological Findings Versus Treatment for Failure

Men with high-risk features following radical prostatectomy have treatment options which may be dictated either by pathological findings at radical prostatectomy or by clinical course after prostatectomy. For surgically treated men who have adverse findings after prostatectomy (typically defined as positive surgical margins, seminal vesicle invasion, or extraprostatic extension), both ADT and radiation therapy immediately after prostatectomy (so-called "adjuvant" approach) have been shown to be associated with reduced risk of biochemical and clinical relapse [68, 69]. However, there are well-known toxicities of both radiation and hormone therapy. Several of the trials demonstrating a survival advantage were done in the pre-PSA era. Thus, monitoring PSA and treating for recurrence have been widely adopted for the past decade [70, 71].

Three recent prospective trials have compared the strategy of immediate adjuvant therapy versus salvage in men with high-risk features after surgery. Their results support the approach of treatment for failure rather than immediate adjuvant therapy. The French GETUG-17, the UK-based RADICALS-RT, and the Australian-based RAVES all randomized men with high-risk features after prostatectomy to receive either immediate radiation and hormonal therapy or close monitoring with "early salvage" which was delivered when the PSA reached a pre-specified level of 0.1 ng/mL (RADICALS) or 0.2 ng/mL (RAVES and GETUG-17).

GETUG-17 found no significant difference in disease relapse (locoregional or metastatic), biochemical progression, or death at five years (HR 0.81, 95% CI 0.48–1.36) but over three times higher rate of grade 2 or worse toxicities in the adjuvant radiotherapy group 27% versus 7% ($p < 0.0001$) [72]. In RADICALS-RT, Parker et al. reported 5-year biochemical progression-free survival was 85% for those in the adjuvant radiotherapy group and 88% for those in the salvage radiotherapy group (HR 1.10, 95% CI 0.81–1.49). Similar to the results from GETUG-17, incontinence and urethral stricture disease were slightly higher in the adjuvant group compared to the early-salvage group. Proportions of men with incontinence and stricture disease were higher in the adjuvant arm of RADICALS-RT compared to the early salvage arm: 6% versus 4% for incontinence and 4.8% versus 4.0% for stricture disease ($p < 0.05$ for both) [73]. Lastly, in RAVES, Kneebone et al. reported 5-year progression-free survival rates of 86% versus 87% in the adjuvant and salvage radiotherapy group (HR 1.12, 95% CI 0.65–1.90) with no difference in genitourinary toxicities [73].

Taken together, these three trials strongly support a policy of close surveillance after radical prostatectomy rather than immediate adjuvant therapy. Timing of salvage therapy is critical. Earlier-salvage RT at PSA levels between 0.01 and 0.20 ng/mL provides better freedom from biochemical free recurrence and metastasis [74].

Regarding the optimal type of treatment in the salvage setting, two recent trials evaluated the role of integrating ADT with RT. GETUG-AFU 16 randomized men with biochemical recurrence after a period of undetectable PSA to either RT alone or ADT plus six months of the LHRH agonist. The authors demonstrate a significantly reduced hazard of clinical or biochemical progression at 5 years 80% vs. 62% ($p < 0.001$) – however it should be noted that only about 1 in 10 study subjects had Gleason 8 or higher [75]. In RTOG 9601, Shipley et al. evaluated the addition of 24 months of the antiandrogen bicalutamide plus RT versus RT and placebo. After a median follow-up of 13 years, the addition of bicalutamide was associated with improved survival and metastasis-free survival. The 12-year of prostate cancer mortality was 5.8% in the ADT groups versus 13.4% in the placebo group [76]. It should be noted that most men in GETUG-AFU 16 had lower PSAs prior to salvage and more favorable parameters prior to radical prostatectomy; thus, the former trial may be more relevant in the high-risk setting [77].

Treatment of Node-Positive Disease

Node-positive disease at the time of surgery does not uniformly portend failure. In a long-term follow-up of a highly selected group of node-positive men treated at Johns Hopkins without adjuvant RT or ADT over a 30-year period, the authors report a 15-year metastases-free and cancer-specific survival of 41.5% and 57.5%, suggesting that some men may indeed be cured with surgery alone [78].

However, metastases at the time of prostatectomy suggest that prostate cancer has already spread outside of the prostate and may therefore benefit from immediate systemic therapy. To assess the benefit of immediate ADT in node-positive disease, the Eastern Cooperative Oncology Group (ECOG) trial 3886 randomized men with node-positive disease at the time of radical prostatectomy to receive either immediate postoperative hormone therapy or hormone therapy upon detection of distant metastases. The authors report that after a median of 11.9 years, men who did not receive immediate ADT had worse hazard of overall survival (HR 1.84, 95% CI 1.01–3.35), prostate cancer-specific survival (HR 4.0, 95% CI 1.76–9.49), and progression-free survival (HR 3.4, 95% CI 1.96–5.98) [79]. The addition of adjuvant

RT also impacts on cure in men with node-positive disease. Lawton et al. published reanalysis of the results of RTOG-8531 and found a marked survival benefit for immediate ADT and RT in node-positive disease (9-year progression rates of 33% versus 4%) [80]. Retrospective studies using both institutional and registry data are mixed regarding benefit for radiation therapy and ADT for men with nodal disease after prostatectomy [81–83].

Surgery After Failure of Radiation Therapy

Recurrence of local prostate cancer after radiation therapy is typically defined based on measurements of serum PSA levels after radiation therapy. This can be complex due to the potential for a "PSA bounce" which can occur in the first 2–3 years after radiation therapy and does not indicate recurrence. In order to standardize the identification of postradiation recurrence, definitions are in use to define PSA recurrence: the American Society for Therapeutic Radiology and Oncology (ASTRO) definition of three consecutive rises after a nadir has been reached with a recurrence date between the nadir and the first raise has been largely replaced by the RTOG-ASTRO Phoenix criteria which is defined as an increase of 2 ng/mL over nadir [84]. While this definition is specific, it may miss some cases of radiorecurrent prostate cancer while still confined to the prostate and surgically curable [85].

When radiorecurrent cancer is caught early enough, data from high-volume centers have demonstrated the potential for durable surgical cure with salvage prostatectomy [86, 87]. This unfortunately comes at the cost of significantly greater morbidity compared to primary radical prostatectomy including a comparatively high rate of rectal injury (7%) and bladder neck contractures (34%) in a large multi-institutional series from Memorial Sloan Kettering. The reports of urinary incontinence and erectile dysfunction were also high, with 88% and 78% of men suffering these complications at six months [88]. Ultimately, the challenge of identifying radiorecurrent disease while still localized and the high side effect profile of this approach are significant barriers to widespread adoption of salvage prostatectomy.

Future Directions

While there is clearly local synergy between conventional ADT and RT, there is also likely an effect of ADT on microscopic metastatic disease which may explain some of the survival benefit. Given the success of ADT plus RT, it is not surprising that investigators began to explore the role of neoadjuvant therapy prior to surgery. Trials looking at conventional ADT with radical prostatectomy in the early 1990s and early 2000s showed that that neoadjuvant chemotherapy may confer a substantial size reduction as well as a reduction in positive margin rate, but it did not improve oncologic outcomes [89]. Similar results have been found in contemporary registry data [90].

The success of systemic agents including both novel hormone therapies and chemohormonal therapies in men with metastatic hormone-sensitive and hormone-resistant disease has revitalized the discussion of whether systemic agents could improve the cure of men with high-risk localized disease in conjunction with surgery or radiation. Results from the PUNCH trial were recently published. This trial randomized men with cT1 to cT3a and biopsy Gleason score of 8–10 or a Kattan preoperative nomogram probability of <60% biochemical progression-free survival to receive neoadjuvant docetaxel plus ADT followed by surgery versus surgery alone. The rate of biochemical-free survival at 8 years was significantly better in the neoadjuvant arm, and there was a non-significant effect toward improved overall survival in patients receiving neoadjuvant chemohormonal therapy (HR 0.66; 95% CI 0.42–1.03) [91].

Some have hypothesized that historical neoadjuvant ADT trials were limited by incomplete androgen ablation. Mostaghel et al. randomized 35 men with localized prostate cancer to goserelin in combination with (1) high-dose dutasteride (ZD), (2) dutasteride plus bicalutamide, or (3) dutasteride plus bicalutamide plus ketoconazole for 3 months before RP [92]. In their study, there was increased suppression of androgen signaling in the combined groups, and there were complete responses seen in one patient each in the two combined groups, but this was not statistically significant given the small numbers of men in these groups.

In castrate-resistant prostate cancer, hormonal signaling remains active in tumors even with castrate testosterone levels, but novel hormonal agents such as abiraterone acetate, enzalutamide, apalutamide, and darolutamide have shown efficacy by inhibiting intratumoral androgens [93–99]. The evaluation of these agents in the neoadjuvant setting is therefore of great interest.

A series of phase II trials examined the efficacy of novel hormone agents in the neoadjuvant setting (Table 4.2). Taplin et al. evaluated the effect of abiraterone acetate on prostate tissue in the neoadjuvant setting among a phase II trial of 58 men with intermediate- to high-risk prostate cancer [100]. Patients who received 24 weeks of abiraterone plus leuprolide (versus 12 weeks) had a higher complete response rate and were less likely to have pT3 disease at prostatectomy. A similar trial of 52 men compared enzalutamide with combined blockade with enzalutamide, leuprolide, and abiraterone and found that 4.3% of men achieved pathological complete response and 13.0% achieved minimal residual disease in the combination therapy group [100, 101]. In a subsequent phase II trial, 75 men were randomized to receive either enzalutamide and leuprolide or enzalutamide, leuprolide, and abiraterone, McKay et al. report pathologic complete response or minimal residual disease rate of 30% in combined group versus 16% in the enzalutamide and leuprolide group ($p = 0.263$) [102].

The endpoint of minimal residual disease appears to correlate with outcome. A pooled analysis of 72 men enrolled in 3 of the phase II trials for neoadjuvant hormone therapy demonstrated that 15.7% had tumor measuring ≤0.5 cm (5.7% with a complete pathologic response and 10.0% with residual tumor measuring 0.1–0.5 cm).

Table 4.2 Selection of recent neoadjuvant trials of novel hormone therapies with primary endpoints and inclusion criteria

Trial	*N*	Selection criteria	Duration	Primary endpoint	Arms	Endpoints		
						Nadir PSA <0.2 ng/mL	*pCR (%)*	*≥ypT3*
TAPS [92]	35	cT1–T3 AND PSA <40 ng/mL AND Gleason 7–10	3 months	Prostatic androgen levels	Goserelin + dutasteride	40%	0%	33%
					Goserelin + dutasteride+ bicalutamide	100%	10%	30%
					Goserelin + dutasteride+ bicalutamide+ ketoconazole	83%	8%	8%
						Nadir PSA <0.2	*pCR (%)*	*CR + MRD*[a]
NeoAbi [100]	58	Positive biopsies (≥3) AND Gleason score ≥7 OR PSA >10 ng/mL OR PSA velocity >2 ng/mL/yr	24 weeks	12-week prostatic androgen levels	12 weeks abiraterone/24 weeks LHRH agonist	82%	4%	4%
					24 weeks abiraterone/24 weeks LHRH agonist	93%	10%	14%
						Median PSA pre-RP	*pCR (%)*	*CR + MRD*[a]
NeoEnza [113]	40	Positive biopsies (≥3) AND PSA >10 ng/mL OR Gleason score ≥7 (4 + 3) T4 excluded	6 months	Pathologic complete response	Enzalutamide	0.51	0%	0
					Enzalutamide + leuprolide + dutasteride	0.04	4%	17%
						Median PSA Pre RP	*pCR (%)*	*CR + MRD*[a]
NeoAbi+Enza [103]	75	Positive biopsies (≥3) AND PSA >20 ng/mL OR Gleason score ≥7 (4 + 3)	6 months	Pathologic complete response	Enzalutamide + LHRH	0.02	8%	16%
					Enzalutamide+ abiraterone + LHRH	0.03	12%	30%

[a]Minimal residual disease

The rate of biochemical-free recurrence among all the men in the trials was 50% compared to 70% predicted using the MSKCC nomogram. Importantly, none of the men with minimal residual disease or complete pathological response had a biochemical failure at 3.4 years follow-up [103]. On the basis of these results, large multi-institutional, phase III trial is currently underway to evaluate apalutamide in the neoadjuvant versus adjuvant setting for men with high-risk localized and locally advanced disease [104].

Radiation and Novel Hormone Therapies

A similar shift to employing novel hormonal agents is also underway in radiotherapy. As is the case in with surgery, there are also several phase II trials utilizing second-generation hormonal agents alongside with radiation therapy. Koontz reported a phase II trial of 37 men with high- and unfavorable intermediate-risk prostate cancer who received abiraterone acetate plus ADT and radiation therapy. The regimen was well tolerated, and 52% of men had undetectable PSA at one year [105]. Similarly, de la Calle et al. recently reported the results of a phase II trial of 16 men treated with leuprolide, enzalutamide, and radiation therapy for high-risk prostate cancer and had no men develop biochemical recurrence at a median follow-up of 28 months [106]. Phase III trials incorporating novel hormonal agents (apalutamide and enzalutamide) with radiation are now underway [107, 108].

Conclusion

High-risk prostate cancer comprises a growing subset of localized disease. Although definitions vary, men with this disease state are characterized by disease which is potentially curable but with a relatively high risk of prostate cancer mortality. Treatment thus often entails the combination of multiple treatment modalities including systemic hormone therapy, radiation, and surgery. Overall, there are several standard-of-care treatments, which must be tailored to individual patients in a multidisciplinary setting. Regarding the future management of high-risk disease, here is considerable promise for integrating systemic therapy with both surgery and radiation therapy, and ongoing phase III trials will determine whether this will become the new standard of care.

References

1. Fletcher SA, von Landenberg N, Cole AP, Gild P, Choueiri TK, Lipsitz SR, et al. Contemporary national trends in prostate cancer risk profile at diagnosis. Prostate Cancer Prostatic Dis. 2019;23(1):81–7. https://doi.org/10.1038/s41391-019-0157-y.

2. Sammon JD, Abdollah F, Choueiri TK, Kantoff PW, Nguyen PL, Menon M, et al. Prostate-specific antigen screening after 2012 US preventive services task force recommendations. JAMA. 2015;314(19):2077–9. https://doi.org/10.1001/jama.2015.7273.
3. Weiner AB, Matulewicz RS, Eggener SE, Schaeffer EM. Increasing incidence of metastatic prostate cancer in the United States (2004–2013). Prostate Cancer Prostatic Dis. 2016;19(4):395–7. https://doi.org/10.1038/pcan.2016.30.
4. Jemal A, Fedewa SA, Ma J, Siegel R, Lin CC, Brawley O, et al. Prostate cancer incidence and PSA testing patterns in relation to USPSTF screening recommendations. JAMA. 2015;314(19):2054–61. https://doi.org/10.1001/jama.2015.14905.
5. Gann PH. Risk factors for prostate cancer. Rev Urol. 2002;4(Suppl 5):S3–S10.
6. D'Amico AV, Moul J, Carroll PR, Sun L, Lubeck D, Chen MH. Cancer-specific mortality after surgery or radiation for patients with clinically localized prostate cancer managed during the prostate-specific antigen era. J Clin Oncol. 2003;21(11):2163–72. https://doi.org/10.1200/JCO.2003.01.075.
7. Eggener SE, Scardino PT, Walsh PC, Han M, Partin AW, Trock BJ, et al. Predicting 15-year prostate cancer specific mortality after radical prostatectomy. J Urol. 2011;185(3):869–75. https://doi.org/10.1016/j.juro.2010.10.057.
8. Bill-Axelson A, Holmberg L, Garmo H, Rider JR, Taari K, Busch C, et al. Radical prostatectomy or watchful waiting in early prostate cancer. N Engl J Med. 2014;370(10):932–42. https://doi.org/10.1056/NEJMoa1311593.
9. Hamilton AS, Fleming ST, Wang D, Goodman M, Wu XC, Owen JB, et al. Clinical and demographic factors associated with receipt of non guideline-concordant initial therapy for nonmetastatic prostate cancer. Am J Clin Oncol. 2016;39(1):55–63. https://doi.org/10.1097/COC.0000000000000017.
10. Mahal BA, Aizer AA, Ziehr DR, Hyatt AS, Sammon JD, Schmid M, et al. Trends in disparate treatment of African American men with localized prostate cancer across National Comprehensive Cancer Network risk groups. Urology. 2014;84(2):386–92. https://doi.org/10.1016/j.urology.2014.05.009.
11. Mahal BA, Aizer AA, Ziehr DR, Hyatt AS, Lago-Hernandez C, Chen YW, et al. The association between insurance status and prostate cancer outcomes: implications for the Affordable Care Act. Prostate Cancer Prostatic Dis. 2014;17(3):273–9. https://doi.org/10.1038/pcan.2014.23.
12. Bratt O, Folkvaljon Y, Hjalm Eriksson M, Akre O, Carlsson S, Drevin L, et al. Undertreatment of men in their seventies with high-risk nonmetastatic prostate cancer. Eur Urol. 2015;68(1):53–8. https://doi.org/10.1016/j.eururo.2014.12.026.
13. D'Amico AV, Whittington R, Malkowicz SB, Schultz D, Blank K, Broderick GA, et al. Biochemical outcome after radical prostatectomy, external beam radiation therapy, or interstitial radiation therapy for clinically localized prostate cancer. JAMA. 1998;280(11):969–74. https://doi.org/10.1001/jama.280.11.969.
14. Payne HA, Gillatt DA. Differences and commonalities in the management of locally advanced prostate cancer: results from a survey of oncologists and urologists in the UK. BJU Int. 2007;99(3):545–53. https://doi.org/10.1111/j.1464-410X.2006.06651.x.
15. Yossepowitch O, Eggener SE, Bianco FJ Jr, Carver BS, Serio A, Scardino PT, et al. Radical prostatectomy for clinically localized, high risk prostate cancer: critical analysis of risk assessment methods. J Urol. 2007;178(2):493–9.; discussion 9. https://doi.org/10.1016/j.juro.2007.03.105.
16. Cooperberg MR, Pasta DJ, Elkin EP, Litwin MS, Latini DM, Du Chane J, et al. The University of California, San Francisco Cancer of the Prostate Risk Assessment score: a straightforward and reliable preoperative predictor of disease recurrence after radical prostatectomy. J Urol. 2005;173(6):1938–42. https://doi.org/10.1097/01.ju.0000158155.33890.e7.
17. Kattan MW, Eastham JA, Stapleton AM, Wheeler TM, Scardino PT. A preoperative nomogram for disease recurrence following radical prostatectomy for prostate cancer. J Natl Cancer Inst. 1998;90(10):766–71.

18. Briganti A, Larcher A, Abdollah F, Capitanio U, Gallina A, Suardi N, et al. Updated nomogram predicting lymph node invasion in patients with prostate cancer undergoing extended pelvic lymph node dissection: the essential importance of percentage of positive cores. Eur Urol. 2012;61(3):480–7. https://doi.org/10.1016/j.eururo.2011.10.044.
19. Albertsen PC, Hanley JA, Barrows GH, Penson DF, Kowalczyk PD, Sanders MM, et al. Prostate cancer and the Will Rogers phenomenon. J Urol. 2005;97(17):1248–53.
20. Cazzaniga W, Garmo H, Robinson D, Holmberg L, Bill-Axelson A, Stattin P. Mortality after radical prostatectomy in a matched contemporary cohort in Sweden compared to the Scandinavian Prostate Cancer Group 4 (SPCG-4) study. BJU Int. 2018;123(3):421–8. https://doi.org/10.1111/bju.14563.
21. Klein EA, Cooperberg MR, Magi-Galluzzi C, Simko JP, Falzarano SM, Maddala T, et al. A 17-gene assay to predict prostate cancer aggressiveness in the context of Gleason grade heterogeneity, tumor multifocality, and biopsy undersampling. Eur Urol. 2014;66(3):550–60. https://doi.org/10.1016/j.eururo.2014.05.004.
22. Cullen J, Brassell SA, Chen Y, Porter C, L'Esperance J, Brand T, et al. Racial/Ethnic patterns in prostate cancer outcomes in an active surveillance cohort. Prostate Cancer. 2011;2011:234519. https://doi.org/10.1155/2011/234519.
23. Klein EA, Yousefi K, Haddad Z, Choeurng V, Buerki C, Stephenson AJ, et al. A genomic classifier improves prediction of metastatic disease within 5 years after surgery in node-negative high-risk prostate cancer patients managed by radical prostatectomy without adjuvant therapy. Eur Urol. 2015;67(4):778–86. https://doi.org/10.1016/j.eururo.2014.10.036.
24. Cuzick J, Berney DM, Fisher G, Mesher D, Moller H, Reid JE, et al. Prognostic value of a cell cycle progression signature for prostate cancer death in a conservatively managed needle biopsy cohort. Br J Cancer. 2012;106(6):1095–9. https://doi.org/10.1038/bjc.2012.39.
25. Hanahan D, Weinberg RA. The hallmarks of cancer. Cell. 2000;100(1):57–70.
26. Norris JM, Simpson BS, Parry MA, Allen C, Ball R, Freeman A, et al. Genetic landscape of prostate cancer conspicuity on multiparametric magnetic resonance imaging: a systematic review and bioinformatic analysis. Eur Urol Open Sci. 2020;20:37–47. https://doi.org/10.1016/j.euros.2020.06.006.
27. Stavrinides V, Giganti F, Trock B, Punwani S, Allen C, Kirkham A, et al. Five-year outcomes of magnetic resonance imaging-based active surveillance for prostate cancer: a large cohort study. Eur Urol. 2020;78(3):443–51. https://doi.org/10.1016/j.eururo.2020.03.035.
28. Albertsen PC, Hanley JA, Fine J. 20-year outcomes following conservative management of clinically localized prostate cancer. JAMA. 2005;293(17):2095–101. https://doi.org/10.1001/jama.293.17.2095.
29. Warde P, Mason M, Ding K, Kirkbride P, Brundage M, Cowan R, et al. Combined androgen deprivation therapy and radiation therapy for locally advanced prostate cancer: a randomised, phase 3 trial. Lancet. 2011;378(9809):2104–11. https://doi.org/10.1016/s0140-6736(11)61095-7.
30. Ward MC, Tendulkar RD, Ciezki JP, Klein EA. Future directions from past experience: a century of prostate radiotherapy. Clin Genitourin Cancer. 2014;12(1):13–20. https://doi.org/10.1016/j.clgc.2013.08.003.
31. Huggins C, Hodges CV. Studies on prostatic cancer I. The effect of castration, of estrogen and androgen injection on serum phosphatases in metastatic carcinoma of the prostate. CA Cancer J Clin. 1972;22(4):232–40.
32. van der Werf-Messing B, Sourek-Zikova V, Blonk DI. Localized advanced carcinoma of the prostate: radiation therapy versus hormonal therapy. Int J Radiat Oncol Biol Phys. 1976;1(11–12):1043–8. https://doi.org/10.1016/0360-3016(76)90074-2.
33. DeWeese TL, Song DY. Current evidence for the role of combined androgen suppression and radiation in the treatment of adenocarcinoma of the prostate. Urology. 2000;55(2):169–74. https://doi.org/10.1016/s0090-4295(99)00419-7.
34. Denmeade SR, Isaacs JT. A history of prostate cancer treatment. Nat Rev Cancer. 2002;2(5):389–96. https://doi.org/10.1038/nrc801.

35. Pilepich MV, Krall JM, Sause WT, Johnson RJ, Russ HH, Hanks GE, et al. Prognostic factors in carcinoma of the prostate–analysis of RTOG study 75-06. Int J Radiat Oncol Biol Phys. 1987;13(3):339–49. https://doi.org/10.1016/0360-3016(87)90007-1.
36. Pilepich MV, Krall JM, John MJ, Rubin P, Porter AT, Marcial VA, et al. Hormonal cytoreduction in locally advanced carcinoma of the prostate treated with definitive radiotherapy: preliminary results of RTOG 83-07. Int J Radiat Oncol Biol Phys. 1989;16(3):813–7. https://doi.org/10.1016/0360-3016(89)90500-2.
37. Pilepich MV, John MJ, Krall JM, McGowan D, Hwang YS, Perez CA. Phase II Radiation Therapy Oncology Group study of hormonal cytoreduction with flutamide and Zoladex in locally advanced carcinoma of the prostate treated with definitive radiotherapy. Am J Clin Oncol. 1990;13(6):461–4. https://doi.org/10.1097/00000421-199012000-00001.
38. Pilepich MV, Krall JM, al-Sarraf M, John MJ, Doggett RL, Sause WT, et al. Androgen deprivation with radiation therapy compared with radiation therapy alone for locally advanced prostatic carcinoma: a randomized comparative trial of the Radiation Therapy Oncology Group. Urology. 1995;45(4):616–23. https://doi.org/10.1016/s0090-4295(99)80053-3.
39. Bolla M, Van Tienhoven G, Warde P, Dubois JB, Mirimanoff R-O, Storme G, et al. External irradiation with or without long-term androgen suppression for prostate cancer with high metastatic risk: 10-year results of an EORTC randomised study. Lancet Oncol. 2010;11(11):1066–73. https://doi.org/10.1016/s1470-2045(10)70223-0.
40. Bolla M, Gonzalez D, Warde P, Dubois JB, Mirimanoff RO, Storme G, et al. Improved survival in patients with locally advanced prostate cancer treated with radiotherapy and goserelin. N Engl J Med. 1997;337(5):295–300. https://doi.org/10.1056/NEJM199707313370502.
41. Bolla M, Collette L, Blank L, Warde P, Dubois JB, Mirimanoff R-O, et al. Long-term results with immediate androgen suppression and external irradiation in patients with locally advanced prostate cancer (an EORTC study): a phase III randomised trial. Lancet. 2002;360(9327):103–8. https://doi.org/10.1016/s0140-6736(02)09408-4.
42. Bolla M, de Reijke TM, Van Tienhoven G, Van den Bergh AC, Oddens J, Poortmans PM, et al. Duration of androgen suppression in the treatment of prostate cancer. N Engl J Med. 2009;360(24):2516–27. https://doi.org/10.1056/NEJMoa0810095.
43. Horwitz EM, Bae K, Hanks GE, Porter A, Grignon DJ, Brereton HD, et al. Ten-year follow-up of radiation therapy oncology group protocol 92-02: a phase III trial of the duration of elective androgen deprivation in locally advanced prostate cancer. J Clin Oncol. 2008;26(15):2497–504. https://doi.org/10.1200/JCO.2007.14.9021.
44. Pilepich MV, Winter K, Lawton CA, Krisch RE, Wolkov HB, Movsas B, et al. Androgen suppression adjuvant to definitive radiotherapy in prostate carcinoma–long-term results of phase III RTOG 85-31. Int J Radiat Oncol Biol Phys. 2005;61(5):1285–90. https://doi.org/10.1016/j.ijrobp.2004.08.047.
45. Leal F, Figueiredo MA, Sasse AD. Optimal duration of androgen deprivation therapy following radiation therapy in intermediate- or high-risk nonmetastatic prostate cancer: a systematic review and metaanalysis. Int Braz J Urol. 2015;41(3):425–34. https://doi.org/10.1590/S1677-5538.IBJU.2014.0412.
46. Chang AJ, Autio KA, Roach M 3rd, Scher HI. High-risk prostate cancer-classification and therapy. Nat Rev Clin Oncol. 2014;11(6):308–23. https://doi.org/10.1038/nrclinonc.2014.68.
47. Widmark A, Klepp O, Solberg A, Damber J-E, Angelsen A, Fransson P, et al. Endocrine treatment, with or without radiotherapy, in locally advanced prostate cancer (SPCG-7/SFUO-3): an open randomised phase III trial. Lancet. 2009;373(9660):301–8. https://doi.org/10.1016/s0140-6736(08)61815-2.
48. Hoskin PJ, Motohashi K, Bownes P, Bryant L, Ostler P. High dose rate brachytherapy in combination with external beam radiotherapy in the radical treatment of prostate cancer: initial results of a randomised phase three trial. Radiother Oncol. 2007;84(2):114–20. https://doi.org/10.1016/j.radonc.2007.04.011.
49. Soumarova R, Homola L, Perkova H, Stursa M. Three-dimensional conformal external beam radiotherapy versus the combination of external radiotherapy with high-dose rate brachytherapy in localized carcinoma of the prostate: comparison of acute toxicity. Tumori. 2007;93(1):37–44.

50. Morris WJ, Tyldesley S, Rodda S, Halperin R, Pai H, McKenzie M, et al. Androgen suppression combined with elective nodal and dose escalated radiation therapy (the ASCENDE-RT Trial): an analysis of survival endpoints for a randomized trial comparing a low-dose-rate brachytherapy boost to a dose-escalated external beam boost for high- and intermediate-risk prostate cancer. Int J Radiat Oncol Biol Phys. 2017;98(2):275–85. https://doi.org/10.1016/j.ijrobp.2016.11.026.
51. Ennis RD, Hu L, Ryemon SN, Lin J, Mazumdar M. Brachytherapy-based radiotherapy and radical prostatectomy are associated with similar survival in high-risk localized prostate cancer. J Clin Oncol. 2018;36(12):1192–8. https://doi.org/10.1200/JCO.2017.75.9134.
52. Kishan AU, Cook RR, Ciezki JP, Ross AE, Pomerantz MM, Nguyen PL, et al. Radical prostatectomy, external beam radiotherapy, or external beam radiotherapy with brachytherapy boost and disease progression and mortality in patients with Gleason score 9-10 prostate cancer. JAMA. 2018;319(9):896–905. https://doi.org/10.1001/jama.2018.0587.
53. Krimphove MJ, Nabi J, Cole AP, Trinh QD, et al. Brachytherapy-based radiotherapy and radical prostatectomy are associated with similar survival in high-risk localized prostate Cancer. J Clin Oncol 2018;36:1192-8: comparative survival analyses of radical prostatectomy and radiation therapy reveal the importance of adequate follow-up time. Eur Urol Oncol. 2019;2(2):222–3. https://doi.org/10.1016/j.euo.2018.08.007.
54. Rodda S, Tyldesley S, Morris WJ, Keyes M, Halperin R, Pai H, et al. ASCENDE-RT: an analysis of treatment-related morbidity for a randomized trial comparing a low-dose-rate brachytherapy boost with a dose-escalated external beam boost for high- and intermediate-risk prostate cancer. Int J Radiat Oncol Biol Phys. 2017;98(2):286–95. https://doi.org/10.1016/j.ijrobp.2017.01.008.
55. Sun M, Cole AP, Hanna N, Mucci LA, Berry DL, Basaria S, et al. Cognitive impairment in men with prostate cancer treated with androgen deprivation therapy: a systematic review and meta-analysis. J Urol. 2018;199(6):1417–25. https://doi.org/10.1016/j.juro.2017.11.136.
56. Krasnova A, Epstein M, Marchese M, Dickerman BA, Cole AP, Lipsitz SR, et al. Risk of dementia following androgen deprivation therapy for treatment of prostate cancer. Prostate Cancer Prostatic Dis. 2020;23(3):410–8. https://doi.org/10.1038/s41391-019-0189-3.
57. Gild P, Cole AP, Krasnova A, Dickerman BA, von Landenberg N, Sun M, et al. Liver disease in men undergoing androgen deprivation therapy for prostate cancer. J Urol. 2018;200(3):573–81. https://doi.org/10.1016/j.juro.2018.03.135.
58. Nguyen PL, Alibhai SM, Basaria S, D'Amico AV, Kantoff PW, Keating NL, et al. Adverse effects of androgen deprivation therapy and strategies to mitigate them. Eur Urol. 2015;67(5):825–36. https://doi.org/10.1016/j.eururo.2014.07.010.
59. D'Amico AV, Chen MH, Renshaw AA, Loffredo M, Kantoff PW. Androgen suppression and radiation vs radiation alone for prostate cancer: a randomized trial. JAMA. 2008;299(3):289–95. https://doi.org/10.1001/jama.299.3.289.
60. D'Amico AV, Chen MH, Renshaw A, Loffredo M, Kantoff PW. Long-term follow-up of a randomized trial of radiation with or without androgen deprivation therapy for localized prostate cancer. JAMA. 2015;314(12):1291–3. https://doi.org/10.1001/jama.2015.8577.
61. Wilt TJ, Brawer MK, Jones KM, Barry MJ, Aronson WJ, Fox S, et al. Radical prostatectomy versus observation for localized prostate cancer. N Engl J Med. 2012;367(3):203–13. https://doi.org/10.1056/NEJMoa1113162.
62. Wilt TJ, Jones KM, Barry MJ, Andriole GL, Culkin D, Wheeler T, et al. Follow-up of prostatectomy versus observation for early prostate cancer. N Engl J Med. 2017;377(2):132–42. https://doi.org/10.1056/NEJMoa1615869.
63. Hamdy FC, Donovan JL, Lane JA, Mason M, Metcalfe C, Holding P, et al. 10-year outcomes after monitoring, surgery, or radiotherapy for localized prostate cancer. N Engl J Med. 2016;375(15):1415–24. https://doi.org/10.1056/NEJMoa1606220.
64. Oxley J, Simpkin A, Goepel J, Varma M, Griffiths D, Grigor K, et al. Gleason drift in the NIHR ProtecT study. Histopathology. 2015;66(3):438–46. https://doi.org/10.1111/his.12549.
65. Berg S, Cole AP, Krimphove MJ, Nabi J, Marchese M, Lipsitz SR, et al. Comparative effectiveness of radical prostatectomy versus external beam radiation therapy plus brachytherapy

in patients with high-risk localized prostate cancer. Eur Urol. 2018;75(4):552–5. https://doi.org/10.1016/j.eururo.2018.10.032.
66. Feldman AS, Meyer CP, Sanchez A, Krasnova A, Reznor G, Menon M, et al. Morbidity and mortality of locally advanced prostate cancer: a population-based analysis comparing radical prostatectomy versus external beam radiation. J Urol. 2017;198(5):1061–8. https://doi.org/10.1016/j.juro.2017.05.073.
67. Gansler T, Fedewa S, Qi R, Lin CC, Jemal A, Moul JW. Most Gleason 8 biopsies are downgraded at prostatectomy-does 4 + 4 = 7? J Urol. 2018;199(3):706–12. https://doi.org/10.1016/j.juro.2017.10.014.
68. Dorff TB, Flaig TW, Tangen CM, Hussain MH, Swanson GP, Wood DP Jr, et al. Adjuvant androgen deprivation for high-risk prostate cancer after radical prostatectomy: SWOG S9921 study. J Clin Oncol. 2011;29(15):2040–5. https://doi.org/10.1200/JCO.2010.32.2776.
69. Thompson IM Jr, Tangen CM, Paradelo J, Lucia MS, Miller G, Troyer D, et al. Adjuvant radiotherapy for pathologically advanced prostate cancer: a randomized clinical trial. JAMA. 2006;296(19):2329–35. https://doi.org/10.1001/jama.296.19.2329.
70. Showalter TN, Ohri N, Teti KG, Foley KA, Keith SW, Trabulsi EJ, et al. Physician beliefs and practices for adjuvant and salvage radiation therapy after prostatectomy. Int J Radiat Oncol Biol Phys. 2012;82(2):e233–8. https://doi.org/10.1016/j.ijrobp.2011.04.003.
71. Taggar A, Alghamdi M, Tilly D, Kostaras X, Kerba M, Husain S, et al. Assessing guideline impact on referral patterns of post-prostatectomy patients to radiation oncologists. Can Urol Assoc J. 2016;10(9–10):314–8. https://doi.org/10.5489/cuaj.3539.
72. Sargos P, Chabaud S, Latorzeff I, Magné N, Benyoucef A, Supiot S, et al. Adjuvant radiotherapy versus early salvage radiotherapy plus short-term androgen deprivation therapy in men with localised prostate cancer after radical prostatectomy (GETUG-AFU 17): a randomised, phase 3 trial. Lancet Oncol. 2020;21(10):1341–52. https://doi.org/10.1016/s1470-2045(20)30454-x.
73. Parker CC, Clarke NW, Cook AD, Kynaston HG, Petersen PM, Catton C, et al. Timing of radiotherapy after radical prostatectomy (RADICALS-RT): a randomised, controlled phase 3 trial. Lancet. 2020;396(10260):1413–21. https://doi.org/10.1016/s0140-6736(20)31553-1.
74. Tendulkar RD, Agrawal S, Gao T, Efstathiou JA, Pisansky TM, Michalski JM, et al. Contemporary update of a multi-institutional predictive nomogram for salvage radiotherapy after radical prostatectomy. J Clin Oncol. 2016;34(30):3648–54. https://doi.org/10.1200/JCO.2016.67.9647.
75. Carrie C, Hasbini A, de Laroche G, Richaud P, Guerif S, Latorzeff I, et al. Salvage radiotherapy with or without short-term hormone therapy for rising prostate-specific antigen concentration after radical prostatectomy (GETUG-AFU 16): a randomised, multicentre, open-label phase 3 trial. Lancet Oncol. 2016;17(6):747–56. https://doi.org/10.1016/S1470-2045(16)00111-X.
76. Shipley WU, Seiferheld W, Lukka HR, Major PP, Heney NM, Grignon DJ, et al. Radiation with or without antiandrogen therapy in recurrent prostate cancer. N Engl J Med. 2017;376(5):417–28. https://doi.org/10.1056/NEJMoa1607529.
77. Spratt DE. Evidence-based risk stratification to guide hormone therapy use with salvage radiation therapy for prostate cancer. Int J Radiat Oncol Biol Phys. 2018;102(3):556–60. https://doi.org/10.1016/j.ijrobp.2018.06.037.
78. Pierorazio PM, Gorin MA, Ross AE, Feng Z, Trock BJ, Schaeffer EM, et al. Pathological and oncologic outcomes for men with positive lymph nodes at radical prostatectomy: the Johns Hopkins Hospital 30-year experience. Prostate. 2013;73(15):1673–80. https://doi.org/10.1002/pros.22702.
79. Messing EM, Manola J, Yao J, Kiernan M, Crawford D, Wilding G, et al. Immediate versus deferred androgen deprivation treatment in patients with node-positive prostate cancer after radical prostatectomy and pelvic lymphadenectomy. Lancet Oncol. 2006;7(6):472–9. https://doi.org/10.1016/S1470-2045(06)70700-8.
80. Lawton CA, Winter K, Grignon D, Pilepich MV. Androgen suppression plus radiation versus radiation alone for patients with stage D1/pathologic node-positive adenocarcinoma of the prostate: updated results based on national prospective randomized trial Radiation

Therapy Oncology Group 85-31. J Clin Oncol. 2005;23(4):800–7. https://doi.org/10.1200/JCO.2005.08.141.
81. Abdollah F, Karnes RJ, Suardi N, Cozzarini C, Gandaglia G, Fossati N, et al. Impact of adjuvant radiotherapy on survival of patients with node-positive prostate cancer. J Clin Oncol. 2014;32(35):3939–47. https://doi.org/10.1200/JCO.2013.54.7893.
82. Rusthoven CG, Carlson JA, Kavanagh BD. External validation of the benefit of adjuvant radiotherapy for pathologic N1M0 prostate cancer. J Clin Oncol. 2015;33(17):1987–8. https://doi.org/10.1200/JCO.2015.60.9404.
83. Kaplan JR, Kowalczyk KJ, Borza T, Gu X, Lipsitz SR, Nguyen PL, et al. Patterns of care and outcomes of radiotherapy for lymph node positivity after radical prostatectomy. BJU Int. 2013;111(8):1208–14. https://doi.org/10.1111/bju.12079.
84. Roach M 3rd, Hanks G, Thames H Jr, Schellhammer P, Shipley WU, Sokol GH, et al. Defining biochemical failure following radiotherapy with or without hormonal therapy in men with clinically localized prostate cancer: recommendations of the RTOG-ASTRO Phoenix Consensus Conference. Int J Radiat Oncol Biol Phys. 2006;65(4):965–74. https://doi.org/10.1016/j.ijrobp.2006.04.029.
85. Stephenson AJ, Eastham JA. Role of salvage radical prostatectomy for recurrent prostate cancer after radiation therapy. J Clin Oncol. 2005;23(32):8198–203. https://doi.org/10.1200/JCO.2005.03.1468.
86. Bianco FJ Jr, Scardino PT, Stephenson AJ, Diblasio CJ, Fearn PA, Eastham JA. Long-term oncologic results of salvage radical prostatectomy for locally recurrent prostate cancer after radiotherapy. Int J Radiat Oncol Biol Phys. 2005;62(2):448–53. https://doi.org/10.1016/j.ijrobp.2004.09.049.
87. Ward JF, Sebo TJ, Blute ML, Zincke H. Salvage surgery for radiorecurrent prostate cancer: contemporary outcomes. J Urol. 2005;173(4):1156–60. https://doi.org/10.1097/01.ju.0000155534.54711.60.
88. Mohler JL, Halabi S, Ryan ST, Al-Daghmin A, Sokoloff MH, Steinberg GD, et al. Management of recurrent prostate cancer after radiotherapy: long-term results from CALGB 9687 (Alliance), a prospective multi-institutional salvage prostatectomy series. Prostate Cancer Prostatic Dis. 2019;22(2):309–16. https://doi.org/10.1038/s41391-018-0106-1.
89. Shelley MD, Kumar S, Wilt T, Staffurth J, Coles B, Mason MD. A systematic review and meta-analysis of randomised trials of neo-adjuvant hormone therapy for localised and locally advanced prostate carcinoma. Cancer Treat Rev. 2009;35(1):9–17. https://doi.org/10.1016/j.ctrv.2008.08.002.
90. McClintock TR, von Landenberg N, Cole AP, Lipsitz SR, Gild P, Sun M, et al. Neoadjuvant androgen deprivation therapy prior to radical prostatectomy: recent trends in utilization and association with postoperative surgical margin status. Ann Surg Oncol. 2018;26(1):297–305. https://doi.org/10.1245/s10434-018-7035-z.
91. Eastham JA, Heller G, Halabi S, Monk P, Clinton SK, Szmulewitz RZ, et al. CALGB 90203 (Alliance): radical prostatectomy (RP) with or without neoadjuvant chemohormonal therapy (CHT) in men with clinically localized, high-risk prostate cancer (CLHRPC). J Clin Oncol. 2019;38(26):3042–50.
92. Mostaghel EA, Nelson PS, Lange P, Lin DW, Taplin ME, Balk S, et al. Targeted androgen pathway suppression in localized prostate cancer: a pilot study. J Clin Oncol. 2014;32(3):229–37. https://doi.org/10.1200/JCO.2012.48.6431.
93. Scher HI, Fizazi K, Saad F, Taplin ME, Sternberg CN, Miller K, et al. Increased survival with enzalutamide in prostate cancer after chemotherapy. N Engl J Med. 2012;367(13):1187–97. https://doi.org/10.1056/NEJMoa1207506.
94. Smith MR, Saad F, Chowdhury S, Oudard S, Hadaschik BA, Graff JN, et al. Apalutamide treatment and metastasis-free survival in prostate cancer. N Engl J Med. 2018;378(15):1408–18. https://doi.org/10.1056/NEJMoa1715546.
95. Hussain M, Fizazi K, Saad F, Rathenborg P, Shore N, Ferreira U, et al. Enzalutamide in men with nonmetastatic, castration-resistant prostate cancer. N Engl J Med. 2018;378(26):2465–74. https://doi.org/10.1056/NEJMoa1800536.

96. Fizazi K, Shore N, Tammela TL, Ulys A, Vjaters E, Polyakov S, et al. Nonmetastatic, castration-resistant prostate cancer and survival with darolutamide. N Engl J Med. 2020;383(11):1040–9. https://doi.org/10.1056/NEJMoa2001342.
97. Ryan CJ, Smith MR, de Bono JS, Molina A, Logothetis CJ, de Souza P, et al. Abiraterone in metastatic prostate cancer without previous chemotherapy. N Engl J Med. 2013;368(2):138–48. https://doi.org/10.1056/NEJMoa1209096.
98. de Bono JS, Logothetis CJ, Molina A, Fizazi K, North S, Chu L, et al. Abiraterone and increased survival in metastatic prostate cancer. N Engl J Med. 2011;364(21):1995–2005. https://doi.org/10.1056/NEJMoa1014618.
99. Beer TM, Armstrong AJ, Rathkopf DE, Loriot Y, Sternberg CN, Higano CS, et al. Enzalutamide in metastatic prostate cancer before chemotherapy. N Engl J Med. 2014;371(5):424–33. https://doi.org/10.1056/NEJMoa1405095.
100. Taplin ME, Montgomery B, Logothetis CJ, Bubley GJ, Richie JP, Dalkin BL, et al. Intense androgen-deprivation therapy with abiraterone acetate plus leuprolide acetate in patients with localized high-risk prostate cancer: results of a randomized phase II neoadjuvant study. J Clin Oncol. 2014;32(33):3705–15. https://doi.org/10.1200/JCO.2013.53.4578.
101. Medivation Inc., Astellas Pharma Inc. Study of enzalutamide (Formerly MDV3100) as a neoadjuvant therapy for patients undergoing prostatectomy for localized prostate cancer. https://ClinicalTrials.gov/show/NCT01547299; 2012
102. McKay RR, Ye H, Xie W, Lis R, Calagua C, Zhang Z, et al. Evaluation of intense androgen deprivation before prostatectomy: a randomized phase II trial of enzalutamide and leuprolide with or without abiraterone. J Clin Oncol. 2019;37(11):923–31. https://doi.org/10.1200/JCO.18.01777.
103. McKay RR, Montgomery B, Xie W, Zhang Z, Bubley GJ, Lin DW, et al. Post prostatectomy outcomes of patients with high-risk prostate cancer treated with neoadjuvant androgen blockade. Prostate Cancer Prostatic Dis. 2018;21(3):364–72. https://doi.org/10.1038/s41391-017-0009-6.
104. Taplin M-E, Gleave M, Evans CP, Efstathiou E, Kantoff PW, Ross A, et al. PROTEUS: a randomized, double-blind, placebo (PBO)-controlled, phase 3 trial of apalutamide (APA) plus androgen deprivation therapy (ADT) versus PBO plus ADT prior to radical prostatectomy (RP) in patients with localized high-risk or locally advanced prostate cancer (PC). J Clin Oncol. 2019;37(15_suppl):TPS5100-TPS. https://doi.org/10.1200/JCO.2019.37.15_suppl.TPS5100.
105. Koontz BF, Hoffman KE, Healy P, George DJ, Harrison MR, Zhang T, et al. Phase II trial of 6 months ADT/abiraterone acetate plus prednisone (AAP) and definitive radiotherapy (AbiRT) for men with intermediate to high risk localized prostate cancer. J Clin Oncol. 2018;36(6_suppl):11. https://doi.org/10.1200/JCO.2018.36.6_suppl.11.
106. Calle CM, Chang A, Rashid G, Wong AC, Choi A, Feng FY, et al. Phase II trial of definitive radiotherapy with leuprolide and enzalutamide in high-risk prostate cancer. J Clin Oncol. 2020;38(6_suppl):323. https://doi.org/10.1200/JCO.2020.38.6_suppl.323.
107. Sandler HM, McKenzie MR, Tombal BF, Baskin-Bey E, Freedland SJ, Roach M, et al. ATLAS: a randomized, double-blind, placebo-controlled, phase 3 trial of apalutamide (ARN-509) in patients with high-risk localized or locally advanced prostate cancer receiving primary radiation therapy. J Clin Oncol. 2016;34(15_suppl):TPS5087-TPS. https://doi.org/10.1200/JCO.2016.34.15_suppl.TPS5087.
108. Williams S, Davis ID, Sweeney C, Stockler MR, Martin AJ, Hague W, et al. Randomised phase 3 trial of enzalutamide in androgen deprivation therapy (ADT) with radiation therapy for high risk, clinically localized prostate cancer: ENZARAD (ANZUP 1303). J Clin Oncol. 2018;36(6_suppl):TPS156-TPS. https://doi.org/10.1200/JCO.2018.36.6_suppl.TPS156.
109. Thompson I, Thrasher JB, Aus G, Burnett AL, Canby-Hagino ED, Cookson MS, et al. Guideline for the management of clinically localized prostate cancer: 2007 update. J Urol. 2007;177(6):2106–31. https://doi.org/10.1016/j.juro.2007.03.003.

110. Heidenreich A, Bellmunt J, Bolla M, Joniau S, Mason M, Matveev V, et al. EAU guidelines on prostate cancer. Part 1: screening, diagnosis, and treatment of clinically localised disease. Eur Urol. 2011;59(1):61–71. https://doi.org/10.1016/j.eururo.2010.10.039.
111. Bahnson RR, Hanks GE, Huben RP, Kantoff P, Kozlowski JM, Kuettel M, et al. NCCN practice guidelines for prostate cancer. Oncology (Williston Park). 2000;14(11A):111–9.
112. Roach M, Lu J, Pilepich MV, Asbell SO, Mohiuddin M, Terry R, et al. Four prognostic groups predict long-term survival from prostate cancer following radiotherapy alone on Radiation Therapy Oncology Group clinical trials. Int J Radiat Oncol Biol Phys. 2000;47(3):609–15. https://doi.org/10.1016/s0360-3016(00)00578-2.
113. Montgomery B, Tretiakova MS, Joshua AM, Gleave ME, Fleshner N, Bubley GJ, et al. Neoadjuvant enzalutamide prior to prostatectomy. Clin Cancer Res. 2017;23(9):2169–76. https://doi.org/10.1158/1078-0432.CCR-16-1357.

Chapter 5
Treatment of Metastatic Hormone-Sensitive Prostate Cancer

Woodson W. Smelser, Christopher J. D. Wallis, and Kelvin A. Moses

Introduction

In both Europe and the United States, prostate cancer remains one of the most prevalent cancers, consistently ranking as the number two cause of male cancer mortality and the second most common malignancy [1, 2]. Of these cases, the majority of patients present with localized prostate cancer, yet 3–8% of men diagnosed in North America and Europe harbor metastatic disease at presentation [3, 4]. Rates of metastatic disease at presentation in Asia are much higher, ostensibly due to lower rates of screening, and have been reported as high as 64% [5].

An understanding of the interplay between prostate cancer progression and metastasis and the male hormonal axis has been described for nearly 90 years. Seminal work by Huggins and Hodges, first reported in 1941, detailed the effect of castration or injection of other anti-androgens on serum phosphatases in metastatic prostate cancer, definitively narrowing scientific focus on the androgen axis as a target for treatment [6]. Thus, androgen deprivation therapy (ADT), through either surgical or medical castration, has remained a mainstay of treatment for nearly 70 years (see Fig. 5.1) [7, 8]. However, even after successful androgen blockade, many men progress to a state of castration-resistant prostate cancer (CRPC) due to myriad tumor adaptations that permit eventual progression of metastatic disease despite castrate levels of testosterone. Historically, median time to progression to castration resistance with either surgical or medical castration was approximately 18–24 months [9]. Men in this space are substantially more likely to die of prostate cancer, and for many years, progression into metastatic castration-resistant prostate cancer (mCRPC) could only be managed with palliation through additional

W. W. Smelser · C. J. D. Wallis · K. A. Moses (✉)
Vanderbilt University Medical Center, Division of Urologic Oncology, Nashville, TN, USA
e-mail: kelvin.a.moses@vumc.org

K. L. Stratton, A. K. Morgans (eds.), *Urologic Oncology*,
https://doi.org/10.1007/978-3-030-89891-5_5

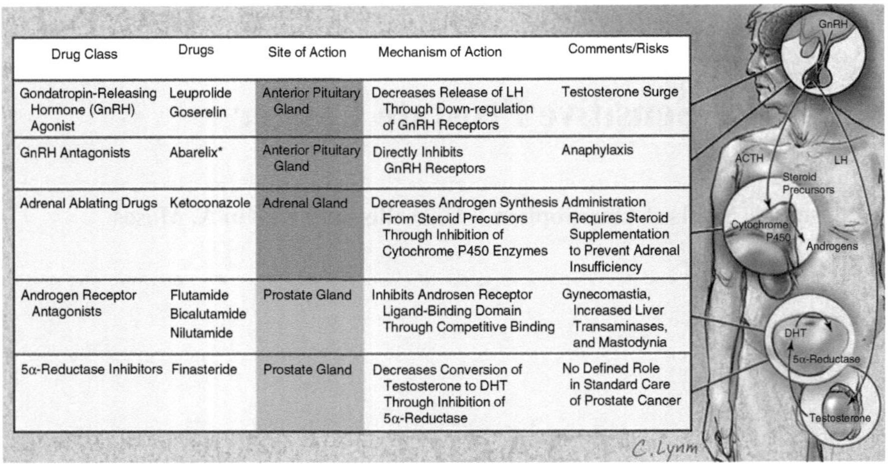

Drug Class	Drugs	Site of Action	Mechanism of Action	Comments/Risks
Gondatropin-Releasing Hormone (GnRH) Agonist	Leuprolide Goserelin	Anterior Pituitary Gland	Decreases Release of LH Through Down-regulation of GnRH Receptors	Testosterone Surge
GnRH Antagonists	Abarelix*	Anterior Pituitary Gland	Directly Inhibits GnRH Receptors	Anaphylaxis
Adrenal Ablating Drugs	Ketoconazole	Adrenal Gland	Decreases Androgen Synthesis From Steroid Precursors Through Inhibition of Cytochrome P450 Enzymes	Administration Requires Steroid Supplementation to Prevent Adrenal Insufficiency
Androgen Receptor Antagonists	Flutamide Bicalutamide Nilutamide	Prostate Gland	Inhibits Androsen Receptor Ligand-Binding Domain Through Competitive Binding	Gynecomastia, Increased Liver Transaminases, and Mastodynia
5α-Reductase Inhibitors	Finasteride	Prostate Gland	Decreases Conversion of Testosterone to DHT Through Inhibition of 5α-Reductase	No Defined Role in Standard Care of Prostate Cancer

Fig. 5.1 Hormonal interventions and endocrine axis in prostate cancer. (*Request permission for use from Springer:* Sharifi [66]. https://doi.org/10.1007/978-1-60327-829-4_9. Chapter 9, Fig. 9.1 Hormonal interventions and endocrine axis in prostate cancer)

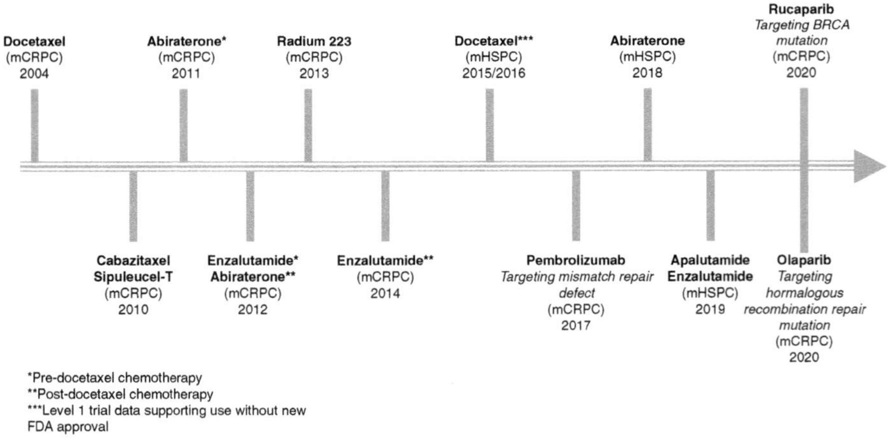

Fig. 5.2 Timeline of approval of therapeutic agents in metastatic prostate cancer. (Original figure)

anti-androgens or mitoxantrone chemotherapy, with median survival as short as 10–12 months [8–12].

Critical advances in the management of CRPC occurred with reports of two studies demonstrating the efficacy of taxane chemotherapy docetaxel in 2004 [13, 14]. Addition of docetaxel with or without estramustine to ADT in CPRC conferred an overall survival (OS) advantage of 1.9–2.4 months when compared to a regimen of mitoxantrone and prednisone [13, 14]. This represented the first improvement in overall survival in advanced prostate cancer since the adoption of ADT. From 2004 to 2018, multiple agents were approved in the CRPC space due to improvements in overall survival. Overall, seven therapeutics ultimately received approval in CRPC during this period (see Fig. 5.2): docetaxel, cabazitaxel (another taxane chemotherapy), sipuleucel-T (an antitumor immunotherapy), abiraterone acetate (an androgen synthesis inhibitor), radium 223 (an alpha-particle-emitting radiotherapy), and enzalutamide and apalutamide (so-called novel anti-androgens) [13–22]. Additionally, three additional agents have been approved for use in the mCRPC space based upon the results of genetic testing: pembrolizumab (for DNA mismatch repair positive tumors), rucaparib (for BRCA-positive tumors), and olaparib (for homologous recombination repair gene mutations) [23].

As a result of the innovation in CRPC, a paradigm shift began to occur, and a new disease space – metastatic hormone-sensitive prostate cancer (mHSPC) – was defined to explore application of novel agents that demonstrated a survival benefit in CRPC. Since 2016, this rapidly evolving landscape has seen the approval of four new agents for treatment of mHSPC: docetaxel, abiraterone acetate, enzalutamide, and apalutamide (see Fig. 5.2). Approval of all of these therapies was based upon demonstrated improvement in overall survival. Each of these agents and the trials demonstrating their efficacy will be discussed in detail below.

Agents Demonstrating Overall Survival Improvement in mHSPC

Docetaxel

Docetaxel is a taxane-based chemotherapy that was an early emerging treatment with evidence of improvement of overall survival in metastatic prostate cancer. Taxanes are diterpene molecules derived from the plant genus *Taxus* or yews. They work by impeding cellular division through inhibition of microtubule formation by stabilizing tubulin bound to guanidine diphosphate (GDP) preventing mitotic division [24]. These agents first demonstrated efficacy in ovarian cancer and later were applied to the metastatic prostate cancer space [24]. Docetaxel was first applied in mCRPC as discussed above and was the first chemotherapy agent to demonstrate an improvement in overall survival when added to standard ADT [13, 14]. The first trial to evaluate the use of docetaxel in addition to ADT in men with mHSPC was the GETUG-AFU 15 trial which reported results in 2013 [25]. From 2004 to 2008, 385 men with pathologically confirmed prostate cancer and metastatic disease proven on radiographic imaging were enrolled at 29 centers in France and 1 in Belgium. Men who had previously received chemotherapy were excluded. Androgen deprivation with either orchiectomy or medical castration was compared to ADT + docetaxel which was administered IV for up to nine total cycles at a dose of 75 mg/m2 every 21 days. Interestingly, this randomized, open-label, phase III trial was negative, demonstrating no improvement in overall survival at a median follow-up of 83 months in patients receiving over ADT + docetaxel versus ADT alone (48.6 months vs 62.1 months, HR 0.88, 95% CI 0.68–1.14, $p = 0.3$). Additionally, no serious adverse events were observed in the ADT group compared to a significant burden of serious side effects in the ADT + docetaxel group, including neutropenia in 21% of patients, febrile neutropenia in 3%, neutropenia with severe infection in 1%, and abnormal liver function tests (LFTs) in 2% [25].

Despite the disappointing outcome of GETUG-AFU 15, the results of two subsequently published trials did demonstrate a significant improvement in overall survival in men with mHSPC who received docetaxel in addition to ADT [25, 26]. First, the results of the Androgen Ablation Therapy With or Without Chemotherapy in Treating Patients With Metastatic Prostate Cancer Trial (CHAARTED) was reported in 2015 in the New England Journal of Medicine [26]. In this randomized controlled trial, 790 men with metastatic prostate cancer were enrolled to receive ADT or ADT plus docetaxel. Like GETUG-AFU 15, patients were included who had a histological diagnosis of prostate cancer, radiographically proven metastatic disease, good to fair (0–2) Eastern Cooperative Oncology Group (ECOG) status, and lack of major organ dysfunction (renal, hepatic, or hematologic). Patients who had prior chemotherapy were excluded, but patients were allowed to have received prior ADT, as long as treatment duration was <2 years or had been initiated within the last 3 months due to newly diagnosed metastatic disease. Again, patients in the ADT arm were allowed either medical or surgical castration, and patients in the experimental arm received ADT plus docetaxel IV 75 mg/m^2 every 21 days [26].

The results of this trial were much more encouraging in favor of addition of docetaxel to standard ADT. Mean age in this trial was 63 years, and median follow-up was 28.9 months, with a median overall survival of 57.6 months in the docetaxel/ADT group versus 44 months in the ADT-only group (HR 0.61, 95% CI 0.47–0.80, $p < 0.0001$). This 13-month overall survival advantage did come at the cost of increased toxicity, with the most common Grade 3 or 4 adverse events observed being febrile neutropenia (6.2%), neutropenia with infection (2.3%), and sensory or motor neuropathy in 0.5%. Additional benefits of docetaxel also included a lower incidence of prostate cancer deaths, longer time to development of castration resistance, and higher rate of PSA decline to <0.2 ng/ml by 12 months post-administration [26]. Furthermore, CHAARTED was also unique to GETUG-AFU 15 in that subgroup analysis was performed stratifying patients by volume of metastatic disease, with high-volume disease (HVD) defined as greater than or equal to 4 bone metastases, with at least one outside of the spine or pelvis and/or visceral metastases. Notably, this classification for volume of metastatic disease would be used in multiple future trials, and an even more substantial benefit was observed with the addition of docetaxel in patients with HVD, with median survival increased by 17 months (HR 0.60, 95% CI 0.45–0.81, $p < 0.0001$) [26].

Like the results of CHAARTED, the data from the STAMPEDE trial also demonstrated an improvement in overall survival with addition of docetaxel to standard ADT [27]. The STAMPEDE trial was a multi-arm, multi-stage randomized controlled trial which was performed in the United Kingdom. This trial examined the use of docetaxel in a 4-arm study, in which men with mCSPC, nodal disease, and high-risk localized prostate cancer were randomized in a 2:1:1:1 ratio to receive either the standard of care, ADT (Arm A), ADT + zoledronic acid (Arm B), ADT+ docetaxel (Arm C), or ADT+ docetaxel + zoledronic acid (Arm E). In total, 2962 men were enrolled, and results were published in 2016. Since this trial enrolled men with high-risk localized and metastatic hormone-sensitive prostate cancer, it is important to note that 61% of participants had metastatic disease at enrollment. When examining the standard of care arm (Arm A) with the group receiving ADT + docetaxel (Arm C), overall survival was improved (HR 0.62, 95% CI 0.51–0.76, $p < 0.0001$). Notably, no survival advantage was noted with the addition of zoledronic acid to either therapy [27].

Given the discrepancy between the results of GETUG-AFU 15 and both CHAARTED and STAMPEDE, the authors of the GETUG-AFU 15 study performed a retrospective subgroup analysis of their trial in 2016, this time stratifying patients by the number and site of metastatic disease using the CHAARTED criteria. In this analysis, they noted an overall survival advantage of 4.7 months in patients with high-volume disease as classified by CHAARTED, affirming the greater benefit seen in patients with HVD [24, 27]. Additionally, the authors and other reviewers of both trials have noted that the baseline characteristics of patients in CHAARTED were different than GETUG-AFU 15 with a higher proportion of patients in CHAARTED having higher median PSA (median >50 in CHAARTED versus median of ~25 in GETUG-AFU 15). Furthermore, more patients in CHAARTED had HVD (64% in ADT arm and 66% in ADT + docetaxel arm) compared to GETUG-AFU 15 (47% in the ADT arm and 48% in the ADT + docetaxel arm). These factors likely explain the discrepancy in outcomes between the initial analysis of both trials [25, 26, 28, 29].

Finally, a systematic review and meta-analysis of all three trials has since been performed to examine the benefits of addition of docetaxel to ADT. In total, the three trials included 2951 men, and the authors examined the benefits on both overall survival and progression-free survival (PFS) of docetaxel in addition to ADT. All three studies demonstrated a statistically significant benefit in OS with docetaxel (HR 0.72, 95% CI 0.06–0.9, $p = 0.0002$). No difference was observed between high- and low-volume diseases in this analysis. Similarly, PFS was improved in men receiving docetaxel in all three studies (HR 0.63, 95% CI 0.57–0.70), with a 27% overall risk reduction of death in all patients with metastatic disease and a further overall risk reduction of 33% in patients with high-volume disease (HR 0.67) [30].

Thus, given the three well-designed trials described above, each of which has shown benefit in overall and progression-free survival in at least some men with mHSPC, docetaxel is being increasingly utilized as a first-line agent. However, addition of chemotherapy to ADT does come at the cost of increased risks of adverse events as demonstrated by all three trials in this space. Namely, the most serious, though uncommon, adverse events in these trials included neutropenia, neutropenia with fever or infection, fatigue, and, in rare cases, death, and patients must be counseled accordingly. Patient selection is critically important in choosing docetaxel as a first-line therapy in mHSPC, as all trial participants were relatively healthy, as men with hematologic, renal, hepatic dysfunction or poor performance status were excluded [25–27]. Nevertheless, in a disease with progression-free survival that was previously measured in months, the addition of docetaxel to ADT has the potential to add substantial survival benefit.

Abiraterone Acetate

Following the level one evidence supporting the use of docetaxel for mHSPC in 2015/2016, the next agent that eventually gained US Food and Drug Administration (FDA) approval specifically for first-line therapy mHSPC was abiraterone acetate. This agent received approval in 2018 on the basis of analysis from two studies: LATITUDE and STAMPEDE [31, 32]. Abiraterone acetate is an orally administered androgen biosynthesis inhibitor that was first developed for use in mCRPC [33–35]. It is well established that prostate cancer overcomes androgen deprivation to develop castration resistance through a number of modifications: changes to the androgen receptor (AR), upregulation of extragonadal androgen sources, cellular modifications to increase intratumoral steroidogenesis despite castrate testosterone levels, and upregulation of nuclear transcription factors to allow androgen receptor-mediated gene transcription [35, 36]. Abiraterone acetate is a prodrug of abiraterone that induces an antitumor response by selectively and irreversibly inhibiting cytochrome P17 (CYP17), resulting in disruption of adrenal androgen biosynthesis [33–35]. Due to disruption of the androgen pathway, and concurrent downstream effects on non-androgen steroids, it is administered with prednisone [22, 33].

LATITUDE, one of the two randomized trials to evaluate abiraterone acetate in mHSPC, was reported in 2017. This multinational, phase III randomized controlled trial enrolled men with mHSPC with at least two of the three high-risk features: at least three bony lesions, visceral metastases, or Gleason score greater than or equal to 8. Patients were stratified by the presence or absence of visceral disease and performance status (ECOG 0 or 1 versus 2). Men were randomized to receive ADT + abiraterone acetate 1000 mg daily +5 mg or prednisone or ADT + placebo. Overall survival was significantly higher in the experimental group at 66% versus 49% in the control group at planned interim analysis with 30.4 months of median follow-up. Median overall survival was not reached in the abiraterone group versus 34.7 months in the placebo group. Relative risk reduction for patients receiving abiraterone acetate in addition to ADT was 38% (HR 0.62, 95% CI 0.51–0.76). The median length of radiographic progression-free survival was 33 months in the abiraterone group compared to only 14.8 months in the placebo group (HR for disease progression or death, 0.47; 95% CI, 0.39 – 0.55; $P < 0.001$) [31]. Adverse events lead to discontinuation in 12% versus 10% of patients in the abiraterone versus placebo group, respectively. Dose interruption or modification occurred in 32% of patients receiving abiraterone compared to only 17% in the placebo group. The most common side effects were hypertension and hypokalemia due to mineralocorticoid effects of abiraterone. Grade 3 or 4 hypertension occurred in 30% of patients in the abiraterone group versus 0.2% of patients in the placebo group. Similarly Grade 3 or 4 hypokalemia occurred in 11% of patients in the abiraterone group versus only 1% of patients receiving placebo [31]. Counseling patients on these anticipated effects and monitoring blood pressure and serum chemistry while on therapy is of paramount importance.

Like LATITUDE, the STAMPEDE trial also evaluated the use of abiraterone acetate in one of the investigational arms of this multi-arm trial. As stated earlier,

STAMPEDE enrolled men with metastatic disease, nodal disease, and high-risk localized prostate cancer. Arm G of the trial evaluated men with these disease characteristics and enrolled them to receive either 100 mg daily of abiraterone acetate +5 mg of prednisone or ADT alone (Arm A). In total, 1917 men were randomized and analyzed, with 52% of patients in this group having metastatic disease. At a median follow-up of 3 years, overall survival was significantly higher in the abiraterone group (Arm G) at 83% compared to 76% in the ADT group (HR 0.63, 95% CI 0.52–0.76, $p < 0.0001$). This was similar to the magnitude of improvement seen in LATITUDE, but with slightly longer follow-up. Side effects were also more prevalent in the abiraterone arm of this trial than in the arm receiving ADT alone, with Grade 3 or greater adverse events observed in 47% of patients versus 33%, respectively [32].

Thus, based upon the level one evidence of benefit of addition of abiraterone with prednisone to standard ADT demonstrated in both LATITUDE and STAMPEDE, current guidelines for management of advanced prostate cancer now recommend consideration of abiraterone acetate plus prednisone and ADT as a first-line option for men with newly diagnosed metastatic hormone-sensitive prostate cancer [37, 38].

Novel Anti-Androgens

Beginning in 2019, new trial data emerged demonstrating the efficacy of a newer class of agents which had also been previously approved in metastatic castration-resistant prostate cancer: novel anti-androgens [18–20]. Novel anti-androgen agents work by targeting multiple sites on the androgen receptor to influence receptor signaling, with minimal to no agonist activity. They accomplish this by impairing DNA binding to the androgen receptor, reducing nuclear translocation of the AR, and decreasing recruitment of co-activators of the AR [39–41].

Two of these agents, apalutamide and enzalutamide, received approval in September and then December 2019, respectively. Each of these therapies is now listed as Category 1 recommendations in the National Comprehensive Cancer Network (NCCN) guidelines for mHSPC [38]. The data supporting their use in this space, as well as considerations regarding side effects, will be discussed individually below.

Apalutamide

Apalutamide is a NAA that was developed as an oral agent for treatment of advanced prostate cancer. As described above, it inhibits the androgen receptor through selective, competitive inhibition without agonist activity [40]. The TITAN trial evaluated the efficacy of apalutamide in mHSPC and was reported in 2019. The TITAN trial was a two-arm, double-blinded, randomized controlled phase III trial in which 1052 men were randomized to receive apalutamide plus ADT ($n = 525$) or ADT plus placebo ($n = 527$). Men were allowed to have received up to six cycles of prior chemotherapy with docetaxel (10.7% of patients), and 16.4% of patients had received prior localized therapy with prostatectomy or radiation, making this a significantly pretreated cohort. Furthermore, 62.7% of patients had high-volume disease as defined by CHAARTED criteria, while 37.3% had low-volume disease (LVD). Ultimately, receipt of apalutamide conferred a 33% lower risk of death over ADT and placebo, with overall survival of 82.4% in the apalutamide group compared to 73.5% in the placebo group at an interim follow-up of 24 months (HR for death 0.67, 95% CI 0.51–0.89, $p = 0.005$). In subgroup analysis, apalutamide demonstrated a consistent survival benefit in groups stratified by receipt of docetaxel, Gleason score, and volume of disease, indicating that apalutamide remained highly active in these men [42]. Apalutamide was overall well tolerated in this study, with no significant difference in the rate of Grade 3 or 4 adverse events between the experimental and placebo groups (42.2% versus 40.8%). Discontinuation occurred due to disease progression most frequently and occurred due to toxicity in on only 8% of patients in the apalutamide group compared to 5.2% in the placebo group. Furthermore, the most commonly observed serious (Grade 3 or >) adverse effect in the apalutamide group was rash, which was seen in 27.1% of patients versus 8.5% in the placebo group [42].

Enzalutamide

Like apalutamide, enzalutamide is another selective, competitive inhibitor of the androgen receptor with no agonist activity [39, 41]. The efficacy of enzalutamide at extending survival in mCRPC had previously been demonstrated [18]. Two trials, both of which were also published in 2019, examined enzalutamide in mHSPC and demonstrated an overall survival advantage [43, 44]. This ultimately has led to FDA approval for use in this indication in December of 2019.

The first notable study of enzalutamide in mHSPC was the ARCHES trial. This trial evaluated 1150 men with mHSPC with good performance status, histologically proven prostate cancer, and radiologic evidence of metastatic disease at the time of enrollment. Like the TITAN trial with apalutamide, men were allowed to enroll if they had received prior localized therapy or if they had received prior docetaxel. In this trial, 17% of men at baseline had received prior docetaxel (versus 10% in TITAN). Men were also allowed to participate if they had received prior ADT as long as they did not have evidence of castration resistance on enrollment labs. Patients were randomized in a 1:1 ratio to receive either enzalutamide 160 mg oral daily plus ADT or ADT plus placebo. Per CHAARTED criteria, 63% of men enrolled had high-volume disease. However, unlike other trials in this space, the primary endpoint was radiographic progression-free survival (rPFS), with imaging performed at screening and then quarterly thereafter during treatment until progression or death. Interim analysis was performed at a median follow-up of 14.4 months, and rPFS was improved in the group receiving enzalutamide over placebo, with a risk reduction of 66% (HR 0.39, 95% CI 0.30–0.50, $p < 0.001$). Importantly, the effect was maintained in subgroup analyses of men who had received prior chemotherapy with docetaxel and in low- and high-volume disease. Additionally, enzalutamide conferred a favorable advantage on secondary endpoints such as time to initiation of new therapies, PSA progression, and rate of undetectable PSA [43]. Overall survival data for this trial is still pending, but given the improvement in all of the aforementioned endpoints favoring enzalutamide, it is now recommended as a first-line option for men with mHSPC [38].

A second trial supporting the use of enzalutamide was also published in 2019, the ENZAMET trial. This was a multinational phase III randomized controlled trial which was published in the New England Journal of Medicine. The study enrolled 1125 men with mHSPC and, like ARCHES, allowed men to have received prior docetaxel and also utilized this as a factor for stratification. Patients who had received docetaxel made up 45% of the total cohort, making this a heavily pretreated group. Patients were randomized to receive either 160 mg of oral enzalutamide daily or a standard nonsteroidal anti-androgen such as bicalutamide, flutamide, or nilutamide in addition to either medical or surgical androgen deprivation therapy. Like similar trials in this space, men in the trial had to have histologically proven prostate cancer, radiographic evidence of metastatic disease, and good performance status. Men were also allowed to have received prior ADT, but it must have been discontinued for at least one year prior to trial enrollment. Unlike ARCHES, which utilized progression-free survival, this trial utilized overall survival as a primary endpoint. At a median follow-up of 34 months, overall survival was greater in the enzalutamide group compared to those receiving standard anti-androgen (HR 0.67, 95% CI 0.52–0.86, $p = 0.0002$). Overall survival estimated via Kaplan-Meier methods at 3 years was 80% in the enzalutamide group compared to 72% in the standard-care group. As in ARCHES, PSA progression-free survival was also improved in the enzalutamide group (HR 0.39, $p < 0.001$). Furthermore, clinical progression-free survival was also improved in the patients receiving enzalutamide (HR 0.40, $p < 0.001$) [44].

In both ARCHES and ENZAMET, toxicity from receipt of enzalutamide was significant, and the most concerning side effects were de novo neurologic effects [43, 44]. Seizures were observed at a significantly higher rate in the enzalutamide group (1% versus 0%) in the ENZAMET trial. Furthermore, receipt of prior docetaxel increased the likelihood of developing grade II or greater peripheral neuropathy (9% versus 0%) compared to patients with no prior docetaxel. Receipt of a longer duration of therapy was also a risk factor for adverse events [44]. Interestingly, in the ARCHES trial, grade III or greater adverse effects were observed in 24.3% of patients in the enzalutamide group compared to 25.6% in the ADT group, without a significantly higher rate of neurologic effects observed [43]. Nevertheless, given the seriousness of possible neurologic adverse events, patients should be thoroughly counseled and then monitored for development while on therapy. Receipt of prior docetaxel is a clinical factor that can identify patients who are at greater risk, particularly for development or progression of peripheral neuropathy (Table 5.1).

Table 5.1 Summary of evidence, dosing, and side effects of agents in metastatic hormone-sensitive prostate cancer

Agent (Trade name)	Level 1 evidence Supporting use	Source	Dosing	Side effects
Docetaxel (Taxotere)	GETUG-AFU15 (2013) CHAARTED (2015) STAMPEDE (2016)	Gravis et al. [25] Sweeney et al. [26] James et al. [27]	75 mg/m^2 every 3 weeks, for 6 cycles	Hair loss Nausea/vomiting Neutropenia Thrombocytopenia Neurotoxicity
Abiraterone acetate (Zytiga)	LATITUDE (2017) STAMPEDE (2017)	Fizazi et al. [31] James et al. [32]	1000 mg daily + prednisone 5 mg twice daily	Hypertension Peripheral edema Hypokalemia Diarrhea Urinary tract infection
Apalutamide (Erleada)	TITAN (2019)	Chi et al. [65]	240 mg daily	Fatigue Rash Diarrhea Nausea Arthralgia Weight loss Falls Interactions with medications due to CYP450 induction
Enzalutamide (Xtandi)	ARCHES (2019) ENZAMET (2019)	Armstrong et al. [43] Davis et al. [44]	160 mg daily	Seizures Fatigue Gynecomastia Diarrhea Hot flashes Headaches Interactions with medications due to CYP450 induction

Agents with No Proven Benefit in mHSPC

Through the intense examination of multiple mechanisms of action to treat metastatic prostate cancer, investigators have identified a number of agents that do not confer a benefit in overall survival. Two classes of agents, bisphosphonates and nonsteroidal anti-inflammatory drugs (NSAIDs), have been well studied, but do not increase survival in men with metastatic prostate cancer.

Bisphosphonates

Bisphosphonates are a class of drugs that, as their name implies, contain two phosphonate groups ($PO(OH)_2$) and are used to treat or prevent osteoporosis [45]. In metastatic prostate cancer, it was hypothesized that they would improve patient survival by preventing or postponing the occurrence of skeletal-related events (SREs) due to the effects of prostate cancer. However, a number of trials examining this hypothesis have been negative. First-generation bisphosphonates such as sodium clodronate were first examined in randomized trials in the early 2000s. In the MRC PR05 trial, 311 men with metastatic prostate cancer were randomized to receive sodium clodronate by mouth or an oral placebo. There is no statistical difference in the overall survival or bone progression-free survival at a median follow-up of 59 months [46]. Furthermore, the STAMPEDE trial utilized various combinations of zoledronic acid, a second-generation bisphosphonate with or without ADT or docetaxel. However, this trial demonstrated no evidence of an overall survival advantage with addition of zoledronic acid to docetaxel (HR 1.06, 95% CI 0.86–1.30, $p = 0.592$).

Focused examination of bisphosphonates in mHSPC was examined in two specific trials, the CALGB 90202 and the ZAPCA trials, neither of which demonstrated an advantage in overall survival [47, 48]. The CALGB 90202 trial was completed in 2014 and randomized men with mHSPC on ADT which had been initiated within the prior 6 months to receive either zoledronic acid at a dose of 4 mg IV every 4 weeks or a placebo. There was no benefit demonstrated in the primary endpoint, which was increased time to first SRE. There was also no improvement seen in bone-related PFS or overall survival in the group receiving zoledronic acid [47]. Similarly, the ZAPCA trial was reported in 2017 and randomized 227 men with mHSPC to receive ADT or ADT in addition to zoledronic acid. Again, no benefit was observed in overall survival, time to treatment failure, clinical progression, skeletal related events, death, or time to discontinuation of treatment with zoledronic acid added to standard therapy. One subgroup, men with a PSA < 200 at enrollment, had an increased time to reaching castration resistance with receipt of zoledronic acid, with time to treatment failure of 23.7 months compared to 9.8 months in the ADT only group (HR 0.58, 95% CI 0.35–0.93, $p = 0.023$).

Based upon the data of the three trials described above, current guidelines support the use of bisphosphonates for maintenance of bone health in men with metastatic prostate cancer, but no data has demonstrated an improvement in overall survival [38]. Nevertheless, bisphosphonates make up an important element of overall supportive management of men with metastatic prostate cancer.

Nonsteroidal Anti-Inflammatory Drugs (NSAIDs)

Like bisphosphonates, examination of cyclo-oxygenase-2 (COX-2) inhibitors such as celecoxib, a subclass of NSAIDS, has not yielded positive results in terms of improvement in survival. The proposed mechanism of action of NSAIDs in the metastatic prostate cancer space is drawn from pre-clinical and population-level studies that have demonstrated elevated levels of prostaglandins due to upregulation of COX-2 in prostate cancer and a lower incidence of prostate cancer in men with higher intake of NSAIDs [49–52]. To this end, the STAMPEDE trial had an early arm (Arm D) that investigated addition of the NSAID celecoxib 400 by mouth twice a day for 1 year or until disease progression. Celecoxib was utilized due to overall better tolerability than some other NSAIDs.

Comparative Efficacy and Sequencing of Agents in mHSPC

With the approval of four new agents with level 1 evidence supporting their use in the mHSPC space, the next challenge facing clinicians has been determining the ideal agent and sequencing of agents, including considerations regarding tailoring therapy to patient performance status, baseline disease burden, and location of metastases. To this end, several meta-analyses have been performed to examine comparative effects of each treatment, though no head-to-head trial of the four agents has been performed (Table 5.2).

The first such study published in 2018 utilized a comparative network meta-analysis to examine the outcomes of GETUG-AFU 15, the docetaxel and abiraterone arms of STAMPEDE, CHAARTED, and LATITUDE. This paper included 6067 patient outcomes from the 5 studies. This trial specifically investigated differences between abiraterone and docetaxel, and indirect comparison between ADT plus docetaxel and ADT plus abiraterone demonstrated no overall survival advantage between the two agents. However, analysis by Bayesian methods with surface

Table 5.2 Summary of meta-analyses comparing clinical and cost-efficacy of therapies in metastatic hormone-sensitive prostate cancer

Source	Year	Number of patients	Agents compared	Key findings
Wallis et al.	2018	6067	Abiraterone, docetaxel	No OS advantage between agents Bayesian analysis predicted with 89% probability that abiraterone is the preferential first-line agent
Sathianathen et al.	2019	8837	Docetaxel, abiraterone, apalutamide, enzalutamide, ADT alone	OS advantage of all 4 agents over ADT alone confirmed SUCRA analysis suggested enzalutamide is the ideal first-line agent
Sathianathen et al.	2019	N/a	Docetaxel, abiraterone	Docetaxel was far superior on cost-efficacy modeling
Marchioni et al.	2020	10,800	Docetaxel, abiraterone, apalutamide, enzalutamide, ADT alone	OS advantage of all 4 agents over ADT alone confirmed No OS advantage demonstrated when comparing docetaxel to anti-androgens Novel anti-androgens enzalutamide and apalutamide demonstrated the best overall safety profile

under the cumulative ranking (SUCRA) scoring suggested with 89% probability that abiraterone is the preferential first-line agent [53]. A 2019 meta-analysis by Sathianathen et al. examined outcomes of novel anti-androgens from the TITAN and ENZAMET studies in addition to the five trials listed above. Not surprisingly, they again demonstrated an overall survival advantage to all four agents approved in mHSPC over ADT alone but no statistically significant benefit of any one agent over the others. In contrast to the study by Wallis et al., this study suggested that enzalutamide may be the optimal agent, again by using SUCRA analysis [54]. This question remains unclear without direct comparisons. Finally, a 2020 meta-analysis by Marchioni et al. examined 13 total trials of novel anti-androgens, docetaxel chemotherapy, and abiraterone using an indirect comparison. The primary outcomes of interest in the meta-analysis were overall survival, progression-free survival, and rate of high-grade adverse events. From this analysis the authors determined that abiraterone, and the novel anti-androgens apalutamide and enzalutamide, though better tolerated with a better safety profile, demonstrated no benefit in overall survival when compared to docetaxel. However, there was a trend towards overall lower mortality with abiraterone, apalutamide, and enzalutamide compared to docetaxel and a statistically significant difference in PFS for the three former treatments. Overall adverse event rate was significantly lower for the novel anti-androgens compared to docetaxel or abiraterone [55]. Further comparisons of these agents, preferably some direct in design, will continue to emerge.

Regarding sequencing of agents for men with metastatic hormone-sensitive prostate cancer, very limited data exists at this time, and performance status and competing comorbidities often act as surrogate decision points influencing the initial and subsequent agents to use. Patients with better performance status are generally eligible for chemotherapy and all of the anti-androgens. Nevertheless, there remains no clear consensus regarding which agent to utilize, and the current NCCN guidelines make no indication of preference [38]. Patient preference may also play a role, as the oral agents that can be administered at home (abiraterone, enzalutamide, and apalutamide) may be preferable over intravenous infusion in a clinic setting. Cost remains a challenge for all of these agents, and patients receiving novel anti-androgens are at risk for financial toxicity due to the high monthly costs of treatment. Though these costs are extremely variable depending upon geographic location, in the United States, retail costs of each of these drugs can easily exceed $350 dollars per day, or more than $11,000 per month, for the lowest-cost regimens as of December 2020 [56]. Clearly, determining optimal drug sequencing has not only significant disease-oriented but also patient-oriented implications, particularly in regard to cost. It is also unclear in the United States and in other developed countries if transition to generic versions of drugs (such as abiraterone which went off patent in 2018) will effectively drive down costs. A comparative health economic cost-effectiveness analysis of docetaxel versus oral agents published in 2019 favored docetaxel by a great margin over abiraterone. This analysis estimated that the monthly cost of abiraterone would have to drop below $3100 per month to be cost-effective when compared to abiraterone [57]. However, the economics of each of these agents remains highly variable, making comparisons of cost-efficacy difficult across jurisdictions. Certainly, additional analysis to determine ideal sequencing is a large unmet need in mHSPC.

Localized Therapies: Surgery, Radiation to the Primary Tumor, and Metastasis-Directed Therapies in Oligometastatic HSPC

In addition to utilization of systemic agents in mHSPC, examination of localized therapies, either towards the primary tumor or metastasis-directed (MDT), has also been performed or is ongoing. There is an important paradigm to acknowledge: the concept of oligometastatic prostate cancer, which represents a previously occult disease state that is now detectable due to increased imaging sensitivity. This has raised several questions regarding benefit of therapy directed at this disease state. Is surgery or radiation directed at the primary site superior when compared to either observation or in some combination with systemic therapy? Is therapy directed at low-volume metastatic sites beneficial either alone or concomitantly with systemic therapy? A 2014 study performed by Culp and colleagues investigated the Surveillance, Epidemiology, and End Results (SEER) database for men diagnosed with metastatic prostate cancer (M1) between 2004 and 2010 who had either undergone treatment of their primary tumor with either radical prostatectomy (RP) or brachytherapy (BT) or received no localized treatment. The authors identified 8185 men who met these criteria, with 245 men having received RP, 129 received BT, and 7811 received no local therapy. Interestingly, receipt of local therapy was significantly associated with improved disease-specific survival (DSS) and overall survival compared to patients receiving no therapy. Overall and disease-specific survival were 67.4% and 75.8%, respectively, in men undergoing RP, compared to 52.6% (OS) and 61.3% (DSS) in men who received BT, and only 22.5% (OS) and 48.7% (DSS) in the men who received no locally directed therapy. Furthermore, receipt of RP or BT was also both associated with a statistically significant decrease in cancer-specific mortality, decreased local/pelvic symptoms, and complications related to disease progression [58].

These findings have generated significant interest in investigating the effect of local therapy in oligometastatic disease, and a high-quality randomized controlled trial, Southwest Oncology Group (SWOG) 1802, is now underway to help answer this question. This trial (NCT03678025) is a phase III randomized controlled trial examining standard systemic therapy (SST) to include ADT with or without the newer agents approved in mHSPC discussed above compared to SST plus definitive local therapy with either radical prostatectomy or external beam radiation therapy (EBRT) within 8 weeks of randomization. The primary outcome is overall survival, and secondary outcomes include rate of symptomatic local progression and progression-free survival. Other important outcomes include comparative quality of life and other patient-oriented outcomes between the groups. This trial was actively accruing at over 250 sites as of December 2020 [59].

Regarding the benefit of radiation therapy directed to the primary tumor in metastatic prostate cancer, in addition to the SEER analysis by Culp that demonstrated benefit with receipt of brachytherapy, two other trials have specifically examined this hypothesis. First, the STAMPEDE trial included a specific arm (Arm H) in its multi-arm, multi-stage design that examined the effect of ADT +/− docetaxel (standard therapy) versus standard therapy plus EBRT to the primary tumor. The authors hypothesized based upon retrospective data that addition of EBRT to standard systemic therapy would improve overall survival, which they utilized as the primary outcome. Important secondary outcomes included failure-free survival, progression-free survival, metastatic progression-free survival, prostate cancer-specific survival, and symptomatic local event-free survival. The results of this arm of the trial were reported in 2018. Overall, 2061 men were randomized to receive either systemic therapy ($n = 1029$) or systemic therapy plus EBRT ($n = 1032$). Importantly, median PSA was high at 97 ng/ml, and 89% of patients had osseous metastatic disease, with 54% having HVD per CHAARTED criteria and 40% having LVD. Overall survival in the group receiving EBRT was no better than in men receiving systemic therapy only (HR 0.92, 95% CI 0.80–1.06, $p = 0.266$). However, EBRT did improve failure-free survival (HR 0·76, 95% CI 0·68–0·84; $p < 0{\cdot}0001$), and subgroup analysis of men with LVD demonstrated improved overall survival (HR 0.68, 95% CI 0.52) [60]. These data underscore the importance of considering overall burden of disease in this evolving treatment paradigm, as oligometastatic disease and more disseminated disease likely behave differently.

Like STAMPEDE, the results of the HORRAD trial were also reported in 2018. This trial randomized men with newly diagnosed metastatic prostate cancer, PSA >20 ng/ml, and osseous metastases to receive ADT or ADT plus EBRT to the prostate. Overall, 432 men underwent randomization from 2004 to 2014, with no difference noted in overall survival between the control and experimental groups at a median survival of 47 months (HR 0.90, 95% CI 0.70–1.14, $p = 0.4$). The negative result of this trial as well as the limited benefit of EBRT in STAMPEDE in all but men with low-volume disease will perhaps be adjudicated by the pending results of SWOG 1802.

Two notable trials have investigated the potential benefit of metastasis-directed therapy with radiation in men with metastatic prostate cancer. The first study by Ost and colleagues was a small phase II trial with 62 patients with biochemical recurrence after prior treatment of primary prostate cancer. Men enrolled in the trial had to have low-volume metastatic disease, with three or fewer lesions, none of which could be cranial. These men were then randomized to receive either observation or MDT with stereotactic body radiation (SBRT). Each group was then surveilled for the presence of metastatic progression or development of new symptoms with serial imaging. The primary outcome was ADT-free survival, and the authors hypothesized that receipt of MDT would prolong time to initiation of ADT due to progression. At a median follow-up of 36 months, the MDT group had superior ADT-free survival at 21 months, compared to 13 months in the observation group (HR 0.60, 80% CI 0.40–0.90). Additionally, overall toxicity from radiation therapy was low compared to observation, and trial participants rated quality of life similarly [61].

This was the first randomized trial to demonstrate a benefit of MDT in prolonging onset of symptoms or development of metastatic progression.

In addition to this study, Palma and colleagues reported on the results of the SABR-COMET trial in 2019. This was an innovative trial across multiple metastatic cancers (i.e., prostate, breast, lung, gastrointestinal/colorectal) that examined the use of stereotactic ablative radiotherapy (SABR) to all metastatic sites. Enrollees in the prostate-cancer arm underwent either best available palliative care or best available palliative care plus SABR to all sites of metastatic disease. Participants were allowed to have up to five metastatic sites, so this trial had participants with both low- and high-volume disease per CHAARTED criteria. In total, 99 patients were enrolled 2:1 to receive either SABR or palliative treatments. The primary outcome was overall survival, which was significantly longer in the experimental group receiving SABR at 41 months compared to 28 months in the control (HR 0.57, 95% CI 0.30–1.10), at median follow-up of 25.5 months. This improvement did come at the cost of higher toxicity, with 29% of patients in the SABR group experiencing Grade 2 or higher adverse events, with pain (12%) being the most frequently reported side effect. There were no deaths related to treatment in the control group, but three patients in the group receiving SABR died of treatment-related complications [62]. Based upon these two small trials, use of MDT with radiation has been demonstrated to lengthen overall survival, increase time to progression, and increase the time to initiation of ADT (Table 5.1).

Emerging Therapies

In addition to trials examining sequencing, synergistic effects, and quality-of-life impact on currently approved therapies in mHSPC, there are also additional novel agents in the research pipeline. The most eminent results will come from the pending ARASENS trial evaluating darolutamide. Darolutamide (ODM-201) is an oral androgen receptor antagonist and has minimal to no agonist activity and high affinity for both the native androgen receptor and androgen receptor variants. Prior Phase 1 and 2 trials in mCRPC, including ARAMIS and ARAFOR, demonstrated good overall tolerability and anticancer activity with darolutamide. The results of the ARAMIS trial demonstrated an improvement in the primary endpoint, metastasis-free survival, of 40.4 months (95% CI: 34.3, not reached) in patients receiving darolutamide compared with 18.4 months in the control group. This has led to the FDA approval for use of darolutamide in non-metastatic castration-resistant prostate cancer (nmCRPC) [63]. The ARASENS trial will examine the addition of the novel agent darolutamide to ADT and docetaxel compared to ADT and docetaxel alone. Patients will receive six cycles of docetaxel following randomization. Patients in the experimental arm will receive oral darolutamide until either symptomatic progression, unacceptable toxicity, or therapeutic class change occurs. This phase III trial is seeking to enroll 1300 patients at 300 sites in 23 countries and began accruing in 2016. The primary endpoint is overall survival, and estimated study conclusion is May 2022 [64].

Conclusions

As recently as two decades ago, men with metastatic prostate cancer were limited to androgen deprivation therapy before almost uniformly developing castration-resistant prostate cancer and early demise. However, since that time numerous agents have been introduced in both castration-resistant and now hormone-sensitive prostate cancer that has led to prolonged overall survival. With addition of docetaxel, abiraterone acetate, apalutamide, and/or enzalutamide, men are now experiencing survival that can approach double or even triple the durations previously observed. Importantly, these agents also decrease symptoms from development of progressive metastatic disease. Clearly, continued study to elucidate the optimal sequencing of agents, as well as the inclusion of possible additional treatments such as radiation or surgery in oligometastatic disease, will be necessary to maximize survivability. Furthermore, consideration of cost-effectiveness, quality of life, and overall treatment toxicity is of critical importance for future investigation. Finally, improvements in imaging and laboratory testing will continue to transform detection of metastatic disease to allow early diagnosis and treatment, potentially extending survival further. Given the rapid progress observed in all of these domains, the landscape of treatment is wholly different today than only a few years ago, a welcome boon of innovation for patients suffering from this life-threatening disease.

Summary of Key Points

- Level 1 evidence supports use of four agents in addition to ADT in mHSPC.
  - Docetaxel.
  - Abiraterone acetate + prednisone.
  - Apalutamide.
  - Enzalutamide.
- Comparative analysis has not demonstrated an overall survival advantage of any of the above four agents over another, though no head-to-head trial data exists.
- Comparative analysis has suggested that docetaxel may be the most cost-effective treatment option, although novel anti-androgens such as apalutamide and enzalutamide may be overall better tolerated.
- Use of localized treatment to the primary tumor with radiation in addition to ADT did not extend overall survival in two trials (HORRAD and STAMPEDE).
- SWOG 1802 is currently examining the use of definitive surgery or radiation in addition to ADT and systemic therapy in men with oligometastatic hormone-sensitive prostate cancer.
- Use of metastasis-directed therapy is potentially promising, but larger, more robust trials are needed to recommend use.
- Additional novel oral androgen inhibitors such as darolutamide (ODM-201) are currently being investigated in large trials for use in mHSPC.

References

1. Torre LA, Bray F, Siegel RL, Ferlay J, Lortet-Tieulent J, Jemal A. Global cancer statistics, 2012. CA Cancer J Clin. 2015;65(2):87–108.
2. Siegel RL, Miller KD, Jemal A. Cancer statistics, 2020. CA Cancer J Clin. 2020;70(1):7–30.
3. Butler SS, Muralidhar V, Zhao SG, Sanford NN, Franco I, Fullerton ZH, et al. Prostate cancer incidence across stage, NCCN risk groups, and age before and after USPSTF Grade D recommendations against prostate-specific antigen screening in 2012. Cancer. 2020;126(4):717–24.
4. Kelly SP, Anderson WF, Rosenberg PS, Cook MB. Past, current, and future incidence rates and burden of metastatic prostate cancer in the United States. Eur Urol Focus. 2018;4(1):121–7.
5. Uemura H, Ye D, Kanesvaran R, Chiong E, Lojanapiwat B, Pu YS, et al. United in Fight against prOstate cancer (UFO) registry: first results from a large, multi-centre, prospective, longitudinal cohort study of advanced prostate cancer in Asia. BJU Int. 2020;125(4):541–52.
6. Huggins C, Hodges CV. Studies on prostatic cancer i. the effect of castration, of estrogen and of androgen injection on serum phosphatases in metastatic carcinoma of the prostate. Cancer Res. 1941;1(4):293–7.
7. Huggins C. The treatment of cancer of the prostate: the 1943 address in surgery before the Royal College of Physicians and Surgeons of Canada. Can Med Assoc J. 1944;50:301–7.
8. Teo MY, Rathkopf DE, Kantoff P. Treatment of advanced prostate cancer. Annu Rev Med. 2019;70(Figure 1):479–99.
9. Eisenberger MA, Blumenstein BA, Crawford ED, Miller G, McLeod DG, Loehrer PJ, et al. Bilateral orchiectomy with or without flutamide for metastatic prostate cancer. J Urol. 1999;339(15):1036–42.
10. Wu JN, Fish KM, Evans CP, Devere White RW, Dallera MA. No improvement noted in overall or cause-specific survival for men presenting with metastatic prostate cancer over a 20-year period. Cancer. 2014;120(6):818–23.
11. Tannock IF, Osoba D, Stockler MR, Ernst DS, Neville AJ, Moore MJ, et al. Chemotherapy with mitoxantrone plus prednisone or prednisone alone for symptomatic hormone-resistant prostate cancer: a Canadian randomized trial with palliative end points. J Clin Oncol. 1996;14(6):1756–64.
12. Kantoff PW, Halabi S, Conaway M, Picus J, Kirshner J, Hars V, et al. Hydrocortisone with or without mitoxantrone in men with hormone- refractory prostate cancer: results of the cancer and leukemia group B 9182 study. J Clin Oncol. 1999;17(8):2506–13.
13. Petrylak DP, Tangen CM, Hussain MHA, Lara PN, Jones JA, Taplin ME, et al. Docetaxel and estramustine compared with mitoxantrone and prednisone for advanced refractory prostate cancer. N Engl J Med. 2004;351(15):1513–20.
14. Tannock IF, de Wit R, Berry WR, Horti J, Pluzanska A, Chi KN, et al. Docetaxel plus prednisone or Mitoxantrone plus prednisone for advanced prostate cancer. N Engl J Med. 2004;351(15):1502–12.
15. De Bono JS, Oudard S, Ozguroglu M, Hansen S, MacHiels JP, Kocak I, et al. Prednisone plus cabazitaxel or mitoxantrone for metastatic castration-resistant prostate cancer progressing after docetaxel treatment: a randomised open-label trial. Lancet. 2010;376(9747):1147–54.
16. Kantoff PW, Higano CS, Shore ND, Berger ER, Small EJ, Penson DF, et al. Sipuleucel-T immunotherapy for castration-resistant prostate cancer. N Engl J Med. 2010;363(5):411–22.
17. Parker C, Nilsson S, Heinrich D, Helle SI, O'Sullivan JM, Fosså SD, et al. Alpha emitter Radium-223 and survival in metastatic prostate cancer. N Engl J Med. 2013;369(3):213–23.
18. Scher HI, Fizazi K, Saad F, Taplin M-E, Sternberg CN, Miller K, et al. Increased survival with enzalutamide in prostate cancer after chemotherapy. N Engl J Med. 2012;367(13):1187–97.
19. Beer TM, Armstrong AJ, Rathkopf DE, Loriot Y, Sternberg CN, Higano CS, et al. Enzalutamide in metastatic prostate cancer before chemotherapy. N Engl J Med. 2014;371(5):424–33.
20. Smith MR, Saad F, Chowdhury S, Oudard S, Hadaschik BA, Graff JN, et al. Apalutamide treatment and metastasis-free survival in prostate cancer. N Engl J Med. 2018;79(1):150–8.

21. Ryan CJ, Smith MR, Fizazi K, Saad F, Mulders PFA, Sternberg CN, et al. Abiraterone acetate plus prednisone versus placebo plus prednisone in chemotherapy-naive men with metastatic castration-resistant prostate cancer (COU-AA-302): final overall survival analysis of a randomised, double-blind, placebo-controlled phase 3 study. Lancet Oncol. 2015;16(2):152–60.
22. Ryan CJ, Smith MR, de Bono JS, Molina A, Logothetis CJ, de Souza P, et al. Abiraterone in metastatic prostate cancer without previous chemotherapy. N Engl J Med. 2013;368(2):138–48.
23. Wallis CJD, Klaasen Z. What is changing in advanced prostate cancer. Everyday Urol Oncol Insights. 2020;5(2). https://www.urotoday.com/journal/everyday-urology-oncology-insights/articles/122176-what-is-changing-inadvanced-prostate-cancer.html.
24. Rowinsky EK. The development and clinical utility of the taxane class of antimicrotubule chemotherapy agents. Annu Rev Med. 1997;48:353–74.
25. Gravis G, Fizazi K, Joly F, Oudard S, Priou F, Esterni B, et al. Androgen-deprivation therapy alone or with docetaxel in non-castrate metastatic prostate cancer (GETUG-AFU 15): a randomised, open-label, phase 3 trial. Lancet Oncol [Internet]. 2013;14(2):149–58. Available from: https://doi.org/10.1016/S1470-2045(12)70560-0
26. Sweeney CJ, Chen Y-H, Carducci M, Liu G, Jarrard DF, Eisenberger M, et al. Chemohormonal therapy in metastatic hormone-sensitive prostate cancer. N Engl J Med. 2015;373(8):737–46.
27. James ND, Sydes MR, Clarke NW, Mason MD, Dearnaley DP, Spears MR, et al. Addition of docetaxel, zoledronic acid, or both to first-line long-term hormone therapy in prostate cancer (STAMPEDE): survival results from an adaptive, multiarm, multistage, platform randomised controlled trial. Lancet. 2016;387(10024):1163–77.
28. Gravis G, Boher JM, Joly F, Soulié M, Albiges L, Priou F, et al. Androgen deprivation therapy (ADT) plus docetaxel versus ADT alone in metastatic non castrate prostate cancer: impact of metastatic burden and long-term survival analysis of the randomized phase 3 GETUG-AFU15 trial. Eur Urol. 2016;70(2):256–62.
29. Hall ME, Huelster HL, Luckenbaugh AN, Laviana AA, Keegan KA, Klaassen Z, et al. Metastatic hormone-sensitive prostate cancer: current perspective on the evolving therapeutic landscape. Onco Targets Ther. 2020;13:3571–81.
30. Tucci M, Bertaglia V, Vignani F, Buttigliero C, Fiori C, Porpiglia F, et al. Addition of docetaxel to androgen deprivation therapy for patients with hormone-sensitive metastatic prostate cancer: a systematic review and meta-analysis. Eur Urol [Internet]. 2016;69(4):563–73. Available from: https://doi.org/10.1016/j.eururo.2015.09.013
31. Fizazi K, Tran N, Fein L, Matsubara N, Rodriguez-Antolin A, Alekseev BY, et al. Abiraterone plus prednisone in metastatic, castration-sensitive prostate cancer. N Engl J Med. 2017;377(4):352–60.
32. James ND, de Bono JS, Spears MR, Clarke NW, Mason MD, Dearnaley DP, et al. Abiraterone for prostate cancer not previously treated with hormone therapy. N Engl J Med. 2017;377(4):338–51.
33. Ryan CJ, Smith MR, Fong L, Rosenberg JE, Kantoff P, Raynaud F, et al. Phase I clinical trial of the CYP17 inhibitor abiraterone acetate demonstrating clinical activity in patients with castration-resistant prostate cancer who received prior ketoconazole therapy. J Clin Oncol. 2010;28(9):1481–8.
34. Fizazi K, Scher HI, Molina A, Logothetis CJ, Chi KN, Jones RJ, et al. Abiraterone acetate for treatment of metastatic castration-resistant prostate cancer: final overall survival analysis of the COU-AA-301 randomised, double-blind, placebo-controlled phase 3 study. Lancet Oncol. 2012;13(10):983–92.
35. Rehman Y, Rosenberg JE. Abiraterone acetate: Oral androgen biosynthesis inhibitor for treatment of castration-resistant prostate cancer. Drug Des Devel Ther. 2012;6:13–8.
36. Klocker H, Culig Z, Hobisch A, Hittmair A, Bartsch G, Peterziel H, et al. Androgen receptor mutations in prostate cancer. Mol Biol Prostate Cancer. 2013:81–8.
37. Oh WK, Resnick M. AUA / ASTRO / SUO Guideline. 2020;(June):1–43.

38. Mohler JL, Antonarakis ES, Armstrong AJ, D'Amico AV, Davis BJ, Dorff T, et al. Prostate cancer, version 2.2019. JNCCN J Natl Compr Cancer Netw. 2019;17(5):479–505.
39. Liu B, Su L, Geng J, Liu J, Zhao G. Developments in nonsteroidal antiandrogens targeting the androgen receptor. ChemMedChem. 2010;5(10):1651–61.
40. Clegg NJ, Wongvipat J, Joseph JD, Tran C, Ouk S, Dilhas A, et al. ARN-509: a novel antiandrogen for prostate cancer treatment. Cancer Res. 2012;72(6):1494–503.
41. Scher HI, Anand A, Rathkopf D, Shelkey J, Morris MJ, Danila DC, et al. Antitumour activity of MDV3100 in castration-resistant prostate cancer: a phase 1-2 study. Lancet [Internet]. 2010;375(9724):1437–46. Available from: https://doi.org/10.1016/S0140-6736(10)60172-9
42. Chi KN, Agarwal N, Bjartell A, Chung BH, Gomes AJPDS, Given R, et al. TITAN trial (apalutamide). N Engl J Med. 2019;381(1):13–24.
43. Armstrong AJ, Szmulewitz RZ, Petrylak DP, Holzbeierlein J, Villers A, Azad A, et al. Arches: a randomized, phase III study of androgen deprivation therapy with enzalutamide or placebo in men with metastatic hormone-sensitive prostate cancer. J Clin Oncol. 2019;37(32):2974–86.
44. Davis ID, Martin AJ, Stockler MR, Begbie S, Chi KN, Chowdhury S, et al. Enzalutamide with standard first-line therapy in metastatic prostate cancer. N Engl J Med. 2019;381(2):121–31.
45. Weinstein RS, Roberson PK, Manolagas SC. Giant osteoclast formation and long-term oral bisphosphonate therapy. N Engl J Med. 2009;360(1):53–62.
46. Dearnaley DP, Sydes MR, Mason MD, Stott M, Powell CS, Robinson ACR, et al. A double-blind, placebo-controlled, randomized trial of oral sodium clodronate for metastatic prostate cancer (MRC PR05 trial). J Natl Cancer Inst. 2003;95(17):1300–11.
47. Smith MR, Halabi S, Ryan CJ, Hussain A, Vogelzang N, Stadler W, et al. Randomized controlled trial of early zoledronic acid in men with castration-sensitive prostate cancer and bone metastases: results of CALGB 90202 (Alliance). J Clin Oncol. 2014;32(11):1143–50.
48. Kamba T, Kamoto T, Maruo S, Kikuchi T, Shimizu Y, Namiki S, et al. A phase III multicenter, randomized, controlled study of combined androgen blockade with versus without zoledronic acid in prostate cancer patients with metastatic bone disease: results of the ZAPCA trial. Int J Clin Oncol. 2017;22(1):166–73.
49. Taketo MM. Cyclooxygenase-2 inhibitors in tumorigenesis (part I). J Natl Cancer Inst. 1998;90(20):1529–36.
50. Mahmud S, Franco E, Aprikian A. Prostate cancer and use of nonsteroidal anti-inflammatory drugs: systematic review and meta-analysis. Br J Cancer. 2004;90(1):93–9.
51. Roberts RO, Jacobson DJ, Girman CJ, Rhodes T, Lieber MM, Jacobsen SJ. A population-based study of daily nonsteroidal anti-inflammatory drug use and prostate cancer. Mayo Clin Proc. 2002;77(3):219–25.
52. Basler JW, Piazza GA. Nonsteroidal anti-inflammatory drugs and cyclooxygenase-2 selective inhibitors for prostate cancer chemoprevention. J Urol. 2004;171(2 Pt 2):S59–62.
53. Wallis CJD, Klaassen Z, Bhindi B, Goldberg H, Chandrasekar T, Farrell AM, et al. Comparison of Abiraterone acetate and docetaxel with androgen deprivation therapy in high-risk and metastatic hormone-naïve prostate cancer: a systematic review and network meta-analysis. Eur Urol. 2018;73(6):834–44.
54. Sathianathen NJ, Koschel S, Thangasamy IA, Teh J, Alghazo O, Butcher G, et al. Indirect comparisons of efficacy between combination approaches in metastatic hormone-sensitive prostate cancer: a systematic review and network meta-analysis. Eur Urol. 2020;77(3):365–72.
55. Marchioni M, Di Nicola M, Primiceri G, Novara G, Castellan P, Paul AK, et al. New antiandrogen compounds compared to docetaxel for metastatic hormone sensitive prostate cancer: results from a network meta-analysis. J Urol. 2020;203(4):751–9.
56. Drugs.com. Drugs.com | Prescription Drug Information, Interactions & Side Effects. 2020.
57. Sathianathen NJ, Alarid-Escudero F, Kuntz KM, Lawrentschuk N, Bolton DM, Murphy DG, et al. A cost-effectiveness analysis of systemic therapy for metastatic hormone-sensitive prostate cancer. Eur Urol Oncol. 2019;2(6):649–55.

58. Culp SH, Schellhammer PF, Williams MB. Might men diagnosed with metastatic prostate cancer benefit from definitive treatment of the primary tumor? A SEER-based study. Eur Urol. 2014;65(6):1058–66.
59. Standard systemic therapy with or without definitive treatment in treating participants with metastatic prostate cancer. [Internet]. Available from: https://clinicaltrials.gov/show/NCT03678025.
60. Parker CC, James ND, Brawley CD, Clarke NW, Hoyle AP, Ali A, et al. Radiotherapy to the primary tumour for newly diagnosed, metastatic prostate cancer (STAMPEDE): a randomised controlled phase 3 trial. Lancet. 2018;392(10162):2353–366.
61. Ost P, Reynders D, Decaestecker K, Fonteyne V, Lumen N, DeBruycker A, et al. Surveillance or metastasis-directed therapy for oligometastatic prostate cancer recurrence: a prospective, randomized, multicenter phase II trial. J Clin Oncol. 2018;36(5):446–53.
62. Palma DA, Olson R, Harrow S, Gaede S, Louie AV, Haasbeek C, et al. Stereotactic ablative radiotherapy versus standard of care palliative treatment in patients with oligometastatic cancers (SABR-COMET): a randomised, phase 2, open-label trial. Lancet. 2019;393(10185):2051–8.
63. Shore ND, Tammela TL, Massard C, Bono P, Aspegren J, Mustonen M, et al. Safety and antitumour activity of ODM-201 (BAY-1841788) in chemotherapy-naïve and CYP17 inhibitor-naïve patients: follow-up from the ARADES and ARAFOR trials. Eur Urol Focus. 2018;4(4):547–53.
64. ODM-201 in addition to standard ADT and docetaxel in metastatic castration sensitive prostate cancer. [Internet]. Available from: https://clinicaltrials.gov/show/NCT02799602.
65. Chi KN, Agarwal N, Bjartell A, Chung BH, Pereira de Santana Gomes AJ, Given R, et al. Re: Apalutamide for metastatic, castration-sensitive prostate cancer. J Urol. 2019;202(4):661.
66. Sharifi N. Androgen deprivation therapy. In: Figg W, Chau C, Small E, editors. Drug management of prostate cancer. New York: Springer; 2010.

Chapter 6
Expanding Options for M0 Castration-Resistant Prostate Cancer (CRPC)

Daniel C. Parker and Michael S. Cookson

Abbreviations

ADT	Androgen deprivation therapy
AR	Androgen receptor
CRPC	Castration-resistant prostate cancer
FDA	Food and Drug Administration
ICECaP	Intermediate Clinical Endpoints in Cancer of the Prostate
MFS	Metastasis-free survival
PET	Positron emission tomography
PSA	Prostate-specific antigen

Introduction

Prostate cancer is the most common non-skin cancer affecting men in the United States [1]. Of the approximately 248,000 new cases of prostate cancer estimated to be diagnosed in 2021, 7% will be diagnosed as late or distant stage [2, 3]. Additionally, as many as 25% of men initially diagnosed and treated for localized disease will unfortunately relapse and develop advanced prostate cancer [4].

D. C. Parker
Department of Urology, University of Oklahoma Health Sciences Center & The Stephenson Cancer Center, Oklahoma City, OK, USA

M. S. Cookson (✉)
Department of Urology and Stephenson Oklahoma Cancer Center at the University of Oklahoma Health Sciences Center, Oklahoma City, OK, USA

Department of Urology, University of Oklahoma Health Sciences Center & The Stephenson Cancer Center, Oklahoma City, OK, USA
e-mail: michael-cookson@ouhsc.edu

K. L. Stratton, A. K. Morgans (eds.), *Urologic Oncology*,
https://doi.org/10.1007/978-3-030-89891-5_6

Advanced prostate cancer is a heterogeneous disease state, and numerous sub-stratifications have been developed to assign patients into the correct therapeutic pathways. These include non-metastatic biochemical recurrence, metastatic castration-sensitive prostate cancer, metastatic castration-resistant prostate cancer, and non-metastatic castration-resistant prostate cancer [5]. Encountering patients in the advanced prostate cancer space is becoming more common. Recently, compiled data from 2003 to 2017 by the Centers for Disease Control and Prevention demonstrated a significantly increased incidence of distant prostate cancer with an average annual percentage change of +2.2% [2]. Conversely, the compiled incidence of localized prostate cancer dropped by an annual percentage change of −3.3%. These data suggest that a stage migration toward more advanced prostate cancer may be in progress.

It is therefore more important now than it has been previously for providers to understand how to properly identify, stage, and treat patients with advanced prostate cancer. This chapter focuses primarily on the non-metastatic castration-resistant prostate cancer space (M0 CRCP). Definitions vary slightly by guideline organization [5, 6], but patients with M0 CRPC are those with a rising prostate-specific antigen (PSA) while continuously exposed to castration levels of androgen deprivation therapy (ADT), but in whom no radiographic evidence of metastatic disease can be identified. A nuance of this criteria that is important to note is that the absence of metastatic disease in M0 CRPC is based on the findings of *conventional* imaging: computed tomography, magnetic resonance imaging, or nuclear medicine bone scan. New positron emission tomography (PET) technologies, both already approved by the Food and Drug Administration (FDA) and in development, are more sensitive in identifying the presence of metastatic disease at ever decreasing volumes [7, 8]. These imaging modalities may have an impact on whether any patients with advanced prostate cancer in the future cannot have the site of their metastatic disease identified. However, the studies leading to FDA approval for agents in the M0 space did not include novel PET imaging, and therefore the results of conventional imaging studies are all that is necessary to categorize the presence or absence of metastasis in prostate cancer [5].

Prior to 2018, the only available strategies to treat patients with M0 CRPC were (1) observation, (2) addition of first-generation anti-androgen agents in order to achieve more potent androgen receptor (AR) blockade, or (3) enrollment in a clinical trial. The addition of AR antagonists in this setting did not provide a durable survival impact [9, 10], and so a new generation of agents aimed at slowing the progression of M0 CRPC to identifiable metastatic disease have been sought. Between 2018 and 2020, three novel therapies passed through phase 3 trial and approval by the FDA: *enzalutamide, apalutamide,* and *darolutamide* (Table 6.1). The success of these therapies was not just profound for patients with M0 CRPC and their providers, but it was also significant for the coordination and design elements investigators imposed which led to rapid publication of novel clinical endpoints and easier comparative analysis between agents.

This chapter will explore each of these agents in detail, the randomized trials which lead to their approval, their comparative efficacy, and side effect profiles, and

Table 6.1 Summary of survival and adverse event outcomes for three anti-androgen agents approved for M0CRPC

	Metastasis-free survival vs. placebo)		Overall survival (vs. placebo)		Discontinued treatment due to AE (%)	No. AEs in > 15% of participants	Deaths attributed to AE (%)	AEs in > 15% of participants
	HR	Months advantage	HR	Months advantage				
Enzalutamide	0.29	22	0.73	11	17	5	5	Fracture, falls, fatigue, musculoskeletal, hypertension
Apalutamide	0.28	24	0.78	14	15	9	3	Hot flashes, fatigue, back pain, diarrhea, weight loss, fall, arthralgia, nausea
Darolutamide	0.41	22	0.69	18	9	0	4	None

provide the reader with a real-world clinical practice guide for how to manage patients with M0 CRPC.

Metastasis-Free Survival (MFS) and Advanced Prostate Cancer Research

An important trend in research of advanced prostate cancer that emerged as a result of the trial designs for the agents discussed below is the use of metastasis-free survival (MFS) as a primary endpoint surrogate for overall survival. Prior to 2018, no network of clinical trials for advanced prostate cancer had been designed to conform to this primary endpoint. Reliance on overall survival as the gold standard of endpoints in prostate cancer, as well as all slowly progressing cancers, leads to long delays between trial completion and publication of the results [11]. Intermediate surrogates for overall survival that measure endpoints with shorter time-to-event intervals have been sought in other diseases with the hopes of speeding up approval for novel therapies [12]. A 2017 landmark study, published in the *Journal of Clinical Oncology* by the Intermediate Clinical Endpoints in Cancer of the Prostate (ICECaP) Working Group, confirmed the appropriateness of MFS as one of these intermediate endpoint surrogates in prostate cancer [13]. In the study, patient-level data was gathered from 28 available randomized clinical trials. Over 12,000 patients were determined to have sufficient data from 19 trials for analyzing the correlation between MFS and overall survival. A Kendall's t correlation of 0.91 was calculated from this individual patient data for MFS, demonstrating a strong correlation. Among the eligible clinical trials, a similar R^2 coefficient was obtained testing the correlation between 8-year overall survival rates with 5-year MFS. The R^2 was 0.83 for MFS, confirming the results of the individual patient data. This explains why, in the trials discussed below, FDA approval was granted based on the preliminary analysis of data that utilized MFS as the primary endpoint and why subsequent publications reported mature overall survival data long after these agents were available to the public.

Therapeutic Options in M0 CRPC

Enzalutamide

Enzalutamide has been approved for use in multiple advanced prostate cancer disease state spaces. Its ability to competitively inhibit not just the AR itself but also downstream AR translocation into the nucleus and interaction with DNA likely explains its ability to slow the progression of prostate cancer and induce cancer cell death at multiple stages of the disease [14]. The experience of medical and urologic oncologists with this agent was first developed in 2012 when results of the AFFIRM study led to its approval for treatment of patients with *metastatic* CRPC following docetaxel exposure [15]. From there, investigators have continued to experiment with enzalutamide at earlier timepoints in the natural history of advanced prostate cancer. In 2014, publication of the PREVAIL study demonstrated improved progression-free survival and delayed time to chemotherapy for metastatic CRPC patients exposed to enzalutamide *before* docetaxel [16]. In 2019, it was brought forth into the metastatic hormone-*sensitive* space following publication of the ENZAMET trial [17]. And at nearly the same time, the success of the 2018 PROSPER trial leads to enzalutamide receiving its first approval for use in non-metastatic prostate cancer [18].

PROSPER was an internationally conducted, placebo-controlled, randomized trial that studied the effects of enzalutamide on MFS in patients with M0 CRPC. Secondary endpoints such as PSA response, time-to-biochemical progression, overall survival, and safety were also measured. All patients in the study had a PSA doubling time of less than 10 months at the time of enrollment. Prior to randomization, patients were stratified by PSA doubling time (greater than or less than 6 months) and by prior exposure to bone mineralization agents such as denosumab or zoledronic acid. In PROSPER, 77% of patients in both the treatment and placebo arms were enrolled with a rapid doubling time of less than 6 months, while only the minority in each group received prior bone-targeting therapy. Patients were then randomized in 2:1 fashion to receive either 160 mg per day of enzalutamide or placebo. In both cases, patients continued to receive ADT during the trial. The study met its recruitment objective for 90% power to detect a hazard ratio of 0.72 or greater, and in total 1401 patients were enrolled (enzalutamide $n = 933$; placebo $n = 468$).

In 2018, the initial results of the PROSPER trial were released including data from the primary endpoint and all secondary endpoints except mature overall survival outcomes [18]. The enzalutamide cohort experienced more than twice the duration of MFS versus placebo (36.6 months vs. 14.7 months), corresponding to a 71% improvement in the risk of metastasis or death during the study period. In absolute terms, at the time of the initial analysis, nearly half of the placebo group had died versus only 23% of the enzalutamide group. Both secondary endpoints of time-to-PSA progression and time to initiation of a subsequent therapeutic alternative were markedly longer in the enzalutamide group. In 2020, mature overall survival results were reported. The enzalutamide group's median overall survival was 67 months versus 56.3 months in the placebo group, corresponding to a 27% improvement in the risk of death during the study period [19].

Apalutamide

Apalutamide is another example of a second-generation nonsteroidal anti-androgen agent that inhibits multiple steps in the AR signaling pathway and has found expanding indications for its use in advanced prostate cancer. Apalutamide is unique in the strength of its adherence to the AR ligand-binding domain, inhibiting transport of the AR signaling complex into the nucleus, blocking DNA binding of the AR, and preventing downstream activation of AR-mediated transcription [20]. In the phase 3 SPARTAN trial published in 2018, investigators randomized 1207 participants with M0 CRPC in 2:1 fashion to receive ADT plus 240 mg per day of apalutamide versus ADT plus placebo [21]. A total of 806 patients ultimately were assigned to receive apalutamide. In similar design to PROSPER, all patients in SPARTAN exhibited PSA doubling times of less than 10 months at the time of enrollment. Once again, MFS was the primary endpoint of the study. At the time of release of the initial results in 2018, apalutamide demonstrated a 72% improvement in the risk of metastasis, with a MFS interval of 40.5 months for the apalutamide group and only 16.2 months for the placebo group. Secondary endpoints of time to metastasis, symptomatic progression-free survival, and radiographic progression-free survival were all significantly improved with the addition of apalutamide. An update to the SPARTAN trial with mature overall survival results was released in 2020, and the addition of apalutamide in M0 CRPC resulted in a 22% improvement in the risk of death, corresponding to 14 months of improved survival versus placebo [22]. Time-to-subsequent chemotherapy with the addition of apalutamide was also markedly improved by 37%. Following the release of these data, which led to apalutamide's first FDA approval for advanced prostate cancer, the agent was subsequently approved for use in metastatic castration-*sensitive* prostate cancer upon release of data from TITAN trial investigators [23].

Darolutamide

Darolutamide is the most recent novel anti-androgen agent to be approved for use in M0 CRPC [24]. Its mechanism of action is similar to that of apalutamide and enzalutamide in terms of its ability to inhibit AR binding, translocation, and AR-activated transcription [25]. However, its unique chemical structure reduces the ability of darolutamide to cross the blood-brain barrier, an effect which may have implications on tolerability and adverse event rate [24]. The phase 3 ARAMIS trial [26] was similarly designed to PROSPER and SPARTAN and examined similar primary as well as secondary endpoints. All patients met M0 CRPC criteria by conventional imaging standards, had a PSA doubling time less than 10 months, were randomized in 2:1 fashion versus placebo, and continued ADT during the trial. Patients in the darolutamide arm received 600 mg by mouth twice daily. The total number of patients included in the study was 1509 (955 in the darolutamide arm versus 554 in the placebo arm). At the planned initial analysis, patients in the darolutamide group received a 22-month MFS advantage over placebo. Secondary endpoints, such as time-to-first symptomatic event, time-to-subsequent chemotherapy, radiographic progression-free survival, and PSA progression-free survival, were all significantly improved with the addition of darolutamide. When mature overall survival data was eventually released, patients taking darolutamide experienced a 31%

decrease in the risk of death while on treatment, corresponding to 6% more patients being alive at 3 years with darolutamide [27].

Agents Under Investigation

A single clinical trial examining the effects of a novel agent in the M0 CRPC space is currently recruiting. NCT03569280 is a phase 1 trial examining the effects of KPG-121 in addition to abiraterone, apalutamide, or enzalutamide in patients with metastatic and non-metastatic CRPC. Target enrollment is 36 patients. KPG-121 is a pharmaceutical agent similar in structure to lenalidomide, which itself is an immunomodulator with known efficacy in multiple myeloma, mantle cell lymphoma, and amyloidosis. KPG-121, compared to lenalidomide, appears to have enhanced effects on tumor proliferation and angiogenesis due to its higher affinity for binding at its target CRBN gene. In vitro and in vivo studies have suggested a synergistic effect of KPG-121 with concurrent anti-androgen therapy or total androgen annihilation [28].

M0 CRPC and Meta-data

While no head-to-head comparative analysis has been performed testing enzalutamide, apalutamide, or darolutamide against each other in randomized fashion, the trial design similarities between PROSPER, SPARTAN, and ARAMIS have given researchers a high-quality path to meta-analysis. Investigators at the University of Florida performed a systematic review and meta-analysis of these three trials' oncologic and adverse event outcomes [29]. In totality, the addition of any agent versus placebo improved MFS by 68%. Apalutamide (HR 0.73) and enzalutamide (HR 0.71) seemed to have superior MFS rates compared with darolutamide, but there was no significant difference when apalutamide and enzalutamide were compared against each other (HR 1.03). The preliminary overall survival results from the three trials were compared against each other prior to release of the mature results. The addition of any agent improved overall survival by 36%. There was no significant overall survival difference between any of the three agents upon indirect comparison. To date, this meta-analysis has not been updated since the release of the PROSPER, SPARTAN, and ARAMIS mature overall survival data.

A second meta-analysis performed by a multinational investigatory team demonstrated similar findings [30]. Using the same three preliminary trial results, the MFS improvement for use of any second-generation anti-androgen agent was 42%. Concordant with findings from the University of Florida, darolutamide had inferior MFS compared with apalutamide and enzalutamide in this study. The highest *P* score, assigned to the agent most likely to have the maximal MFS benefit, went to apalutamide (*P* score, 0.8809), while enzalutamide came in a close second (*P* score, 0.7852).

Adverse Events and Side Effects in M0 CRPC Treatment

With the three agents currently approved for M0 CRPC having similar efficacy at prolonging time to metastasis, radiographic progression, PSA progression, and overall survival, the next question naturally raised has become how to select the most appropriate agent for patients who are candidates for any one of the three. Again, we currently lack randomized head-to-head comparative studies to guide us, and one approach has been to select the treatment based on the adverse effect profiles gleaned from each of the phase 3 trials. This, however, should be interpreted with caution as it lacks the rigor and standardization of a true comparative analysis.

A surrogate for adverse event severity measured across PROPSER, SPARTAN, and ARAMIS were the treatment discontinuation rates due to adverse events. For enzalutamide, 17% (n = 158) of patients in the intervention arm discontinued therapy citing an adverse event as the primary reason. A total of 51 patients (5% of the enzalutamide cohort) were determined to have died due to an adverse event [19]. This compares with apalutamide, which saw 15% (n = 120) treatment discontinuation due to adverse events. Fewer patients in the SPARTAN trial died due to an adverse event on apalutamide (3.0%, n = 24) [22]. Darolutamide appears to carry the lowest rate of treatment discontinuation due to an adverse event, with an overall attrition rate of 8.9% [27].

Since adverse events are a relatively rare cause for patients to be unsuccessful with treatment, another strategy is to compare the common side effect profiles of each agent against the patient's comorbidities and choose the option of best fit [31]. Of the three agents, darolutamide appears to be the best tolerated. In the final report of the ARAMIS trial, no recorded adverse event was exhibited in greater than 15% of enrolled patients, and only fatigue crossed the 10% threshold. Rates of coronary artery disorder and heart failure were all under 5%, and only 7.3% of patients developed a cardiac arrhythmia. Possibly due to its low propensity for crossing the blood-brain barrier, seizures and mental impairment were extremely rare events for patients randomized to darolutamide (0.2%, 2.0%, respectively) [27]. This compares to the intervention arm in SPARTAN in which fatigue, falls, hypertension, and diarrhea all had adverse event rates >20% [22]. Fractures, falls, and hypertension were the most serious common adverse events encountered with enzalutamide in the PROSPSER trial (all 18%) [19].

It should be noted that as of this writing, several clinical trials examining the effects of currently approved therapies on toxicity are open for enrollment. APA-CARDIO1 (NCT04567875) is an observational study seeking to examine the effects of apalutamide on hypertension and cardiovascular disease. The ARACOG trial (NCT04335682) will examine the cognitive and quality of life effects of treatment with darolutamide and enzalutamide in patients with M0 CRPC. Finally, the DAROL study (NCT04122976) follows patients with M0 CRPC who have been selected for treatment with darolutamide and will follow them prospectively for real-world safety and efficacy outcomes.

Managing M0 CRPC in Clinical Practice

Treatment of patients with M0 CRPC disease continues to evolve. Recognizing that the disease space exists because of our current technological limitations in radiographic staging, future recommendations will have to reconcile efficacy and outcomes in the setting of micro-metastatic disease. The ability to detect small volume metastatic disease continues to improve with advances in position emission technology. Currently, we advocate for treatment of M0 CRPC in patients with a PSA doubling time of 10 months or less. Among those patients with slow PSA doubling times, we recommend observation and periodic restaging and PSA monitoring. We do not add first-generation AR antagonists in these scenarios. The decision to treat and choice of agent in the M0 CRPC space must also take into account patient-specific factors given the limitations of comparative data. For example, if the patient has a history of stroke, dementia, or another intracranial comorbidity, darolutamide may be the most appropriate choice. In addition, if the patient has a history of rash, psoriasis, or another integumentary disorder, enzalutamide or darolutamide might be preferred. Enzalutamide should probably be avoided in patients with a history of osteoporosis, osteopenia, or falls. Risk for cardiovascular related toxicity needs to be diligently assessed regardless of therapy on an ongoing basis [32]. In agreement with the Advanced Prostate Cancer Guidelines from the American Urological Association, ADT is continued during treatment with enzalutamide, apalutamide, or darolutamide [5]. Patients are restaged with serum PSA and total testosterone levels every 3 to 6 months and with conventional imaging every 6 to 12 months. Finally, frequent involvement of our multidisciplinary care team consisting of colleagues from medical and radiation oncology and clinical research support staff is paramount to ensuring these complex patients receive evidence-based and guideline concordant care while having access to the latest clinical trials.

References

1. Siegel RL, Miller KD, Jemal A. Cancer statistics, 2020. CA Cancer J Clin. 2020;70(1):7–30.
2. Siegel DA, O'Neil ME, Richards TB, Dowling NF, Weir HK. Prostate cancer incidence and survival, by stage and race/ethnicity – United States, 2001–2017. MMWR Morb Mortal Wkly Rep. 2020;69(41):1473–80.
3. Farhad, Islami Elizabeth M, Ward Hyuna, Sung Kathleen A, Cronin Florence K L, Tangka Recinda L, Sherman Jingxuan, Zhao Robert N, Anderson S Jane, Henley K Robin, Yabroff Ahmedin, Jemal Vicki B, Benard, 2021. Annual Report to the Nation on the Status of Cancer

Part 1: National Cancer Statistics. JNCI: Journal of the National Cancer Institute. https://doi.org/10.1093/jnci/djab131.
4. Smith MR, Kabbinavar F, Saad F, Hussain A, Gittelman MC, Bilhartz DL, et al. Natural history of rising serum prostate-specific antigen in men with castrate nonmetastatic prostate cancer. J Clin Oncol. 2005;23(13):2918–25.
5. Lowrance W, Breau R, Chou R. www DJAH, 2020. Advanced prostate cancer: AUA/ASTRO/SUO guideline. Auanetorg.
6. Cornford P, Bellmunt J, Bolla M, Briers E, De Santis M, Gross T, et al. EAU-ESTRO-SIOG guidelines on prostate cancer. Part II: treatment of relapsing, metastatic, and castration-resistant prostate cancer. Eur Urol. 2017;71(4):630–42.
7. Giovacchini G, Incerti E, Mapelli P, Kirienko M, Briganti A, Gandaglia G, et al. [^{11}C]Choline PET/CT predicts survival in hormone-naive prostate cancer patients with biochemical failure after radical prostatectomy. Eur J Nucl Med Mol Imaging. 2015;42(6):877–84.
8. Calais J, Fendler WP, Eiber M, Gartmann J, Chu F-I, Nickols NG, et al. Impact of 68Ga-PSMA-11 PET/CT on the Management of Prostate Cancer Patients with biochemical recurrence. J Nucl Med. 2018;59(3):434–41.
9. Lodde M, Lacombe L, Fradet Y. Salvage therapy with bicalutamide 150 mg in nonmetastatic castration-resistant prostate cancer. Urology. 2010;76(5):1189–93.
10. Suzuki H, Okihara K, Miyake H, Fujisawa M, Miyoshi S, Matsumoto T, et al. Alternative nonsteroidal antiandrogen therapy for advanced prostate cancer that relapsed after initial maximum androgen blockade. J Urol. 2008;180(3):921–7.
11. ICECaP Working Group, Sweeney C, Nakabayashi M, Regan M, Xie W, Hayes J, et al. The development of intermediate clinical endpoints in cancer of the prostate (ICECaP). J Natl Cancer Inst. 2015;107(12):djv261.
12. Sargent DJ, Wieand HS, Haller DG, Gray R, Benedetti JK, Buyse M, et al. Disease-free survival versus overall survival as a primary end point for adjuvant colon cancer studies: individual patient data from 20,898 patients on 18 randomized trials. J Clin Oncol. 2005;23(34):8664–70.
13. Xie W, Regan MM, Buyse M, Halabi S, Kantoff PW, Sartor O, et al. Metastasis-free survival is a strong surrogate of overall survival in localized prostate cancer. J Clin Oncol. 2017;35(27):3097–104.
14. Tran C, Ouk S, Clegg NJ, Chen Y, Watson PA, Arora V, et al. Development of a second-generation antiandrogen for treatment of advanced prostate cancer. Science. 2009;324(5928):787–90.
15. Scher HI, Fizazi K, Saad F, Taplin M-E, Sternberg CN, Miller K, et al. Increased survival with enzalutamide in prostate cancer after chemotherapy. Cabot RC, Harris NL, Rosenberg ES, Shepard J-AO, Cort AM, Ebeling SH, et al., editors. N Engl J Med. 2012;367(13):1187–97.
16. Beer TM, Armstrong AJ, Rathkopf DE, Loriot Y, Sternberg CN, Higano CS, et al. Enzalutamide in metastatic prostate cancer before chemotherapy. N Engl J Med. 2014;371(5):424–33.
17. Davis ID, Martin AJ, Stockler MR, Begbie S, Chi KN, Chowdhury S, et al. Enzalutamide with standard first-line therapy in metastatic prostate cancer. N Engl J Med. 2019;381(2):121–31.
18. Hussain M, Fizazi K, Saad F, Rathenborg P, Shore N, Ferreira U, et al. Enzalutamide in men with nonmetastatic, castration-resistant prostate cancer. N Engl J Med. 2018;378(26):2465–74.
19. Sternberg CN, Fizazi K, Saad F, Shore ND, De Giorgi U, Penson DF, et al. Enzalutamide and survival in nonmetastatic, castration-resistant prostate cancer. N Engl J Med. 2020;382(23):2197–206.
20. Clegg NJ, Wongvipat J, Joseph JD, Tran C, Ouk S, Dilhas A, et al. ARN-509: a novel antiandrogen for prostate cancer treatment. Cancer Res. 2012;72(6):1494–503.
21. Smith MR, Saad F, Chowdhury S, Oudard S, Hadaschik BA, Graff JN, et al. Apalutamide treatment and metastasis-free survival in prostate cancer. N Engl J Med. 2018;378(15):1408–18.
22. Smith MR, Saad F, Chowdhury S, Oudard S, Hadaschik BA, Graff JN, et al. Apalutamide and overall survival in prostate cancer. Eur Urol. 2021;79(1):150–8.
23. CHI KN, Agarwal N, Bjartell A, Chung BH, Pereira de Santana Gomes AJ, Given R, et al. Apalutamide for metastatic, castration-sensitive prostate cancer. N Engl J Med. 2019;381(1):13–24.

24. Aragon-Ching JB. Darolutamide: a novel androgen-signaling agent in nonmetastatic castration-resistant prostate cancer. Asian J Androl. 2020;22(1):76–8.
25. Scott LJ. Darolutamide: a review in non-metastatic castration-resistant prostate cancer. Target Oncol. 2020;15(6):791–9.
26. Fizazi K, Shore N, Tammela TL, Ulys A, Vjaters E, Polyakov S, et al. Darolutamide in non-metastatic, castration-resistant prostate cancer. N Engl J Med. 2019;380(13):1235–46.
27. Fizazi K, Shore N, Tammela TL, Ulys A, Vjaters E, Polyakov S, et al. Nonmetastatic, Castration-resistant prostate cancer and survival with Darolutamide. N Engl J Med. 2020;383(11):1040–9.
28. Ge C, Zhang L, Liao B. Abstract 5327: KPG-121, a novel CRBN modulator, potently inhibits growth of metastatic castration resistant prostate cancer as a single agent or in combination with androgen receptor signaling inhibitors both in vitro and in vivo. Cancer Res. 2020;80(16 Suppl):5327.
29. Kumar J, Jazayeri SB, Gautam S, Norez D, Alam MU, Tanneru K, et al. Comparative efficacy of apalutamide darolutamide and enzalutamide for treatment of non-metastatic castrate-resistant prostate cancer: a systematic review and network meta-analysis. Urol Oncol. 2020;38(11):826–34.
30. Mori K, Mostafaei H, Pradere B, Motlagh RS, Quhal F, Laukhtina E, et al. Apalutamide, enzalutamide, and darolutamide for non-metastatic castration-resistant prostate cancer: a systematic review and network meta-analysis. Int J Clin Oncol. 2020;25(11):1892–900.
31. Heidegger I, Brandt MP, Heck MM. Treatment of non-metastatic castration resistant prostate cancer in 2020: what is the best? Urol Oncol. 2020;38(4):129–36.
32. Morgans AK, Shore N, Cope D, McNatty A, Moslehi J, Gomella L, et al. Androgen receptor inhibitor treatments: cardiovascular adverse events and comorbidity considerations in patients with non-metastatic prostate cancer. Urol Oncol. 2021;39(1):52–62.

Chapter 7
Immunotherapy for Metastatic Prostate Cancer

Mohammad Atiq and Ravi Madan

Abbreviations

bRFS	Biochemical recurrence-free survival
Cas9	CRISPR associated protein 9
CDK12	Cyclin-dependent kinase 12
CRISPR	Clustered Regularly Interspaced Short Palindromic Repeats
CTLA-4	Cytotoxic T-lymphocyte-associated protein 4
DDR	DNA Damage Repair
DMFS	Distant metastasis-free survival
dMMR	Deficient mismatch repair
ECOG	Eastern Cooperative Oncology Group
HRR	Homologous recombination repair
IL-23	Interleukin 23
IL-8	Interleukin 8
mCRPC	Metastatic castration-resistant prostate cancer
MDSC	Myeloid-derived suppressor cells
MSI	Microsatellite instability
MSI-H	Microsatellite instability high
PARP	Poly ADP-ribose polymerase inhibitor
PCSS	Prostate cancer-specific survival
PD-1	Programmed cell death protein 1
PD-L1	Programmed death-ligand 1

M. Atiq
National Cancer Institute, Bethesda, MD, USA

R. Madan (✉)
Genitourinary Malignancy Branch, National Cancer Institute, Bethesda, MD, USA
e-mail: madanr@mail.nih.gov

K. L. Stratton, A. K. Morgans (eds.), *Urologic Oncology*,
https://doi.org/10.1007/978-3-030-89891-5_7

PD-L2	Programmed death-ligand 2
PMN	Polymorphonuclear
RCC	Renal Cell Carcinoma
RECIST	Response Evaluation Criteria in Solid Tumors
RP	Radical prostatectomy
TMB	Tumor mutational burden

Introduction

Immunotherapy has not been as clinically impactful in prostate cancer when compared to other genitourinary malignancies such as renal cell cancer and bladder cancer. Currently, there are two immune-based therapies with established roles for usage in the metastatic castration-resistant setting: sipuleucel-T and pembrolizumab. There is not a current role for immunotherapy in metastatic castration-naïve prostate cancer, nor is there one in earlier disease (e.g., neoadjuvant or adjuvant settings). Nevertheless, there have been trials conducted on the usage of immunotherapy in prostate cancer outside of the aforementioned treatments, with many demonstrating potential antitumor activity. Moreover, trials have been done using combinations of immunotherapeutic agents with other treatment modalities, and there are additional data suggesting new possible directions of development in prostate cancer. This includes potential novel targets outside of the traditional focus of immunotherapy in this disease.

Approved Immunotherapies for Prostate Cancer

Sipuleucel-T

The first foray of immunotherapy in prostate cancer started with sipuleucel-T (Provenge). Sipuleucel-T is an autologous cellular immunotherapy made from peripheral blood mononuclear cells. These cells are removed from a patient by apheresis and then exposed to prostatic acid phosphatase and granulocyte macrophage colony-stimulating factor before being reinfused into the patient [1]. The dosing schedule for this is every 2 weeks for a total of three doses. A multicenter phase III, double-blind study randomized 512 patients in a 2:1 ratio to sipuleucel-T or placebo using the dosing schedule previously described. This study showed that sipuleucel-T did prolong overall survival with a median survival 4.1 months longer than the placebo group [2]. It was associated with a 22% relative risk reduction of death as compared with the placebo group (hazard ratio, 0.78; $p = 0.03$). Also, the rate of 3-year survival was improved in the treatment group compared to the placebo (31.7% in the sipuleucel-T group versus 23.0% in the placebo group). However, sipuleucel-T did not have an effect on the time to disease progression (3.7 months in the sipuleucel-T group as compared to 3.6 months in the placebo group). In addition, PSA reductions of at least 50% on repeat visits were seen in 2.6% of patients in the sipuleucel-T group as compared to 1.3% in the placebo group making it hard for patients and physicians to discern clinical benefit in the short term. It should be noted that sipuleucel-T was relatively well tolerated with only 0.9% of patients in the treatment group unable to receive all three infusions because of infusion-related adverse events. There were no reports of autoimmune-related adverse events or anaphylaxis. Most commonly, the adverse events experienced were felt to be related to cytokine release (e.g., chills, fatigue, pyrexia).

Sipuleucel-T is currently approved for metastatic castration-resistant prostate cancer (mCRPC) that is asymptomatic or minimally symptomatic. The study only enrolled patients with prostate adenocarcinoma, and therefore, sipuleucel-T is not recommended for use in patients with neuroendocrine prostate cancer. Additionally, patients with visceral metastases were excluded from the trial, and consequently, the therapy is not recommended for these patients. A subgroup analysis of the phase III study highlights that patients in the quartile with lowest PSA values had the greatest benefit, perhaps suggesting that patients with the lowest tumor burden are most appropriate for this treatment [3]. The overall survival hazard ratio was 0.51 (95% CI 0.31–0.85) for patients in the quartile with the lowest baseline PSA versus 0.84 (95% CI 0.55–1.29) for patients in the quartile with the highest baseline PSA. Estimated improvement in median survival favored those in the lowest baseline PSA quartile compared to those in the highest (13.0 months and 2.8 months, respectively). Also, those in the lowest PSA quartile had an estimated 3-year survival of 62.6% compared to 41.6% for control patients.

Another patient population that may benefit more from sipuleucel-T is African Americans with mCRPC as was suggested in an exploratory analysis of the PROCEED registry [4]. The PROCEED registry is a prospective observational study of men with advanced prostate cancer who at the time of enrollment were either planned to receive sipuleucel-T or had undergone their first leukapheresis for production of sipuleucel-T 6 months or less prior to enrollment. The study analyzing the registry compared the overall survival in African American and Caucasian men who had received at least one infusion of sipuleucel-T in both an all-patient set and a baseline PSA-matched set. The hazard ratios for overall survival were 0.81 (95% CI 0.68–0.97, $p = 0.03$) and 0.70 (95% CI 0.57–0.86, $p < 0.001$) between African American and Caucasian men in the all-patient and baseline PSA-matched sets, correspondingly. Median OS was 35.3 months for African American men compared to 25.8 months for Caucasian men in the PSA-matched set. It was similar in the all-patient set: 35.2 months for African American men and 29.9 months for Caucasian men.

Future directions for sipuleucel-T may include usage in the neoadjuvant setting or in combination with other therapies. The phase II study NeoACT took patients with localized prostate cancer who received sipuleucel-T prior to radical prostatectomy (RP) and looked for immunologic effects of treatment on prostate tissue [5, 6]. Patients were treated with three infusions of sipuleucel-T prior to RP. Most of the adverse events prior to RP were Grade 1–2 with the most frequent adverse events within 1 day after infusion being fatigue, headache, and myalgia. There did not seem to be any effect on operative complications, procedure time, or estimated blood loss. Compared to the pretreatment biopsy, there were > threefold increases in infiltrating CD3+, CD3+/CD4+, and CD3+/CD8+ T cell populations in the RP tissues ($p = 0.0001$ for all populations). Importantly, 12 concurrent cases that were not treated with neoadjuvant sipuleucel-T did not have the same level of T cell infiltration. Further exploratory analysis of this study showed sipuleucel-T treatment was associated with increased expression of Th1-associated genes as well as upregulation of immune inhibitory checkpoints, including CTLA-4 [7] . Declines in PSA while on treatment were associated with induction of Th1 response. PSA progression on treatment was correlated with an upregulation of genes of inhibitory checkpoints, including CTLA-4. This provides a basis for trials combining checkpoint inhibition with sipuleucel-T, which are currently being conducted.

Immunotherapy Based on Biomarkers in Prostate Cancer

Understanding biomarkers for response to immunotherapy is crucial to its success. In trying to discover biomarkers for response to immunotherapy in several settings, there are data that have centered around high microsatellite instability (MSI-H)/ deficient mismatch repair (dMMR), cyclin-dependent kinase 12 (*CDK12*) status, and tumor mutational burden (TMB). All three of these biomarkers relate to treatments with PD-1/PD-L1 inhibitors.

Currently, pembrolizumab is approved for treatment across solid tumors that are MSI-H/dMMR or with tumor mutational burden-high (TMB-H) status ($\geq$10 mutations per megabase (mut/MB)). Abida et al. performed a retrospective analysis of prostate cancer patients treated at Memorial Sloan Kettering Cancer Center from 2015 to 2018 [8]. Eleven patients with MSI-H/dMMR castration-resistant prostate cancer were treated with anti-PD-1/PD-L1 therapy, out of which six (54.5%) had PSA responses of greater than 50%. Four of these six also had radiographic response. At the time of analysis, five of the six responders were still on therapy with the longest ongoing response being 89 weeks. Particularly interesting about this study is that two of six patients who underwent longitudinal tumor profiling acquired the MSI-H/dMMR phenotype somatically. A second retrospective study looking at the response to anti-PD-1/PD-L1 therapy in dMMR/MSI-H metastatic prostate cancer also demonstrated benefit [9]. All of these patients were initially treated with medical/surgical castration. PSA response of 50% was seen in eight of 15 patients treated with pembrolizumab. Median PFS was not reached, and seven of the eight responders remained on treatment without progression at a median follow-up of 12 months. These studies support the treatment of MSI-H/dMMR metastatic prostate cancer with pembrolizumab, although it is noteworthy that responses are not universal.

Initial data revealing the potential benefit of immunotherapy in mCRPC patients with *CDK12* mutations were presented in a genomic analysis by Wu et al. [10]. The study showed a statistically significant increase in the frequency of biallelic *CDK12* loss in mCRPC (6.9%) as compared to primary prostate cancer (1.2%). *CDK12* mutant cases were associated with elevated neoantigen burden and increased tumor

T cell infiltration. Eleven patients with *CDK12* mutations were identified in the Michigan Oncology Sequencing (Mi-ONCOSEQ) program. Five of these patients who were pretreated had subsequent exposure to anti-PD-1 inhibitors. Four of these five were analyzed, and two patients were noted to have significant decreases in PSA after being treated with anti-PD-1 inhibitors.

A more recent retrospective study by Antonarakis et al. looked at patients with at least monoallelic *CDK12* alterations to further characterize the clinical features and responses to various therapies in patients with somatic loss-of-function *CDK12* mutations [11]. Of the nine men with mCRPC who received a PD-1 inhibitor (either pembrolizumab or nivolumab), 33% had a PSA response and the median progression-free survival was 5.4 months. It should be noted that these patients were heavily pretreated and were receiving the PD-1 inhibitor as a fourth- to sixth-line systemic therapy. Still, this benefit in a mCRPC population that had seen many treatments already is noteworthy given the median PFS of 5.3 months and 3.8 months for abiraterone/enzalutamide and taxane, respectively, when used in the same population but in the first-line setting. Interestingly enough, even though the PFS was similar between the abiraterone/enzalutamide and PD-1 inhibitor groups, the PSA response in the patients treated with first-line abiraterone/enzalutamide was higher at 41%, which may relate to how PSA responses and survival can be discordant when patients are treated with immunotherapy, as seen with sipuleucel-T [2].

Tumor mutational burden is a biomarker that may have utility in predicting response to PD-1 inhibitors as monotherapy and in combination with the anti-CTLA-4 inhibitor, ipilimumab. Currently, pembrolizumab is FDA-approved for the treatment of any solid tumor with high TMB (defined as >10 mutations/megabase) that have progressed on prior treatments and do not have alternative treatment options. The approval was based on results from KEYNOTE-158. This prospective phase II study enrolled patients with advanced incurable solid tumors who had progression on at least one line of standard therapy, ECOG 0 or 1, and measurable disease per RECIST [12]. All of these patients were treated with pembrolizumab 200 mg every 3 weeks for up to 35 cycles. There were objective responses in 29% of the TMB-high group and 6% of the non-TMB-high group. Interestingly, the predictive value of TMB was independent of PD-L1 and microsatellite status. It is important to note it is unclear how many prostate cancer patients were treated on this trial as the prostate cancer patients with MSI-H disease were included in a cohort of mixed tumor types, and the published data did not list the number of patients per tumor type. Also, the cohort these patients were included in, cohort K, was not included in the analysis. Concerning toxicity, 15% of patients had a grade 3–5 treatment-related adverse event. More data on tumor mutational burden would clearly define the benefit of checkpoint inhibitors in prostate cancer patients meeting this criteria for treatment.

In a retrospective study of metastatic prostate cancer specimens, whole genome sequencing was done to try and identify patients more likely to respond to immune checkpoint blockade [13]. Twelve patients were found to have high TMB (>10 mut. MB). The patients were treated with anti-PD-1 checkpoint inhibitors as a monotherapy and 7/12 patients with high TMB had >50% decline in PSA. While the approval for pembrolizumab in the TMB-H setting is based on data that did not include prostate cancer, the effectiveness across tumor types, irrespective of MSI/PD-L1 expression, and the results of the retrospective analysis are encouraging for similar results with pembrolizumab monotherapy in a subset of patients with metastatic prostate cancer.

Evaluations of Immunotherapy in Unselected Patients

Ipilimumab

Ipilimumab, a cytotoxic T-lymphocyte-associated protein 4 (CTLA-4) antibody, has been studied in various settings regarding prostate cancer, both as a monotherapy and in combination with other agents. As for its use as a monotherapy, there are two phase III trials that address the utility of ipilimumab in both the post-chemotherapy and chemotherapy-naïve settings. The first trial by Kwon et al. that reported results included patients with mCRPC who had progressed after treatment with docetaxel [14]. These patients were randomized to bone-directed radiotherapy (8 Gy in one fraction to up to five lesions for potential immune synergy) followed by ipilimumab or placebo every 3 weeks for up to four doses. Those who did not progress could continue to receive ipilimumab or placebo every 3 months until disease progression. Posttreatment PSA reduction of 50% or more was seen in 13.1% of the ipilimumab group as compared to 5.2% of the placebo group. The progression-free survival in the ipilimumab group was 4.0 months as compared to 3.1 months in the placebo group (HR 0.70, $p < 0.0001$). There was a nonsignificant difference in median overall survival, with mOS of 11.2 months in the ipilimumab group versus 10 months in the placebo group (HR 0.85, $p = 0.053$). A subgroup analysis of patients with favorable features (classified based on alkaline phosphatase, hemoglobin, and absence of visceral metastases) did have a median overall survival of 22.7 months with ipilimumab versus 15.8 months with placebo (HR 0.62, $p = 0.0038$), suggesting that there may be a subset of post-chemotherapy mCRPC patients that may benefit from ipilimumab. Nevertheless, it is important to note that 26% of the patients in the ipilimumab group had grade 3–4 immune-related adverse events as compared to 3% of patients in the placebo group, highlighting the concern of toxicity with this agent. A final analysis of this trial was published in early 2020 after an additional 2 years of follow-up from the primary analysis [15]. Although the study did not meet its primary endpoint, this additional analysis showed statistically substantial differences in overall survival at 2 years, 3 years, 4 years, and 5 years favoring the iplimumab arm over placebo.

A second phase III trial was conducted with asymptomatic or minimally symptomatic mCRPC patients in the chemotherapy-naïve setting [16]. Notably, this trial excluded patients with visceral metastases but was otherwise conducted similarly to the trial in patients who had progressed on docetaxel as far as the treatment schedule and dosing of ipilimumab, although radiation therapy was not administered [14].

For the study in chemotherapy-naïve patients, PSA response rate was 23% in the ipilimumab arm versus 8% with placebo. The median progression-free survival was 5.6 months versus 3.8 months in ipilimumab and placebo arms, respectively (HR 0.67 95.87% CI, 0.55 to 0.81) [16]. While the PSA response rate and median progression-free survival in the ipilumumab-treated patients suggest some antitumor activity in this specific patient population of pre-chemotherapy mCRPC patients, ipilumumab was not associated with improved median overall survival, with mOS of 28.7 months in the ipilimumab group versus 29.7 months in the placebo arm (HR 1.11, $p = 0.3667$). The percentage of grade 3 to 4 adverse events (31% in the ipilimumab arm vs. 2% with placebo) was similar to that of the trial conducted in the post-chemotherapy setting. Though the results of these two trials highlight potential antitumor activity of ipilimumab in mCRPC, the significant toxicity from immune-related adverse events and lack of strong improvements in OS have not led to the use of ipilimumab as a monotherapy for mCRPC.

Pembrolizumab

Another immunotherapy being evaluated as a monotherapy is the anti-programed death receptor-1 (PD-1) checkpoint inhibitor pembrolizumab. As noted above, pembrolizumab is approved for use in patients with MSI-H and TMB-H tumors. Additional analyses were performed specifically in mCRPC patients in the phase II study KEYNOTE-199. In this study pembrolizumab was evaluated in five cohorts of mCRPC patients defined by their prior treatment exposures and location of metastatic disease. In all cohorts pembrolizumab was administered every 3 weeks for a maximum of 35 infusions, barring specific withdrawal or discontinuation criteria. Patients in cohorts 1–3 were treated with pembrolizumab, while cohorts 4–5 evaluated patients treated with pembrolizumab in combination with enzalutamide. Cohorts 1–3 have been analyzed in a paper by Antonarakis et al. [17]. These patients were all previously treated with one to two chemotherapy regimens, one of which had to include docetaxel, and one or more targeted endocrine therapies. The patients in cohorts 1 and 2 had measurable disease as per RECIST v1.1. Additionally, cohort 1 patients had PD-L1-positive disease and cohort 2 patients had PD-L1-negative disease. Cohort 3 consisted of patients, irrespective of PD-L1 status, who had bone metastases detectable by whole-body bone scintigraphy and no measurable by tumors by RECIST criteria.

PSA response, measured as a decrease in PSA level from baseline by 50% or greater, across all three cohorts was 6%. Individual analysis of the cohorts shows similar percentages in cohorts 1 and 2 (6% and 8%, respectively) and a noticeably lower percentage (2%) in cohort 3. The results from cohorts 1 and 2 suggest that the PSA response was independent of PD-L1 status. Additionally, 9% of all patients had stable PSA, which may point to an antitumor effect that is more involved in disease control. The objective response rate (ORR) was 5% for cohort 1, 3% for cohort 2, and 5% for these two cohorts combined. The median overall survival was

9.5 months in cohort 1, 7.9 months in cohort 2, and 14.1 months in cohort 3. The investigators of this study expressed optimism regarding the OS, but randomized trials are needed to confirm these findings. In terms of toxicity across cohorts, 15% of the patients experienced grade 3 to 5 treatment-related adverse events with 5% of the patients discontinuing pembrolizumab because of a treatment-related adverse event. The trial is limited by its lack of a control arm, and the main conclusion to be drawn is that pembrolizumab has limited clinical efficacy in an unselected population.

Investigating Combinations of Immunotherapy in Prostate Cancer

Ipilimumab and Nivolumab

Ipilimumab and nivolumab have established roles in melanoma and renal cell carcinoma (RCC). In regard to prostate cancer, ipilimumab and nivolumab were evaluated in combination with CheckMate 650 [18]. This phase II study looked at mCRPC patients with an ECOG of 1 or less and separated these patients into asymptomatic/minimally symptomatic patients who had progressed after at least one second-generation hormone therapy but had not seen chemotherapy in the mCRPC setting (cohort 1) and patients who had progressed after cytotoxic chemotherapy in the mCRPC setting (cohort 2). The co-primary endpoints were objective response rate and median rPFS. Objective response rates were 25% and 10%, while median rPFS was 5.5 months and 3.8 months for cohorts 1 and 2, respectively. The secondary endpoint of overall survival showed a median of 19.0 months in cohort 1 and 15.2 months in cohort 2.

Safety was assessed as a secondary endpoint as well. Grade 3–4 treatment-related adverse events were seen in 42.2% of patients in cohort 1 and 53.3% of patients in cohort 2. Looking at this further, at the time of the data cutoff, there were only 3/90 patients between both cohorts who were on study treatment. The majority of patients (71%) discontinued treatment during combination dosing with ipilimumab and nivolumab, while most of the remaining patients (25.6%) discontinued treatment during the maintenance phase with monotherapy nivolumab. There were two main reasons for discontinuation: toxicity from treatment (51.1% from cohort 1 and 44.4% from cohort 2) and disease progression (33.3% in cohort 1 and 44.4% in cohort 2). These safety data show that the regimen used for this combination is not tolerable for mCRPC patients.

There are data on the utility of using TMB to select patients when combining anti-CTLA-4 antibodies and anti-PD-1 antibodies. A subpopulation of 44 patients with quality-controlled whole-exome sequencing data were found to have a median TMB of 74.5 mutations/patient. Patients were divided into those above versus below the median. The objective response rate was 50.0% for those with TMB above the median versus 5.3% for those below. This pattern favoring the patients with TMB above the median versus those below was seen across PSA response rate (30.0% vs. 5.9%), median rPFS (7.4 vs. 2.4 months), and median overall survival (19.0 vs. 10.1 months). In addition to the exploratory analysis regarding TMB mentioned above, this study also examined patients in regard to status with homologous recombination deficiency, DNA damage repair (DDR), and PD-L1 expression. There was no clear association between these biomarkers and clinical activity.

Enzalutamide and PD-1/PD-L1 Inhibitors

In addition to combinations of checkpoint inhibitors with each other, checkpoint inhibitors, specifically PD-1/PD-L1 inhibitors, have been studied in combination with the second-generation anti-androgen, enzalutamide. A phase II study looked at the combination of enzalutamide with pembrolizumab in men with mCRPC who were progressing on enzalutamide monotherapy [19]. These patients were treated with four doses of pembrolizumab given every 3 weeks. Five of the 28 patients in this study (18%) had a PSA decline of at least 50%. Median overall survival for all patients on the study was 21.9 months compared to 41.7 months in the responders. Out of the three responders who had baseline biopsies, none of them had detectable PD-L1 expression and only one had MSI high disease with mutations consistent with DNA-repair defects. This was a particularly interesting point as it suggested that tumors did not have to express PD-L1 or harbor DNA-repair defects to respond to treatment.

This phase II study with pembrolizumab was followed by a randomized phase III study that looked at the combination of atezolizumab and enzalutamide versus enzalutamide alone in mCRPC who had progressed on abiraterone and docetaxel or were not candidates for a taxane regimen [20]. Patients were randomized 1:1 to either the atezolizumab plus enzalutamide group or the enzalutamide alone group. Median OS was 15.2 months in the atezolizumab plus enzalutamide group and 16.6 months in the enzalutamide group. This study did not meet its primary endpoint of overall survival as there was no significant difference in overall survival between the two groups [stratified HR, 1.12, $p = 0.28$). The percentage of patients with grade 3–4 treatment-related AEs was 28.3% in the combination group versus 9.6% in the enzalutamide monotherapy group. As this study did not show an improvement in overall survival in the atezolizumab plus enzalutamide group compared to those treated with enzalutamide alone, it was terminated early.

Cabozantinib and Atezolizumab

Cabozantinib targets MET, vascular endothelial growth factor receptor-2, KIT, AXL, and FLT3 [21]. The role of cabozantinib in prostate cancer to date has been largely defined by two phase III trials: COMET-1 and COMET-2. COMET-1 was a phase III study that randomly assigned men with mCRPC who progressed on docetaxel and abiraterone and/or enzalutamide to treatment with cabozantinib or prednisone [22]. Median OS was 11.0 months in the cabozantinib group and 9.8 months in the prednisone group (HR 0.90; 95% CI 0.76 to 1.06; stratified log-rank $p = 0.213$) showing that cabozantinib did not significantly improve OS compared to prednisone in the post-chemotherapy and post-second-generation anti-androgen mCRPC setting. It also did not improve PSA outcomes. COMET-2 was a randomized phase III trial in men with mCRPC and narcotic-dependent pain from bone metastases who had progressed on docetaxel and either abiraterone or enzalutamide [23]. Patients were treated with cabozantinib or mitoxantrone plus prednisone. The primary endpoint was pain response at week 6 confirmed at week 12. The study ceased enrollment early due to the lack of survival benefit from COMET-1. In COMET-2, 15% of the cabozantinib group and 17% of the mitoxantrone-prednisone group had a pain response (−2% difference, 95% CI −16% to 11%, $p = 0.8$). As the difference in pain response was not statistically significant, it was concluded cabozantinib did not provide better pain relief compared to mitoxantrone plus prednisone in mCRPC patients with symptomatic bone metastases who had progressed on docetaxel and a second-generation anti-androgen.

COSMIC-021 is a trial that is studying the potential from a combination of a PD-L1 checkpoint inhibitor (atezolizumab) with cabozantinib in solid tumors. Cohort 6 of this study enrolled mCRPC patients with radiographic soft tissue progression after enzalutamide/abiraterone, measurable disease, and an ECOG of 1 or less [24]. After starting treatment, patients were assessed with scans every 6 weeks for the first year and then every 12 weeks. The objective response rate for the 44 included patients was 32% and 48% of patients had stable disease. Overall, this meant that the combination achieved a disease control rate of 80%. The duration of response for all patients was 8.3 months. Tumor PD-L1 expression is planned to be reported. The treatment-related adverse events included fatigue (50%), nausea (43%), decreased appetite (39%), diarrhea (39%), dysgeusia (34%), and palmar-plantar erythrodysesthesia (32%). The results show meaningful activity, and the reporting of additional data on PD-L1 expression will provide insight into the potential utility of this as a biomarker of response to the combination of cabozantinib and atezolizumab.

Olaparib and Durvalumab

Another immunotherapy combination studied in mCRPC patients used the PD-L1 inhibitor, durvalumab, and the poly(ADP-ribose) polymerase inhibitor (PARP), olaparib [25]. The study evaluated the combination of olaparib and durvalumab in patients with and without somatic and germline DDR mutations. The analysis reported here is of the mCRPC cohort of this study. The patients on this study had all previously received enzalutamide and/or abiraterone. Out of the 17 patients enrolled, seven patients had been treated with vaccine therapy (sipuleucel-T and/or PROSTVAC). No patients were allowed to enroll if they had been previously treated with a checkpoint inhibitor. Nine out of 17 patients had a radiographic and/or PSA response with a decline of at least 50%. Median rPFS for all patients was 16.1 months with a 12-month rPFS of 51.5%. The median rPFS was the same for patients with alterations in DDR genes (16.1 months). Comparing the 12-month PFS probability in patients with DDR gene alterations versus those without showed a significant advantage in those with DDR gene alterations (83.3% vs. 36.4%, $p = 0.031$). As for toxicity, no patients had to be taken off the trial for toxicity and nausea was the only nonhematologic grade 3 or 4 toxicity, occurring in 2/17 patients. The rate of hematologic grade 3 or 4 adverse events was 24% in anemia and 12% in lymphopenia. Four of the 17 patients had immune-related adverse events of any grade. Moreover, there was only one grade 4 toxicity seen in all the patients which was lymphopenia.

Still, a potentially important mechanistic finding of this study was the activity of this regimen among patients without biallelic inactivation in DDR pathways. There were early changes in innate and adaptive immunity that were associated with response as well: Patients with a baseline percentage of myeloid-derived suppressor cells (MDSC) among total viable cells that was less than or equal to the median had prolonged PFS. Future studies are required to better understand the clinical ramifications of these findings.

Future Directions

Immunotherapy has not had the same success in prostate cancer as compared to other cancers. However, success with specific subgroups and with some combination approaches necessitates further exploration into potential clinically relevant avenues. One new direction to investigate is PD-L2. A study by Zhao et al. analyzed gene expression data from a mix of 7826 prospectively collected prostatectomy samples and 1567 retrospective samples [26]. The primary outcome measured was distant metastasis-free survival (DMFS), while secondary outcomes included biochemical recurrence-free survival (bRFS), prostate cancer-specific survival (PCSS), and overall survival. Among other variables, the study assessed four immune checkpoints (CTLA-4, PD-1, PD-L1, PD-L2) that are currently targeted by clinically utilized therapies. Notably, PD-L1 was found not to be prognostic. PD-L2, which was expressed at higher levels than PD-L1 across all the samples in the study, was associated with worse bRFS (HR 1.17, $p = 0.01$), DMFS (HR 1.25, $p = 0.01$), and PCSS (HR 1.45, $p = 0.003$). Prostate cancer tumors with higher expression of PD-L2 had worse outcomes without postoperative radiation therapy. However, tumors treated with postoperative radiation therapy that had high PD-L2 expression had equivalent outcomes to tumors with low PD-L2 expression not treated with postoperative radiation. The data from this study suggest that tumors with higher PD-L2 expression are more aggressive. Although the patients studied here did not have metastatic prostate cancer, the findings still present an area for further inspection when discussing potential new targets in immunotherapy.

Antibodies able to select for multiple targets with a single construct have also been studied in prostate cancer. Two examples include bi-specific T-cell engagers (BiTEs) and tri-specific killer engagers (TriKEs). Both treatments are essentially polyspecific antibodies that target for two to three antigens on either T cells or natural killer cells, respectively. A phase I study of pasotuxizumab, a PSMA BiTE, was conducted in advanced CRPC patients (stage III/IV) who had treatment failure after at least one taxane and were refractory to abiraterone/enzalutamide or refused any other standard of care option [27]. The once daily subcutaneous maximum tolerated dose was 172.0 μg/d. There were 9/47 PSA responders (PSA reductions >50% relative to baseline) to the subcutaneous dosage. All patients discontinued treatment with the most common reason being radiologic disease progression. All patients had treatment-emergent adverse events (TEAEs) with the most common in descending order being fever, injection site reaction, chills, and fatigue. As for TEAEs of grade ≥3, these were seen in 87% of the subcutaneous cohort and the most common was anemia and decreased lymphocyte count. While the safety has been determined, further evaluation of efficacy is needed.

TriKEs have been evaluated at the preclinical level in prostate cancer cell lines. In a preclinical study utilizing a TriKE that targeted EpCAM on tumor cells, the TriKE was shown to augment antibody-dependent cell-mediated cytotoxicity and improve the proliferation and activation of natural killer cells across multiple solid tumor cell lines, including prostate cancer cell lines [28]. TriKEs are being analyzed in clinical trials for hematological malignancies but have not yet made it to clinical analysis in the prostate cancer setting. Further preclinical studies are ongoing.

The immunotherapies covered so far in this chapter utilize mechanisms that are predominantly T-cell focused. In the olaparib plus durvalumab study by Karzai et al., baseline fraction of MDSCs was found to be associated with PFS. Other preclinical data in support of further investigation into MDSCs suggest targeting cytokines as a different way to affect the tumor microenvironment. Preclinical work by Lopez-Bujanda et al. examined cancer cells from castration-sensitive and castration-resistant prostate tumors [29]. They saw that castration led to significant secretion of IL-8, which caused intratumoral infiltration with polymorphonuclear (PMN) MDSCs, stimulating tumor progression. The role of IL-8 was further delineated when removing it from prostate cancer cells with CRISPR/Cas9 resulted in a decrease in intratumoral PMN-MDSC infiltration, as did utilizing antibodies to the IL-8 receptor. The decrease in PMN-MDSC infiltration made the prostate tumors more responsive to immune checkpoint blockage. A murine model from this study tested a therapeutic approach that blocked the IL-8 receptor at the time of ADT, but this was not effective [29]. However, combining blockade of the IL-8 receptor with an anti-CTLA-4 antibody at the time of ADT resulted in significantly increased survival as compared to ADT by itself and anti-CTLA-4 antibody monotherapy in this preclinical setting (citation). The results from this study are the basis for an ongoing phase Ib/II trial of nivolumab with ADT versus nivolumab and an anti-IL-8 monoclonal antibody with ADT in patients with hormone-sensitive prostate cancer. Another potential cytokine target that relates to MDSCs is IL-23. A study by Calcinotto et al. looked at the role of IL-23 in driving the development of metastatic castration-resistant prostate cancer [30]. Tumor samples from patients with mCRPC had increased intratumoral myeloid-derived suppressor cell (MDSC) infiltration and blood IL-23 concentration. IL-23 made by MDSCs sustained androgen receptor signaling contributing to androgen-independent tumorigenesis. Mice who were castration-resistant were treated with anti-IL-23 antibodies and enzalutamide. These mice had normalization of prostate glands affected by cancer, as there were decreases in both tumor volume and proliferation. This showed that treatment of castration-resistant mice with anti-IL-23 antibodies made them sensitive to androgen deprivation therapy again. These studies support further investigation into cytokine-targeted regimens in the treatment of metastatic castration-resistant prostate cancer.

Conclusion

The trials we have covered in this chapter all point toward antitumor activity of the multiple immunotherapies, although for the most part, survival benefits were largely lacking. Certain subsets of mCRPC patients, other than those currently able to receive immunotherapy under FDA-approved indications, did seem to have higher degrees of antitumor activity compared to the general mCRPC population (Table 7.1). As a type of cancer traditionally thought to be immunogenically "cold," the data from these trials would suggest that identifying biomarkers for selecting metastatic prostate cancer patients for treatment may result in more robust responses just as promoting a higher degree of immunogenic stimulation to the treatment may produce more substantial results. This may be achieved with combinations of existing treatments or by treatments focused on new targets and must also balance toxicity with efficacy. Additionally, examination of novel avenues, such as targeting additional checkpoints, immune cells beyond T cells, and utilizing polyspecific antibodies offer potential for expanding the therapeutic armament in prostate cancer treatment.

Table 7.1 Summary of clinical immunotherapy studies in prostate cancer. Studies are listed in the order of citation in the chapter. All studies are done in the metastatic castration-resistant prostate cancer setting

Reference #	Treatment	Population	Key outcome(s)
[2]	Sipuleucel-T	No visceral metastases	Prolonged OS by 4.1 months vs. placebo No effect on PFS/PSA response
[8]*	Anti-PD-1/PD-L1	MSI-H/dMMR	6/11 with PSA response Longest ongoing response: 89 weeks
[9]*	Anti-PD-1/PD-L1	MSI-H/dMMR	8/15 with PSA response 7/8 responders on treatment at median 12mo f/u
[10]*	Anti-PD-1 inhibitor	*CDK12* mutated	2/4 with significant decreases in PSA
[11]*	Anti-PD-1 inhibitor (pembrolizumab/ nivolumab)	*CDK12* mutated; ≥ 4 systemic therapy	Median PFS 5.4 months
[14]	Single fraction radiotherapy followed by ipilimumab	Post-docetaxel	OS: 11.2 months with ipilimumab vs. 10 months with placebo (HR 0.85, $p = 0.053$)
[16]	Ipilimumab	Chemo-naïve	OS: 28.7 months with ipilimumab vs. 29.7 months with placebo (HR 1.11, $p = 0.3667$)
[17]	Pembrolizumab	Post-chemo and targeted endo therapy; PD-L1 +/− (no control arm)	Median OS: 9.5 months cohort 1, 7.9 months cohort 2, 14.1 months cohort 3
[18]	Nivolumab + ipilimumab	≥1 second-generation hormone, pre/ post-chemo	Cohort 1: OS 19.0 months; G3–4 tRAE 42.2% Cohort 2: OS 15.2 months; G3-G4 tRAE 53.3%
[19]	Pembrolizumab + enzalutamide	Progressed on enza	41.7-month median OS in responders
[20]	Atezolizumab + enzalutamide	Progressed on abi and docetaxel	OS: 15.2 months with atezo + enza vs. 16.6 months with enza (HR 1.12, $p = 0.28$)
[24]	Cabozantinib + atezolizumab	Progressed on enza/ abi	ORR: 32% Duration of response: 8.3 months
[25]	Durvalumab + olaparib	+/− DDR mutations	Median rPFS: 16.1 months in all patients and in patients with DDR mutations

*Denotes retrospective analysis. Studies without an asterisk are prospective studies

References

1. Bilusic M, Einstein DJ, Karzai FH, Dahut WL, Gulley JL, Aragon-Ching JB, et al. The potential role for immunotherapy in biochemically recurrent prostate cancer. Urol Clin North Am. 2020;47(4):457–67.
2. Kantoff PW, Higano CS, Shore ND, Berger ER, Small EJ, Penson DF, et al. Sipuleucel-T immunotherapy for castration-resistant prostate cancer. N Engl J Med. 2010;363(5):411–22.
3. Schellhammer PF, Chodak G, Whitmore JB, Sims R, Frohlich MW, Kantoff PW. Lower baseline prostate-specific antigen is associated with a greater overall survival benefit from sipuleucel-T in the Immunotherapy for Prostate Adenocarcinoma Treatment (IMPACT) trial. Urology. 2013;81(6):1297–302.
4. Sartor O, Armstrong AJ, Ahaghotu C, McLeod DG, Cooperberg MR, Penson DF, et al. Survival of African-American and Caucasian men after sipuleucel-T immunotherapy: outcomes from the PROCEED registry. Prostate Cancer Prostatic Dis. 2020;23(3):517–26.
5. Fong L, Carroll P, Weinberg V, Chan S, Lewis J, Corman J, et al. Activated lymphocyte recruitment into the tumor microenvironment following preoperative sipuleucel-T for localized prostate cancer. J Natl Cancer Inst. 2014;106(11)
6. Fong L, Weinberg V, Chan S, Corman J, Amling C, Stephenson RA, Simko J, Sims RB, Carroll P, Small EJ. 939P- neoadjuvant Sipuleucel-T in localized prostate cancer: effects on immune cells within the prostate tumor microenvironment. Ann Oncol. 2012;23(Suppl 9):ix310.
7. Hagihara K, Chan S, Zhang L, Oh DY, Wei XX, Simko J, et al. Neoadjuvant sipuleucel-T induces both Th1 activation and immune regulation in localized prostate cancer. Onco Targets Ther. 2019;8(1):e1486953.
8. Abida W, Cheng ML, Armenia J, Middha S, Autio KA, Vargas HA, et al. Analysis of the prevalence of microsatellite instability in prostate cancer and response to immune checkpoint blockade. JAMA Oncol. 2019;5(4):471–8.
9. Graham LS, Montgomery B, Cheng HH, Yu EY, Nelson PS, Pritchard C, et al. Mismatch repair deficiency in metastatic prostate cancer: response to PD-1 blockade and standard therapies. PLoS One. 2020;15(5):e0233260.
10. Wu YM, Cieslik M, Lonigro RJ, Vats P, Reimers MA, Cao X, et al. Inactivation of CDK12 delineates a distinct immunogenic class of advanced prostate cancer. Cell. 2018;173(7):1770–82.e14.
11. Antonarakis ES, Isaacsson Velho P, Fu W, Wang H, Agarwal N, Sacristan Santos V, et al. CDK12-altered prostate cancer: clinical features and therapeutic outcomes to standard systemic therapies, poly (ADP-ribose) polymerase inhibitors, and PD-1 inhibitors. JCO Precis Oncol. 2020;4:370–81.
12. Marabelle A, Fakih M, Lopez J, Shah M, Shapira-Frommer R, Nakagawa K, et al. Association of tumour mutational burden with outcomes in patients with advanced solid tumours treated with pembrolizumab: prospective biomarker analysis of the multicohort, open-label, phase 2 KEYNOTE-158 study. Lancet Oncol. 2020;21(10):1353–65.
13. Mehra N, van Riet J, Smith M, et al. In-depth assessment of metastatic prostate cancer with high tumour mutational burden. Ann Oncol. 2018;29:viii274.
14. Kwon ED, Drake CG, Scher HI, Fizazi K, Bossi A, van den Eertwegh AJ, et al. Ipilimumab versus placebo after radiotherapy in patients with metastatic castration-resistant prostate cancer that had progressed after docetaxel chemotherapy (CA184-043): a multicentre, randomised, double-blind, phase 3 trial. Lancet Oncol. 2014;15(7):700–12.
15. Fizazi K, Drake CG, Beer TM, Kwon ED, Scher HI, Gerritsen WR, et al. Final analysis of the Ipilimumab versus placebo following radiotherapy phase III trial in Postdocetaxel metastatic castration-resistant prostate cancer identifies an excess of long-term survivors. Eur Urol. 2020;78(6):822–30.
16. Beer TM, Kwon ED, Drake CG, Fizazi K, Logothetis C, Gravis G, et al. Randomized, double-blind, phase III trial of Ipilimumab versus placebo in asymptomatic or minimally symptomatic

patients with metastatic chemotherapy-naive castration-resistant prostate cancer. J Clin Oncol. 2017;35(1):40–7.
17. Antonarakis ES, Piulats JM, Gross-Goupil M, Goh J, Ojamaa K, Hoimes CJ, et al. Pembrolizumab for treatment-refractory metastatic castration-resistant prostate cancer: multicohort, open-label phase II KEYNOTE-199 study. J Clin Oncol. 2020;38(5):395–405.
18. Sharma P, Pachynski RK, Narayan V, Flechon A, Gravis G, Galsky MD, et al. Nivolumab plus Ipilimumab for metastatic castration-resistant prostate cancer: preliminary analysis of patients in the CheckMate 650 trial. Cancer Cell. 2020;38(4):489–99 e3.
19. Graff JN, Beer TM, Alumkal JJ, Slottke RE, Redmond WL, Thomas GV, et al. A phase II single-arm study of pembrolizumab with enzalutamide in men with metastatic castration-resistant prostate cancer progressing on enzalutamide alone. J Immunother Cancer. 2020;8(2):e000642.
20. Sweeney CJ, Gillessen S, Rathkopf D, Matsubara N, Drake C, Fizazi K, et al. Abstract CT014: IMbassador250: a phase III trial comparing atezolizumab with enzalutamide vs enzalutamide alone in patients with metastatic castration-resistant prostate cancer (mCRPC). 2020;80(16 Suppl):CT014-CT.
21. Pinto A. Cabozantinib: a novel agent with a dual mechanism of action for castration-resistant prostate carcinoma. Cancer Chemother Pharmacol. 2014;73(2):219–22.
22. Smith M, De Bono J, Sternberg C, Le Moulec S, Oudard S, De Giorgi U, et al. Phase III study of Cabozantinib in previously treated metastatic castration-resistant prostate cancer: COMET-1. J Clin Oncol. 2016;34(25):3005–13.
23. Basch EM, Scholz M, de Bono JS, Vogelzang N, de Souza P, Marx G, et al. Cabozantinib versus Mitoxantrone-prednisone in symptomatic metastatic castration-resistant prostate cancer: a randomized phase 3 trial with a primary pain endpoint. Eur Urol. 2019;75(6):929–37.
24. Agarwal N, Loriot Y, McGregor BA, Dreicer R, Dorff TB, Maughan BL, et al. Cabozantinib in combination with atezolizumab in patients with metastatic castration-resistant prostate cancer: results of cohort 6 of the COSMIC-021 study. J Clin Oncol. 2020;38(15_suppl):5564.
25. Karzai F, VanderWeele D, Madan RA, Owens H, Cordes LM, Hankin A, et al. Activity of durvalumab plus olaparib in metastatic castration-resistant prostate cancer in men with and without DNA damage repair mutations. J Immunother Cancer. 2018;6(1):141.
26. Zhao SG, Lehrer J, Chang SL, Das R, Erho N, Liu Y, et al. The immune landscape of prostate cancer and nomination of PD-L2 as a potential therapeutic target. J Natl Cancer Inst. 2019;111(3):301–10.
27. Hummel HD, Kufer P, Grullich C, Seggewiss-Bernhardt R, Deschler-Baier B, Chatterjee M, et al. Pasotuxizumab, a BiTE((R)) immune therapy for castration-resistant prostate cancer: phase I, dose-escalation study findings. Immunotherapy. 2021;13(2):125–41.
28. Schmohl JU, Felices M, Taras E, Miller JS, Vallera DA. Enhanced ADCC and NK cell activation of an Anticarcinoma bispecific antibody by genetic insertion of a modified IL-15 cross-linker. Mol Ther. 2016;24(7):1312–22.
29. Lopez-Bujanda ZA, Haffner MC, Chaimowitz MG, Chowdhury N, Venturini NJ, Obradovic A, et al. Castration-mediated IL-8 promotes myeloid infiltration and prostate cancer progression. Nat Cancer. 2021;2:803–18, 651083.
30. Calcinotto A, Spataro C, Zagato E, Di Mitri D, Gil V, Crespo M, et al. IL-23 secreted by myeloid cells drives castration-resistant prostate cancer. Nature. 2018;559(7714):363–9.

Chapter 8
Advances in Prostate Cancer Imaging

Ali Aria Razmaria, Heiko Schoder, and Michael J. Morris

Introduction

The imaging of prostate cancer at different disease states has undergone a series of quantum leaps in the past decade. Imaging in prostate cancer serves, in part, the purpose of staging and risk-stratifying patients to formulate the most effective treatment plan with the least adverse side effects. However, traditional imaging techniques could only serve this role with significant limitations. Computed tomography (CT), for instance, has a size criterion of 1 cm for lymph nodes as threshold of raising suspicion for malignancy, which would not detect sub-centimeter or microscopic nodal disease often encountered on pathologic specimens. Traditional Tc-99 m methylene diphosphonate (MDP) bone scan limited by inherent single photon emission scintigraphic spatial resolution in the 1 cm range would fall short of delineating early bone metastases. Magnetic resonance imaging (MRI), despite its exquisite soft tissue resolution, faces challenges in identifying malignant lymph nodes in sub-centimeter range. To compensate for the shortcomings of standard imaging, statistical tools such as nomograms function as decision support in patient management in prostate cancer. Nomograms offer predictions based on population statistics to an individual on the risk of extraprostatic disease at diagnosis, the risk of relapse after primary therapy, or the risk of developing metastatic disease at biochemical relapse.

However, contemporary molecular imaging modalities can now more accurately depict a patient's distribution of disease on an individual level. This additional insight can supplement information from predictive models to better tailor treatment plans to an individual patient's cancer and can translate into superior treatment

A. A. Razmaria (✉) · H. Schoder · M. J. Morris
Memorial Sloan Kettering Cancer Center, New York, NY, USA
e-mail: razmaria@mskcc.org; morrism@mskcc.org

K. L. Stratton, A. K. Morgans (eds.), *Urologic Oncology*,
https://doi.org/10.1007/978-3-030-89891-5_8

plans based on a more accurate understanding of a patient's disease. Tailored treatment plans can be devised by detailed knowledge of the disease characteristics and its distribution. The new paradigm of molecular imaging allows for detection of disease at a molecular level, at a stage where often no macroscopic structural abnormalities can be demonstrated. It holds the promise of answering questions not sufficiently addressed by conventional imaging and better characterizes prostate cancer at its different stages. New methods have been successfully deployed to validate these new imaging modalities and establish reference standards for comparison.

This chapter introduces different positron emission tomography (PET) imaging probes in use for prostate cancer and their mechanisms of action. Subsequently, by way of following the clinical state model of prostate cancer, we will appraise data supporting the use of different imaging modalities in each disease state, addressing challenges in clinical trial design in each instance. An emphasis will be put on PET imaging techniques with molecular imaging principles.

PET Imaging Techniques for Prostate Cancer

F-18 Sodium Fluoride PET/CT or PET/MRI Bone Scan (F-18 NaF PET Bone Scan)

The F-18-NaF PET bone scan has a mechanism of action similar to the MDP bone scan: chemisorption to hydroxyl apatite crystals in the extracellular matrix, as an indicator of osteoblastic bone turnover in response to metastatic lesions [1]. As a result, it is not the cancer but the osteoblastic activity of the bone surrounding the cancer that is imaged.

As compared to the planar single photon emission tomographic method used in the MDP bone scan, positron emission tomographic (PET) technology combined with companion low-dose CT or MRI offers better spatial resolution and immediate anatomic correlation. F-18-NaF PET/CT has superior diagnostic performance characteristics compared to a conventional MDP bone scans [2]. In addition to diagnostic advantages, F-18 NaF PET bone scan offers more patient convenience with faster study completion time (1 hour vs. typically 3 hours with an MDP bone scan), comparable radiation exposure, and only moderately increased cost [3]. However, the US Centers for Medicare and Medicaid Services does not cover this modality at the current time [4, 5].

F-18 Fluorodeoxyglucose (FDG) PET

FDG is the most commonly used PET tracer in oncology. FDG is a glucose analog and is transferred by cell membrane glucose transporters (GLUT) into the cell, where it is phosphorylated by hexokinase and trapped [6]. Many cancers have upregulated glycolytic metabolism with overexpression of glucose transporters. While early states of prostate cancer predominantly rely on non-glycolytic metabolism (and FDG is therefore not suitable for disease staging or characterization), advanced states of the disease and high-grade tumors exhibit increased glucose metabolism [7, 8]. In the latter scenario FDG has a potential role as a prognostic biomarker and indicator of response to therapy [9–12].

C-11 Choline or F-18-Choline PET

Choline, a major component of cell membrane phospholipids, is internalized into the cell by choline transporters and metabolized by choline kinase, an enzyme overexpressed in several malignancies including prostate cancer [13–15]. The C11 isotope has a short half-life of 20 minutes, requiring on-site cyclotron production, whereas F-18, with a half-life of 110 minutes, offers logistical advantages like central radiopharmacy production and distribution. Otherwise, both tracers have similar imaging characteristics and detection rates [16]. Variable degrees of physiologic radiotracer activity in bone marrow and urinary tract, including the bladder, may interfere with the detection of early bone, pelvic nodal, and prostatic bed recurrent disease. Additional delayed post-void images may mitigate diagnostic limitations in the pelvis.

F-18 Fluciclovine

F-18 fluciclovine (anti-1-amino-3-F-18-fluorocyclobutane-1-carboxylic acid, also known as anti-F-18-FACBC) is a radiolabeled synthetic amino acid PET tracer (a leucine analog) used for the imaging of upregulated amino acid metabolism in tumors including prostate cancer [17, 18]. The tracer enters the cell by amino acid transporters including alanine, serine, cysteine transporter 2 (ASCT2), and L-type amino acid transporter 1 (LAT1), with the latter being overexpressed in high-grade prostate cancer [19, 20]. F-18 fluciclovine is not metabolized once inside the cell and can leave the cell through the same transporters. In order to optimize distribution and also because of rapid influx and efflux of the tracer into and out of prostate cancer cells, imaging must start within 3–5 minutes of the injection of radiotracer [21–23].

The advantage of low urinary excretion makes this tracer desirable for prostate cancer imaging and constitutes an advantage over other available PET tracers. A disadvantage, however, is the relatively high skeletal, muscle, and bone marrow uptake [24]. The latter can interfere with detection of osseous metastases. In addition, prostate cancer cannot be ruled out in sclerotic bone lesions seen only on CT without radiotracer activity, since dense osteoblastic lesions may lack increased F-18 fluciclovine uptake [25].

Ga-68 or F-18 Prostate-Specific Membrane Antigen (PSMA)

Prostate-specific membrane antigen (PSMA) is a transmembrane protein highly expressed on benign prostatic tissue and overexpressed by 100–1000-fold in malignant prostate epithelial cells. The PSMA gene was cloned in the research laboratory of Dr. Warren Heston at Memorial Sloan Kettering Cancer Center in 1993 [26–28]. Unlike prostate-specific antigen (PSA), which is truly prostate specific, other normal tissues like the brush border epithelium of the duodenum and small intestine, renal proximal tubule epithelium, salivary glands, as well as ganglions in nervous system also express PSMA [29–30]. Several other cancers express PSMA, including urothelial cancer of bladder, neo-vasculature of clear cell renal cancer, or endometrial cancer, albeit to a lesser extent than prostate cancer [30–34]. PSMA is a type 2 transmembrane glycoprotein enzyme involved in folate metabolism and is also known as folate hydrolase 1 [35, 36]. In the nervous system, PSMA increases the excitatory neurotransmitter glutamate and is also referred to as glutamate carboxypeptidase II (GCPII) [37]. PSMA activity in peripheral ganglionic tissue may pose a pitfall in interpretation of clinical scans. It is hypothesized that overexpression of this enzyme in malignancies may provide a growth advantage in low folate environments; other proposed functions are involvement in signal transduction and cell migration [38, 39].

The extent of PSMA overexpression in prostate adenocarcinoma correlates with Gleason grade [40, 41]. PSMA is also overexpressed in castration-resistant prostate cancer; cell lines with decreasing androgen sensitivity demonstrate increasing levels of PSMA expression [42]. Androgen-receptor-mediated signaling and PSMA expression are interconnected, and there is an inverse relationship between androgen levels and PSMA gene expression in experimental models [43, 44]. Preclinical studies demonstrate that androgen deprivation therapy (ADT) induces an increase in PSMA expression, although the ultimate effect of androgen deprivation is shrinkage in cell size and apoptosis [43]. Small-sized clinical studies appear to confirm the preclinical data with the difference that in castration-sensitive prostate cancer the rapid involutory effect of ADT appears to outweigh the initial increase in PSMA expression with the net effect of decreased detectability of lesions on PSMA scans [45]. Conversely, castration-resistant prostate cancer may display a more sustained PSMA overexpression or "PSMA flare" at further androgen manipulation with second-generation antiandrogens [46, 45]. However, larger studies in more defined prostate cancer phenotypes are required to confirm these initial observations.

Initial attempts to image prostate cancer using PSMA targeted the intracellular epitope (7E11) with indium-111-conjugated monoclonal antibodies (indium-111 capromab pendetide, ProstaScint ®). This tracer found only limited use due to multiple factors, including the difficulty of the large antibody conjugate reaching the intracellular epitope, which is only exposed in necrotic cells with membrane disruption, as well as its suboptimal imaging properties.

The desired sensitivity and specificity for imaging was subsequently achieved with the development of monoclonal antibodies and especially small molecule ligands to the extracellular domain, particularly the active catalytic site of PSMA [36]. Among monoclonal antibodies, J591 has been most investigated in clinical trials showing good tumor localization [47]. In general, imaging with monoclonal antibodies poses several potential disadvantages, however. First, antibodies have a relatively long circulation time, resulting in a low signal-to-noise ratio due to delayed blood clearance and nonspecific background activity. The delayed blood clearance requires longer times after injection of radiotracer before imaging can be performed with an acceptable signal-to-noise ratio. These properties imply that antibodies must be tagged with longer-lived isotopes, and patients must return typically 3–5 days after the injection for the actual imaging. Available isotopes with long half-lives such as zirconium-89 (Zr-89; physical half-life 78.4 hours) meet this need, but the logistical inconvenience to patients of a multiday study remains. An additional theoretical disadvantage pertains to tumor penetration by the relatively large-sized antibody protein. Use of antibody fragments (like single-chain fragments) might be a possible solution for both challenges [48, 49].

Among several clinically introduced PSMA-targeting small molecule compounds, Ga-68 PSMA–N,N′-bis-[2-hydroxy-5-(carboxyethyl)benzyl]ethylenediamine-N,N′-diacetic acid (68Ga-HBED-CC) also known as Ga-68 PSMA 11 is probably the best studied and most widely clinically used radiotracer (Fig. 8.1). Also, a robust body of literature exists for fluorine-18-conjugated PSMA compounds N-[N-[(S)-1,3-dicarboxypropyl]carbamoyl]-4-18F-fluorobenzyl-l-cysteine, also

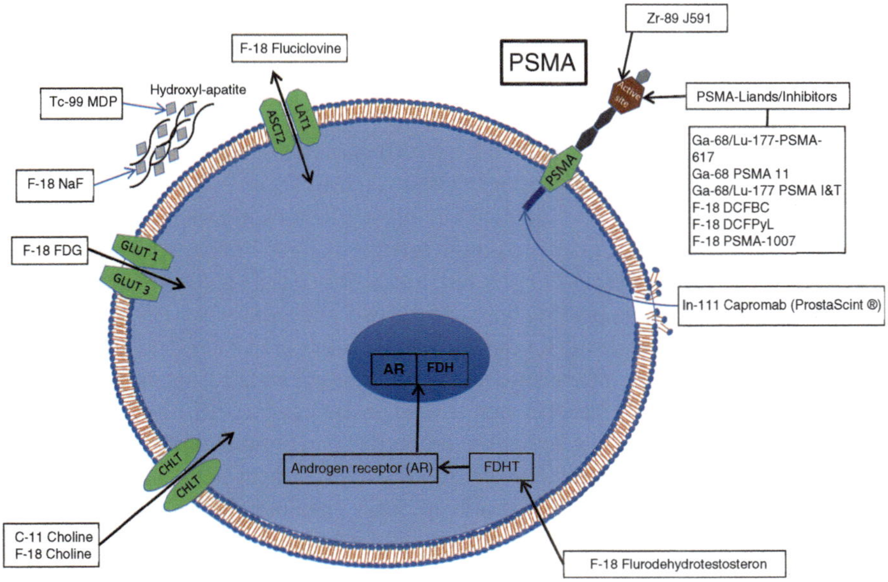

Fig. 8.1 Radiotracer distribution and targets at cellular level. *PSMA* Prostate-specific membrane antigen, *CHLT* Choline transporter, *FDG* Fluorodeoxyglucose, *GLUT* Glucose transporter, *NaF* Sodium fluoride, *MDP* Methylene diphosphonate, *ASCT2* Alanine, serine, cysteine transporter 2, *LAT1* L-type amino acid transporter 1

known as F-18 DCFBC, and the newer iteration 2-(3-[1-carboxy-5-[(6-fluoro-pyridine-3-carbonyl)-amino]-pentyl]-ureido)-pentanedioic, also known as F-18 DCFPyL [50–53]. Ga-68 PSMA 11 and F-18 DCFPyL appear to have similar imaging characteristics and share the mode of urinary excretion posing challenges in the detection of cancer in prostate fossa and in the vicinity of the bladder or ureters. Some centers utilize additional postvoid pelvic images with or without use of a diuretic to mitigate sometimes-faced diagnostic difficulties in the pelvis. Newer PSMA ligands without urinary excretion like F-18 PSMA-1007 or rh-PSMA-7 are promising, but limited data is available on these compounds at the current time [54, 55].

Although PSMA-11 has strong chelating properties for Ga-68, it does not bind the therapeutic radionuclides lutetium-177 (Lu-177) or yittrium-90 (Y-90) with the same stability. Other PSMA ligands including PSMA-671 or PSMA I&T [56] provide more stable binding for the therapeutic radionuclides. The PSMA-617 ligand can be conjugated with Ga-68 for imaging and with Lu-177 for therapy and is the agent used in recent randomized therapeutic clinical trials [57–59]. PSMA-617 features reduced kidney uptake when compared to PSMA-11, which might be of benefit in the therapeutic scenario; however, it also features urinary mode of excretion with slightly slower tracer kinetics than PSMA-11, rendering it less favorable for imaging [60]. PSMA I&T can also be conjugated with Ga-68 and with Lu-177 and demonstrates reduced hepatic uptake, but has lower lesion binding and higher background activity than PSMA-11 with the same mode of urinary excretion [61].

F-18 Fluorodehydrotestosterone PET (F-18 FDHT PET)

Investigational use of F-18 FDHT PET has also garnered special interest in the setting of advanced metastatic prostate cancer. Androgen receptor (AR) signaling plays a crucial role in the development and progression of metastatic prostate cancer. AR expression can be assessed noninvasively by F-18 FDHT, which is an analog of dihydrotestosterone (DHT) [62, 63]. Since FDHT is an analog of endogenous DHT, there is competitive binding between the two molecules for AR, similar to the relation between FDG and high levels of plasma glucose in FDG PET/CT. Therefore, this agent is used in the androgen-deprived or castrate state to obtain good target binding of the tracer. F-18 FDHT enters the cell by passive diffusion through the cell membrane because of its lipophilic properties and combines with AR in cytoplasm before translocating to the nucleus. Of note, treatment with androgen receptor blockers such as apalutamide, bicalutamide, or enzalutamide should be avoided to prevent interference with F-18 FDHT binding to AR [64]. F-18 FDHT has not yet been approved by the FDA for routine clinical use.

A cell-level depiction of distribution and targets of different tracers used in prostate cancer imaging can be found in Fig. 8.1.

Localized Disease/Initial Staging

The difficulty of imaging prostate cancer is in part explained by its often-multifocal presentation on histology within the prostate gland and confounding factors including commonly present benign prostatic hyperplasia or prostatitis. This is why an initial diagnosis is, in many cases, established by systematic sampling of the entire prostate gland as opposed to targeted biopsy of a suspicious lesion, as is the case in many other malignancies. The clinical questions in localized prostate cancer pertain to the presence of unifocal versus multifocal disease, extracapsular extension, seminal vesicle invasion, and neurovascular bundle involvement. In cases of nomogram-predicted high probability of metastasis (intermediate- and high-risk disease), evaluation for metastatic sites, including nodal and osseous disease, becomes relevant at initial staging. The presence of metastatic disease has direct implications for treatment planning and can change the approach from localized treatment to systemic therapy or a combination of both.

The paucity of high-quality data in this realm is in part explained by challenges in trial design, which apply to imaging trials at all stages of prostate cancer but are most tangible in the setting of localized disease. Patients diagnosed with prostate cancer with low risk of metastasis based on elevated PSA who subsequently obtained standard systematic biopsy will undergo radical prostatectomy and template pelvic nodal dissection. Consequently, proposed new imaging modalities in this setting will always be compared to histology as gold standard. As a result, an imaging tool with a technical resolution limit in millimeter range will be compared to microscopy with resolution in micrometer range. Hence, the diagnostic performance of macroscopic imaging modalities invariably suffers in sensitivity; historically, for many clinicians, this has implied a lack of utility. Clinics are increasingly adopting the perspective that not all prostate cancers require treatment and not each microscopic focus is clinically relevant, sparking renewed interest in distinguishing specifically clinically relevant disease. The implementation of new outcome measures in imaging trials — such as the detection of dominant focus of disease, high-grade disease, specificity, or correct localization — has opened new avenues in imaging trial design. Although new molecular imaging probes narrow the gap between macroscopic and microscopic disease, and molecular tracers can overcome size constraints by high levels of target expression, the resolution boundaries of imaging instrumentation and hardware remain a limitation.

Magnetic Resonance Imaging (MRI)

Multiparametric MRI (mpMRI) has changed the imaging landscape of localized prostate cancer by improving on the detection rates of high-grade tumors offered by ultrasound or computed tomography (CT). Due to its high soft tissue resolution,

MRI can also delineate locally advanced disease with relative accuracy, with a sensitivity and specificity for extraprostatic extension of 49% and 82% and for seminal vesicle involvement of 45% and 96% [65, 66]. This anatomical characterization can inform subsequent treatment planning.

In a retrospective study of 150 prostate cancer patients, investigators evaluated the detection of clinically significant prostate cancer (Gleason score ≥4 + 3) by mpMRI and correlated imaging findings with whole mount pathology mapping from subsequent prostatectomy. Using the Prostate Imaging Reporting and Data System version 2 (PI-RADSv2), 94% (118/125) of peripheral zone and 95% (42/44) of transition zone tumors with a tumor volume equal or greater than 0.5 mL were detected. However, only 26% (7/27) of peripheral zone and 20% (2/10) of transition zone tumors with a Gleason score ≥4 + 3, but less than 0.5 mL tumor volume, were identified, pointing out the limited sensitivity in small-volume intermediate- to high-grade lesions [67]. As a result of data like these and others [68], prostate biopsies are increasingly performed based on MRI or as MRI-guided biopsies, in addition to systematic sampling of the prostate. At the current time mpMRI remains the imaging standard of choice for detection and localization of tumor within prostate gland and assessment of extracapsular extension or seminal vesicle involvement.

PET Imaging Probes

Limited data exists evaluating the application of PET agents for intra-gland localization of prostate cancer. Furthermore, many PET agents show similar uptake in prostate cancer, benign prostatic hyperplasia, and prostatitis reducing the ability to localize disease within the prostate. Nevertheless, preliminary data combining newer PET imaging agents with pelvic MRI for primary tumor localization (T-staging) suggest a beneficial effect in diagnostic performance. In a small prospective study of 21 men with prostate cancer, serial 3 Tesla mpMRI of the prostate and F-18 fluciclovine PET/CT within 6-month interval were obtained to evaluate for localization of cancer within prostate. All patients underwent radical prostatectomy for histological confirmation. When all tumors where included, sensitivities and specificities of 67% and 66%, for F-18 fluciclovine PET/CT, and 73% and 79%, for MRI, respectively, were demonstrated. When localization of dominant tumors was assessed, both imaging modalities achieved 90% sensitivity. The combination of both modalities yielded a positive predictive value (PPV) of 82% for localization of any tumor within prostate, a value higher than each modality separately [69].

One can compellingly argue that the most important component of staging is not detection of disease in the prostate, which will be done by biopsy, but the detection of extraglandular disease. For most patients, the pelvic nodes represent the boundary between locoregional and systemic disease and the potential for cure rather than chronic management. Hence, PET imaging has extensively been explored for the purposes of initial staging, with a particular toward assessing the status of the pelvic nodes. There is some prospective evidence for metabolic PET probes like choline

(C-11 or F-18) or F-18 fluciclovine in the setting of initial staging of intermediate- to high-risk prostate cancer. In a prospective study of 210 patients with intermediate- to high-risk prostate cancer, Poulsen et al. evaluated the presence of nodal metastases at initial staging using F-18 choline with histological confirmation by pelvic node dissection. A sensitivity of 73.2% and specificity of 87.6% in per-patient nodal staging was demonstrated. Incidental bone lesions in 18 patients, consistent with metastases, not detected on standard bone scintigraphy, were noted. No central scan reporting or measure of inter-reader agreement was included [70].

Beheshti et al. evaluated F-18 choline PET in a prospective cohort of 130 patients with intermediate- to high-risk prostate cancer. With pathologic confirmation in 111 (85%) patients, a per-patient nodal staging sensitivity and specificity of 45% and 96%, respectively, was found. Interestingly, for lymph node metastases of 5 mm or larger in diameter, an improved sensitivity of 66% (unchanged specificity) was shown. Incidental detection of occult bone metastases in 13 patients was also reported. No central independent reporting or blinding to clinical history of readers was incorporated in the study design [71].

Using F-18 fluciclovine PET/MRI for preoperative lymph node staging in high-risk prostate cancer, Selnaes et al. prospectively evaluated a small cohort of 28 patients and compared findings of PET and MR images, interpreted by separate readers, using 3 Tesla MRI as scan equipment and the mpMRI protocol to assess the prostate. An extended pelvic lymph node dissection was carried out in 26 patients, who comprised the final study cohort. Patient-based sensitivity/specificity for detection of pelvic lymph node metastases was 40%/87.5% for MRI and 40%/100% for F-18 fluciclovine, respectively [72]. No independent central reporting or measure of inter-reader agreement was employed. Although small in size, this study suggests a higher specificity for F-18 fluciclovine than MRI at a similar sensitivity.

Finally, in a meta-analysis of both C-11 and F-18 choline PET, Evangelista et al. evaluated ten studies, the majority of which were prospective small- to moderate-sized cohorts (12–130 patients) including the study by Beheshti et al. (overall 441 patients). In the setting of initial staging of intermediate- to high-risk prostate cancer and employing histological confirmation, a pooled sensitivity of 49% and pooled specificity of 95% was reported [73].

More robust, regulatory-quality contemporary data is available on PET agents that target the prostate-specific membrane antigen (PSMA) for initial staging. The FDA approved Ga-68 PSMA-11 PET in December 2020 and F-18 DCFPyl in May 2021, multiplying the options for FDA-approved agents in the setting of initial staging of prostate cancer with increased risk for metastasis [74, 75]. Both PSMA PET agents appear to have similar imaging characteristics with direct comparisons between the two agents currently lacking. A summary of select studies with emphasis on pivotal trials leading to regulatory approvals of PET agents for initial staging of prostate cancer is provided in Table 8.1.

In the OSPREY study, a prospective multicenter trial, Pienta et al. evaluated the diagnostic performance with sensitivity and specificity as co-primary endpoints of F-18 DCFPyL PET in 252 patients with high-risk prostate cancer undergoing radical prostatectomy with pelvic lymphadenectomy (cohort A). In a separate cohort B,

Table 8.1 Summary of selected studies with emphasis on trials leading to FDA approval of PET agents in initial staging of high-risk prostate cancer

	Total patients	PSA (ng/mL)	Primary endpoint	Central read	Sensitivity (SE) Specificity (SP)	Histopathologic confirmation	Nodal tumor size
Ga-68 PSMA 11							
Hope et al. 2020 [77]	633	Median (range) 11.1 (0.04–147)	SE/SP Detection of PLNM	Yes	SE 40% SP 95%	277 patients (44%)	Average 10 mm in TP Average 4 mm in FN
F-18 DCFPyL							
Osprey, Pienta et al. 2021 [76]	268	Median (range) 9.7 (1.2–125.3)	SE/SP Detection of PLNM	Yes	SE 40.3% SP 97.9%	252 patients (94%)	For >5 mm SE 60% SP 97.9%
F-18 Choline							
Beheshti et al. 2010 [71]	130	Range 0.25–462	SE/SP Detection of PLNM	No	SE 45% SP 96%	111 patients (85%)	For ≥5 mm SE 66% SP 97.9%
3 Tesla MRI							
von Below et al. 2016 [68]	40	Range 10–20	SE/SP Detection of PLNM	No	SE 55% SP 90%	40 patients (100%)	Average 12.3 mm in TP Average 5.2 mm in FN

FN False negative, *TP* True positive, *SE* Sensitivity, *SP* Specificity, *PSMA* Prostate-specific membrane antigen, *PLNM* Pelvic nodal metastasis, *PET* Positron emission tomography

93 evaluable prostate cancer patients with suspected recurrence or metastases on conventional imaging undergoing biopsies were enrolled. Central independent reporting of scans with blinding to clinical information was obtained and measures of inter-reader and intra-reader agreement provided. In cohort A, a median specificity of 97.9% and median sensitivity of 40.3% (the latter not meeting the prespecified endpoint for sensitivity) was reported. In a post hoc sensitivity analysis of cohort A, exploring detection of nodal metastases larger than 5 mm, assuming that smaller tumor foci are below PET detection limits, resulted in a sensitivity of 60%

(unchanged high specificity), meeting the prespecified confidence bounds for sensitivity. For cohort B, the median sensitivity and PPV for extraprostatic lesions were 95.8% and 81.9%, respectively. F-18 DCFPyL PET, although similar in sensitivity to conventional imaging, including CT and MRI, demonstrated consistently higher specificity and PPVs in the setting of initial staging of high-risk prostate cancer [76].

Similarly, Hope et al. evaluated the sensitivity and specificity of Ga-68 PSMA PET for nodal detection in a prospective multicenter cohort of 633 patients with intermediate- to high-risk prostate cancer. Scans were read by independent central readers blinded to clinical information. A majority rule was applied for final consensus interpretation. With histopathologic confirmation by way of pelvic nodal dissection in 277 patients (44%), a per-patient sensitivity of 40% and specificity of 95% were demonstrated. Also in this trial, the size of nodal involvement was associated with detectability with an average node size of 10 mm in true-positive patients as compared to 4 mm in false-negative patients [77].

In the proPSMA trial, a prospective multicenter randomized study with crossover design, authors investigated the accuracy of Ga-68 PSMA PET as first-line imaging compared to CT and bone scan for detection of pelvic nodal and distant metastases in patients with high-risk prostate cancer. Patients either underwent curative-intent surgery or radiotherapy. A predefined reference standard including histopathology, imaging, and biochemistry at 6-month follow-up was applied. Scans were reported by central independent readers in addition to local readers, and high measures of inter-reader agreement were reported. Of 339 assessed patients for eligibility, 302 men were randomly assigned equally to the two study arms. Patients crossed over unless three or more distant metastases were identified. Of 295 (98%) men with follow-up, 87 (30%) had pelvic nodal or distant metastatic disease. Conventional imaging including CT and bone scan had lower sensitivity (38% vs. 85%) and lower specificity (91% vs. 98%) compared with PSMA PET-CT. In addition, management changes occurred more frequently with PSMA PET as compared to conventional imaging (28% vs. 15%), and PSMA PET conveyed less equivocal findings than conventional imaging (7% vs. 23%). Furthermore, in patients with second-line imaging following crossover, more management changes ensued after second-line PSMA PET versus second-line conventional imaging in 27% versus 5%, respectively. The authors concluded that PSMA PET is a suitable replacement for combined CT and bone scan in initial staging of high-risk prostate cancer [78].

The proPSMA trial provided compelling high-quality evidence that PSMA PET can replace bone scan and CT in the initial staging of high-risk prostate cancer and can be considered practice-changing. However, the initial T-staging of high-risk prostate cancer will continue to rely on mpMRI, due to the shortcomings of currently available PSMA PET agents in the evaluation of the prostate gland, which relate in part to urine PSMA excretion and normal mild PSMA expression in prostatic tissue.

Biochemical Recurrent (BCR) Prostate Cancer

Biochemical recurrence follows initial definitive treatment with curative intent, either with radical prostatectomy or radiation therapy. This crucial disease state represents recurrence without radiographic evidence of disease by standard techniques. Biochemical recurrence is defined as when prostate-specific antigen (PSA) values rise above 0.2 ng/mL after radical prostatectomy or rise 2 ng/mL or more above the nadir PSA following definitive radiation therapy of the prostate (ASTRO Phoenix consensus definition) [79]. About 20–40% of patients after radical prostatectomy [80–82] and 30–50% after radiation therapy [83] develop biochemical recurrence 10 years after treatment. The importance of this disease state and interest in more accurate imaging modalities rests on the assumption that early accurate detection of recurrent disease constitutes a window of opportunity for curative or "salvage" treatment. For instance, the RADICALS-RT randomized prospective phase III trial, comparing adjuvant radiation therapy versus salvage radiation in 1396 men after prostatectomy with high-risk features for progression (i.e., pT3/4 disease, Gleason score 7–10, positive margins, or preoperative PSA level >10 ng/mL), supported early salvage radiation therapy over adjuvant radiation [84]. The results of this trial further increased the interest of clinicians in better characterization of recurrent disease at low PSA values.

While the patterns of recurrence are variable, some clinicopathological characteristics can help predict sites of recurrent disease which in turn can guide treatment decisions. For example, in patients with positive surgical margins after radical prostatectomy, local recurrence is more common [85]. On the other hand, biochemical recurrence within 6 months of radical prostatectomy, short PSA doubling time, and unsurprisingly nodal involvement on pathology are predictors of metastasis [86–88].

Historically, patients with BCR underwent imaging with abdominopelvic computed tomography and bone scan. However, these imaging modalities have limited sensitivity. For instance, a standard bone scan is positive for metastatic disease in less than 5% of cases if the PSA value is below 7 ng/mL in the biochemical recurrence setting [89–91]. Similarly, CT studies in men experiencing BCR after surgery with a mean PSA value in the range of 2.4–33.1 ng/mL detect disease in only 11–14% of patients [92, 93].

One conundrum in clinical trial design in this setting in developing new imaging modalities is the establishment of a reference standard or gold standard. Often, the ideal scenario of obtaining histological confirmation in lesions detected by imaging is not feasible or possible due to small size, location, multiplicity, or patient preference. In such situations, many well-designed studies establish a composite reference of "truth" based on subsequent imaging or PSA response to targeted therapy. As in the setting of initial staging of prostate cancer, the utility of F-18 FDG PET and F-18 NaF PET is not well established in the biochemical recurrence setting and has not been tested in well-designed prospective trials.

In the following section, FDA-approved PET agents in the biochemical recurrent setting will be discussed.

C-11 Choline or F-18 Choline PET

In the setting of BCR prostate cancer after radical prostatectomy or radiation therapy, the US Food and Drug Administration (FDA) approved in 2012 the use of C-11 choline PET after noninformative conventional imaging.

In a retrospective study of 176 patients with biochemical recurrence and a median PSA of 7.2 ng/mL, investigators evaluated the detection of recurrent disease by C-11 choline PET. Patients had undergone either a radical prostatectomy, radiation therapy, or cryoablation as initial treatment. Studies were reported as clinical reads by local readers with access to clinical information and prior imaging. No measures of inter-reader agreement were investigated. Histological confirmation was obtained in 73 patients (41%) with conventional imaging (CT, bone scan, and MRI) serving as confirmation in remaining cases. A per-patient sensitivity of 93%, specificity of 76%, PPV of 91%, and an overall detection rate of 75% (132/176) were reported. Sites of detection were in the pelvic lymph nodes (68 of 132, 51.5%), prostatectomy bed (38 of 132, 38.8%), skeleton (26 of 132, 19.7%), mediastinum (3 of 132, 2.3%), and prostate (14 of 132, 10.6%). Detection rates based on PSA value were 31% at less than 0.5 ng/mL, 56% for 0.5–1.0 ng/mL, 68% for 1.1–2.0 ng/mL, 84% for 2.1–5.0 ng/mL, and 89% above 5 ng/mL. The value of 2 ng/mL was proposed as the best cutoff to distinguish a positive scan from a negative scan with a probability value of 0.73. Findings on C-11 choline PET were deemed clinically useful and lead to a management change in 56% [94].

In a retrospective cohort of 358 patients with biochemical recurrence (mean PSA 3.77 ng/mL) after radical prostatectomy, the diagnostic performance of C-11 choline and detection rates for C-11 choline at different PSA values were studied. PET/CT findings were validated using histological criteria in 13% (46/358) of patients and follow-up clinical and imaging criteria in 87% (312/358). Scans were interpreted by local readers independently with knowledge of clinical history and consensus resolutions of discrepancies. An interobserver agreement of 94% was reported. Sensitivity, specificity, PPV, negative predictive value, and overall accuracy were 85%, 93%, 91%, 87%, and 89%, respectively. Overall detection rate was 45% (161/358) with detection rate per anatomical region of 66% in lymph nodes, 34% in prostatectomy bed, and 29% in skeleton [95]. Detection rates correlated with PSA value, with 13% in PSA equal or less than 0.6 ng/ml, 29% for 0.6–1 ng/mL, 46% for 1–2 ng/mL, 60% for 2–5 ng/mL, and 83% above 5 ng/mL.

In a more contemporary retrospective cohort of 287 patients with biochemical recurrence (median PSA 0.94 ng/mL) after surgery or radiotherapy, investigators used C-11 choline PET for localization of recurrent disease. Two local readers, one blinded to clinical information and one unblinded, reported separately on each study utilizing a 3-point scale (0 = negative, 1 = equivocal, 2 = positive), with a consensus read constituting the final designation. Intra-reader and inter-reader concordance were 86% and 76%, respectively. When scores 1 and 2 were considered positive, an overall detection rate of 66% was found, and PSA level detection rates of 45% for less than 0.5 ng/mL, 56% for 0.5–0.99 ng/mL, 70% for 1.0–1.99 ng/mL, and 90%

for equal or greater than 2.0 ng/mL were obtained. Considering only scores of 2 as positive, the overall detection rate was 54%, and PSA cutoff detection rates were of 28%, 46%, 62%, and 81%, PSA less than 0.5 ng/mL, 0.5–0.99 ng/mL, 1.0–1.99 ng/mL, and equal or greater than 2.0 ng/mL, respectively, were reported. In the final consensus read, 47 (16.4%) scans were equivocal. Histological confirmation was obtained in 49 patients (17%). Patterns of recurrence were overall 20.3% in the prostate bed, 48% in the pelvic nodes, 5.6% in the extrapelvic lymph nodes, 10.5% in bone, and 1.4% in visceral metastases (17.8% extrapelvic metastases). Recurrent sites outside the initial treatment field were observed in 28% of patients [96].

A meta-analysis of 18 in majority retrospective studies including two of studies mentioned above, with a total of 2126 patients, demonstrated a pooled detection rate of 62% and a pooled sensitivity and specificity of 89% and 89%, respectively [97]. The studies varied in inclusion of patients after radical prostatectomy, radiation therapy, or both as well as in PSA value at time of imaging with a mean and median PSA ranging from 0.9 ng/ml to 21.1 ng/ml and 0.5 ng/ml to 10.7 ng/ml, respectively. Reporting of scans varied across studies and some studies used readers blinded to clinical history to interpret results. All studies used a composite reference standard including histology (in average 26%), other imaging (CT, MRI, and bone scan), and clinical follow-up for more than 12 months, including repeated imaging after treatment. Pooled detection rates among studies were 27% for local recurrence, 36% for nodal metastasis, and 25% for bone metastasis.

F-18 Fluciclovine

The diagnostic performance of F-18 fluciclovine in comparison to In-111 capromab pendetide was evaluated in a prospective single-center cohort of 50 patients with BCR (mean PSA 6.62 ng/mL) after definitive therapy for prostate cancer including prostatectomy and radiation therapy. Studies were each interpreted by two local readers with disagreement resolved by consensus. No measures of interobserver agreement were explored. The reference standard was a combination of tissue correlation in 18% (9/50), imaging, laboratory, and clinical data. F-18 fluciclovine had a disease detection sensitivity and specificity in the prostate bed of 89% and 67% and a sensitivity of 100% and specificity of 100% in extraprostatic recurrence. F-18 fluciclovine was more sensitive than In-111 capromab pendetide SPECT/CT in the detection of recurrent prostate carcinoma [98]. One might argue that the comparison to In-111 capromab pendetide, which is FDA approved in BCR setting, is not clinically relevant.

In a multicenter retrospective study including 596 patients with BCR after initial therapy, including prostatectomy and radiation therapy, an overall detection rate of 67.7% by F-18 fluciclovine was reported [99]. Image interpretation was based on clinical reads without utilization of central blinded readers. Anatomic site-specific detection rates were 38.7% in the prostate/prostate bed, 32.6% in pelvic lymph nodes, and 26.2% for metastatic involvement outside the pelvis. The overall detection rate based on PSA level was 41.4% in the PSA range of 0.79 ng/ml or less, approximately 60% (45% for extraprostatic disease) in the range 0.8–2.03 ng/ml, approximately 75% (45% for extraprostatic disease) in the range 2.04–6.00 ng/ml, and approximately 85% (approximately 60% for extraprostatic disease) for PSA above 6 ng/mL. Based on histological confirmation in 143 patients, a lesion-based overall PPV of 62.2% with site-specific PPV of 92.3% for extraprostatic lesions and 71.8% for prostate/prostate bed involvement was described. Patient-based sensitivity, specificity, and PPV were, 91%, 40%, and 82%. The authors associate the suboptimal specificity and PPV with confounding factors that occur when the prostate is still in place, caused by overlap of activity with prostatitis and BPH as well as, in part, sampling errors for histology. This assumption is supported by the relatively high proportion of patients after radiotherapy for prostate cancer in the cohort and discrepantly low lesion-based PPV for prostate/prostate bed lesions as compared to extraprostatic sites of disease.

In the LOCATE trial, a prospective multicenter study of 213 patients in BCR setting (median PSA 1.0 ng/mL), the authors evaluated as a primary endpoint the change in planned treatment. The study results were based on clinical reads without central readers or blinding of interpreters to clinical information. No routine histological confirmation was pursued, and diagnostic test performance was not the primary goal of the study. A detection rate of F-18 fluciclovine-avid lesions in 122 patients (57%) was reported. The detection rate was 30% in the prostate/prostate bed and 38% outside the prostate, i.e., 29% in lymph nodes, 2.3% in soft tissue, and 11% in bone.

Detection rates based on PSA values in this trial were 31% for PSA ranges of 0–0.5 ng/ml, 50% for PSA 0.5–1.0 ng/ml, 66% for PSA 1.0–2.0 ng/ml, approximately 75% for PSA 2.0–5.0 ng/mL, and approximately 87% above 5 ng/mL. A change in management after the scan was instated in 59% of patients [100].

The differences in detection rate between the different studies are explained by their different populations — e.g., radical prostatectomy patients versus patients after radiation therapy with prostate gland in situ — as well as different PSA cutoff values. A recent systematic review and meta-analysis reported a pooled sensitivity of 0.79 (95% CI 0.60–0.91) and a pooled specificity of 0.69 (95% CI 0.59–0.77) for F-18 fluciclovine for BCR prostate cancer [101].

The higher diagnostic yield by F-18 fluciclovine PET compared to conventional imaging including CT, bone scan, or MRI has repercussions in assessment of eligibility for and planning of radiation therapy (RT). The EMPIRE-1 study, a single-center, phase II/III trial, randomized 165 patients with biochemical recurrence and negative conventional imaging to either standard template-based RT versus RT informed by F-18 fluciclovine PET [102]. All patients had prior radical prostatectomy with a median PSA of 0.34 ng/mL at time of recurrence. Radiation fields included the prostate bed, with or without inclusion of pelvic lymph nodes. The primary outcome was 3-year event-free survival, defined as biochemical recurrence or progression, or initiation of systemic therapy. Four patients in the F-18 fluciclovine PET group were deemed ineligible for RT due to extrapelvic or skeletal lesions. With a median follow-up of 3.5 years, a significant difference in event-free survival of 63.0% (95% confidence interval 49.2–74.0) in the conventional imaging group versus 75.5% (95% confidence interval 62.5–84.6) in the F-18 fluciclovine PET group (difference 12.5; 95% confidence interval 4.3–20.8; $p = 0.0028$) was observed. This study indicates that beyond improvements in diagnostic test performance, this new-generation PET agent translates into tangible clinical benefit. Similar maturing radiation therapy clinical trials evaluating PSMA-PET tracers and comparing PSMA PET to F-18 fluciclovine PET are underway and will likely better inform indication and planning of radiation therapy for BCR prostate cancer.

Ga-68 or F-18 Prostate-Specific Membrane Antigen (PSMA)

Based on FDA approval of Ga-68 PSMA-11 PET in December 2020 and F-18 DCFPyl in May 2021 also in the BCR setting, concomitant with time of compilation of this book chapter, the choices of FDA-approved agents in this disease state of prostate cancer have further expanded [74, 75]. Both PSMA PET agents appear to have also similar imaging characteristics in BCR scenario with head-to-head comparisons currently not available.

A prospective multicenter trial of Ga-68 PSMA evaluated 635 patients with biochemical recurrence (median PSA 2.1 ng/mL) after radical prostatectomy or radiation therapy with the endpoints of PPV, detection rate, and inter-reader reproducibility, using central readers with three independent reads per study and blinding of readers to clinical information or prior imaging. Lesions were validated by histopathologic analysis in 87 patients and a composite reference standard in remaining cases. An overall detection rate of 75% and site-specific detection rate of 26% in prostate bed/prostate, 38% in pelvic lymph nodes (N1 disease), 17% in extrapelvic lymph nodes or visceral organs (M1a/M1c disease), 16% in bones (M1c disease), and 7% in multiple sites (Multiple M1) were reported [103]. Overall, 35% had pelvic-only disease and 49% extrapelvic involvement. Detection rates based on PSA cutoffs were 38% for PSA values less than 0.5 ng/mL, 57% for PSA 0.5–1.0 ng/mL, 84% for PSA 1.0–2.0 ng/mL, 86% for PSA 2.0–5.0 ng/mL, and 97% for PSA values above 5.0 ng/mL. A patient-based PPV of 84% by histopathologic validation was demonstrated and 92% by composite reference standard where no histopathologic confirmation was available. Interestingly, several cases of false-positive interpretation were intraprostatic lesions after radiation therapy [103].

The CONDOR trial, a prospective multicenter study of F-18 DCFPyL PSMA PET, evaluated 208 men after primary therapy including prostatectomy and radiation therapy for prostate cancer, who were experiencing biochemical relapse (median PSA 0.8 ng/mL) without evidence of disease on conventional imaging [53]. The primary endpoint of the study was correct localization rate (CLR), a term that corresponds to PPV with the additional requirement of anatomical colocalization. This endpoint as corresponded to the F-18 DCFPyL PET-positive lesions that met the criteria of the study's composite standard of truth. The reference standard of truth consisted of histopathology in 31 patients, correlative imaging in 100 patients, and PSA response after radiation therapy in one patient. Central independent readers blinded to clinical information as well as local readers were utilized. A CLR of 84.8–87.0% was reported. This finding translates to a 13.0–15.2% false-positive rate. Region-based PPVs were 79.5% for prostate/prostatic bed, 70.9% for pelvic lymph nodes, 67.4% for extrapelvic metastasis (M1), 61.5% for extrapelvic lymph nodes (M1a), 62.5% for bone (M1b), and 28.6% for visceral disease. The overall detection rate was 59–66% and rose with PSA values, with 36% at less than 0.5 ng/mL, 51% for 0.5–1.0 ng/mL, 67% for 1.0–2.0 ng/mL, 85% for 2.0–5.0 ng/mL, and 97% for 5.0 ng/mL and above. A change in intended management occurred in 63.9% of evaluable patients. A high inter-reader and intra-reader agreement was achieved.

There is a paucity of data comparing C-11 choline/F-18 choline, F-18 fluciclovine, and Ga-68 PSMA-11/F-18 PSMA DCFPyL in the setting of BCR prostate cancer. In a small prospective study of 50 patients with BCR after radical prostatectomy undergoing F-18 fluciclovine and C-11 choline PET scans, overall detection rates were 34% versus 22% (37 lesions vs. 23 lesions, respectively, p-value < 0.0001) [104]. Site-specific detection rates for F-18 fluciclovine and C-11 choline were 10% versus 6% for local recurrence (5 vs. 3 lesions, p-value < 0.0001), 20% versus 10% for nodal disease (15 vs. 6 lesions, p-value < 0.0001), and 10% versus 8% for bone metastasis (17 vs. 14 lesions, p-value < 0.0001), respectively. Detection rates based on PSA cutoff values were 21% versus 14% below 1 ng/mL, 20% versus 13% for 1–2 ng/mL, 33% versus 17% for 2–3 ng/mL, and 60% versus 40% above 3 ng/mL. It is hypothesized that the suggested superiority of F-18 fluciclovine over C-11 choline may have biological underpinnings. For example, in prostate cancer cell lines, fluciclovine uptake is higher than choline, acetate, or methionine uptake [105, 106].

Another small, prospective study comparing Ga-68 PSMA-11 to F-18 fluciclovine demonstrated higher detection rates with PSMA-11 PET, especially in the low PSA range. A head-to-head comparison of 50 patients experiencing biochemical recurrence after prostatectomy and with PSA range of 2 ng/mL or less demonstrated an overall detection rate of 56% for Ga-68 PSMA-11 versus 26% for F-18 fluciclovine (Odds ratio of 4.8, 95% CI 1.6–19.2; p-value = 0.0026) [107]. In the same study, site-specific detection rates of Ga-68 PSMA-11 and F-18 fluciclovine were 30% versus 8% (Odds ratio 12.0, 95% CI 1·8–513·0, p = 0·0034) for pelvic nodal disease and 16% versus 0% for any extrapelvic lesions (Odds ratio and CI non-estimable, p-value = 0·0078), respectively. Of note, detection of local recurrence in the prostate bed suggested a trend towards superior detection with F-18 fluciclovine (14% vs. 18%), although this finding remains hypothesis-generating and in need of further evaluation.

In the absence of high-quality comparative evidence, it appears prudent to combine pelvic MRI with PSMA PET (if available) for local pelvic evaluation of disease in the BCR setting. In fact, based on physiologic excretion of Ga-68 PSMA and F-18 PSMA PET agents, evaluation of local recurrence in prostatic fossa may be compromised. Furthermore, PSMA PET has limited sensitivity in detection of recurrent prostate cancer within prostate gland after radiation therapy, likely due to false-positive PSMA activity in postradiation inflammatory prostate gland changes [103]. F-18 fluciclovine is the only approved PET agent in the BCR setting with no or limited urinary excretion and may be considered as a tracer to evaluate suspected or equivocal findings in the prostatic surgical bed.

The advent of new targeted molecular imaging tracers like PSMA that can better detect disease will serve to redefine disease states. For example, patients considered to have non-metastatic castration-resistant prostate cancer (nmCRPC) based on conventional imaging will likely be reclassified with better imaging tools, as having metastatic disease. A vivid demonstration of this stage migration was published in a retrospective review of 200 patients classified as nmCRPC based on conventional imaging at six different centers who then underwent PSMA PET imaging. Central review revealed that 196 patients had positive scans, with 55% reclassified as having M1 disease despite negative conventional imaging [108]. This stage migration has significant implications for clinical trial design in terms of defining both eligibility criteria and relapse.

Approximately 5–10% of prostate cancers do not express PSMA to a significant degree on immunohistochemistry (IHC) [109]. These cancers are as expected PSMA-PET negative [110, 111]. Furthermore, there is heterogeneity in the intensity and extent of PSMA expression in primary tumors and to a lesser degree also in lymph node metastases on IHC [112, 113]. Although prior reports show strong associations between tumor grade and PSMA expression, even high-grade and high-volume metastatic disease can be PSMA-negative [113]. There appears to be a correlation between PSMA expression in the primary tumor (or percentage of tumor negative for PSMA) and nodal metastasis, which is associated with PSMA-PET detectability [113].

An illustration of different PET tracers commonly used in biochemical settings is provided in Fig. 8.2. Table 8.2 summarizes select studies with an emphasis on pivotal trials leading to regulatory approvals of PET agents for BCR prostate cancer.

Metastatic Prostate Cancer

In the United States, 5% of patients present with a diagnosis of metastatic disease, versus 77% with localized and 11% with regional disease [114]. Approximately, 15% of patients with localized disease treated with curative intent primary therapy develop metastatic disease with most frequent sites in lymph nodes (38.2%) and bones (36.8%) [115]. In the United States, a 5-year survival for metastatic prostate cancer improved from 28.7% from 2001–2005 to 32.3% from 2011–2016 [114]. This is at least in part related to expanded effective treatment strategies.

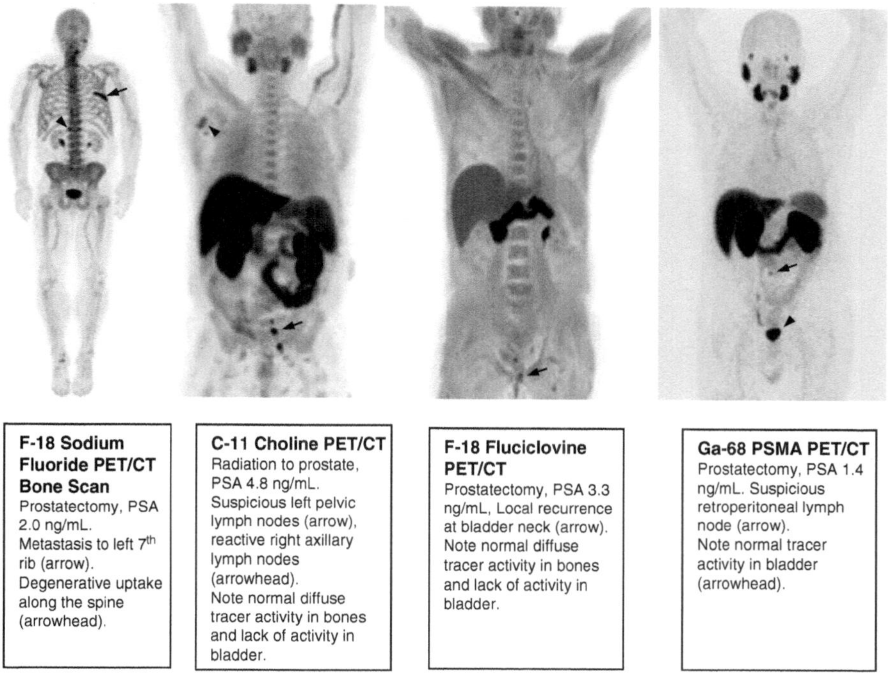

Fig. 8.2 Use of different PET probes in biochemical recurrence prostate cancer. *PET* Positron emission tomography, *CT* Computed tomography, *PSA* Prostate-specific antigen

Treatment Response

The purpose of imaging in advanced metastatic disease is to describe the extent of disease, provide information on response to therapy, and define the etiology of clinical symptoms, such as pathologic fractures or cord compression. Cornerstones of imaging at this stage remain conventional imaging, including bone scan, CT, and MRI. Computed tomography is of value to delineate nodal disease and visceral involvement. MRI is helpful in better characterizing visceral disease with the probable exception of lung and early bone metastases. The standard MDP bone scan remains relevant in the metastatic setting and is included in the recommendations of the Prostate Cancer Clinical Trial Working Group 3 (PCWG 3) for assessment of osseous metastatic disease in clinical trials [116]. These criteria for defining radiographic progression in metastatic prostate cancer are a prospectively validated measure of progression that correlates well with overall survival and has therefore earned regulatory recognition for the purposes of new drug approval [117–119]. According to PCWG 3 recommendations, progression of osseous disease is confirmed only if two or more lesions appear on first bone scan after initiation of therapy and at least an additional two lesions are seen on the subsequent bone scan at least 6 weeks later. At later time points in the course of treatment, osseous progression is established if at least two new confirmed lesions appear relative to the first

Table 8.2 Summary of select studies with emphasis on trials leading to FDA approval of PET agents in BCR prostate cancer

	Total patients	Study design	PSA (ng/mL)	Primary outcome	Initial treatment	Central read	Detection rate (overall/ per region)	Detection Rate by PSA (ng/mL) stratification		Pathologic confirmation
F-18/C-11 choline										
Mitchell et al. 2013 [94]	176	Retro	Median (range) 7.2 (2.2–1028.0)	SE, SP, DR	RP, RT, Cryo	No	75% PR: 10.6% PB: 38.8% PLN: 51.5% Bone: 19.7% Visc: 2.3%	<0.5 0.5–1.0 1.1–2.0 2.1 to 5.0 >5.0	31% 56% 68% 84% 89%	73 pts. (41%)
Michaud et al. 2020 [96]	287	Retro	Median (range) 0.94 (0.15–89.9)	DR	RP, RT	No	66% PB: 20.3% PLN: 48%% EPLN: 5.6% Bone: 10.5% Visc: 1.4% EP: 17.8%	<0.5 0.5–0.99 1.0–1.99 ≥2.0	45% (28%)[a] 56% (46%)[a] 70% (62%)[a] 90% (81%)[a]	49 pts. (17%)
F-18 Fluciclovine										
Schuster et al. 2011 [98]	50	Pros	Mean (range) 6.62 (0.11–44.74)	SE, SP, DR	RP, RT, Cryo, HIFU	No	PB: 74% SE: 89% SP: 67% EPD: 24% SE: 100% SP: 100%	N/A		PB: 46 pts. (92%) EPD: 9 pts. (18%)
Bach-Gansmo et al., 2017 [99]	596	Retro	Median (range) 2.0 (0.05–82.0)	DR, SE, SP, PPV	RP, RT, other	No	DR: 67.7% PR/PB: 38.7% PLN: 32.6% EP: 26.2%	≤0.79 0.8–2.03 2.04–6.00 >6	41.4% 60% 75% 85%	143 pts. (24%)

LOCATEAndriole et al. 2019 [100]	213	Pros	Median (range) 1.0 (0.2–93.5)	DR, change in management	RP, RT, Cryo, HIFU	No	DR: 57% PR/PB: 30% LN: 29% Bone: 11% Visc: 2.3% EPD: 38%	0–0.5 0.5–1.0 1.0–2.0 2.0–5.0 > 5	31% 50% 66% 75% 87%	N/A
Ga-68 PSMA 11										
Fendler et al. 2019 [103]	635	Pros	Median (range) 2.1 (0.1–1154)	AC	RP, RT	Yes	DR: 75% PR/PB: 26% PLN: 38% EPLN/Visc: 17% Bone: 16% Multiple sites: 38% EPD: 49%	<0.5 0.5 to <1.0 1.0 to <2.0 2.0 to <5.0 ≥5.0	38% 57% 84% 86% 97%	87 pts. (13.7%)
F-18 DCFPyL-PSMA										
CONDOR Morris et al. 2020 [131]	208	Pros	Median (range) 0.8 (0.17–98.4)	CLR, PPV	RP, RT	Yes	DR 59–66% PPV per region: PR/PB: 79.5% PLN: 70.9% EP: 67.4% EPLN: 61.5% Bone: 62.5% Visc: 28.6%	< 0.5 0.5 to <1.0 1.0 to <2.0 2.0 to <5.0 ≥5.0	36% 51% 67% 85% 97%	31 pts. (14.9%)

[a]When equivocal reads considered negative

RP Radical prostatectomy, *RT* Radiation therapy, *Cryo* Cryosurgery, *Retro* Retrospective, *Pros* Prospective, *SE* Sensitivity, *SP* Specificity, *DR* Detection rate, *CLR* Correct localization rate, *AC* Accuracy, *PPV* Positive predictive value, *PB* Prostate bed, *PR* Prostate, *PLN* Pelvic lymph nodes, *EPLN* Extrapelvic lymph nodes, *LN* Lymph nodes, *Visc* Visceral, *EP* Extrapelvic metastasis, *EPD* Extraprostatic disease, *PET* Positron emission tomography, *HIFU* High-intensity modulated ultrasound, pts. Patients, *N/A* Not available on-treatment scan [116]. These recommendations avoid misinterpreting a flare after initiation of therapy as progression or transient benign osseous foci as disease. However, few prospective studies have examined, much less validated, a definition for response assessments for new imaging modalities.

F-18 NaF bone scan has capabilities similar to the MDP bone scan, with increased sensitivity and more precise quantification stemming from the addition of improved resolution based on PET technology. Several studies demonstrate the value of NaF-PET bone scan for quantification of osseous metastatic burden, response to therapy, and differentiation between flare phenomena and true progression in bone-only metastatic prostate cancer [120, 121]. Nonetheless, F-18 NaF is still limited to imaging bone, rather than any quality of the tumor itself.

In all likelihood, PSMA will be used to assess treatment response for metastatic disease; however, studies validating how a meaningful change on a PSMA scan manifests have yet to be performed.

Biologic Characterization

FDG-PET provides prognostic information on dedifferentiating prostate cancer with high glycolytic activity [7, 11, 12] and is frequently used at some centers in this stage of disease. It has received increasing scrutiny for its potential role in identifying aggressive cancers that may have undergone treatment-emergent lineage plasticity, which occurs as a complex adaptive process involving both genomic and epigenetic factors when prostate cancers are subjected to androgen signaling inhibition [122–126]. Preliminary studies have indicated that FDG has a role in identifying neuroendocrine prostate cancer on a lesional level [127]; even more provocatively, FDG has been combined with FDHT to directly image for the presence of androgen receptor expression with an intact ligand binding domain. In a cohort of 133 men with metastatic castration-resistant prostate cancer (mCRPC) who were naïve to androgen receptor signaling inhibitors (ARSi), Fox et al. performed serial FDG PET/CT and FDHT PET/CT scans evaluating for glycolysis and androgen receptor expression patterns with correlation to overall survival. In 2405 lesions, the following imaging phenotypes emerged: 71.2% with both FDG and FDHT avidity, 16.0% with FDHT but not FDG avidity, and 12.7% with FDG but not FDHT avidity. The latter group would be expected to have the most similarities to a population undergoing lineage plasticity, and indeed these patients had the worst prognosis of any group. The study demonstrated that the heterogeneity of the PET/CT phenotype has clinical relevance on a lesion and patient level. Most lesions expressed androgen receptors, consistent with the initial benefit of second-line ARSi drugs in the mCRPC setting. At the same time, on a patient level, 49% had at least one lesion without FDHT uptake and with FDG uptake — the imaging phenotype with the most negative effect on survival, possibly due to ARSi resistance [128]. This work must be considered preliminary, with future studies comparing imaging findings and biologic correlates.

The ability to noninvasively assess AR expression can be used as part of drug development as a pharmacodynamic marker. FDHT was indeed used in the original dose-finding studies for both enzalutamide and apalutamide to establish AR saturation and occupancy and can be used for the development of new classes of AR-degrading agents or inhibitors for pre-treatment stratification, planning of clinical trials, and response assessment [129, 130].

Theranostics

With the advent of new therapeutic avenues using PSMA-targeting radionuclide therapies, the use of molecular imaging to determine PSMA expression as part of a theranostic approach in advanced prostate cancer will grow increasingly relevant in the near future. Emerging data support the use of lutetium-177 PSMA-targeted therapy in the setting of advanced metastatic prostate cancer. In the TheraP trial, a randomized phase II multicenter trial evaluating lutetium-177 PSMA-617 (Lu-177 PSMA) versus cabazitaxel in patients with metastatic castration-resistant prostate cancer [59], 200 patients underwent Ga-68 PSMA-11 PET as well as F-18 FDG PET imaging as part of their eligibility assessment. Patients included in the study were those with PSMA-expressing disease and no sites of metastatic disease with discordant FDG-positivity and PSMA-negative findings. A case of discordant PSMA PET and FDG PET is illustrated in Fig. 8.3. PSA responses were significantly more frequent among patients in the Lu-177 PSMA arm than in the cabazitaxel arm: 65% versus 37% (66% vs. 37% by intention to treat; difference 29% [95% CI 16–42; $p < 0{\cdot}0001$; and 66% vs. 44% by treatment received; difference 23% [95% CI 9–37; $p = 0{\cdot}0016$]).

The international VISION trial, a randomized open-label phase III study evaluating Lu-177 PSMA-617 plus standard of care (SOC) in men with PSMA-positive mCRPC versus SOC alone, recently reported similarly positive outcomes with significantly improved primary endpoint of overall survival in the Lu-177 PSMA-617 group (median OS, 15.3 vs. 11.3 months; HR, 0.62 [95% CI: 0.52, 0.74]; $p < 0.001$, one-sided). The other primary endpoint, radiologic progression-free survival (rPFS), was also strongly positive, with a 60% reduction in the risk of radiographic progression or death and a 5-month improvement in time to rPFS (HR = 0.40, $p < 0.001$, median 8.7 vs. 3.4 months). These patients were selected only on the basis of Ga-68 PSMA 11 scans alone with no FDG imaging. Eighty-seven percent of the patients were allowed into the study on the basis of a positive PSMA PET scan, with only 13% screen-failing by imaging criteria. These data would suggest that FDG imaging may not be necessary to identify patients who will clinically benefit from therapeutic lutetium-based PSMA-directed radioligand therapy. Whether or not FDG further improves outcomes, or PSMA alone is sufficient, or even the relationship between either imaging modality or a treatment benefit from Lu-177 PSMA-617 is not known. These areas will all require further study. These recent therapy trials suggest that the novel radioligand therapy with Lu-177 PSMA-617 will soon enter the

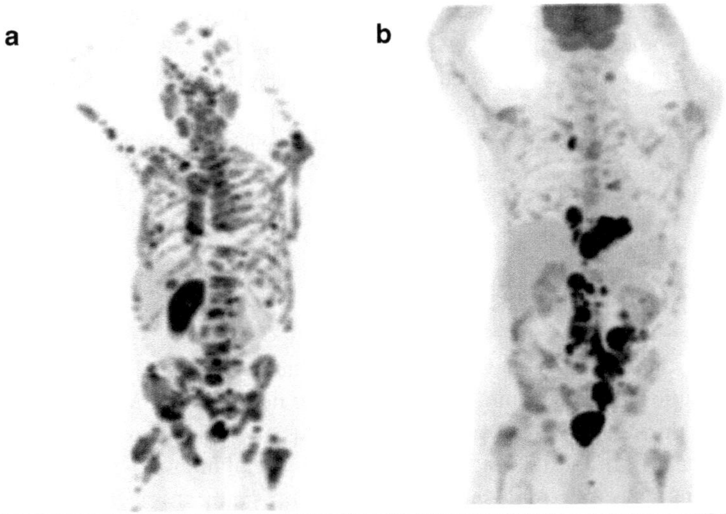

Ga-68 PSMA PET (Panel A) and FDG PET (Panel B) in a patient with metastatic castration resistant prostate Cancer (PSA 361 ng/mL) within 1-week interval. Intense PSMA activity in osseous and hepatic metastasis without significant activity in FDG avid pulmonary metastasis, thoracoabdominal adenopathy and masses encasing left upper urinary tract. Lack of tracer activity in left kidney due to obstructive nephropathy.

Fig. 8.3 Concurrent use of FDG PET and Ga-68 PSMA PET in advanced prostate cancer. *PSMA* Prostate-specific membrane antigen, *FDG* Fluorodeoxyglucose, *PET* Positron emission tomography

clinical practice for the treatment of advanced prostate cancer and that PSMA PET imaging will play a key role in determining the eligibility of patients for this treatment.

In summary, imaging of prostate cancer at its various stages is undergoing a transformation. The fight against prostate cancer will benefit broadly from molecular imaging paradigms. The abundance of available choices in imaging options, as compared to a decade ago, approaches the metaphor of a transition from famine to feast. Responsibility now lies in the hands of experienced clinicians and imaging experts to tailor the optimal imaging approach, in full awareness of strengths and shortcomings of each modality, meeting clinical need along the spectrum of disease stages in prostate cancer.

Ultimately, new imaging modalities, beyond diagnostic test performance, ideally need to demonstrate improved patient outcomes. Initial high-level evidence demonstrates the benefit in such outcomes achieved by new-generation PET imaging tools. Ongoing and future studies will potentially further substantiate the translation of better imaging characterization of prostate cancer to improved patient outcomes.

References

1. Czernin J, Satyamurthy N, Schiepers C. Molecular mechanisms of bone 18F-NaF deposition. J Nucl Med. 2010;51(12):1826–9.
2. Grant FD, Fahey FH, Packard AB, Davis RT, Alavi A, Treves ST. Skeletal PET with 18F-fluoride: applying new technology to an old tracer. J Nucl Med. 2008;49(1):68–78.
3. Mick CG, James T, Hill JD, Williams P, Perry M. Molecular imaging in oncology: (18) F-sodium fluoride PET imaging of osseous metastatic disease. AJR Am J Roentgenol. 2014;203(2):263–71.
4. Centers For Medicare & Medicaid Services. Decision Memo for Positron Emission Tomography (NaF-18) to Identify Bone Metastasis of Cancer (CAG-00065R2); 2015. Available from: https://www.cms.gov/medicare-coverage-database/details/nca-decision-memo.aspx?NCAId=279.
5. American College Of Radiology. CMS Refuses Medicare Coverage of NaF PET Scans 2018.
6. Macheda ML, Rogers S, Best JD. Molecular and cellular regulation of glucose transporter (GLUT) proteins in cancer. J Cell Physiol. 2005;202(3):654–62.
7. Jadvar H. Imaging evaluation of prostate cancer with 18F-fluorodeoxyglucose PET/CT: utility and limitations. Eur J Nucl Med Mol Imaging. 2013;40 Suppl 1:S5–10.
8. Beauregard JM, Blouin AC, Fradet V, Caron A, Fradet Y, Lemay C, et al. FDG-PET/CT for pre-operative staging and prognostic stratification of patients with high-grade prostate cancer at biopsy. Cancer Imaging. 2015;15:2.
9. Fox JJ, Morris MJ, Larson SM, Schoder H, Scher HI. Developing imaging strategies for castration resistant prostate cancer. Acta Oncol. 2011;50 Suppl 1:39–48.
10. Scher HI, Morris MJ, Larson S, Heller G. Validation and clinical utility of prostate cancer biomarkers. Nat Rev Clin Oncol. 2013;10(4):225–34.
11. Meirelles GS, Schoder H, Ravizzini GC, Gonen M, Fox JJ, Humm J, et al. Prognostic value of baseline [18F] fluorodeoxyglucose positron emission tomography and 99mTc-MDP bone scan in progressing metastatic prostate cancer. Clin Cancer Res. 2010;16(24):6093–9.
12. Fox JJ, Gavane SC, Blanc-Autran E, Nehmeh S, Gonen M, Beattie B, et al. Positron emission tomography/computed tomography-based assessments of androgen receptor expression and glycolytic activity as a prognostic biomarker for metastatic castration-resistant prostate cancer. JAMA Oncol. 2018;4(2):217–24.
13. Schoder H, Larson SM. Positron emission tomography for prostate, bladder, and renal cancer. Semin Nucl Med. 2004;34(4):274–92.
14. Michel V, Yuan Z, Ramsubir S, Bakovic M. Choline transport for phospholipid synthesis. Exp Biol Med (Maywood). 2006;231(5):490–504.
15. Ramirez de Molina A, Rodriguez-Gonzalez A, Gutierrez R, Martinez-Pineiro L, Sanchez J, Bonilla F, et al. Overexpression of choline kinase is a frequent feature in human tumor-derived cell lines and in lung, prostate, and colorectal human cancers. Biochem Biophys Res Commun. 2002;296(3):580–3.
16. von Eyben FE, Kairemo K. Meta-analysis of (11)C-choline and (18)F-choline PET/CT for management of patients with prostate cancer. Nucl Med Commun. 2014;35(3):221–30.
17. Shoup TM, Olson J, Hoffman JM, Votaw J, Eshima D, Eshima L, et al. Synthesis and evaluation of [18F]1-amino-3-fluorocyclobutane-1-carboxylic acid to image brain tumors. J Nucl Med. 1999;40(2):331–8.
18. Schuster DM, Votaw JR, Nieh PT, Yu W, Nye JA, Master V, et al. Initial experience with the radiotracer anti-1-amino-3-18F-fluorocyclobutane-1-carboxylic acid with PET/CT in prostate carcinoma. J Nucl Med. 2007;48(1):56–63.
19. Oka S, Okudaira H, Yoshida Y, Schuster DM, Goodman MM, Shirakami Y. Transport mechanisms of trans-1-amino-3-fluoro[1-(14)C]cyclobutanecarboxylic acid in prostate cancer cells. Nucl Med Biol. 2012;39(1):109–19.
20. Segawa A, Nagamori S, Kanai Y, Masawa N, Oyama T. L-type amino acid transporter 1 expression is highly correlated with Gleason score in prostate cancer. Mol Clin Oncol. 2013;1(2):274–80.

21. Gusman M, Aminsharifi JA, Peacock JG, Anderson SB, Clemenshaw MN, Banks KP. Review of (18)F-Fluciclovine PET for detection of recurrent prostate cancer. Radiographics. 2019;39(3):822–41.
22. Blue Earth Diagnostics. Axumin prescription information; 2016. Available from: https://www.axumin.com/sites/default/files/2018-03/Axumin_PI_08_2016_Clean.pdf.
23. Nanni C, Zanoni L, Bach-Gansmo T, Minn H, Willoch F, Bogsrud TV, et al. [(18)F]Fluciclovine PET/CT: joint EANM and SNMMI procedure guideline for prostate cancer imaging-version 1.0. Eur J Nucl Med Mol Imaging. 2020;47(3):579–91.
24. Schuster DM, Nanni C, Fanti S, Oka S, Okudaira H, Inoue Y, et al. Anti-1-amino-3-18F--fluorocyclobutane-1-carboxylic acid: physiologic uptake patterns, incidental findings, and variants that may simulate disease. J Nucl Med. 2014;55(12):1986–92.
25. Lowentritt BH, Kipper MS. Understanding and improving (18)F-Fluciclovine PET/CT reports: a guide for physicians treating patients with biochemical recurrence of prostate cancer. Prostate Cancer. 2020;2020:1929565.
26. Israeli RS, Powell CT, Fair WR, Heston WD. Molecular cloning of a complementary DNA encoding a prostate-specific membrane antigen. Cancer Res. 1993;53(2):227–30.
27. Israeli RS, Powell CT, Corr JG, Fair WR, Heston WD. Expression of the prostate-specific membrane antigen. Cancer Res. 1994;54(7):1807–11.
28. O'Keefe DS, Bacich DJ, Huang SS, Heston WDW. A perspective on the evolving story of PSMA biology, PSMA-based imaging, and endoradiotherapeutic strategies. J Nucl Med. 2018;59(7):1007–13.
29. Ristau BT, O'Keefe DS, Bacich DJ. The prostate-specific membrane antigen: lessons and current clinical implications from 20 years of research. Urol Oncol. 2014;32(3):272–9.
30. Mhawech-Fauceglia P, Zhang S, Terracciano L, Sauter G, Chadhuri A, Herrmann FR, et al. Prostate-specific membrane antigen (PSMA) protein expression in normal and neoplastic tissues and its sensitivity and specificity in prostate adenocarcinoma: an immunohistochemical study using mutiple tumour tissue microarray technique. Histopathology. 2007;50(4):472–83.
31. Silver DA, Pellicer I, Fair WR, Heston WD, Cordon-Cardo C. Prostate-specific membrane antigen expression in normal and malignant human tissues. Clin Cancer Res. 1997;3(1):81–5.
32. Thorek DL, Watson PA, Lee SG, Ku AT, Bournazos S, Braun K, et al. Internalization of secreted antigen-targeted antibodies by the neonatal Fc receptor for precision imaging of the androgen receptor axis. Sci Transl Med. 2016;8(367):367ra167.
33. Kinoshita Y, Kuratsukuri K, Landas S, Imaida K, Rovito PM Jr, Wang CY, et al. Expression of prostate-specific membrane antigen in normal and malignant human tissues. World J Surg. 2006;30(4):628–36.
34. Samplaski MK, Heston W, Elson P, Magi-Galluzzi C, Hansel DE. Folate hydrolase (prostate-specific membrane [corrected] antigen) 1 expression in bladder cancer subtypes and associated tumor neovasculature. Mod Pathol. 2011;24(11):1521–9.
35. Pinto JT, Suffoletto BP, Berzin TM, Qiao CH, Lin S, Tong WP, et al. Prostate-specific membrane antigen: a novel folate hydrolase in human prostatic carcinoma cells. Clin Cancer Res. 1996;2(9):1445–51.
36. Maurer T, Eiber M, Schwaiger M, Gschwend JE. Current use of PSMA-PET in prostate cancer management. Nat Rev Urol. 2016;13(4):226–35.
37. Hlouchova K, Barinka C, Klusak V, Sacha P, Mlcochova P, Majer P, et al. Biochemical characterization of human glutamate carboxypeptidase III. J Neurochem. 2007;101(3):682–96.
38. Ghosh A, Heston WD. Tumor target prostate specific membrane antigen (PSMA) and its regulation in prostate cancer. J Cell Biochem. 2004;91(3):528–39.
39. Rajasekaran AK, Anilkumar G, Christiansen JJ. Is prostate-specific membrane antigen a multifunctional protein? Am J Physiol Cell Physiol. 2005;288(5):C975–81.
40. Bostwick DG, Pacelli A, Blute M, Roche P, Murphy GP. Prostate specific membrane antigen expression in prostatic intraepithelial neoplasia and adenocarcinoma: a study of 184 cases. Cancer. 1998;82(11):2256–61.

41. Marchal C, Redondo M, Padilla M, Caballero J, Rodrigo I, Garcia J, et al. Expression of prostate specific membrane antigen (PSMA) in prostatic adenocarcinoma and prostatic intraepithelial neoplasia. Histol Histopathol. 2004;19(3):715–8.
42. Denmeade SR, Sokoll LJ, Dalrymple S, Rosen DM, Gady AM, Bruzek D, et al. Dissociation between androgen responsiveness for malignant growth vs. expression of prostate specific differentiation markers PSA, hK2, and PSMA in human prostate cancer models. Prostate. 2003;54(4):249–57.
43. Evans MJ, Smith-Jones PM, Wongvipat J, Navarro V, Kim S, Bander NH, et al. Noninvasive measurement of androgen receptor signaling with a positron-emitting radiopharmaceutical that targets prostate-specific membrane antigen. Proc Natl Acad Sci U S A. 2011;108(23):9578–82.
44. Bakht MK, Oh SW, Youn H, Cheon GJ, Kwak C, Kang KW. Influence of androgen deprivation therapy on the uptake of PSMA-targeted agents: emerging opportunities and challenges. Nucl Med Mol Imaging. 2017;51(3):202–11.
45. Emmett L, Yin C, Crumbaker M, Hruby G, Kneebone A, Epstein R, et al. Rapid modulation of PSMA expression by androgen deprivation: serial (68)Ga-PSMA-11 PET in men with hormone-sensitive and castrate-resistant prostate cancer commencing androgen blockade. J Nucl Med. 2019;60(7):950–4.
46. Ettala O, Malaspina S, Tuokkola T, Luoto P, Loyttyniemi E, Bostrom PJ, et al. Prospective study on the effect of short-term androgen deprivation therapy on PSMA uptake evaluated with (68)Ga-PSMA-11 PET/MRI in men with treatment-naive prostate cancer. Eur J Nucl Med Mol Imaging. 2020;47(3):665–73.
47. Tagawa ST, Beltran H, Vallabhajosula S, Goldsmith SJ, Osborne J, Matulich D, et al. Anti-prostate-specific membrane antigen-based radioimmunotherapy for prostate cancer. Cancer. 2010;116(4 Suppl):1075–83.
48. Holland JP, Divilov V, Bander NH, Smith-Jones PM, Larson SM, Lewis JS. 89Zr-DFO-J591 for immunoPET of prostate-specific membrane antigen expression in vivo. J Nucl Med. 2010;51(8):1293–300.
49. Wiehr S, Buhler P, Gierschner D, Wolf P, Rolle AM, Kesenheimer C, et al. Pharmacokinetics and PET imaging properties of two recombinant anti-PSMA antibody fragments in comparison to their parental antibody. Prostate. 2014;74(7):743–55.
50. Cho SY, Gage KL, Mease RC, Senthamizhchelvan S, Holt DP, Jeffrey-Kwanisai A, et al. Biodistribution, tumor detection, and radiation dosimetry of 18F-DCFBC, a low-molecular-weight inhibitor of prostate-specific membrane antigen, in patients with metastatic prostate cancer. J Nucl Med. 2012;53(12):1883–91.
51. Chen Y, Pullambhatla M, Foss CA, Byun Y, Nimmagadda S, Senthamizhchelvan S, et al. 2-(3-{1-Carboxy-5-[(6-[18F]fluoro-pyridine-3-carbonyl)-amino]-pentyl}-ureido)-pen tanedioic acid, [18F]DCFPyL, a PSMA-based PET imaging agent for prostate cancer. Clin Cancer Res. 2011;17(24):7645–53.
52. Rowe SP, Macura KJ, Mena E, Blackford AL, Nadal R, Antonarakis ES, et al. PSMA-based [(18)F]DCFPyL PET/CT is superior to conventional imaging for lesion detection in patients with metastatic prostate cancer. Mol Imaging Biol. 2016;18(3):411–9.
53. Morris MJ, Rowe SP, Gorin MA, Saperstein L, Pouliot F, Josephson DY, et al. Diagnostic performance of (18)F-DCFPyL-PET/CT in men with biochemically recurrent prostate cancer: results from the CONDOR phase 3, multicenter study. Clin Cancer Res. 2021.
54. Kuten J, Fahoum I, Savin Z, Shamni O, Gitstein G, Hershkovitz D, et al. Head-to-head comparison of (68)Ga-PSMA-11 with (18)F-PSMA-1007 PET/CT in staging prostate cancer using histopathology and immunohistochemical analysis as a reference standard. J Nucl Med. 2020;61(4):527–32.
55. Eiber M, Kroenke M, Wurzer A, Ulbrich L, Jooss L, Maurer T, et al. (18)F-rhPSMA-7 PET for the detection of biochemical recurrence of prostate cancer after radical prostatectomy. J Nucl Med. 2020;61(5):696–701.
56. Weineisen M, Schottelius M, Simecek J, Baum RP, Yildiz A, Beykan S, et al. 68Ga- and 177Lu-labeled PSMA I&T: optimization of a PSMA-targeted theranostic concept and first proof-of-concept human studies. J Nucl Med. 2015;56(8):1169–76.

57. Afshar-Oromieh A, Hetzheim H, Kratochwil C, Benesova M, Eder M, Neels OC, et al. The theranostic PSMA ligand PSMA-617 in the diagnosis of prostate cancer by PET/CT: biodistribution in humans, radiation dosimetry, and first evaluation of tumor lesions. J Nucl Med. 2015;56(11):1697–705.
58. Morris M. Phase III study of lutetium-177-PSMA-617 in patients with metastatic castration-resistant prostate cancer (VISION). J Clin Oncol, 2021;39:(suppl 15; abstr LBA4) 2021. Available from: https://meetinglibrary.asco.org/record/196661/abstract.
59. Hofman MS, Emmett L, Sandhu S, Iravani A, Joshua AM, Goh JC, et al. [(177) Lu]Lu-PSMA-617 versus cabazitaxel in patients with metastatic castration-resistant prostate cancer (TheraP): a randomised, open-label, phase 2 trial. Lancet. 2021.
60. Farolfi A, Calderoni L, Mattana F, Mei R, Telo S, Fanti S, et al. Current and emerging clinical applications of PSMA PET diagnostic imaging for prostate cancer. J Nucl Med. 2021;62(5):596–604.
61. Herrmann K, Bluemel C, Weineisen M, Schottelius M, Wester HJ, Czernin J, et al. Biodistribution and radiation dosimetry for a probe targeting prostate-specific membrane antigen for imaging and therapy. J Nucl Med. 2015;56(6):855–61.
62. Liu A, Dence CS, Welch MJ, Katzenellenbogen JA. Fluorine-18-labeled androgens: radiochemical synthesis and tissue distribution studies on six fluorine-substituted androgens, potential imaging agents for prostatic cancer. J Nucl Med. 1992;33(5):724–34.
63. Larson SM, Morris M, Gunther I, Beattie B, Humm JL, Akhurst TA, et al. Tumor localization of 16beta-18F-fluoro-5alpha-dihydrotestosterone versus 18F-FDG in patients with progressive, metastatic prostate cancer. J Nucl Med. 2004;45(3):366–73.
64. Bonasera TA, O'Neil JP, Xu M, Dobkin JA, Cutler PD, Lich LL, et al. Preclinical evaluation of fluorine-18-labeled androgen receptor ligands in baboons. J Nucl Med. 1996;37(6):1009–15.
65. Silva RC, Sasse AD, Matheus WE, Ferreira U. Magnetic resonance image in the diagnosis and evaluation of extra-prostatic extension and involvement of seminal vesicles of prostate cancer: a systematic review of literature and meta-analysis. Int Braz J Urol. 2013;39(2):155–66.
66. Wibmer AG, Vargas HA, Hricak H. Role of MRI in the diagnosis and management of prostate cancer. Future Oncol. 2015;11(20):2757–66.
67. Vargas HA, Hotker AM, Goldman DA, Moskowitz CS, Gondo T, Matsumoto K, et al. Updated prostate imaging reporting and data system (PIRADS v2) recommendations for the detection of clinically significant prostate cancer using multiparametric MRI: critical evaluation using whole-mount pathology as standard of reference. Eur Radiol. 2016;26(6):1606–12.
68. von Below C, Daouacher G, Wassberg C, Grzegorek R, Gestblom C, Sorensen J, et al. Validation of 3 T MRI including diffusion-weighted imaging for nodal staging of newly diagnosed intermediate- and high-risk prostate cancer. Clin Radiol. 2016;71(4):328–34.
69. Turkbey B, Mena E, Shih J, Pinto PA, Merino MJ, Lindenberg ML, et al. Localized prostate cancer detection with 18F FACBC PET/CT: comparison with MR imaging and histopathologic analysis. Radiology. 2014;270(3):849–56.
70. Poulsen MH, Bouchelouche K, Hoilund-Carlsen PF, Petersen H, Gerke O, Steffansen SI, et al. [18F]fluoromethylcholine (FCH) positron emission tomography/computed tomography (PET/CT) for lymph node staging of prostate cancer: a prospective study of 210 patients. BJU Int. 2012;110(11):1666–71.
71. Beheshti M, Imamovic L, Broinger G, Vali R, Waldenberger P, Stoiber F, et al. 18F choline PET/CT in the preoperative staging of prostate cancer in patients with intermediate or high risk of extracapsular disease: a prospective study of 130 patients. Radiology. 2010;254(3):925–33.
72. Selnaes KM, Kruger-Stokke B, Elschot M, Willoch F, Storkersen O, Sandsmark E, et al. (18) F-Fluciclovine PET/MRI for preoperative lymph node staging in high-risk prostate cancer patients. Eur Radiol. 2018;28(8):3151–9.
73. Evangelista L, Guttilla A, Zattoni F, Muzzio PC, Zattoni F. Utility of choline positron emission tomography/computed tomography for lymph node involvement identification in intermediate- to high-risk prostate cancer: a systematic literature review and meta-analysis. Eur Urol. 2013;63(6):1040–8.

74. United States Food & Drug Administration. FDA Approves First PSMA-Targeted PET Imaging Drug for Men with Prostate Cancer; 2020. Available from: https://www.fda.gov/news-events/press-announcements/fda-approves-first-psma-targeted-pet-imaging-drug-men-prostate-cancer.
75. United States Food & Drug Administration. FDA approves second PSMA-targeted PET imaging drug for men with prostate cancer; 2021. Available from: https://www.fda.gov/drugs/drug-safety-and-availability/fda-approves-second-psma-targeted-pet-imaging-drug-men-prostate-cancer.
76. Pienta KJ, Gorin MA, Rowe SP, Carroll PR, Pouliot F, Probst S, et al. A phase 2/3 prospective multicenter study of the diagnostic accuracy of prostate-specific membrane antigen PET/CT with (18)F-DCFPyL in prostate cancer patients (OSPREY). J Urol. 2021:101097JU0000000000001698.
77. Hope TA, Armstrong WR, Murthy V, Heath CL, Behr S, Barbato F, et al. Accuracy of 68Ga-PSMA-11 for pelvic nodal metastasis detection prior to radical prostatectomy and pelvic lymph node dissection: a multicenter prospective phase III imaging study. J Clin Oncol. 2020;38(15_suppl):5502.
78. Hofman MS, Lawrentschuk N, Francis RJ, Tang C, Vela I, Thomas P, et al. Prostate-specific membrane antigen PET-CT in patients with high-risk prostate cancer before curative-intent surgery or radiotherapy (proPSMA): a prospective, randomised, multicentre study. Lancet. 2020;395(10231):1208–16.
79. Roach M 3rd, Hanks G, Thames H Jr, Schellhammer P, Shipley WU, Sokol GH, et al. Defining biochemical failure following radiotherapy with or without hormonal therapy in men with clinically localized prostate cancer: recommendations of the RTOG-ASTRO Phoenix Consensus Conference. Int J Radiat Oncol Biol Phys. 2006;65(4):965–74.
80. Han M, Partin AW, Pound CR, Epstein JI, Walsh PC. Long-term biochemical disease-free and cancer-specific survival following anatomic radical retropubic prostatectomy. The 15-year Johns Hopkins experience. Urol Clin North Am. 2001;28(3):555–65.
81. Hull GW, Rabbani F, Abbas F, Wheeler TM, Kattan MW, Scardino PT. Cancer control with radical prostatectomy alone in 1,000 consecutive patients. J Urol. 2002;167(2 Pt 1):528–34.
82. Freedland SJ, Humphreys EB, Mangold LA, Eisenberger M, Dorey FJ, Walsh PC, et al. Risk of prostate cancer-specific mortality following biochemical recurrence after radical prostatectomy. JAMA. 2005;294(4):433–9.
83. Kupelian PA, Mahadevan A, Reddy CA, Reuther AM, Klein EA. Use of different definitions of biochemical failure after external beam radiotherapy changes conclusions about relative treatment efficacy for localized prostate cancer. Urology. 2006;68(3):593–8.
84. Parker CC, Clarke NW, Cook AD, Kynaston HG, Petersen PM, Catton C, et al. Timing of radiotherapy after radical prostatectomy (RADICALS-RT): a randomised, controlled phase 3 trial. Lancet. 2020;396(10260):1413–21.
85. Yossepowitch O, Briganti A, Eastham JA, Epstein J, Graefen M, Montironi R, et al. Positive surgical margins after radical prostatectomy: a systematic review and contemporary update. Eur Urol. 2014;65(2):303–13.
86. Lange PH, Ercole CJ, Lightner DJ, Fraley EE, Vessella R. The value of serum prostate specific antigen determinations before and after radical prostatectomy. J Urol. 1989;141(4):873–9.
87. Patel A, Dorey F, Franklin J, deKernion JB. Recurrence patterns after radical retropubic prostatectomy: clinical usefulness of prostate specific antigen doubling times and log slope prostate specific antigen. J Urol. 1997;158(4):1441–5.
88. Moschini M, Sharma V, Zattoni F, Quevedo JF, Davis BJ, Kwon E, et al. Natural history of clinical recurrence patterns of lymph node-positive prostate cancer after radical prostatectomy. Eur Urol. 2016;69(1):135–42.
89. Beresford MJ, Gillatt D, Benson RJ, Ajithkumar T. A systematic review of the role of imaging before salvage radiotherapy for post-prostatectomy biochemical recurrence. Clin Oncol (R Coll Radiol). 2010;22(1):46–55.

90. Gomez P, Manoharan M, Kim SS, Soloway MS. Radionuclide bone scintigraphy in patients with biochemical recurrence after radical prostatectomy: when is it indicated? BJU Int. 2004;94(3):299–302.
91. Dotan ZA, Bianco FJ Jr, Rabbani F, Eastham JA, Fearn P, Scher HI, et al. Pattern of prostate-specific antigen (PSA) failure dictates the probability of a positive bone scan in patients with an increasing PSA after radical prostatectomy. J Clin Oncol. 2005;23(9):1962–8.
92. Kane CJ, Amling CL, Johnstone PA, Pak N, Lance RS, Thrasher JB, et al. Limited value of bone scintigraphy and computed tomography in assessing biochemical failure after radical prostatectomy. Urology. 2003;61(3):607–11.
93. Johnstone PA, Tarman GJ, Riffenburgh R, Rohde DC, Puckett ML, Kane CJ. Yield of imaging and scintigraphy assessing biochemical failure in prostate cancer patients. Urol Oncol. 1997;3(4):108–12.
94. Mitchell CR, Lowe VJ, Rangel LJ, Hung JC, Kwon ED, Karnes RJ. Operational characteristics of (11)c-choline positron emission tomography/computerized tomography for prostate cancer with biochemical recurrence after initial treatment. J Urol. 2013;189(4):1308–13.
95. Giovacchini G, Picchio M, Coradeschi E, Bettinardi V, Gianolli L, Scattoni V, et al. Predictive factors of [(11)C]choline PET/CT in patients with biochemical failure after radical prostatectomy. Eur J Nucl Med Mol Imaging. 2010;37(2):301–9.
96. Michaud L, Touijer KA, Mauguen A, Zelefsky MJ, Morris MJ, Lyashschenko SK, et al. (11) C-choline PET/CT in recurrent prostate cancer: retrospective analysis in a large U.S. patient series. J Nucl Med. 2020;61(6):827–33.
97. Fanti S, Minozzi S, Castellucci P, Balduzzi S, Herrmann K, Krause BJ, et al. PET/CT with (11)C-choline for evaluation of prostate cancer patients with biochemical recurrence: meta-analysis and critical review of available data. Eur J Nucl Med Mol Imaging. 2016;43(1):55–69.
98. Schuster DM, Savir-Baruch B, Nieh PT, Master VA, Halkar RK, Rossi PJ, et al. Detection of recurrent prostate carcinoma with anti-1-amino-3-18F-fluorocyclobutane-1-carboxylic acid PET/CT and 111In-capromab pendetide SPECT/CT. Radiology. 2011;259(3):852–61.
99. Bach-Gansmo T, Nanni C, Nieh PT, Zanoni L, Bogsrud TV, Sletten H, et al. Multisite experience of the safety, detection rate and diagnostic performance of fluciclovine ((18)F) positron emission tomography/computerized tomography imaging in the staging of biochemically recurrent prostate cancer. J Urol. 2017;197(3 Pt 1):676–83.
100. Andriole GL, Kostakoglu L, Chau A, Duan F, Mahmood U, Mankoff DA, et al. The impact of positron emission tomography with 18F-fluciclovine on the treatment of biochemical recurrence of prostate cancer: results from the LOCATE trial. J Urol. 2019;201(2):322–31.
101. Kim SJ, Lee SW. The role of (18)F-fluciclovine PET in the management of prostate cancer: a systematic review and meta-analysis. Clin Radiol. 2019;74(11):886–92.
102. Jani AB, Schreibmann E, Goyal S, Halkar R, Hershatter B, Rossi PJ, et al. (18)F-fluciclovine-PET/CT imaging versus conventional imaging alone to guide postprostatectomy salvage radiotherapy for prostate cancer (EMPIRE-1): a single centre, open-label, phase 2/3 randomised controlled trial. Lancet. 2021;397(10288):1895–904.
103. Fendler WP, Calais J, Eiber M, Flavell RR, Mishoe A, Feng FY, et al. Assessment of 68Ga-PSMA-11 PET accuracy in localizing recurrent prostate cancer: a prospective single-arm clinical trial. JAMA Oncol. 2019;5(6):856–63.
104. Nanni C, Schiavina R, Brunocilla E, Boschi S, Borghesi M, Zanoni L, et al. 18F-Fluciclovine PET/CT for the detection of prostate cancer relapse: a comparison to 11C-choline PET/CT. Clin Nucl Med. 2015;40(8):e386–91.
105. Okudaira H, Oka S, Ono M, Nakanishi T, Schuster DM, Kobayashi M, et al. Accumulation of trans-1-amino-3-[(18)F]fluorocyclobutanecarboxylic acid in prostate cancer due to androgen-induced expression of amino acid transporters. Mol Imaging Biol. 2014;16(6):756–64.
106. Schuster DM, Nanni C, Fanti S. Evaluation of prostate cancer with radiolabeled amino acid analogs. J Nucl Med. 2016;57(Suppl 3):61S–6S.

107. Calais J, Ceci F, Eiber M, Hope TA, Hofman MS, Rischpler C, et al. (18)F-fluciclovine PET-CT and (68)Ga-PSMA-11 PET-CT in patients with early biochemical recurrence after prostatectomy: a prospective, single-centre, single-arm, comparative imaging trial. Lancet Oncol. 2019;20(9):1286–94.
108. Fendler WP, Weber M, Iravani A, Hofman MS, Calais J, Czernin J, et al. Prostate-specific membrane antigen ligand positron emission tomography in men with nonmetastatic castration-resistant prostate cancer. Clin Cancer Res. 2019;25(24):7448–54.
109. Minner S, Wittmer C, Graefen M, Salomon G, Steuber T, Haese A, et al. High level PSMA expression is associated with early PSA recurrence in surgically treated prostate cancer. Prostate. 2011;71(3):281–8.
110. Yaxley JW, Raveenthiran S, Nouhaud FX, Samaratunga H, Yaxley WJ, Coughlin G, et al. Risk of metastatic disease on (68) gallium-prostate-specific membrane antigen positron emission tomography/computed tomography scan for primary staging of 1253 men at the diagnosis of prostate cancer. BJU Int. 2019;124(3):401–7.
111. Maurer T, Gschwend JE, Rauscher I, Souvatzoglou M, Haller B, Weirich G, et al. Diagnostic efficacy of (68)gallium-PSMA positron emission tomography compared to conventional imaging for lymph node staging of 130 consecutive patients with intermediate to high risk prostate cancer. J Urol. 2016;195(5):1436–43.
112. Woythal N, Arsenic R, Kempkensteffen C, Miller K, Janssen JC, Huang K, et al. Immunohistochemical validation of PSMA expression measured by (68)Ga-PSMA PET/CT in primary prostate cancer. J Nucl Med. 2018;59(2):238–43.
113. Ferraro DA, Ruschoff JH, Muehlematter UJ, Kranzbuhler B, Muller J, Messerli M, et al. Immunohistochemical PSMA expression patterns of primary prostate cancer tissue are associated with the detection rate of biochemical recurrence with (68)Ga-PSMA-11-PET. Theranostics. 2020;10(14):6082–94.
114. Siegel DA, O'Neil ME, Richards TB, Dowling NF, Weir HK. Prostate cancer incidence and survival, by stage and race/ethnicity – United States, 2001–2017. MMWR Morb Mortal Wkly Rep. 2020;69(41):1473–80.
115. Pascale M, Azinwi CN, Marongiu B, Pesce G, Stoffel F, Roggero E. The outcome of prostate cancer patients treated with curative intent strongly depends on survival after metastatic progression. BMC Cancer. 2017;17(1):651.
116. Scher HI, Morris MJ, Stadler WM, Higano C, Basch E, Fizazi K, et al. Trial design and objectives for castration-resistant prostate cancer: updated recommendations from the prostate cancer clinical trials working group 3. J Clin Oncol. 2016;34(12):1402–18.
117. Rathkopf DE, Beer TM, Loriot Y, Higano CS, Armstrong AJ, Sternberg CN, et al. Radiographic progression-free survival as a clinically meaningful end point in metastatic castration-resistant prostate cancer: the PREVAIL randomized clinical trial. JAMA Oncol. 2018;4(5):694–701.
118. Morris MJ, Molina A, Small EJ, de Bono JS, Logothetis CJ, Fizazi K, et al. Radiographic progression-free survival as a response biomarker in metastatic castration-resistant prostate cancer: COU-AA-302 results. J Clin Oncol. 2015;33(12):1356–63.
119. Kluetz PG, Ning YM, Maher VE, Zhang L, Tang S, Ghosh D, et al. Abiraterone acetate in combination with prednisone for the treatment of patients with metastatic castration-resistant prostate cancer: U.S. Food and Drug Administration drug approval summary. Clin Cancer Res. 2013;19(24):6650–6.
120. Weisman AJ, Harmon SA, Perk TG, Eickhoff J, Choyke PL, Kurdziel KA, et al. Quantification of bone flare on (18)F-NaF PET/CT in metastatic castration-resistant prostate cancer. Prostate Cancer Prostatic Dis. 2019;22(2):324–30.
121. Harmon SA, Perk T, Lin C, Eickhoff J, Choyke PL, Dahut WL, et al. Quantitative assessment of early [(18)F]sodium fluoride positron emission tomography/computed tomography response to treatment in men with metastatic prostate cancer to bone. J Clin Oncol. 2017;35(24):2829–37.

122. Beltran H, Tomlins S, Aparicio A, Arora V, Rickman D, Ayala G, et al. Aggressive variants of castration-resistant prostate cancer. Clin Cancer Res. 2014;20(11):2846–50.
123. Beltran H, Wyatt AW, Chedgy E, Donoghue A, Annala M, Warner E, et al. Impact of therapy on genomics and transcriptomics in high-risk prostate cancer treated with neoadjuvant docetaxel and androgen deprivation therapy. Clin Cancer Res. 2017.
124. Beltran H, Prandi D, Mosquera JM, Benelli M, Puca L, Cyrta J, et al. Divergent clonal evolution of castration-resistant neuroendocrine prostate cancer. Nat Med. 2016;22(3):298–305.
125. Dardenne E, Beltran H, Benelli M, Gayvert K, Berger A, Puca L, et al. N-Myc induces an EZH2-mediated transcriptional program driving neuroendocrine prostate cancer. Cancer Cell. 2016;30(4):563–77.
126. Mu P, Zhang Z, Benelli M, Karthaus WR, Hoover E, Chen CC, et al. SOX2 promotes lineage plasticity and antiandrogen resistance in TP53- and RB1-deficient prostate cancer. Science. 2017;355(6320):84–8.
127. Spratt DE, Gavane S, Tarlinton L, Fareedy SB, Doran MG, Zelefsky MJ, et al. Utility of FDG-PET in clinical neuroendocrine prostate cancer. Prostate. 2014;74(11):1153–9.
128. Fox JJ, Autran-Blanc E, Morris MJ, Gavane S, Nehmeh S, Van Nuffel A, et al. Practical approach for comparative analysis of multilesion molecular imaging using a semiautomated program for PET/CT. J Nucl Med. 2011;52(11):1727–32.
129. Rathkopf DE, Morris MJ, Fox JJ, Danila DC, Slovin SF, Hager JH, et al. Phase I study of ARN-509, a novel antiandrogen, in the treatment of castration-resistant prostate cancer. J Clin Oncol. 2013;31(28):3525–30.
130. Scher HI, Beer TM, Higano CS, Anand A, Taplin ME, Efstathiou E, et al. Antitumour activity of MDV3100 in castration-resistant prostate cancer: a phase 1–2 study. Lancet. 2010;375(9724):1437–46.
131. Morris MJ, Rowe SP, Gorin MA, Saperstein L, Pouliot F, Josephson D, et al. Diagnostic performance of (18)F-DCFPyL-PET/CT in men with biochemically recurrent prostate cancer: results from the CONDOR phase III, multicenter study. Clin Cancer Res. 2021.

Chapter 9
Bone Health Management

Zineb Hamilou and Fred Saad

Introduction

Prostate cancer is the most frequent non-skin cancer and the third leading cause of death from cancer in men in the United States [1]. Consistent advances in prostate cancer treatments led to considerable improvement in survival of these patients. Indeed, when localized, the prognosis is excellent with a recently reported 1.5 deaths per 1000 person-years (CI 0.7–3.0) at 10 years of median follow-up [2]. For the proportion of 5–10% of patients presenting with metastatic disease, the addition of novel androgen receptor axis-targeted therapies (ARAT) or early chemotherapy to androgen deprivation therapy (ADT) improved greatly their median overall survival now reaching 6.6 years [3]. By 2024, it is estimated that prostate cancer survivors in the United States will exceed four million in number [4]. Increasingly, clinical trials are now incorporating health-related quality of life data and patient-reported outcome measures to capture treatment late effects.

ADT is the frontline of systemic treatment for prostate cancer across all stages, whether it is prescribed transiently in patients with localized disease, intermittently in nonmetastatic patients, or indefinitely in metastatic patients [5–7]. Despite the need for this therapy, its multiple side effects can impact the quality of life of patients and cause secondary late physical complications. These side effects are also associated with significant economic costs to the health system.

Z. Hamilou (✉)
Department of Medicine, Division on Hematology Oncology, Centre Hospitalier de l'Université de Montréal, Montreal, QC, Canada
e-mail: zineb.hamilou.chum@ssss.gouv.qc.ca

F. Saad
Department of Surgery, Division of Urology, Centre Hospitalier de l'Université de Montréal, Montreal, QC, Canada
e-mail: fred.saad@umontreal.ca

K. L. Stratton, A. K. Morgans (eds.), *Urologic Oncology*,
https://doi.org/10.1007/978-3-030-89891-5_9

Bone health is particularly important for men with prostate cancer as the bone is the primary site of metastasis in 90% of the cases [8]. Skeletal integrity is thus impacted by the disease itself and by ADT. By reducing bone mineral density (BMD), ADT increases the risk of osteoporotic fragility fractures [9–11]. It was estimated that osteoporotic skeletal fractures occur in up to 20% of men within 5 years of starting ADT [10]. Moreover, reduction in BMD combined with the occurrence of bone metastases raises the occurrence of skeletal-related events (SREs), defined as fractures, spinal cord compressions, need for bone surgery, or radiation therapy. In addition to bone metastasis reducing quality of life, SREs are a main cause of morbidity in these patients and are associated with a 6.6-fold mortality risk compared to patients without metastasis or SREs [12]. For many years, bone loss remained underdiagnosed and undertreated. This chapter is dedicated to reviewing the factors regulating bone homeostasis, the pathophysiology of bone loss secondary to ADT, its clinical complications, and pharmacological and non-pharmacological options offered to these patients.

Physiology of Bone Remodeling

Bone remodeling is a continuous physiological process under the strict regulation of osteoclast and osteoblast activity in response to mechanical strain, microcracks, and hormonal changes in the bone environment. After bones have completed their longitudinal growth, 10% of the bone is remodeled per year [13]. In order to keep a stable bone mass, multiple signaling pathways regulate this process. Despite this balance, gradual bone loss still occurs throughout the years, its degree being related to genetic predisposition, lifestyle, and comorbidities [14].

Advanced age is a main risk factor of loss of BMD. Independently of sex steroid hormone levels, different mechanisms contribute to normal aging of the bone. They include increased oxidative stress, increased apoptosis of osteoblasts and osteocytes, and alterations in decreased efficiency of macroautophagy mechanisms [15, 16]. The rate of loss of cortical bone mass is estimated at 0.5–1%/year in healthy men.

Sex steroid hormones are essential for bone growth and maturation [17]. They reduce excessive oxidative stress and slow down the rate of bone turnover, thus protecting against osteoporosis. First, testosterone is converted to dihydrotestosterone (DHT), the most active androgen in the prostate via 5-alpha-reductase enzyme. Second, via aromatase activity in the adipose tissue, testosterone is also converted to estradiol. While DHT binds to the androgen receptor (AR) of osteoblasts in cortical and trabecular bone, estradiol binds to the estrogen receptor in the osteoblasts and osteoclasts and is mainly implicated in the trabecular bone remodeling [17, 18]. More precisely, testosterone and DHT upregulate osteoblast AR expression, promote their differentiation, and inhibit the interaction of receptor activator of nuclear factor-kappa B ligand (RANK-L) with its receptor consequently regulating osteoclast activity [19]. Androgens and estradiol prevent osteoblast apoptosis, stimulate osteoclast apoptosis, and decrease osteoclastogenesis. Therefore, sex steroids help increase cortical bone formation resulting in the attainment of the peak of the bone mass in the first three decades of life [20]. Levels of sex steroids diminish with aging and so does their protective effect on bone remodeling. First, there is an increase in sex hormone-binding globulin, directly reducing the bioavailability of these hormones. Also, production of testosterone and activity of follicle-stimulating hormone (FSH) and luteinizing hormone (LH) are reduced [21].

With normal aging, the cortical compartment of the bone is increasingly remodeled compared to the trabecular compartment, leading to increased cortical porosity and thinning [21].

In the last decades, some lifestyle factors have been recognized to directly influence bone mineral density. Sufficient supply of calcium, vitamin D, and sun exposure are strongly recommended to prevent osteoporosis. Vitamin D acts conjointly with parathyroid hormone to regulate calcium and phosphate levels [22]. Deficiency of calcium and phosphate impairs bone formation and mineralization and decreases muscular mass and strength raising the risk of falls. Physical activity also prevents osteoporosis by different mechanisms. It decreases oxidative stress and triggers osteocyte-bone remodeling by putting mechanical pressure and load on the entire musculoskeletal system. Chronic, excessive intake of alcohol in turn decreases BMD and inhibits new bone formation, thereby increasing the risk of fractures. Finally, there is a clear association between cigarette smoking and a deficit in BMD [14].

Evaluation of Bone Mineral Density

Osteoporosis is diagnosed clinically if a fragility fracture at the spine, hip, wrist, humerus, or pelvis is present. In the absence of a fracture, osteoporosis is diagnosed according to the World Health Organization (WHO) guidelines by the standard modality of dual-energy X-ray absorptiometry (DXA) (Table 9.1) [23]. Among other techniques available to evaluate BMD, DXA is the only technology that can

Table 9.1 Diagnostic categories for osteoporosis and low bone mass based upon BMD measurement by DXA

Category	Bone mass
Normal	A value for BMD within 1.0 standard deviation (SD) of the young adult reference mean (T-score greater than or equal to −1.0 SD)
Low bone mass (osteopenia)	A value of BMD more than 1.0 but less than 2.5 SD below the young adult reference mean (T-score less than −1 and greater than −2.5 SD)
Osteoporosis	A value for BMD 2.5 or more SD below the young adult reference mean (T-score less than or equal to −2.5 SD)
Severe (established) osteoporosis	A value for BMD more than 2.5 SD below the young adult reference mean in the presence of one or more fragility fractures

Data from WHO scientific group on the assessment of osteoporosis at the primary health care level: summary meeting report, 2004

Table 9.2 Clinical risk factors of osteoporosis included in FRAX risk assessment tool

Age (increasing age is at higher risk)
Gender (female at greater risk than male)
Low body mass index
Personal history of fragility fracture
Glucocorticoid therapy
Parental history of hip fracture
Current cigarette smoking
Excessive alcohol consumption (3 or more units per day)
Rheumatoid arthritis

be used for both diagnostic classification and serial evaluation of the patients. Moreover, many studies established a correlation between low BMD measured by DXA and osteoporotic fractures [24, 25]. Overall, there is an approximately twofold increase in risk of such fractures for each standard deviation decrease in BMD.

However, many patients present with fractures without a diagnosis of osteoporosis according to a T-score of −2.5 or less, stressing the importance of clinical risk factors [26].

The University of Sheffield launched in 2008 Fracture Risk Assessment Tool (FRAX) based on data collected from large prospective, observational studies of men and women of different ethnicities and world regions [13]. FRAX tool estimates the 10-year probability of hip fracture and major osteoporotic fracture for untreated patients between ages 40 and 90 years by combining clinical risk factors for fracture with femoral neck BMD (g/cm^2, using dual-energy X-ray absorptiometry [DXA]), when available (Table 9.2). Unlike other clinical models, FRAX has been validated in approximately 26 independent cohorts, mainly comprised of women [27].

Pathophysiology of Bone Metastasis in Prostate Cancer

In 1889, Stephen Paget hypothesized in his "seed-and-soil" theory that cancer cells metastasize to a site where the local microenvironment is favorable [28]. Indeed, bone tissue offers an environment rich with several growth factors such as transforming growth factor B, insulin-like growth factors I and II, fibroblast growth factors, platelet-derived growth factors, bone morphogenetic proteins, and calcium. These growth factors are all released during bone remodeling induced by the metastasis and allow its growth. In addition, the bone/bone marrow compartment may produce factors and certain vascular growth factor types favoring bone tumor growth. In turn, tumor cells produce adhesive molecules that bind them to marrow stromal cells and bone matrix [29].

Bone metastases are described as osteolytic or osteoblastic, and often cancers present one way or another along this continuum of bone remodeling [30].

Except for multiple myeloma where metastases are exclusively osteolytic, a patient may have either pattern. Unlike osteolytic metastases, mechanisms of osteoblastic metastasis and factors involved are less recognized [30].

In prostate cancer, bone metastases are mostly osteoblastic even if markers of bone resorption are also increased, suggesting a degree of osteolysis [31]. Prostate cancer cells produce several factors responsible for the vicious cycle behind osteoblastic metastases such as urokinase-type plasminogen activator and PSA, a kallikrein serine protease. These factors can block tumor-induced bone resorption and activate osteoblastic growth factors such as IGF-I and IGF-II or TGF-B to promote metastatic growth [32].

Treatment-Related Bone Loss

In addition to androgen suppression, many patients with advanced prostate cancer are exposed to glucocorticoids. Indeed, prednisone is a part of many regimens for men with metastatic prostate cancer, including use with chemotherapy agents docetaxel and cabazitaxel and abiraterone acetate [33, 34–38]. Depending on the disease state, prednisone is prescribed at 5–10 mg per day with these therapies.

Consequences of Glucocorticoids

Glucocorticoid-induced osteoporosis is the most common secondary cause of osteoporosis, and vertebral fractures are characteristic of glucocorticoid-induced osteoporosis. Interestingly, bone loss is seen after only 3–6 months of initiation of glucocorticoids and is dose related [39]. In a large database, fracture incidence rate was estimated at 5–9/1000 person years even with doses under a prednisone equivalent of 15 mg/day [40].

Glucocorticoids are associated with decreased bone formation and a transient early increase of bone resorption creating a negative remodeling balance through many mechanisms. Upregulation of peroxisome proliferator-activated receptor gamma receptor 2 (PPARy2) favors the differentiation of pluripotent precursor cells to adipocytes in preference to osteoblasts. Increased expression of sclerostin inhibits Wnt signaling resulting in reduced differentiation of osteoblast and increased apoptosis of osteoblasts and osteocytes [41]. Glucocorticoids also increase the production of macrophage colony-stimulating factor (M-CSF) and RANKL and decrease production of osteoprotegerin (OPG) by osteoblastic cells and osteocytes amplifying the number and activity of osteoclasts [42].

Glucocorticoids also contribute to bone loss via indirect effects. They are a cause of hypogonadism, increased renal and intestinal losses of calcium, reduced physical activity, myopathy, and increased risk of falls.

Consequences of Androgen Deprivation Therapy

Prostate cancer is an androgen-driven disease, and androgen deprivation therapy is the backbone of all therapies currently employed for patients affected with prostate cancer. ADT is carried out in two ways, either by gonadotropin-releasing hormone (GnRH) agonists or GnRH antagonists. After initiation of ADT, testosterone falls to castrate levels rapidly, reaching a nadir within 2 to 4 weeks [43, 44].

Consequences on Bone Metabolism

ADT reduces cortical and trabecular bone most rapidly during the first year of its initiation with a reported 5–10% loss of bone marrow density. Thus even patients with short-term ADT experience reduction in BMD. This effect continues as long as sex steroid levels are diminished. Earlier data estimated that without bone protective treatment, approximately 3000 excess fractures per year would be attributable to the use of GnRH-directed treatment [10].

Previous data already showed biochemical evidence of hypogonadism in up to 50% of men with hip fractures and a fivefold increase in hip fracture risk compared to men with eugonadal function. Moreover, orchiectomy in men with prostate cancer results in a 7-year cumulative fracture incidence of 13.6% versus 1.1% in noncastrate men [45]. Small prospective trials revealed that six out of 12 patients treated with GnRH agonist treatment had a statistically significant decrease in femoral BMD of 6.6% [46]. Later, one of the first trials examined BMD in 60 patients with prostate cancer receiving GnRH agonist therapy and compared it to 197 healthy controls of similar age. Significantly lower BMD was found at the lateral spine, total hip, and forearm (all $p < 0.01$) [47]. Urinary N-telopeptide and bone-specific alkaline phosphatase were elevated in the group under GnRH translating an increase in bone turnover [47]. The same authors examined prospectively the timing of bone loss under ADT in 152 men with prostate cancer. After 12 months, men who received ADT for less than 6 months had a significant reduction in BMD just like men who received ADT for 6 months and more [44]. This BMD reduction was present at multiple skeletal sites, and loss of BMD was most significant in the first year after ADT initiation. After 3 years of testosterone suppression, radius bone loss continued, suggesting that preventive measures should be implemented without delay and BMD should be monitored as long as patients are castrated [44].

In 2005, a large study recruited nonmetastatic prostate cancer men from a claims-based cohort to characterize the relationship between GnRH agonists and risk for clinical fractures [48]. A group of 3887 patients were compared to a control group of 7774 patients who did not receive ADT. The rate of any clinical fracture was 7.88 per 100 person-years at risk compared to 6.51 per 100 person-years (RR 1.21; 95% CI, 1.14 to 1.29; $p < 0.001$). The risk of vertebral fractures was also increased (RR 1.45; 95% CI, 1.19 to 1.75; $p < 0.001$). In a multivariate analysis, men who received less than 1 year of GnRH agonist had no significant increase in fracture risk compared to men who never received this therapy [48].

Contemporaneously, records from 50,613 men from the Surveillance, Epidemiology, and End Results program (SEER) and Medicare program were retrieved to examine the occurrence of fracture under GnRH agonist therapy [10]. During 12–60 months after diagnosis, 19.4% of patients in the ADT group had a fracture compared to 12.6% patients in the control group ($p < 0.001$). In addition, 5.2% of patients in the treatment group were hospitalized because of fracture compared to 2.4% ($p < 0.001$). There was a linear trend to the relative risk of the occurrence of any fracture or a fracture that resulted in a hospitalization with increasing number of doses of GnRH agonist therapy ($p < 0.001$). Finally, fracture risk was higher in older patients and in patients who received more doses of GnRH agonist therapy. As an example, the number needed to harm for the occurrence of any fracture in this study was 74 among patients 66–69 years of age who received four doses, whereas it was only 12 among those 80 years of age who received nine or more doses.

Management of Bone Health and Bone Metastases (Tables 9.3 and 9.4; Fig. 9.1)

It is established now that ADT affects the bone health of men living with prostate cancer across many stages. Early on bisphosphonates and later denosumab proved to be valuable agents for the prevention of osteoporosis-related fragility fractures and skeletal-related events in patients with prostate cancer. Multiple randomized controlled trials demonstrated their effectiveness, and clinical practice guidelines from different societies such as European Association of Urology (EAU), European Society for Medical Oncology (ESMO), American Society of Clinical Oncology (ASCO), National Comprehensive Cancer Network (NCCN), and Ontario's Critical Care are now available for therapists caring for these patients [49–51].

Patients under long-term ADT and thus at high risk of osteoporosis must have their risk of fracture estimated according to a recognized tool such as the FRAX evaluation tool. Baseline bone mineral density conventional dual-energy X-ray absorptiometry should ideally be offered to patients before the start of ADT and repeated according to the T-score of the patient and current guidelines, either annually if T-score is between −2.5 and −1.0 or, every 2 years if it is greater than −1.0 [49–51]. Supplemental intake of at least 1000 mg of calcium daily and 800 IU of vitamin D daily is endorsed by many expert panels, all the more in patients receiving denosumab or bisphosphonates [52]. Non-pharmacological interventions for the prevention of ADT-induced osteoporosis include also smoking cessation, alcohol intake limitation, and physical exercise [49–51]. In this matter, small trials compared exercise programs with usual care or group exercise versus personal training. Despite minor changes in lean body mass, no significant improvement in area BMD was found. These trials were all limited by very small cohorts (under 100 patients) and short study periods [53–55]. One positive trial investigated the effect of recreational football intervention on BMD in patients with prostate cancer on ADT. Patients who

Tables 9.3 and 9.4 Summary of clinical guidelines for management of bone health in prostate cancer

Prevention of androgen deprivation therapy-related osteoporosis and fracture
Target population: Men with nonmetastatic prostate cancer at high risk of fracture receiving ADT/men with metastatic hormone-sensitive prostate cancer/men with nonmetastatic castrate prostate cancer
BMD assessment with DXA combined with risk prediction tool such as FRAX at the initiation of ADT Monitoring of BMD according to initial T-score/WHO guidelines Smoking/alcohol counseling Exercise Calcium at least 1000 mg per day/vitamin D at least 800 UI per day Initiate bone-targeted therapy if T-score <2.0 or high FRAX score[a]: Denosumab preferentially, bisphosphonates if denosumab contraindicated or not available Monitoring of calcium, renal function Dental evaluation before start of bone-targeted therapies Counseling on osteonecrosis of the jaw Optimal duration of treatment not clear, up to 36 months
Prevention of skeletal-related events
Target population: Men with metastatic castration-resistant prostate cancer
Initiate monthly treatment with denosumab or zoledronic acid at SRE prevention dosages as early as possible Monitoring of calcium, renal function Calcium at least 1000 mg per day/vitamin D at least 800 UI per day Dental evaluation before initiation of bone-targeted therapies Counseling on osteonecrosis of the jaw and dental exam before start of bone-targeted therapies Optimal duration of treatment not clear, maximum of 24 months based on trials Radiotherapy when indicated to palliate pain and prevent bone complications

[a]The current National Osteoporosis Foundation Guide recommends treating patients with FRAX 10-year risk scores of > or = 3% for hip fracture or > or = 20% for major osteoporotic fracture, to reduce their fracture risk

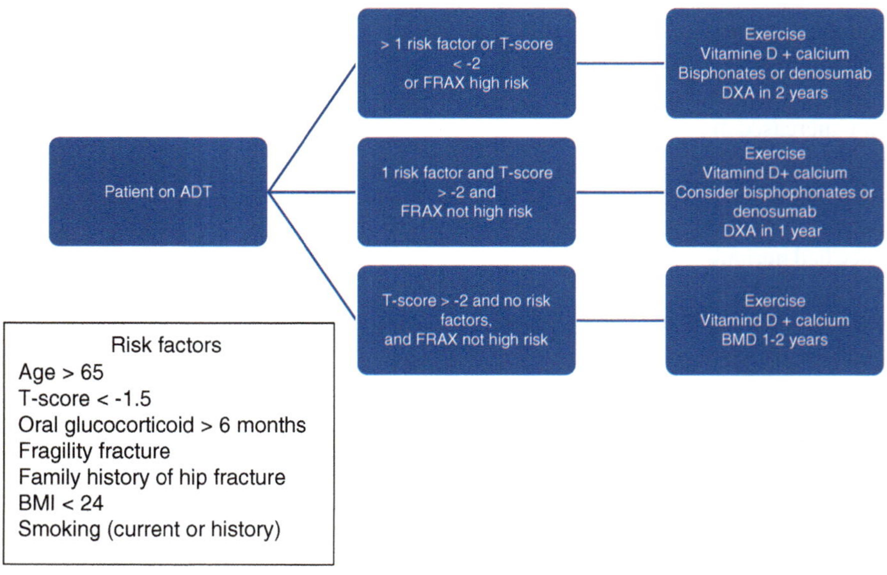

Fig. 9.1 Proposed approach for men on ADT

participated in the football intervention arm had a significant 2.1% difference at the lumbar spine ($p = 0.0144$), a 1.7% difference at the femoral neck ($p = 0.078$), and 1.7% difference at the hip ($p = 0.015$) as compared with standard of care arm [56].

Bone-Targeted Agents: Bisphosphonates and Denosumab (Table 9.5)

Bisphosphonates are pyrophosphate analogs that attach to hydroxyapatite binding sites of active bone metabolism and inhibit osteoclastic bone resorption [21]. When osteoclasts cause resorption of a bone impregnated with bisphosphonate, the agent released impairs osteoclast adhesion and production of the protons necessary for continued bone resorption. Bisphosphonates also decrease osteoclast progenitor development and recruitment and promote their apoptosis. Less importantly, they may prevent osteocyte and osteoblast apoptosis. Bisphosphonates are classified as nitrogen-containing (zoledronic acid, risedronate, ibandronate, alendronate) or not (etidronate, clodronate, tiludronate), the first group being more potent. Nitrogen-containing bisphosphonates inhibit the enzyme farnesyl pyrophosphate (FPP) synthase, disrupting protein prenylation. This process creates cytoskeletal abnormalities in the osteoclast, promotes its detachment from the bone, and results in reduced resorption [57, 58]. Bisphosphonates are available orally and in intravenous preparations. Orally, they are poorly absorbed, only in 1–5% of the total dose. With a half-life of approximately 1 hour, they are cleared rapidly from the plasma but may persist in the bone for the patient's lifetime [59].

Denosumab is a monoclonal antibody agent against the receptor activator of nuclear factor-kappa B ligand (RANKL) and thus blocks osteoclast activity [21]. RANKL activates osteoclast precursors and osteolysis promoting the release of bone-derived growth factors. Denosumab binds to RANKL and blocks the interaction between RANKL and RANK preventing osteoclast formation. Denosumab onset of action is quite rapid. It decreases markers of bone resorption by 85% within 3 days with maximal reductions observed at 1 month.

Table 9.5 Recommended doses and administration schedules for bone-targeted agents

Drug	Indication	Recommended dosage
Denosumab[a]	ADT-osteoporosis	60 mg subcutaneous injection every 6 months
	SRE prevention	120 mg subcutaneous injection every 4 weeks
Zoledronic acid	ADT-osteoporosis	5 mg intravenous infusion once per year[b]
	SRE prevention	4 mg intravenous infusion every 3–4 weeks[b]
Pamidronate	ADT-osteoporosis	60 mg intravenous infusion every 3 months
Alendronate	ADT-osteoporosis	70 mg per os once weekly
Risedronate	ADT-osteoporosis	35 mg once weekly

[a]Denosumab. Should not be given to patients with preexisting hypocalcemia until it is corrected. Patients with conditions predisposing to hypocalcemia should be monitored closely

[b]Zoledronic acid, pamidronate, alendronate, and risedronate are not recommended below creatinine clearance of 30 ml/min or less and should be adjusted in cases of renal insufficiency

Prevention and Treatment of Osteoporosis and Fragility Fractures

Nonmetastatic prostate cancer patients at high risk of fracture receiving ADT have access to denosumab which proved a benefit in reducing risk of fracture. Alternatively, if this therapy is contraindicated or not available, bisphosphonates showed also a clear benefit in improving BMD without reduction in the risk of fracture. For this indication, denosumab is prescribed at a dose of 60 mg subcutaneously twice a year. While optimal duration is unknown, studies provided data up until 36 months of therapy [49–51].

In a multicenter randomized double-blind placebo-controlled trial, 1468 patients undergoing ADT received denosumab at a dose of 60 mg subcutaneously compared to 734 patients in the placebo group. All patients took daily supplements of calcium and vitamin D. At 25 months, denosumab increased significantly bone mineral density at all measured sites. Denosumab was also associated with decreased incidence of new vertebral fracture at 12, 24, and 36 months, and levels of biochemical markers of bone turnover decreased significantly in the treatment group [60].

In the early 2000s, many bisphosphonates, such as pamidronate, alendronate, neridronate, and zoledronate, have been shown in some randomized controlled trials to prevent bone loss associated with ADT in nonmetastatic prostate cancer patients. A systematic meta-analysis reviewed data from 1017 participants across ten trials. The analysis evaluated both bone mineral density as an intermediate outcome and the more clinically important endpoint that is the occurrence of new fractures. Pooled results showed that there was no significant effect of treatment on fractures for participants in 1 year despite statistically improved BMD at different sites (lumbar spine, femoral neck, and total hip) [61].

The majority of trials addressed osteoporosis prevention in nonmetastatic hormone-sensitive prostate cancer. Patients with metastatic hormone-sensitive prostate cancer were rarely included. These patients may also benefit from treatment with denosumab or bisphosphonates at the osteoporosis-indicated dosage, especially if a low T-score is diagnosed or if the FRAX score suggests an elevated risk of developing fragility fracture.

Prevention of Skeletal-Related Events

Both denosumab and zoledronic acid are recommended for patients with metastatic castrate-resistant prostate cancer (mCRPC) to delay SREs.

For men with mCRPC, trials including early-generation bisphosphonates such as pamidronate did not prove a reduction in skeletal-related events for this population. In contrast, a phase III double-blind trial of 643 patients with mCRPC demonstrated benefit associated with zoledronic acid in preventing SREs [62]. In this study, men with mCRPC received placebo or 8 mg zoledronic acid initially that was reduced later to 4 mg because of renal toxicity. This trial demonstrated an 11% reduction in

≥1 SRE associated with zoledronic acid when compared with placebo ($p = 0.021$). Median time to first SRE was 321 for patients on placebo and was not reached for patients taking zoledronic acid ($p = 0.011$). Long-term results confirmed this benefit. Among 122 patients who completed a total of 24 months on study, fewer patients in the 4 mg zoledronic acid group than in the placebo group had at least one SRE (11% difference, $p = 0.028$). Median time to first SRE was significantly reduced from 488 days to 321 days in the placebo group ($p = 0.09$). Finally, zoledronic acid also reduced the risk of ongoing SREs by 36% ($p = 0.002$).

Less than a decade later, denosumab was compared to standard of care zoledronic acid for the prevention of SRE in men with mCRPC. In a multicenter randomized phase III trial, 1904 patients were randomized to denosumab 120 mg subcutaneously every 4 weeks and to 4 mg intravenous zoledronic acid [63]. Denosumab increased significantly bone mineral density in all sites within 1 month and the effect continued at 24 months. It was also associated with a significant 62% decrease of cumulative incidence of new vertebral fractures ($p = 0.006$). Finally, median time to first on-study SRE was 20.7 with denosumab versus 17.1 months with zoledronic acid ($p = 0.008$ for superiority) [63].

In regard to nonmetastatic CRPC, denosumab increased bone metastasis-free survival (MFS) by a median of 4.2 months compared to placebo ($p = 0.028$) and time to first bone metastasis (33.2 vs. 29.5 months, $p = 0.032$) [64]. Given the relatively short prolongation of MFS, the lack of any survival advantage, and the risks related to ONJ with long-term exposure, denosumab was not approved for metastasis prevention for men with nmCRPC.

Recently there have been disease-directed treatment advances in the management of hormone-sensitive metastatic prostate cancer with the addition of upfront docetaxel or novel ARATs to ADT. The pioneer multi-arm multistage STAMPEDE trial contributed greatly to the improvement of overall survival of men presenting with metastasis, regardless of their risk and tumor burden.

Under the STAMPEDE umbrella, two arms investigated zoledronic association with standard of care. First, the addition of ZA to ADT in arm B (with or without docetaxel) failed to improve time to SRE in the whole cohort and in the men with only bone metastases (HR 0.94, $p = 0.564$) [65]. In a second analysis, addition of ZA in 1245 randomized to ADT with ZA, celecoxib, both, or neither did not affect time to development of symptomatic SREs (HR 0.58, $p = 0.162$) [66].

CALGB 90202 is another trial that tested early treatment with zoledronic acid in 643 men with castration-sensitive metastatic prostate cancer [67]. Patients with mCSPC were randomized in a 1:1 ratio to receive zoledronic acid or placebo and followed for a primary endpoint of developing SRE. At disease progression to castration-resistant status, all patients received open-label ZA. Similar to STAMPEDE data, median time to first SRE was not statistically different between the groups (31.9 in ZA group vs. 29.8 months in placebo group, $P = 0.39$).

Zoledronic acid and denosumab are prescribed on a monthly basis for the prevention of SREs. Because of the long-term impregnation in the bone of bone-targeted agents, the optimal dosing interval and duration has been questioned. In a non-inferiority randomized trial, 263 patients (60.8% breast and 39.2% prostate) were randomized to 12-weekly and 4-weekly therapy. Patients in this trial received denosumab ($n = 148$), zoledronate ($n = 63$), and pamidronate ($n = 19.8\%$). There was no difference in health-related quality of life as a primary endpoint nor in the symptomatic skeletal event (SSE) rates and time to SSEs as secondary outcomes between the arms [68]. REDUSE is a phase III non-inferiority trial investigating whether or not denosumab efficacy is maintained at every 12 weeks compared to standard 4-week dosing. In this larger trial, 1380 patients with bone metastases will be randomized, among which 680 are mCRPC patients. The primary endpoint is time to first symptomatic skeletal event, and results are eagerly awaited (NCT02051218).

Safety of Bone-Targeted Agents

While hypocalcemia is more frequent with denosumab, zoledronic acid needs to be adjusted according to kidney function and may cause acute phase reactions. The most important adverse event associated with bone-targeted therapies is osteonecrosis of the jaw (ONJ). The natural history and the management of this complication evolved since it was first reported. ONJ is more frequently described in patients receiving intravenous bisphosphonates compared to oral formulation. While it can occur spontaneously, recent dental procedures increase the risk. Symptoms of ONJ include pain, swelling, and infection of soft tissues, loosening of teeth, drainage, and numbness of the jaw. The American Association of Oral and Maxillofacial Surgeons (AAOMS) recommends conservative management of this complication using antibiotics, oral rinses, and/or limited debridement. Bone resection is limited for more severe stages. Indeed, in 2011, authors presented an integrated analysis from three blinded active-controlled phase III trials in order to define the incidence, risk factors, and outcomes of ONJ in a cohort of 5723 patients [69]. The three trials encompassed in this analysis compared denosumab with zoledronic acid and included safety as a secondary outcome. Overall, 1.6% of the population were diagnosed with confirmed ONJ with no significant difference between treatment groups (1.3% ZA vs. 1.8% denosumab, $p = 0.13$). ONJ occurred between 4 and 30 months after the first dose of the drug. Jaw pain was reported in nearly three quarters of the patients with ONJ, and prior tooth extraction occurred in nearly 2/3 of ONJ events. In total 54% of the patients were treated conservatively, 41% underwent limited debridement, and four patients underwent resection of the affected bone.

Other Therapies and Combinations

Radium-223 Dichloride

Radium-223 dichloride (Ra223) is a targeted α-emitting radiopharmaceutical agent that preferentially binds to newly formed bone matrix. It acts by delivering short-range α-particle radiation, inducing irreparable double-stranded DNA breaks in target osteoblastic metastatic lesions.

Radium-223 is approved for the treatment of men with mCRPC with symptomatic bone metastases and without visceral metastases based on improved overall survival when compared with best supportive care in the ALSYMPCA trial. This trial investigated the effect of radium-223 on survival of 921 patients who were ineligible or refused docetaxel chemotherapy. In addition to improving disease control outcomes, time to SSE was also significantly longer in a post hoc analysis (median 14.7 vs. 8.1 months, $p < 0.0001$). Moreover, patients who received bisphosphonates at baseline had a longer time to SSE with radium-223 (HR 0.49; 95% CI 0.33–0.74; $p = 0.00048$) versus placebo (HR 0.77; 95% CI 0.0.58–1.02; $p = 0.07$) and a decreased risk of SSE in a multivariate analysis (HR 0.49; 95% CI 0.38–0.64; $p < 0.001$) [70].

Various guidelines strongly recommend use of bone-targeted agents for the prevention of SRE in patients with mCRPC. However, optimal timing for starting them, optimal dose and frequency, and optimal duration of treatment have not yet been defined. In addition, no recommendations on how to most effectively combine these agents with cancer-directed therapies such as ARAT or radium-223 are available [71].

Different post hoc analyses from several clinical trials questioned a potential effect on survival when bone-targeted agents were combined with other therapies. This evidence has yet to be validated prospectively. One post hoc analysis from COU-AA 302 study revealed that concomitant use of bisphosphonates or denosumab with abiraterone acetate (AA) improved OS ($n = 353$ patients; HR 0.75; 95% CI 0.60–0.94; $p = 0.012$) [72]. In contrast, this was not demonstrated when these agents were combined with enzalutamide in a post hoc analysis from PREVAIL trial [73].

ARAT's enzalutamide and abiraterone acetate modified the outcome of patients with mCRPC. Because of their effectiveness and tolerability, almost all patients with mCRPC are exposed to one of these agents. Recently, trials combining enzalutamide or AA with other therapies such as radium-223 have been conducted to improve patients' outcome. In this regard, ERA 223 phase III RCT randomized men with mCRPC to AA with or without radium-223 to determine whether this was associated with a decreased rate of symptomatic skeletal events (citation). Separately, EORTC 1333/PEACE III randomized patients with mCRPC to enzalutamide with or without Ra223 with a primary endpoint of radiographic progression-free survival. ERA 223 trial was unblinded early due to an imbalance in the incidence of deaths and fractures in patients receiving the abiraterone plus radium-223 combination when compared to patients receiving AA alone (39% vs. 36% and 29% vs. 11%, for deaths and fractures in the combination vs. abiraterone alone arms, respectively) [74]. Following this data, ESMO clinical guidelines recommended the use of a bone-targeted agent for all men with mCRPC treated with Ra223. Authors from phase 3 PEACE-III trial reported their data before and after ESMO recommendation: In the 45% patients treated without bone-protecting agent, the cumulative risk of fracture with enzalutamide at 1 year was at 12.4% and increased to 37.4% when Ra223 was added. After mandatory addition of a bone-protecting agent, the cumulative risk of fracture at 1 year fell drastically to 0% in enzalutamide group versus 2.2% with the combination arm [75].

Conclusion

There have been significant advances in the understanding of bone metabolism in men living with prostate cancer. Surely, preserving bone health is crucial for these patients. In the last two decades, the addition of bisphosphonates or denosumab has become standard of care for patients with nonmetastatic hormone-naïve prostate cancer and for those with metastatic castrate prostate cancer. In addition to preventing SREs, they are indicated in the prevention of osteoporosis and fracture for any patient, including men with hormone-sensitive prostate cancer and nmCRPC, who is at elevated risk of fracture and on long-term ADT. Furthermore, bone-protecting agents prove to be essential as new combinations of therapies are currently evaluated in large trials.

References

1. Bray F, Ferlay J, Soerjomataram I, Siegel RL, Torre LA, Jemal A. Global cancer statistics 2018: GLOBOCAN estimates of incidence and mortality worldwide for 36 cancers in 185 countries. CA Cancer J Clin. 2018;68(6):394–424.
2. Hamdy FC, Donovan JL, Lane JA, Mason M, Metcalfe C, Holding P, et al. 10-year outcomes after monitoring, surgery, or radiotherapy for localized prostate cancer. N Engl J Med. 2016;375(15):1415–24.
3. James ND, Rush H, Clarke N, Attard G, Cook A, Dearnaley D. 611O Abiraterone acetate plus prednisolone for hormone-naïve prostate cancer (PCa): long-term results from metastatic (M1) patients in the STAMPEDE randomised trial (NCT00268476). Ann Oncol. 2020;31:S509.
4. DeSantis CE, Lin CC, Mariotto AB, Siegel RL, Stein KD, Kramer JL, et al. Cancer treatment and survivorship statistics, 2014. CA Cancer J Clin. 2014;64(4):252–71.
5. Bolla M, Collette L, Blank L, Warde P, Dubois JB, Mirimanoff RO, et al. Long-term results with immediate androgen suppression and external irradiation in patients with locally advanced prostate cancer (an EORTC study): a phase III randomised trial. Lancet. 2002;360(9327):103–6.
6. Hussain M, Tangen CM, Berry DL, Higano CS, Crawford ED, Liu G, et al. Intermittent versus continuous androgen deprivation in prostate cancer. N Engl J Med. 2013;368(14):1314–25.
7. Huggins C, Hodges CV. Studies on prostatic cancer. I. the effect of castration, of estrogen and androgen injection on serum phosphatases in metastatic carcinoma of the prostate. CA Cancer J Clin. 1972;22(4):232–40.
8. Parker C, Nilsson S, Heinrich D, Helle SI, O'Sullivan JM, Fossa SD, et al. Alpha emitter radium-223 and survival in metastatic prostate cancer. N Engl J Med. 2013;369(3):213–23.
9. Mittan D, Lee S, Miller E, Perez RC, Basler JW, Bruder JM. Bone loss following hypogonadism in men with prostate cancer treated with GnRH analogs. J Clin Endocrinol Metab. 2002;87(8):3656–61.
10. Shahinian VB, Kuo YF, Freeman JL, Goodwin JS. Risk of fracture after androgen deprivation for prostate cancer. N Engl J Med. 2005;352(2):154–64.
11. Lassemillante AC, Doi SA, Hooper JD, Prins JB, Wright OR. Prevalence of osteoporosis in prostate cancer survivors: a meta-analysis. Endocrine. 2014;45(3):370–81.
12. Norgaard M, Jensen AO, Jacobsen JB, Cetin K, Fryzek JP, Sorensen HT. Skeletal related events, bone metastasis and survival of prostate cancer: a population based cohort study in Denmark (1999 to 2007). J Urol. 2010;184(1):162–7.
13. Kanis JA, Johnell O. Requirements for DXA for the management of osteoporosis in Europe. Osteoporos Int. 2005;16(3):229–38.

14. Hendrickx G, Boudin E, Van Hul W. A look behind the scenes: the risk and pathogenesis of primary osteoporosis. Nat Rev Rheumatol. 2015;11(8):462–74.
15. Callaway DA, Jiang JX. Reactive oxygen species and oxidative stress in osteoclastogenesis, skeletal aging and bone diseases. J Bone Miner Metab. 2015;33(4):359–70.
16. Jilka RL, O'Brien CA, Roberson PK, Bonewald LF, Weinstein RS, Manolagas SC. Dysapoptosis of osteoblasts and osteocytes increases cancellous bone formation but exaggerates cortical porosity with age. J Bone Miner Res. 2014;29(1):103–17.
17. Vanderschueren D, Vandenput L, Boonen S, Lindberg MK, Bouillon R, Ohlsson C. Androgens and bone. Endocr Rev. 2004;25(3):389–425.
18. Chen JF, Lin PW, Tsai YR, Yang YC, Kang HY. Androgens and androgen receptor actions on bone health and disease: from androgen deficiency to androgen therapy. Cell. 2019;8(11).
19. Huber DM, Bendixen AC, Pathrose P, Srivastava S, Dienger KM, Shevde NK, et al. Androgens suppress osteoclast formation induced by RANKL and macrophage-colony stimulating factor. Endocrinology. 2001;142(9):3800–8.
20. Manolagas SC, O'Brien CA, Almeida M. The role of estrogen and androgen receptors in bone health and disease. Nat Rev Endocrinol. 2013;9(12):699–712.
21. Bienz M, Saad F. Androgen-deprivation therapy and bone loss in prostate cancer patients: a clinical review. Bonekey Rep. 2015;4:716.
22. Eisman JA, Bouillon R. Vitamin D: direct effects of vitamin D metabolites on bone: lessons from genetically modified mice. Bonekey Rep. 2014;3:499.
23. Cosman F, de Beur SJ, LeBoff MS, Lewiecki EM, Tanner B, Randall S, et al. Clinician's guide to prevention and treatment of osteoporosis. Osteoporos Int. 2014;25(10):2359–81.
24. Johnell O, Kanis JA, Oden A, Johansson H, De Laet C, Delmas P, et al. Predictive value of BMD for hip and other fractures. J Bone Miner Res. 2005;20(7):1185–94.
25. Leslie WD, Tsang JF, Caetano PA, Lix LM, Manitoba Bone Density P. Effectiveness of bone density measurement for predicting osteoporotic fractures in clinical practice. J Clin Endocrinol Metab. 2007;92(1):77–81.
26. Cranney A, Jamal SA, Tsang JF, Josse RG, Leslie WD. Low bone mineral density and fracture burden in postmenopausal women. CMAJ. 2007;177(6):575–80.
27. Marques A, Ferreira RJ, Santos E, Loza E, Carmona L, da Silva JA. The accuracy of osteoporotic fracture risk prediction tools: a systematic review and meta-analysis. Ann Rheum Dis. 2015;74(11):1958–67.
28. Akhtar M, Haider A, Rashid S, Al-Nabet A. Paget's "seed and soil" theory of cancer metastasis: an idea whose time has come. Adv Anat Pathol. 2019;26(1):69–74.
29. Hauschka PV, Mavrakos AE, Iafrati MD, Doleman SE, Klagsbrun M. Growth factors in bone matrix. Isolation of multiple types by affinity chromatography on heparin-Sepharose. J Biol Chem. 1986;261(27):12665–74.
30. Roodman GD. Mechanisms of bone metastasis. N Engl J Med. 2004;350(16):1655–64.
31. Roudier MP, Vesselle H, True LD, Higano CS, Ott SM, King SH, et al. Bone histology at autopsy and matched bone scintigraphy findings in patients with hormone refractory prostate cancer: the effect of bisphosphonate therapy on bone scintigraphy results. Clin Exp Metastasis. 2003;20(2):171–80.
32. Achbarou A, Kaiser S, Tremblay G, Ste-Marie LG, Brodt P, Goltzman D, et al. Urokinase overproduction results in increased skeletal metastasis by prostate cancer cells in vivo. Cancer Res. 1994;54(9):2372–7.
33. Oudard S. TROPIC: phase III trial of cabazitaxel for the treatment of metastatic castration-resistant prostate cancer. Future Oncol. 2011;7(4):497–506.
34. Tannock IF, de Wit R, Berry WR, Horti J, Pluzanska A, Chi KN, et al. Docetaxel plus prednisone or mitoxantrone plus prednisone for advanced prostate cancer. N Engl J Med. 2004;351(15):1502–12.
35. Fizazi K, Tran N, Fein L, Matsubara N, Rodriguez-Antolin A, Alekseev BY, et al. Abiraterone plus prednisone in metastatic, castration-sensitive prostate cancer. N Engl J Med. 2017;377(4):352–60.

36. James ND, de Bono JS, Spears MR, Clarke NW, Mason MD, Dearnaley DP, et al. Abiraterone for prostate cancer not previously treated with hormone therapy. N Engl J Med. 2017;377(4):338–51.
37. Fizazi K, Scher HI, Molina A, Logothetis CJ, Chi KN, Jones RJ, et al. Abiraterone acetate for treatment of metastatic castration-resistant prostate cancer: final overall survival analysis of the COU-AA-301 randomised, double-blind, placebo-controlled phase 3 study. Lancet Oncol. 2012;13(10):983–92.
38. Ryan CJ, Smith MR, Fizazi K, Saad F, Mulders PF, Sternberg CN, et al. Abiraterone acetate plus prednisone versus placebo plus prednisone in chemotherapy-naive men with metastatic castration-resistant prostate cancer (COU-AA-302): final overall survival analysis of a randomised, double-blind, placebo-controlled phase 3 study. Lancet Oncol. 2015;16(2):152–60.
39. Compston J. Glucocorticoid-induced osteoporosis: an update. Endocrine. 2018;61(1):7–16.
40. Balasubramanian A, Wade SW, Adler RA, Lin CJF, Maricic M, O'Malley CD, et al. Glucocorticoid exposure and fracture risk in patients with new-onset rheumatoid arthritis. Osteoporos Int. 2016;27(11):3239–49.
41. Sato AY, Cregor M, Delgado-Calle J, Condon KW, Allen MR, Peacock M, et al. Protection from glucocorticoid-induced osteoporosis by anti-catabolic signaling in the absence of sost/sclerostin. J Bone Miner Res. 2016;31(10):1791–802.
42. Swanson C, Lorentzon M, Conaway HH, Lerner UH. Glucocorticoid regulation of osteoclast differentiation and expression of receptor activator of nuclear factor-kappaB (NF-kappaB) ligand, osteoprotegerin, and receptor activator of NF-kappaB in mouse calvarial bones. Endocrinology. 2006;147(7):3613–22.
43. Handforth C, D'Oronzo S, Coleman R, Brown J. Cancer treatment and bone health. Calcif Tissue Int. 2018;102(2):251–64.
44. Greenspan SL, Coates P, Sereika SM, Nelson JB, Trump DL, Resnick NM. Bone loss after initiation of androgen deprivation therapy in patients with prostate cancer. J Clin Endocrinol Metab. 2005;90(12):6410–7.
45. Daniell HW. Osteoporosis after orchiectomy for prostate cancer. J Urol. 1997;157(2):439–44.
46. Maillefert JF, Sibilia J, Michel F, Saussine C, Javier RM, Tavernier C. Bone mineral density in men treated with synthetic gonadotropin-releasing hormone agonists for prostatic carcinoma. J Urol. 1999;161(4):1219–22.
47. Stoch SA, Parker RA, Chen L, Bubley G, Ko YJ, Vincelette A, et al. Bone loss in men with prostate cancer treated with gonadotropin-releasing hormone agonists. J Clin Endocrinol Metab. 2001;86(6):2787–91.
48. Smith MR, Lee WC, Brandman J, Wang Q, Botteman M, Pashos CL. Gonadotropin-releasing hormone agonists and fracture risk: a claims-based cohort study of men with nonmetastatic prostate cancer. J Clin Oncol. 2005;23(31):7897–903.
49. Alibhai SMH, Zukotynski K, Walker-Dilks C, Emmenegger U, Finelli A, Morgan SC, et al. Bone health and bone-targeted therapies for prostate cancer: a programme in evidence-based care – Cancer Care Ontario Clinical Practice Guideline. Clin Oncol (R Coll Radiol). 2017;29(6):348–55.
50. Coleman R, Body JJ, Aapro M, Hadji P, Herrstedt J, Group EGW. Bone health in cancer patients: ESMO clinical practice guidelines. Ann Oncol. 2014;25 Suppl 3:iii124–37.
51. Saylor PJ, Rumble RB, Tagawa S, Eastham JA, Finelli A, Reddy PS, et al. Bone health and bone-targeted therapies for prostate cancer: ASCO Endorsement of a Cancer Care Ontario Guideline. J Clin Oncol. 2020;38(15):1736–43.
52. Tang BM, Eslick GD, Nowson C, Smith C, Bensoussan A. Use of calcium or calcium in combination with vitamin D supplementation to prevent fractures and bone loss in people aged 50 years and older: a meta-analysis. Lancet. 2007;370(9588):657–66.
53. Cormie P, Galvao DA, Spry N, Joseph D, Chee R, Taaffe DR, et al. Can supervised exercise prevent treatment toxicity in patients with prostate cancer initiating androgen-deprivation therapy: a randomised controlled trial. BJU Int. 2015;115(2):256–66.

54. Galvao DA, Nosaka K, Taaffe DR, Spry N, Kristjanson LJ, McGuigan MR, et al. Resistance training and reduction of treatment side effects in prostate cancer patients. Med Sci Sports Exerc. 2006;38(12):2045–52.
55. Winters-Stone KM, Dobek JC, Bennett JA, Maddalozzo GF, Ryan CW, Beer TM. Skeletal response to resistance and impact training in prostate cancer survivors. Med Sci Sports Exerc. 2014;46(8):1482–8.
56. Uth J, Hornstrup T, Christensen JF, Christensen KB, Jorgensen NR, Schmidt JF, et al. Efficacy of recreational football on bone health, body composition, and physical functioning in men with prostate cancer undergoing androgen deprivation therapy: 32-week follow-up of the FC prostate randomised controlled trial. Osteoporos Int. 2016;27(4):1507–18.
57. Rodan GA, Fleisch HA. Bisphosphonates: mechanisms of action. J Clin Invest. 1996;97(12):2692–6.
58. Sato M, Grasser W, Endo N, Akins R, Simmons H, Thompson DD, et al. Bisphosphonate action. Alendronate localization in rat bone and effects on osteoclast ultrastructure. J Clin Invest. 1991;88(6):2095–105.
59. Fleisch H. Pharmacokinetics. Biphosphonates in bone disease: from the laboratory to the patient, 1993.
60. Smith MR, Egerdie B, Hernandez Toriz N, Feldman R, Tammela TL, Saad F, et al. Denosumab in men receiving androgen-deprivation therapy for prostate cancer. N Engl J Med. 2009;361(8):745–55.
61. Ding H, Yang L, Du W, Teng Y, Fu SJ, Tao Y, et al. Bisphosphonates for osteoporosis in nonmetastatic prostate cancer patients receiving androgen-deprivation therapy: a systematic review and meta-analysis. Asian Pac J Cancer Prev. 2013;14(5):3337–43.
62. Saad F, Gleason DM, Murray R, Tchekmedyian S, Venner P, Lacombe L, et al. A randomized, placebo-controlled trial of zoledronic acid in patients with hormone-refractory metastatic prostate carcinoma. J Natl Cancer Inst. 2002;94(19):1458–68.
63. Fizazi K, Carducci M, Smith M, Damiao R, Brown J, Karsh L, et al. Denosumab versus zoledronic acid for treatment of bone metastases in men with castration-resistant prostate cancer: a randomised, double-blind study. Lancet. 2011;377(9768):813–22.
64. Smith MR, Saad F, Coleman R, Shore N, Fizazi K, Tombal B, et al. Denosumab and bone-metastasis-free survival in men with castration-resistant prostate cancer: results of a phase 3, randomised, placebo-controlled trial. Lancet. 2012;379(9810):39–46.
65. James ND, Sydes MR, Clarke NW, Mason MD, Dearnaley DP, Spears MR, et al. Addition of docetaxel, zoledronic acid, or both to first-line long-term hormone therapy in prostate cancer (STAMPEDE): survival results from an adaptive, multiarm, multistage, platform randomised controlled trial. Lancet. 2016;387(10024):1163–77.
66. Mason MD, Clarke NW, James ND, Dearnaley DP, Spears MR, Ritchie AWS, et al. Adding celecoxib with or without Zoledronic acid for hormone-naive prostate cancer: long-term survival results from an adaptive, multiarm, multistage, platform. Randomized Controlled Trial J Clin Oncol. 2017;35(14):1530–41.
67. Smith MR, Halabi S, Ryan CJ, Hussain A, Vogelzang N, Stadler W, et al. Randomized controlled trial of early zoledronic acid in men with castration-sensitive prostate cancer and bone metastases: results of CALGB 90202 (alliance). J Clin Oncol. 2014;32(11):1143–50.
68. Clemons M, Ong M, Stober C, Ernst S, Booth C, Canil C, et al. A randomised trial of 4- versus 12-weekly administration of bone-targeted agents in patients with bone metastases from breast or castration-resistant prostate cancer. Eur J Cancer. 2021;142:132–40.
69. Saad F, Brown JE, Van Poznak C, Ibrahim T, Stemmer SM, Stopeck AT, et al. Incidence, risk factors, and outcomes of osteonecrosis of the jaw: integrated analysis from three blinded active-controlled phase III trials in cancer patients with bone metastases. Ann Oncol. 2012;23(5):1341–7.
70. Hoskin P, Sartor O, O'Sullivan JM, Johannessen DC, Helle SI, Logue J, et al. Efficacy and safety of radium-223 dichloride in patients with castration-resistant prostate cancer and symptomatic bone metastases, with or without previous docetaxel use: a prespecified sub-

group analysis from the randomised, double-blind, phase 3 ALSYMPCA trial. Lancet Oncol. 2014;15(12):1397–406.
71. Saad F, Sternberg CN, Mulders PFA, Niepel D, Tombal BF. The role of bisphosphonates or denosumab in light of the availability of new therapies for prostate cancer. Cancer Treat Rev. 2018;68:25–37.
72. Saad F, Shore N, Van Poppel H, Rathkopf DE, Smith MR, de Bono JS, et al. Impact of bone-targeted therapies in chemotherapy-naive metastatic castration-resistant prostate cancer patients treated with abiraterone acetate: post hoc analysis of study COU-AA-302. Eur Urol. 2015;68(4):570–7.
73. Beer TM, Armstrong AJ, Rathkopf DE, Loriot Y, Sternberg CN, Higano CS, et al. Enzalutamide in metastatic prostate cancer before chemotherapy. N Engl J Med. 2014;371(5):424–33.
74. Radium-223-dichloride (Xofigo): Increased risk of death and fractures in a randomised clinical trial with Xofigo used in combination with abiraterone acetate and prednisolone/prednisone, 2017.
75. Tombal F LY, Saad F. Decreased fracture rate by mandating bone protecting agents in the EORTC 1333/PEACE III trial comparing enzalutamide and Ra223 versus enzalutamide alone; an interim safety analysis. ASCO; Chicago, IL, 2019.

Chapter 10
Radiotherapy for Advanced Prostate Cancer

Soumyajit Roy and Daniel E. Spratt

Introduction

All cancers in the human body are assigned using various methods to prognostic groups. Classically this is performed using TNM staging and/or histologic grading systems [1]. Prostate cancer is no exception, and accurate risk stratification is paramount to appropriately guide therapy for men with prostate cancer. Traditionally, the treatment of localized or non-metastatic malignancies includes radical local therapy with either radiotherapy or surgery [2]. In contrast, the role of local therapy with patients with metastatic disease was limited – mainly intended for palliation of advanced symptoms, such as pain, bleeding, or addressing spinal cord compression. In absence of optimal systemic therapy, it was challenging to demonstrate isolated benefit of local therapy to primary or metastatic sites [3, 4]. However, with advancement of systemic treatment, there has been rekindled interest in the role of local therapy in patients with metastatic malignancies. As demonstrated in breast cancer, the benefit of local therapy is more pronounced in presence of effective systemic therapies [5]. Similar advancements have been noticed in prostate cancer. From the approval of docetaxel in the early 2000s, to the surge of newer anti-androgen and chemotherapeutic options in the last few years, there now is an unprecedented arsenal of highly effective life-prolonging systemic therapies for men with advanced prostate cancer [6–15]. This begs the question to what the current role of local therapy in men with advanced prostate cancer is.

S. Roy
Department of Radiation Oncology, Rush University Medical Center, Chicago, IL, USA

D. E. Spratt (✉)
Department of Radiation Oncology, University Hospitals Seidman Cancer Center, Cleveland, OH, USA
e-mail: daniel.spratt@uhhospitals.org

K. L. Stratton, A. K. Morgans (eds.), *Urologic Oncology*,
https://doi.org/10.1007/978-3-030-89891-5_10

In this chapter, we review the historical role of both external beam and systemic radionuclide forms of radiotherapy for men with advanced prostate cancer. Additionally, guideline-concordant indications for radiotherapy are reviewed. Finally, emerging roles of external beam and novel systemic radionuclide forms of radiotherapy for advanced prostate cancer are discussed.

Palliative Radiotherapy for Advanced Prostate Cancer

Radiotherapy can be given for solely palliative intent and/or to improve oncologic outcomes (i.e., progression-free survival or overall survival). In this section we will review the uses of radiotherapy in advanced prostate cancer in settings in which the primary or sole intent is to provide palliation and improve quality of life.

External Beam Radiotherapy

Radiotherapy is commonly used as a highly effective form of palliation for patients with metastatic cancer. Common indications include palliation of biologic pain, bleeding, obstruction, brain metastases, and epidural spinal cord compression (Table 10.1) [16]. In prostate cancer, given the most common site of metastases is the bone, palliative radiotherapy is commonly used for palliation of skeletal pain in this patient population. In fact, a common mode by which patients in clinical trials of advanced prostate cancer experience a "progression" event is by experiencing clinical progression in a way that necessitates treatment with palliative external beam radiotherapy.

Table 10.1 Indications of palliative radiotherapy by symptoms in advanced prostate cancers

Symptoms/Indications	Etiology
Pain	Skeletal metastasis Visceral metastasis Spinal cord compression Nerve impingement
Obstructive symptoms such as hesitancy in urination, poor or intermittent urinary stream, prolonged micturition, anuria	Bladder infiltration or bladder outlet obstruction
Bleeding such as hematuria or blood in the stool	Hematuria from bladder infiltration Rectal wall infiltration leading to rectal bleeding
Neurologic symptoms such as headache, seizure, neurologic dysfunction	Brain or dural-based metastasis Spinal cord compression
Post-surgical fixation or instrumentation	Stabilization of pathologic fracture

The optimal control of pain in cancer patients relies on understanding the underlying pathophysiology and molecular mechanisms of the pain experience and is best achieved through multidisciplinary management [17]. Palliative external beam radiotherapy is most effective for biologic or oncologic sources of pain. The hallmarks of biologic pain are pain at rest, especially during nighttime or early morning that can occur even without movements. Such pain is associated with a diurnal variation in systemic corticosteroid levels and is directly related to the local inflammation caused by remodeling of the bones by active tumors [18]. A recent meta-analysis demonstrated that palliative external beam radiotherapy results in overall response rate in terms of pain control of more than 60%, independent of number of fractions. Additionally, complete response in pain control in which patients no longer require systemic treatment for pain is noted in approximately 1/4th of patients [19].

Another common cause of pain in cancer patients is mechanical. Such pain usually originates from a pathologic or non-pathologic fracture. Palliative radiotherapy is unlikely to improve this pain, but rather mechanical stabilization is likely to improve symptoms. Mechanical pain is most commonly exacerbated by movement and is relieved by rest. Although there is often a mixed component of biologic and mechanical pain, radiotherapy is not effective in alleviating the mechanical component of the pain, whereas surgical fixation or procedures such as vertebroplasty or kyphoplasty have been proven to be beneficial [20].

Another common indication for palliative radiotherapy is malignant epidural spinal cord compression. This is an alarming sequela of spine metastases that have been left untreated and therefore have progressed to the point of cortical destruction and compression of the thecal sac. This can either be an acute or chronic process. Early detection is the key to reverse the potential neurological consequences of malignant spinal cord compression with treatment. Depending on the level of the spinal cord or cauda equina that is being compressed, patients may complain of pain, focal weakness or paraplegia, sensory loss, or loss of bowel or bladder function. Having neurologic symptoms for more than 72 hours before initiating treatment significantly reduces the chances of restoring complete neurological function in a patient [21].

Prostate cancer represents a moderately radiosensitive tumor; therefore, external beam radiotherapy provides a durable local control and optimal decompression for spinal cord compression originating from prostate cancer. The acuity and severity of the compression helps guide the decision of whether to proceed with immediate surgical decompression followed by a re-exploration combined with postoperative radiotherapy or proceed with radiotherapy alone. If the latter is chosen, more advanced radiotherapy techniques such as stereotactic body radiotherapy (SBRT) are not used in the presence of significant epidural or intramedullary disease. In such cases standard conventional radiotherapy, commonly in 10 fractions, 3 Gy per fraction to a total of 30 Gy, is used [21].

Fortunately, prostate cancer rarely causes brain metastases. When they occur, brain metastases usually originate from the more aggressive subtypes of prostate cancer such as small cell variant or neuroendocrine prostate cancer. Thus, new onset of headaches, blurry vision, or other neurologic deficits in these patients that cannot readily be explained should prompt imaging of the brain, preferably with an MRI with and without contrast. When present these are treated most commonly with stereotactic radiosurgery alone or in combination with resection or whole brain radiotherapy depending on the size and number of lesions [22].

In advanced prostate cancer, especially before 2018, it was uncommon for patients who presented with de novo metastatic disease to receive treatment to their prostate. However, an untreated prostate cancer can continue to progress locally despite several lines of systemic therapy and result in significant deterioration in quality of life. This is most often related to local obstruction of the urinary tract from either direct compression or extension into the urethra or invasion or compression into the bladder and ureteral orifices. This leads to the requirement for either temporary intermittent self-catheterization, permanent Foley or suprapubic catheterization, or often repeated transurethral resections of the prostate. Similarly, although less common, a locally advanced primary can cause compression or infiltration into the rectum leading to obstruction, fistula, or bleeding. Palliative local radiotherapy can ameliorate these symptoms. Early institution of palliative local radiotherapy when the tumor is small allows for safe delivery of optimum dose to address these symptoms and to avoid any undue radiation-induced morbidity. Therefore, multidisciplinary care including input from urology is important to have prior to proceeding with palliative local radiotherapy. Various dose fractionation schedules can be used, but typically something less than a definitive dose of radiotherapy is used to minimize the risk of side effects.

Bleeding is a common manifestation from local invasion of prostate cancer, and radiotherapy is an effective method to reduce bleeding if the source of the bleed can be identified [23, 24]. Various schedules have been studied. This ranges from an abbreviated course, termed "quad-shot", of two treatments given in the same day 6–8 hours apart, 2 days in a row to other common palliative schedules of 4 Gy x 5 fractions or 3 Gy x 10 fractions.

Radionuclides

Various radionuclides have been and are currently used for the primary purpose of palliation of symptoms in oncology. Strontium-89 and samarium-153 were the two most commonly used and studied in advanced prostate cancer for palliation.

Strontium-89 has a physical half-life of 50.6 days and emits beta radiation. Strontium emits a small fraction of gamma photons and thus poses minimal radiation exposure risk to those in contact with the patient. This radioisotope is preferentially taken up by the bone with metastatic prostate cancer at a ratio of 10:1 compared to healthy normal bone and can remain in these metastatic lesions for up to 100 days. Strontium undergoes urinary excretion. Strontium-89 is most commonly administered with an activity of 1.48–2.22 MBq (40–60 μCi per kilogram of body weight, approximately 4 mCi [148 MBq] for standard weight) given by intravenous infusion over several minutes.

There is evidence to support the use of strontium, including a phase III placebo-controlled randomized controlled trial that evaluated conventional palliative radiotherapy ± strontium-89. This trial used a single injection of 10.8 mCi of strontium or placebo in 126 patients with metastatic castration-resistant prostate cancer (mCRPC). There was an improvement in complete pain relief at 3 months with strontium-89 compared to placebo (40% vs. 23%) and a significant reduction in the need for subsequent and continued analgesic use ($P < 0.05$). A significantly smaller proportion of patients treated with strontium experienced new sites of pain compared with placebo ($P < 0.002$). Finally, treatment with strontium resulted in a longer disease-free interval and longer interval before subsequent retreatment with radiotherapy (35 weeks vs. 20 weeks) [25]. Another 2x2 factorial randomized clinical trial investigated the clinical efficacy and cost-effectiveness of strontium-89 with or without docetaxel and/or zoledronic acid in metastatic castrate-resistant prostate cancer. Cox regression analysis adjusted for all stratification variables showed benefit of strontium-89 on clinical progression-free survival (HR 0.85; 95%CI, 0.73–0.99; $P = 0.03$). However, there was no additional advantage of strontium-89 with respect to overall survival [26].

Samarium-153 has a short physical half-life of 46.3 hours and emits both beta and gamma radiation. The gamma radiation can be used for a low-resolution bone scan. Samarium is bound to ethylenediamine tetramethylene phosphonic acid (EDTMP) which confers bone-seeking properties. Samarium-153 lexidronam is most commonly administrated with an activity of 37.0 MBq (1.0 mCi) per kilogram of body weight and given intravenously over several minutes.

The use of samarium-153 was evaluated in a phase III randomized controlled trial of 152 patients with mCRPC and randomized patients to samarium-153 at 1 mCi/kg vs. nonradioactive samarium-152. This study demonstrated that use of samarium-153 led to a significant improvement in pain scale scores by week 1 and pain intensity visual analogue scale scores by week 2 compared to the nonradioactive samarium-152. There was also a significant reduction in opioid consumption by week 3 with samarium-153 use [27]. There are two major sources of toxicity from samarium-153 treatment: targeting of sites other than the bone and due to the presence of unchelated samarium. Sm3+ metal has been found to distribute to the liver, lungs, and spleen. Thus, it is paramount that the amount of unchelated Sm3+ is as low as possible to avoid uptake by the liver and hepatotoxicity [28]. Additionally, bone marrow toxicity is often observed during samarium-153 therapy. Furthermore, significant radiation from 153Sm is often delivered to the bladder wall and kidneys [28]. Samarium-153 and strontium-89 emit high-energy beta particles and result in bone marrow toxicity [29]. This is why radium-223, an alpha emitter, has gained popularity in recent times. We have reviewed radium-223 later in this chapter.

Radiotherapy with Oncologic Intent for Advanced Prostate Cancer

Traditionally radiotherapy has been used with palliative intent in advanced prostate cancer as described in the previous section. However, several seminal randomized studies over the past decade have demonstrated substantial improvement in oncological outcome with use of radiotherapy with definitive intent in advanced prostate

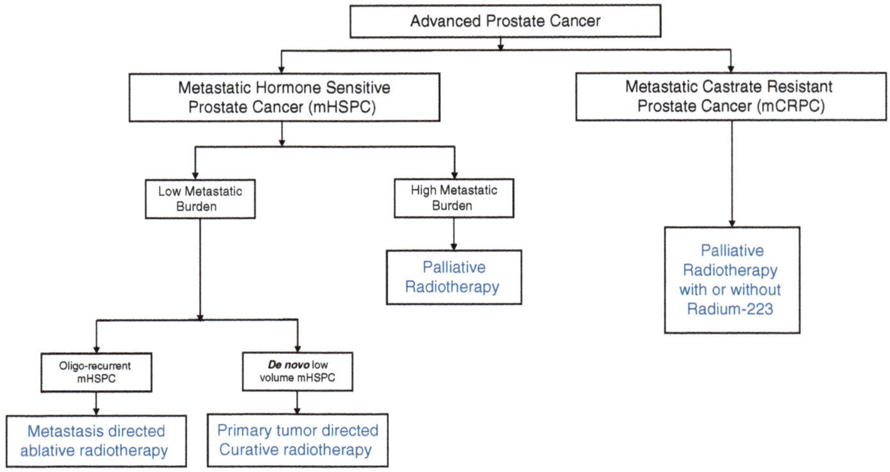

A simple algorithm for radiotherapeutic management of advanced prostate cancer

cancer. These include primary tumor-directed radiotherapy in metastatic hormone-sensitive prostate cancer (mHSPC) with low metastatic volume, ablative radiotherapy to metastatic sites in oligometastatic HSPC or oligorecurrent HSPC, and finally systemic radionuclide therapy with radium-223 in metastatic castrate-resistant prostate cancer (Table 10.2).

Treatment of the Primary

Combination of androgen deprivation therapy with local radiotherapy has been a well-established modality to treat high-risk localized, locally advanced, or clinically node-positive prostate cancer [2, 30–34]. However, because of no specified requirement of baseline imaging as a part of trial protocol and poor sensitivity and specificity of conventional imaging when these trials were conducted, a notable proportion of the enrolled patients presumably harbored metastatic disease and benefitted from this combined modality treatment. This hypothesis was tested in multiple retrospective studies. A large non-randomized registry-based study demonstrated that treatment to the primary with radiotherapy in mHSPC patients significantly improvement overall survival on multivariable and propensity score matched analysis (HR 0.62, 95% CI, 0.55–71, $p < 0.001$) [35].

Subsequently a number of randomized studies investigated this hypothesis. The first reported phase III randomized trial was the HORRAD trial. This was a relatively small randomized trial in men with mHSPC (n = 432). Patients were randomly allocated to either ADT alone or ADT in conjunction with prostate-directed radiotherapy. Radiotherapy was delivered to the prostate and base of the seminal vesicles with a 1 cm margin to a total dose of 70 Gy in 35 fractions using conventional fractionation or 57.76 Gy in 19 fractions using moderate hypofractionation. At a median follow-up of almost 4 years, the primary endpoint of overall survival

Table 10.2 Selected randomized evidence supporting definitive role of radiotherapy and systemic radionuclide therapy in advanced prostate cancer

Trial	Patient population	Treatment arms	Endpoint	Findings	Toxicity
Metastatic hormone-sensitive prostate cancer					
STAMPEDE Arm H (Phase III)	Newly diagnosed metastatic castrate-sensitive prostate cancer (pre-planned stratification into low volume vs. high volume metastatic burden based on CHAARTED definition)	Standard of care systemic therapy (ADT±Docetaxel) Vs. Systemic therapy + primary tumor directed radiotherapy (55 Gy in 20 fractions over 4 weeks or 36 Gy in 6 fractions over 6 weeks) 1:1 Randomization	Primary: OS Secondary: FFS Toxicity	For the entire study cohort: Control vs. radiotherapy: Improvement in FFS (median: 13 months vs. 17 months; HR: 0.76, 95% CI: 0.68–0.84) No improvement in OS (Median: 46 months vs. 48 months; HR: 0.92, 95% CI: 0.80–1.06) Low metastatic burden: Improvement in OS with radiotherapy (3-year OS: 73% vs. 81% HR: 0.68, 95% CI: 0.52–0.90) High metastatic burden: No Improvement in OS with radiotherapy (HR: 1.07, 95% CI: 0.90–1.28)	Late grade ≥3 adverse events: At 6 months (control vs. radiotherapy): 21% vs. 22% At 12 months (control vs. radiotherapy): 12% vs. 13% At 24 months (control vs. radiotherapy): 15% vs. 13%

(continued)

Table 10.2 (continued)

Trial	Patient population	Treatment arms	Endpoint	Findings	Toxicity
ORIOLE	Oligo-recurrent hormone-sensitive prostate cancer ≤3 metastases detectable by conventional imaging who had not received ADT within 6 months of enrollment or 3 or more years total	SABR vs. observation 2:1 randomization	Primary: Progression at 6 months Progression included biochemical, symptomatic, clinical, or radiographic progression, or death or initiation of ADT, or withdrawal after randomization	Proportion of disease progression at 6 months (control vs. SABR): 61% (95% CI: 38.5-79.6) vs. 19% (95% CI: 9.6-35.4) ($P = 0.005$) Median PFS (control vs. SABR): 5.8 months vs. NR (HR: 0.30, 95% CI: 0.11-0.81, $P = 0.002$)	No grade 3 or higher adverse events were identified New Grade 2 adverse events at 90 days (control vs. SABR): 0% vs. 9% New Grade 2 adverse events at 180 days (control vs. SABR): 0% vs. 6%
STOMP	Oligorecurrent prostate cancer with up to 3 metastases as detected by choline PET-CT and controlled primary	MDT of all detected lesions (with metastasectomy or SBRT) vs. surveillance 1:1 randomization	Primary: ADT-free survival, defined as the time between random assignment and the start of palliative ADT or death because of any cause. The indication to start ADT was symptomatic progression, progression to more than three metastases, or local progression of metastases	MDT vs. surveillance arm: 5-year ADT-free survival: 34% vs. 8%, HR: 0.57, 80% CI: 0.38–0.84, $P = 0.06$ (tests were performed two-sided; $P < 0.20$ was deemed significant)	Six patients developed grade 1 toxicity in the MDT arm. No grade 2 or higher toxicity was observed. Patient-reported QoL findings were similar between the two arms

SABR COMET (Phase II)	Patients with controlled primary tumor and one to five metastatic lesions (multiple tumor types enrolled; included patients with prostate cancer)	Palliative standard of care Vs. Metastasis-directed stereotactic ablative radiotherapy (30–60 Gy in three to eight fractions) Single fractions of 16–24 Gy were permitted for targets in the brain and vertebrae 2:1 randomization	Primary: OS Secondary: PFS Toxicity QoL	Control vs. ablative radiotherapy: 5-year OS: 17.7% (95% CI: 6% to 34%) vs. 42.3% (95% CI: 28% to 56%); (HR: 0.47, 95% CI: 0.27–0.81, stratified log-rank $P = 0.006$) Median PFS: 5.4 months (95% CI: 3.2–6.8) vs. 11.6 months (95% CI: 6.1–23.4); (HR: 0.48, 95% CI: 0.31–0.76, stratified log-rank test $P = 0.001$)	Grade ≥2 adverse events: Control vs. ablative radiotherapy: 9% vs. 29% 3 (4.5%) treatment-related deaths in the ablative radiotherapy group No differences in patient-reported QoL between treatment groups
Metastatic castrate-resistant prostate cancer					
ALSYMPCA	Treatment-resistant castration-resistant metastatic prostate cancer with ≥2 bone metastases detected on skeletal scintigraphy and no visceral metastases and had received docetaxel, were not fit for, or declined docetaxel, or it was not available	Six injections of radium-223 (at a dose of 50 kBq per kilogram of body weight IV) or matching placebo 2:1 Randomization	Primary: OS Secondary: Time to the first symptomatic skeletal event and various biochemical end points	Radium-223 vs. placebo: Median OS: 14.9 months vs. 11.3 months (HR: 0.70, 95% CI: 0.58–0.83) Median time to the first symptomatic skeletal event: 15.6 months vs. 9.8 months (HR: 0.66, 95% CI: 0.52–0.83)	No difference in the grade ≥3 hematologic (25% vs. 18%) or non-hematologic side effects between the Radium-223 vs. placebo group

was not statistically significantly different between arms (HR, 0.90, 95% CI, 0.70–1.14). On an unplanned subgroup analysis based on the metastatic burden or volume of disease, patients with ≤5 metastases had a greater relative benefit compared to patients with >5 metastases. This potential treatment-volume interaction suggested that patients with low-volume disease would preferentially benefit from definitive treatment of the primary tumor [36].

Shortly after the HORRAD trial was published, the large Systemic Therapy for Advanced or Metastatic Prostate cancer: Evaluation of Drug Efficacy (STAMPEDE) trial, arm H, reported its results. This trial enrolled men with mHSPC and investigated the use of standard systemic therapy with or without treatment of the primary tumor with definitive radiotherapy. Standard systemic therapy consisted of ADT or combination of ADT and docetaxel. The study enrolled nearly 2000 patients and had a primary endpoint of overall survival. Radiotherapy was delivered to the prostate gland with a margin of 10 mm (8 mm posteriorly). Two fractionation schedules were permitted, including a moderate hypofractionation schedule of 55 Gy in 20 fractions or an ultra-hypofractionation schedule of 36 Gy in 6 weekly fractions. Considering the treatment-volume interaction seen in the HORRAD trial, the investigators integrated a detailed prespecified subgroup analysis plan to assess the primary and secondary endpoints based on volume of disease. This was done prior to unblinding. Approximately 40% of men had low-volume disease (per the CHAARTED definition) and the proportion was near identical in the two treatment arms.

There was no significant difference in overall survival in the overall cohort (HR 0.92, 95% CI, 0.80–1.06; p = 0.266). Failure-free survival was significantly improved by the addition of radiotherapy to the primary (HR 0.76, 95% CI, 0.68–0.84). In the prespecified subgroup analysis, patients with low-volume disease had an improvement in both failure-free survival and overall survival (HR 0.68, 95% CI, 0.52–0.90; $p = 0.007$) with primary tumor-directed radiotherapy. However, there was no overall survival benefit of prostate-directed radiotherapy in the high-volume subgroup (HR 1·07, 95% CI, 0·90–1·28). Notably, there was no evidence that use of docetaxel had an impact on the magnitude of benefit with prostate-directed radiotherapy. Furthermore, there was no significant increase in time to toxicity or long-term rates of grade 3+ toxicity with radiotherapy to the primary [37].

Treatment of Metastatic Lesions

In the last decade or so, there has been a significant interest in using radiotherapy to consolidate metastatic sites. The goal of metastasis-directed radiotherapy (MDT) is to delay the need for systemic therapy, improve progression-free survival, and potentially improve overall survival. Although we are still in the incipient phase of demonstrating benefit of MDT with respect to oncologically robust endpoints such as overall survival, improvement in endpoints such as progression-free survival has been noticed with MDT in a number of randomized clinical studies.

Stereotactic body radiotherapy (SBRT) and stereotactic ablative body radiotherapy (SABR) are terms that describe a method of external beam radiotherapy that accurately delivers a high irradiation dose to an extracranial target in 5 or few treatment fractions. SBRT has been commonly adopted as a preferred method of MDT over conventionally fractionated (longer-course) radiotherapy or other ablative or surgical techniques. This is in part due to the convenience and noninvasive nature, but also due to the radiobiologic rationale that prostate cancer has a low α/β ratio. This means that for an equal risk of normal tissue damage one can have greater tumor cell kill with high dose per fraction. Moreover, such ablative dose of radiotherapy also portends microvascular damage which has a substantial effect on the tumor cell kill. Based on different systematic reviews and meta-analyses, SBRT maximizes the therapeutic ratio as it confers excellent local control (80–90%) and portends low rates of moderate to severe toxicity (<10% and < 5%, respectively) [21, 38, 39].

There is emerging and growing data to support the role of MDT in both prostate cancer and other cancer types. Non-small cell lung cancer has appreciated the largest oncologic benefits from MDT. To date, two trials have shown overall survival benefits with metastasis-directed radiotherapy, despite their small sample size and phase II nature. Gomez et al. randomized patients with ≤3 metastases to maintenance systemic therapy with or without total consolidation of local tumor and MDT. The trial stopped early after enrolling 49 patients due to the early overall survival benefit seen from radiotherapy on interim analysis [40]. SABR-COMET was another phase II randomized trial investigating the benefit of metastasis-directed ablative radiotherapy in oligometastatic malignancies regardless of the primary site, and approximately 15% of patients enrolled had prostate cancer. This trial randomized patients to standard systemic therapy with or without MDT for patients with oligometastatic cancer (≤5 metastases). In their initial report, SBRT-based MDT led to significant prolongation of progression-free survival (6 months in control group vs. 12 months in the SBRT group (HR 0.47, 95% CI, 0.30–0.76; stratified log-rank $p = 0.0012$)) [41]. After a median follow-up of 51 months, the 5-year OS rate was 17.7% in the control group (95% CI, 6–34%) versus 42.3% in SBRT group (95%CI, 28–56%; stratified log-rank $P = 0.006$). However, MDT was also associated with increased risk of grade 2 or higher adverse events (9% in the control group vs. 29% in MDT group, $P = 0.03$). There were three deaths (4.5%) in the SABR arm that were possibly, probably, or definitely related to treatment [42].

Two small phase II randomized trials have evaluated the role of MDT in metastatic prostate cancer. There is a wealth of retrospective data and single-arm trials, but this will not be discussed. STOMP was a randomized phase II trial, which randomized 62 patients to observation +/− MDT with a primary endpoint of ADT-free survival. Importantly, this trial had prespecified indications for initiation of ADT. Patients enrolled had oligorecurrent prostate cancer based on PET choline imaging with ≤3 metastases, and thus these patients were more akin to biochemically recurrent disease than de novo M1 disease by conventional imaging. MDT was given as SBRT in most patients (25 of 31), and at a median 3-year follow-up, the use of MDT improved median ADT-free survival from 13 to 21 months and median time to PSA-progression from 6 to 10 months [43]. There was no clinically or statistically meaningful between-arm difference in the mean change in score from baseline to 3 months and 1 year. For example, mean (95% CI) difference between the arms for change in global health status score from baseline to 3 months was 0 (−7 to 6). The same for baseline to 1 year was 2 (−9 to 6) [43]. The second phase II trial was the Observation verus Stereotactic Ablative Radiation for Oligometastatic Prostate Cancer (ORIOLE), which enrolled 54 men with oligorecurrent prostate cancer, but unlike STOMP which was a 1:1 randomization, ORIOLE was a 2:1 randomization of observation +/− MDT with SBRT. The primary endpoint was progression by 6 months, which was a composite endpoint including ADT initiation, PSA progression, symptomatic progression, or death. The primary endpoint was improved with SBRT (19% vs. 61%; HR 0.30, 95% CI, 0.11–0.81; $P = 0.002$). There was no grade 3 or higher adverse events from MDT [44].

Radionuclide Therapy

Radium-223 dichloride is currently the most common form of systemic radionuclide therapy for the treatment of prostate cancer. Radium is a bone-seeking calcium analogue that has a half-life of 11.4 days and emits high-energy alpha particles. Unlike samarium and strontium, the alpha particles from radium-223 have a high biologic effectiveness and linear energy transfer. However, alpha particles have a short path length of <10 cell lengths. This short length of trajectory helps in minimizing bone marrow toxicity with alpha particle-based treatment. However, this is one of the reasons for which Ra-223 is unable to reach tumor extension beyond the bone. Radium-223 is primarily cleared through the intestine [45]. Radium-223 is most commonly given as a monthly (q4 week) injection (50 kBq/kg intravenous) for a total of six cycles.

Radium-223 has FDA approval for the treatment of symptomatic bone metastases from mCRPC. However, unlike samarium-153 and strontium-89, radium-223 has been shown to improve both pain and overall survival. This finding was from the multinational phase III, double-blind, randomized controlled trial of 922 men with symptomatic mCRPC. Patients were randomized to six injections of radium-223 (50 kBq/kg) versus placebo. The trial was stopped early at a planned interim analysis after an overall survival benefit was reached (median overall survival with radium-223 treatment was 14.0 vs. 11.2 months; $P = 0.0019$; HR 0.695, 95% CI, 0.552–0.875). Additionally, radium-223 resulted in a lower incidence of skeletal-related events ($P = 0.016$). Radium-223 was generally well tolerated (grade 3–4 neutropenia of 1.8% vs. 0.8%, and thrombocytopenia 4% vs. 2%, respectively) [15].

An important discussion point that is often overlooked is that when radium-223 was tested in the landmark phase III trial, other novel androgen signaling inhibitors (ARSIs) had not gained FDA approval yet. Thus, radium-223 was generally used early in the treatment course of mCRPC. In contrast, since the approval of enzalutamide, abiraterone, and other agents, radium-223 is commonly a 3rd- or fourth-line therapy. Such delay in the use of this radioisotope has been found to portend poor compliance, and this in turn brings down the expected benefit from this radioisotope therapy. Furthermore, it becomes increasingly less likely that these patients harbor isolated osseous disease without any extension to periosseous soft tissue or epidural extension, potentially limiting the efficacy of radium-223 [46].

Future Indications of Radiotherapy for Advanced Prostate Cancer

Radiotherapy is a critically important tool to be used in men with advanced prostate cancer to prolong life and improve quality of life. However, there are even further areas that radiotherapy has the potential to improve outcomes for men in this patient population. The use of SBRT as MDT has its primary evidence in oligorecurrent prostate cancer. Ongoing trials are evaluating the role of radiotherapy to sites of metastases in both de novo mHSPC in the next arm of the STAMPEDE trial (arm M) and in mCRPC (e.g., FORCE trial, NCT03556904). These trials will help to establish additional contexts where MDT with radiotherapy may become part of the routine standard of care. There is also interest in understanding if treatment of the primary with radiotherapy may have benefit in high-volume metastatic disease when used concurrently with treatment of the metastases, in essence to functionally render these patients more akin to low-volume disease.

Additionally, other radionuclides are being studied. The most exciting are based on targeting prostate-specific membrane antigen (PSMA). The molecules are linked commonly to the beta-emitter, lutetium-177, which has shown promise. 177Lu-PSMA-617 delivers beta-particle radiation selectively to PSMA-positive cells and the surrounding microenvironment. Several new alpha-particle emitting agents such as actinium-225, bismuth-212, terbium-149, astatin-211 are being actively evaluated for PSMA-based targeted alpha particle therapy [47]. Moreover, in the recently presented phase III randomized VISION trial, addition of lutetium-177-PSAM-617(LuPSMA) to standard of care in men with PSMA-avid metastatic castrate-resistant prostate cancer was associated with a 38% reduction in the risk of death (HR 0.62, 95%CI, 0.52–0.74) and a 4-month improvement in overall survival. Furthermore, LuPSMA combined with standard of care treatment significantly improved radiographic progression-free survival (rPFS) by a median of 5.3 months (median rPFS, 8.7 vs. 3.4 months; HR 0.40, 99.2% CI, 0.29–0.57; $p < 0.001$, one-sided). There was a higher rate of high-grade (grade 3–5) treatment-related adverse events with LuPSMA (28.4% vs. 3.9%). Additionally, there were five deaths attributable to the experimental treatment. In terms of specific adverse events, treatment with LuPSMA was associated with increased rates of bone marrow suppression, xerostomia, and nausea and vomiting [48, 49]. Note should be made of the fact that only about 1/2 of the patients in both arms received one or two taxane-based regimens before being given trial regimen. Hence there remains a doubt on the actual efficacy of the LuPSMA therapy in patients heavily pre-treated with taxane-based regimens.

Conclusion

Radiotherapy is now used in the vast majority of patients with advanced prostate cancer. This ranges from palliation (e.g., bone pain, urinary or rectal obstruction or bleeding, or epidural spinal cord compression) to treatment of the primary or metastases for oncologic benefit. Palliation can be accomplished with both external beam radiotherapy or radionuclides, such as strontium or samarium. These radionuclides have largely been replaced by radium-223, which not only provides palliation of pain but also prolongs survival. External beam radiotherapy directed to primary tumor has been shown to confer survival advantage in low-volume mHSPC. PSMA ligand-based radionuclide therapy has also demonstrated survival advantage in metastatic castrate-resistant prostate cancer. Furthermore, MDT using SBRT has been shown to delay progression and forestall use of ADT in men with oligorecurrent mHSPC. Trials are ongoing or maturing to further establish the oncologic benefit of MDT in de novo mHSPC, use of MDT in patients with >5 metastases. Given the critical role radiotherapy has in the multidisciplinary management of advanced prostate cancer, incorporation of radiation oncology and nuclear medicine into the care team is paramount for optimizing overall outcome in this patient population.

References

1. AJCC – Cancer Staging Manual. https://cancerstaging.org/references-tools/deskreferences/Pages/default.aspx. Accessed 18 Jan 2021.
2. Mohler JL, Antonarakis ES, Armstrong AJ, et al. Prostate cancer, version 2.2019. JNCCN J Natl Compr Cancer Netw. 2019;17(5):479–505. https://doi.org/10.6004/jnccn.2019.0023.
3. Lutz ST, Chow EL, Hartsell WF, Konski AA. A review of hypofractionated palliative radiotherapy. Cancer. 2007;109(8):1462–70. https://doi.org/10.1002/cncr.22555.
4. Lutz S, Korytko T, Nguyen J, Khan L, Chow E, Corn B. Palliative radiotherapy: when is it worth it and when is it not? Cancer J. 2010;16(5):473–82. https://doi.org/10.1097/PPO.0b013e3181f28b4d.
5. Jutzy JMS, Lemons JM, Luke JJ, Chmura SJ. The evolution of radiation therapy in metastatic breast cancer: from local therapy to systemic agent. Int J Breast Cancer. 2018;2018 https://doi.org/10.1155/2018/4786819.
6. Davis ID, Martin AJ, Stockler MR, et al. Enzalutamide with standard first-line therapy in metastatic prostate cancer. N Engl J Med. 2019;381(2):121–31. https://doi.org/10.1056/nejmoa1903835.
7. Sweeney CJ, Chen Y-H, Carducci M, et al. Chemohormonal therapy in metastatic hormone-sensitive prostate cancer. N Engl J Med. 2015;373(8):737–46. https://doi.org/10.1056/NEJMoa1503747.
8. Fizazi K, Tran N, Fein L, et al. Abiraterone plus prednisone in metastatic, castration-sensitive prostate cancer. N Engl J Med. 2017;377(4):352–60. https://doi.org/10.1056/NEJMoa1704174.
9. James ND, de Bono JS, Spears MR, et al. Abiraterone for prostate cancer not previously treated with hormone therapy. N Engl J Med. 2017;377(4):338–51. https://doi.org/10.1056/NEJMoa1702900.
10. James ND, Sydes MR, Clarke NW, et al. Addition of docetaxel, zoledronic acid, or both to first-line long-term hormone therapy in prostate cancer (STAMPEDE): survival results

from an adaptive, multiarm, multistage, platform randomised controlled trial. Lancet. 2016;387(10024):1163–77. https://doi.org/10.1016/S0140-6736(15)01037-5.
11. De Bono JS, Oudard S, Ozguroglu M, et al. Prednisone plus cabazitaxel or mitoxantrone for metastatic castration-resistant prostate cancer progressing after docetaxel treatment: a randomised open-label trial. Lancet. 2010;376(9747):1147–54. https://doi.org/10.1016/S0140-6736(10)61389-X.
12. Chi KN, Agarwal N, Bjartell A, et al. Apalutamide for metastatic, castration-sensitive prostate cancer. N Engl J Med. 2019;381(1):13–24. https://doi.org/10.1056/nejmoa1903307.
13. Beer TM, Armstrong AJ, Rathkopf DE, et al. Enzalutamide in metastatic prostate cancer before chemotherapy. N Engl J Med. 2014;371(5):424–33. https://doi.org/10.1056/NEJMoa1405095.
14. Tannock IF, de Wit R, Berry WR, et al. Docetaxel plus prednisone or mitoxantrone plus prednisone for advanced prostate cancer. N Engl J Med. 2004;351(15):1502–12. https://doi.org/10.1056/nejmoa040720.
15. Parker C, Nilsson S, Heinrich D, et al. Alpha emitter Radium-223 and survival in metastatic prostate cancer. N Engl J Med. 2013;369(3):213–23. https://doi.org/10.1056/nejmoa1213755.
16. Spencer K, Parrish R, Barton R, Henry A. Palliative radiotherapy. BMJ. 2018;360 https://doi.org/10.1136/bmj.k821.
17. Raphael J, Ahmedzai S, Hester J, et al. Cancer pain: part 1: pathophysiology; oncological, pharmacological, and psychological treatments: a perspective from the British pain society endorsed by the UK association of palliative medicine and the royal college of general practitioners. Pain Med. 2010;11(5):742–64. https://doi.org/10.1111/j.1526-4637.2010.00840.x.
18. Lozano-Ondoua AN, Symons-Liguori AM, Vanderah TW. Cancer-induced bone pain: mechanisms and models. Neurosci Lett. 2013;557:52–9. https://doi.org/10.1016/j.neulet.2013.08.003.
19. Rich SE, Chow R, Raman S, et al. Update of the systematic review of palliative radiation therapy fractionation for bone metastases. Radiother Oncol. 2018;126(3):547–57. https://doi.org/10.1016/j.radonc.2018.01.003.
20. Zajączkowska R, Kocot-Kępska M, Leppert W, Wordliczek J. Bone pain in cancer patients: mechanisms and current treatment. Int J Mol Sci. 2019;20(23) https://doi.org/10.3390/ijms20236047.
21. Spratt DE, Beeler WH, de Moraes FY, et al. An integrated multidisciplinary algorithm for the management of spinal metastases: an international spine oncology consortium report. Lancet Oncol. 2017;18(12):e720–30. https://doi.org/10.1016/S1470-2045(17)30612-5.
22. Brown PD, Ahluwalia MS, Khan OH, Asher AL, Wefel JS, Gondi V. Whole-brain radiotherapy for brain metastases: evolution or revolution? J Clin Oncol. 2018;36(5):483–91. https://doi.org/10.1200/JCO.2017.75.9589.
23. Cameron MG, Kersten C, Vistad I, et al. Palliative pelvic radiotherapy for symptomatic incurable prostate cancer – a prospective multicenter study. Radiother Oncol. 2015;115(3):314–20. https://doi.org/10.1016/j.radonc.2015.05.021.
24. Carl J, Rades D, Doemer C, Setter C, Dunst J, Holländer NH. Palliative radiotherapy to dominant symptomatic lesion in patients with hormone refractory prostate cancer (PRADO). Radiat Oncol. 2019;14(1):3. https://doi.org/10.1186/s13014-019-1209-0.
25. Porter AT, McEwan AJB, Powe JE, et al. Results of a randomized phase-III trial to evaluate the efficacy of strontium-89 adjuvant to local field external beam irradiation in the management of endocrine resistant metastatic prostate cancer. Int J Radiat Oncol Biol Phys. 1993;25(5):805–13. https://doi.org/10.1016/0360-3016(93)90309-J.
26. James ND, Pirrie SJ, Pope AM, et al. Clinical outcomes and survival following treatment of metastatic castrate-refractory prostate cancer with docetaxel alone or with strontium-89, zoledronic acid, or both: the TRAPEZE randomized clinical trial. JAMA Oncol. 2016;2(4):493–9. https://doi.org/10.1001/jamaoncol.2015.5570.
27. Sartor O, Reid RH, Hoskin PJ, et al. Samarium-153-lexidronam complex for treatment of painful bone metastases in hormone-refractory prostate cancer. Urology. 2004;63(5):940–5. https://doi.org/10.1016/j.urology.2004.01.034.
28. Anderson P. Samarium for osteoblastic bone metastases and osteosarcoma. Expert Opin Pharmacother. 2006;7(11):1475–86. https://doi.org/10.1517/14656566.7.11.1475.

29. Morgan SC. Radium-223 in metastatic castration-resistant prostate cancer: clinical development and use in contemporary practice. J Med Imaging Radiat Sci. 2019;50(4):S26–30. https://doi.org/10.1016/j.jmir.2019.05.006.
30. Widmark A, Klepp O, Solberg A, et al. Endocrine treatment, with or without radiotherapy, in locally advanced prostate cancer (SPCG-7/SFUO-3): an open randomised phase III trial. Lancet (London, England). 2009;373(9660):301–8. https://doi.org/10.1016/S0140-6736(08)61815-2.
31. Mason MD, Parulekar WR, Sydes MR, et al. Final report of the intergroup randomized study of combined androgen-deprivation therapy plus radiotherapy versus androgen-deprivation therapy alone in locally advanced prostate cancer. J Clin Oncol. 2015;33:2143. https://doi.org/10.1200/JCO.2014.57.7510.
32. Bolla M, Van Tienhoven G, Warde P, et al. External irradiation with or without long-term androgen suppression for prostate cancer with high metastatic risk: 10-year results of an EORTC randomised study. Lancet Oncol. 2010;11(11):1066–73. https://doi.org/10.1016/S1470-2045(10)70223-0.
33. Pilepich MV, Winter K, Lawton CA, et al. Androgen suppression adjuvant to definitive radiotherapy in prostate carcinoma—long-term results of phase III RTOG 85–31. Int J Radiat Oncol Biol Phys. 2005;61(5):1285–90. https://doi.org/10.1016/J.IJROBP.2004.08.047.
34. Roach M, Bae K, Speight J, et al. Short-term neoadjuvant androgen deprivation therapy and external-beam radiotherapy for locally advanced prostate cancer: long-term results of RTOG 8610. J Clin Oncol. 2008;26(4):585–91. https://doi.org/10.1200/JCO.2007.13.9881.
35. Rusthoven CG, Jones BL, Flaig TW et al. Improved Survival With Prostate Radiation in Addition to Androgen Deprivation Therapy for Men With Newly Diagnosed Metastatic Prostate Cancer. J Clin Oncol. 2016;34(24):2835–42. https://doi.org/10.1200/JCO.2016.67.4788
36. Boevé LMS, Hulshof MCC, Vis AN et al. Effect on Survival of Androgen Deprivation Therapy Alone Compared to Androgen Deprivation Therapy Combined with Concurrent Radiation Therapy to the Prostate in Patients with Primary Bone Metastatic Prostate Cancer in a Prospective Randomised Clinical Trial: Data from the HORRAD Trial. Eur Urol. 2019;75(3):410-418. doi: 10.1016/j.eururo.2018.09.008.
37. Parker CC, James ND, Brawley CD, et al. Radiotherapy to the primary tumour for newly diagnosed, metastatic prostate cancer (STAMPEDE): a randomised controlled phase 3 trial. Lancet. 2018;392(10162):2353–66. https://doi.org/10.1016/S0140-6736(18)32486-3.
38. Alongi F, Arcangeli S, Filippi AR, Ricardi U, Scorsetti M. Review and uses of stereotactic body radiation therapy for oligometastases. Oncologist. 2012;17(8):1100–7. https://doi.org/10.1634/theoncologist.2012-0092.
39. Spencer KL, Van Der Velden JM, Wong E, et al. Systematic review of the role of stereotactic radiotherapy for bone metastases. J Natl Cancer Inst. 111:1023. https://doi.org/10.1093/jnci/djz101.
40. Gomez DR, Tang C, Zhang J, et al. Local consolidative therapy vs. maintenance therapy or observation for patients with oligometastatic non–small-cell lung cancer: long-term results of a multi-institutional, phase II, randomized study. J Clin Oncol. 2019;37(18):1558–65. https://doi.org/10.1200/JCO.19.00201.
41. Palma DA, Olson R, Harrow S, et al. Stereotactic ablative radiotherapy versus standard of care palliative treatment in patients with oligometastatic cancers (SABR-COMET): a randomised, phase 2, open-label trial. Lancet. 2019;393(10185):2051–8. https://doi.org/10.1016/S0140-6736(18)32487-5.
42. Palma DA, Olson R, Harrow S, et al. Stereotactic ablative radiotherapy for the comprehensive treatment of oligometastatic cancers: long-term results of the SABR-COMET phase II randomized trial. J Clin Oncol. 2020;38(25):2830–8. https://doi.org/10.1200/JCO.20.00818.
43. Ost P, Reynders D, Decaestecker K, et al. Surveillance or metastasis-directed therapy for oligometastatic prostate cancer recurrence: a prospective, randomized, multicenter phase II trial. J Clin Oncol. 2018;36(5):446–53. https://doi.org/10.1200/JCO.2017.75.4853.
44. Phillips R, Shi WY, Deek M, et al. Outcomes of observation vs stereotactic ablative radiation for oligometastatic prostate cancer: the ORIOLE phase 2 randomized clinical trial. JAMA Oncol. 2020;6(5):650–9. https://doi.org/10.1001/jamaoncol.2020.0147.

45. Dauer LT, Williamson MJ, Humm J, et al. Radiation safety considerations for the use of 223 RaCl 2 DE in men with castration-resistant prostate cancer HHS public access author manuscript. Health Phys. 2014;106(4):494–504. https://doi.org/10.1097/HP.0b013e3182a82b37.
46. Parker C, Heidenreich A, Nilsson S, Shore N. Current approaches to incorporation of radium-223 in clinical practice. Prostate Cancer Prostatic Dis. 2018;21(1):37–47. https://doi.org/10.1038/s41391-017-0020-y.
47. Juzeniene A, Stenberg VY, Bruland ØS, Larsen RH. Preclinical and clinical status of psma-targeted alpha therapy for metastatic castration-resistant prostate cancer. Cancers (Basel) 2021;13:1–25. https://doi.org/10.3390/cancers13040779.
48. Morris MJ, De Bono JS, Chi KN, et al. Phase III study of lutetium-177-PSMA-617 in patients with metastatic castration-resistant prostate cancer (VISION). J Clin Oncol. 2021;39(18_suppl):LBA4. https://doi.org/10.1200/JCO.2021.39.15_suppl.LBA4.
49. Sartor O, Bono J de, Chi KN, Fizazi K, Herrmann K, Rahbar K, et al. Lutetium-177–PSMA-617 for Metastatic Castration-Resistant Prostate Cancer. https://doi.org/101056/NEJMoa2107322 2021.

Chapter 11
Optimizing Perioperative Treatment for Kidney Cancer

Wesley H. Chou, Daniel Lin, Viraj Master, and Sarah P. Psutka

Introduction

Complications After Surgery for Localized/Advanced Renal Cell Carcinoma

Surgery remains the mainstay of treatment in patients with localized or locally advanced renal cell carcinoma (RCC), as well as in select patients with advanced/metastatic RCC (mRCC). Five-year relative survival rates in the United States for RCC patients have improved from 47% in 1977 to 76% (2009–2015) [1]. However, these rates vary substantially based on cancer stage, with 5-year relative survival in patients with localized, regional, and distant RCC being 93%, 70%, and 12%, respectively [2]. Procedures for RCC remain associated with substantial perioperative morbidity. Inpatient complication and mortality rates in patients undergoing nephrectomy for nonmetastatic RCC are 19% and 1% versus 27% and 2.4% in those undergoing cytoreductive nephrectomy for mRCC [3]. Patients with tumor thrombus experience major complications in 30% of cases, and 90-day postoperative mortality is reported in 6% [4].

W. H. Chou
Harvard Medical School, Boston, MA, USA

D. Lin · S. P. Psutka (✉)
Department of Urology, University of Washington, Seattle, WA, USA

Seattle Cancer Care Alliance, Seattle, WA, USA
e-mail: spsutka@uw.edu

V. Master
Department of Urology, Emory School of Medicine, Atlanta, GA, USA

Winship Cancer Institute, Atlanta, GA, USA

K. L. Stratton, A. K. Morgans (eds.), *Urologic Oncology*,
https://doi.org/10.1007/978-3-030-89891-5_11

Potential perioperative complications include hemorrhage, infection, or damage to surrounding structures, including the pleura, great vessels and surrounding vasculature, intestines, and other surrounding viscera, such as the liver and adrenal gland on the right and the spleen, pancreas, and adrenal gland on the left. Cardiopulmonary complications including myocardial infarction, stroke, and venous thromboembolism; complications related to major abdominal surgery, such as lymphoceles, postoperative ileus, and adhesion-related small bowel obstructions; and incisional hernias or other wound-healing complications may occur.

In the case of partial nephrectomy, vascular fistula or pseudoaneurysm can develop in the healing nephrorrhaphy, potentially leading to delayed postoperative hemorrhage. Urinary leaks can also occur from incomplete or insufficient repairs of injuries to the collecting system or renal pelvis. For these reasons, nephron-sparing surgery is associated with a higher rate of complications and reoperation compared to radical nephrectomy [5]. The unusual predilection of RCC for vascular invasion also raises the possibility of intraoperative embolization from tumor thrombus with subsequent cardiopulmonary collapse, a potentially devastating complication [6].

Decision-Making: When to Operate

Due to the potential complications that may arise from procedures for RCCs, surgical decision-making is paramount. This is especially relevant in several settings specific to RCC where there may be other viable therapeutic options, such as active surveillance or percutaneous thermal ablation for small renal masses, or in the setting of metastatic disease, where frontline therapy is heavily weighted toward systemic therapy, and localized treatment of metastases may include embolization, thermal ablation, and radiation, in addition to surgical extirpation.

In the United States, the average age at diagnosis with RCC is 64 years [2]. Furthermore, patients with RCC have a high burden of comorbidities, with a median of eight chronic comorbid conditions compared to only four in age-matched controls [7]. As such, decisions regarding whether to operate, or in cases where surgery may be staged with systemic therapy options, become complex. These decisions require a detailed evaluation of the oncologic potential of the tumor and the various risks associated with the surgery, including the competing risks associated with comorbidities, baseline renal reserve, nutrition, and functional status or frailty, in addition to patient preference and priorities. While guideline-based algorithms provide recommendations for optimal evidence-based care, patient-specific factors may dictate a more nuanced approach. Trade-offs between oncologic benefits and treatment risks and competing risks of death are challenging to evaluate in an objective fashion.

The objective of this chapter is to review tools that can aid in this risk stratification process and provide an outline of best practices to optimize perioperative outcomes for patients undergoing surgical management of RCC (Fig. 11.1).

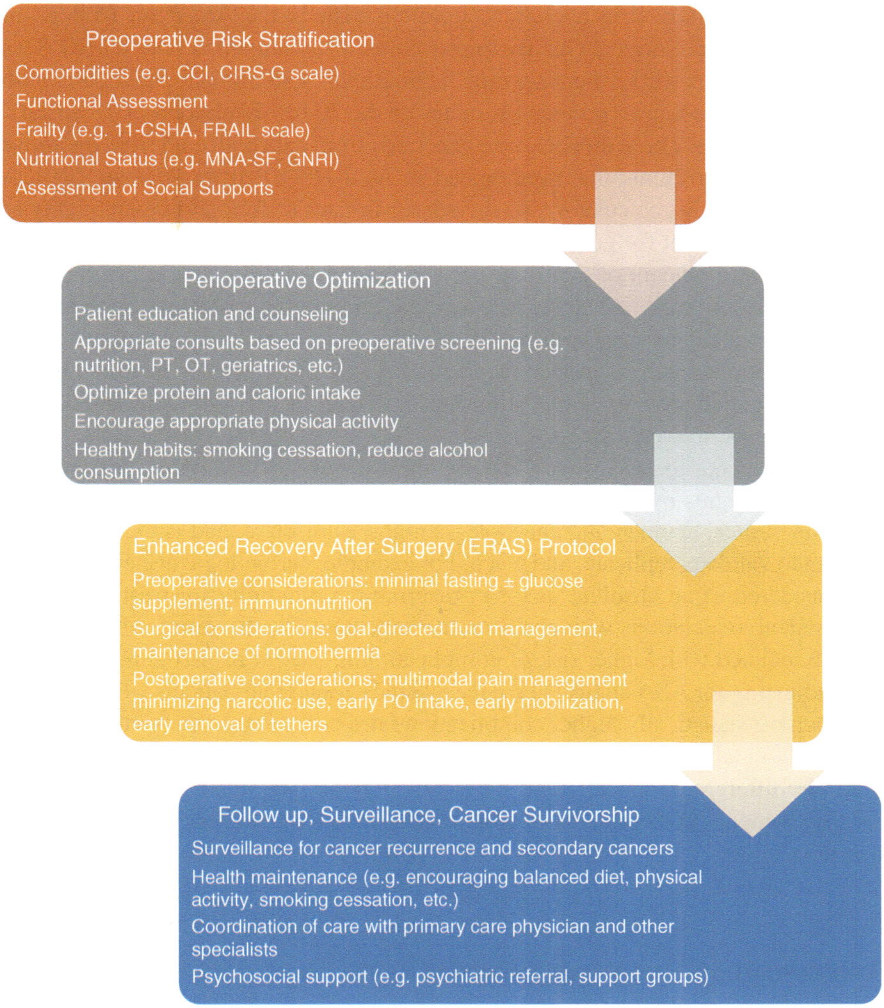

Fig. 11.1 Suggested workflow for patients with RCC spanning from preoperative evaluation through follow-up

Preoperative Risk Stratification

While tumor characteristics (e.g., TNM staging) are key prognostic factors, the focus of this discussion is patient-specific prognostic factors that can aid with risk stratification, also described as "host factors." Importantly, while some of these factors are fixed, others are potentially modifiable. Therefore, these factors may be potentially optimized in the pre- and perioperative period.

Numerous risk calculators have been developed to estimate the predicted risk of short- and long-term complications and may be helpful when reviewing a specific patient's individual predicted risks with a specific procedure. One candidate tool that may be employed in a clinic counseling visit is the American College of Surgeons National Surgical Quality Improvement Program (ACS NSQIP) [8]. This calculator combines 20 patient-specific demographic and clinical parameters with the planned procedure to provide estimates of the 30-day likelihood of 18 specific adverse outcomes. These models were generated from data collected from operative data from 855 hospitals that participated in ACS NSQIP from 2015 to 2019. A recent update to this calculator also includes estimates of four additional quality of life outcomes salient for geriatric patients including risk of development of a pressure ulcer, development of delirium, need for a new mobility device, or functional decline. This tool may be helpful as a baseline for gauging a patient's general level of risk; the calculator has been noted to underestimate rates of complication for some operations such as partial nephrectomy [9, 10]. Thus it is important to acknowledge that the output are estimates alone with incorporating these risks into shared decision-making.

Our aim is not to exhaustively catalog the various tools available, but rather to provide paradigms by which surgeons can move beyond the "eyeball" test, which relies on clinical acumen and anecdote, is highly subjective, and is therefore challenging to validate, replicate, and teach. For example, chronologic age alone cannot be considered as an absolute factor in determining eligibility for treatment given inconsistent associations with perioperative outcomes. To this point, while age has been associated with higher risk of complication in radical or partial nephrectomy after adjusting for ASA status [11], a recent study found that patients ≥65 years old did not have statistically higher complication rates compared to the younger group, even without adjusting for ASA grade or comorbidities [12]. Herein we will review multiple different parameters and tools that may be integrated into perioperative risk assessments to define a more comprehensive and nuanced assessment of perioperative risk.

Assessment of Comorbidity Burden

Common assessments of comorbidity burden include the Charlson Comorbidity Index (CCI), Elixhauser Comorbidity Index (EI), and the ASA Physical Status Classification System (ASA) score (Table 11.1). CCI has been shown to predict overall complication rates in patients undergoing robotic partial nephrectomy, as well as major complications in the setting of radical nephrectomy and thrombectomy [13, 14]. Conversely, a Surveillance, Epidemiology, and End Results (SEER)-based study demonstrated that that CCI was not associated with overall complication rates in patients undergoing local tumor ablation for RCC. Similar inconsistencies are found with respect to ASA scores [13–15]. It should be noted that while CCI is a common covariate used in perioperative assessment, the index was initially developed to determine 10-year survival rates, not perioperative outcomes [16]. Thus, while these indices can provide valuable data on a patient's comorbidity burden, other measures should be taken into account as well. A final point when actually assessing comorbidity burden in practice is that while many of these tools have been operationalized and widely adopted to convey comorbidity for research purposes,

Table 11.1 Selected comorbidity, performance status, and frailty assessments

Assessment tool	Criteria
Comorbidity burden	
Charlson comorbidity index (CCI) [16]	1. Age (<50, 50–59, 60–69, 70–79, ≥80 years): 1 point for each decade beginning from 50 to 59 years 2. Myocardial infarction: 1 point 3. Congestive heart failure: 1 point 4. Peripheral vascular disease: 1 point 5. Stroke or transient ischemic attack: 1 point 6. Dementia: 1 point 7. Chronic obstructive pulmonary disease: 1 point 8. Connective tissue disease: 1 point 9. Peptic ulcer disease: 1 point 10. Liver disease: 1 point for mild disease, 3 points for moderate to severe disease 11. Diabetes mellitus: 1 point for uncomplicated disease, 2 points with end-organ damage 12. Hemiplegia: 2 points 13. Moderate to severe chronic kidney disease: 2 points 14. Solid tumor: 2 points for localized disease, 6 points for metastases 15. Leukemia: 2 points 16. Lymphoma: 2 points 17. AIDS: 6 points ***Predicts 10-year survival for hospitalized patients***
Elixhauser comorbidity index (EI) [114]	1. Congestive heart failure: 7 points 2. Cardiac arrhythmias: 5 points 3. Valvular disease: −1 point 4. Pulmonary circulation disorders: 4 points 5. Peripheral vascular disorders: 2 points 6. Hypertension: 0 points 7. Paralysis: 7 points 8. Neurodegenerative disorders: 6 points 9. Chronic pulmonary disease: 3 points 10. Diabetes (with or without chronic complications): 0 points 11. Hypothyroidism: 0 points 12. Renal failure: 5 points 13. Liver disease: 11 points 14. Peptic ulcer disease, no bleeding: 0 points 15. AIDS/HIV: 0 points 16. Lymphoma: 9 points 17. Metastatic cancer: 12 points 18. Solid tumor without metastasis: 4 points 19. Rheumatoid arthritis/collagen vascular disease: 0 points 20. Coagulopathy: 3 points 21. Obesity: −4 points 22. Weight loss: 6 points 23. Fluid and electrolyte disorders: 5 points 24. Blood loss anemia: −2 points 25. Deficiency anemia: −2 points 26. Alcohol abuse: 0 points 27. Drug abuse: −7 points 28. Psychosis: 0 points 29. Depression: −3 points ***Predicts likelihood of inhospital death***

(continued)

Table 11.1 (continued)

Assessment tool	Criteria
CIRS-G[17]	Each category graded from 0–4 points 1. Heart: Increasing severity based on angina, MI, CHF, etc. 2. Vascular; increasing severity based on hypertension, hyperlipidemia, atherosclerosis, aortic aneurysm, etc. 3. Hematopoietic: Increasing severity of anemia, leukopenia, or hematologic cancer 4. Respiratory: Increasing severity based on infection, asthma, smoking history, COPD, etc. 5. Eyes, ears, nose, throat, and larynx: Increasing severity of visual or hearing impairment, sinonasal complaints, vertigo, etc. 6. Upper GI: Increasing severity of heartburn, ulcer disease, dysphagia, etc. 7. Lower GI: Increasing severity of constipation, hemorrhoids, diverticulitis, etc. 8. Liver, pancreas, and biliary: Increasing severity of hepatitis, LFTs, etc. 9. Renal: Increasing severity of kidney stones, pyelonephritis, chronic kidney disease, etc. 10. Genitourinary: Increasing severity of urinary incontinence, UTIs, etc. 11. Musculoskeletal and skin: Increasing severity of arthritis, skin cancers, joint deformity, etc. 12. Neurologic: Increasing severity of headaches, history of stroke, etc. 13. Endocrine and breast: Increasing severity of diabetes mellitus, obesity, hormone replacement, etc. 14. Psychiatric illness: Increasing severity of psychiatric illness, dementia, substance use disorder, etc. ***Predicts higher severity of disease burden in elderly patients***
Performance status metrics	
ASA Score [115]	I: A normal healthy patient II: A patient with mild systemic disease III: A patient with severe systemic disease IV: A patient with severe systemic disease that is a constant threat to life V: A moribund patient who is not expected to survive without the operation VI: A declared brain-dead patient whose organs are being removed for donor purposes
Eastern cooperative oncology group (ECOG) Score [18]	0: Fully active, able to carry on all predisease activities without restriction 1: Restricted in strenuous activity, ambulatory, and able to do light work 2: Capable of all self-care, but no work activities, out of bed >50% of day 3: Capable of limited self-care, confined to bed or chair >50% of day 4: Completely disabled, no self-care, confined to bed or chair 5: Dead

Table 11.1 (continued)

Assessment tool	Criteria
Karnofsky performance Status [116]	100: Normal, no complaints, no evidence of disease 90: Able to carry on normal activity; minor signs or symptoms of disease 80: Normal activity with effort, some signs or symptoms of disease 70: Cares for self but unable to carry on normal activity or to do active work 60: Requires occasional assistance but is able to care for most of personal needs 50: Requires considerable assistance and frequent medical care 40: Disabled; requires special care and assistance 30: everely disabled; hospitalization is indicated although death is not imminent 20: Very ill; hospitalization and active supportive care necessary 10: Moribund 0: Dead
Frailty metrics	
Fried frailty phenotype [30]	1. Unintentional weight loss (>10 lb. over 1 year) 2. Sarcopenia 3. Weakness: Grip strength in lowest 20% based on gender and BMI 4. In slowest 20% for gait based on gender and height 5. Lowest 20% kcal/week with regard to activity * ≥ ***3 criteria = frailty*** ***1–2 criteria = pre-frail***
Canadian study of health and aging frailty index [31]	Assessment of 70 variables that measure comorbidity burden, ADL ability, and physical/neurological signs based on examination of mobility, function, and self-rated health
FRAIL scale [33]	1. Do you feel worn out/tired? 2. Ability to climb one flight of stairs 3. Ability to walk 100 m 4. >5% weight loss 5. At least five conditions from the following: Dementia, heart disease, depression, arthritis, asthma, bronchitis/emphysema, diabetes, hypertension, osteoporosis, stroke * ≥ ***3 points = frail***
Clinical frailty scale [117]	1. Very fit: Robust individuals and who exercise regularly 2. Well: Without active disease but less fit that those in category 1 3. Well, with treated comorbid disease: Disease symptoms well-controlled 4. Apparently vulnerable: Not frankly dependent, but with disease symptoms or experiencing being "slowed" up by comorbidities 5. Mildly frail: Limited dependence on others for IADL(s) 6. Moderately frail: Help needed with both IADL and ADL 7. Severely frail: Completely dependent on others for ADLs, or terminally ill

(continued)

Table 11.1 (continued)

Assessment tool	Criteria
Modified frailty index [118]	1. Functional health status before surgery (partially dependent, totally dependent) 2. Diabetes mellitus 3. Chronic obstructive pulmonary disease 4. Congestive heart failure 5. History of myocardial infarction within 6 months 6. Prior cardiac surgery 7. Hypertension 8. Impaired sensorium 9. History of TIA 10. History of stroke 11. Peripheral vascular disease requiring surgery or with active claudication present ***Index = number of present factors/11; pre-frail defined as 0.09–0.19; frail defined as ≥ 0.27***
Simplified frailty index [119]	1. Diabetes 2. Functional status 3. Chronic obstructive pulmonary disease 4. Congestive heart failure 5. Hypertension ***Scored as 1, 2, or ≥ 3 risk factors***

they remain underutilized in general clinical practice. One potential additional factor to consider when assessing a patient's burden of comorbidity is how severely each of the comorbidities impacts or interferes with a patient's day-to-day quality of life. A candidate classification system that attempts to communicate not only the number of comorbidities but also their perceived impact is the Cumulative Illness Rating Scale-Geriatric (CIRS-G) scale [17], which is predictive of hospital outcomes and short-term mortality in older adults, but has yet to be validated in RCC. Given the patient-reported element of this scale, it may be more relevant for use in the evaluation of an individual during clinical assessment and can be assessed during history-taking, but is not widely adopted at this point in urologic oncology practice.

Functional Status

Conventionally, the Eastern Cooperative Oncology Group performance status (ECOG-PS) has been used to assess function in patients (Table 11.1) [18], such as within the University of California Integrated Staging System (UISS) for localized RCC [19]. The Karnofsky Performance Status (KPS) scale is a similar, older system analogous to the ECOG-PS [18]. While fairly simple to determine and validated as prognostic factors, these scales have their shortcomings. The ECOG-PS has been criticized for poor sensitivity. For example, in one study of older patients with cancer, over half of those with ECOG-PS of 0–1 needed help with activities of daily living (ADLs) [20]. In patients undergoing partial nephrectomy, ECOG-PS also did not correlate with length of stay or overall complication [13]. Similarly, in a study of older patients with cancer, KPS did not predict mortality [21]. Furthermore, data from Bergerot and colleagues suggested that there are substantial discrepancies in how patients and physicians characterize performance status, such that clinicians more frequently characterized patients as having an ECOG PS of 0 compared to patients themselves (92.4% vs. 64.1%; $p = 0.001$), highlighting the potential subjectivity of this assessment [22]. Finally, while KPS is widely used in risk stratification models for mRCC [23–25], the scale has been less robustly studied in localized disease.

Current guidelines from the ACS NSQIP/American Geriatrics Society (AGS) recommend explicitly screening patient ability to perform ADLs, as well as documenting any recent falls or impairments in vision, hearing, or swallowing [26]. This screening can be supplemented by a functional assessment such as the Timed Up-and-Go Test (TUGT), a simple test for walking speed that has been correlated with postoperative complications and mortality [27].

Frailty

Frailty is a multidimensional concept distinct from traditional comorbidity scores and absolute age that may help address these shortcomings that has gained considerable traction in the urologic literature recently. Frailty is defined as "a medical syndrome with multiple causes and contributors that is characterized by diminished strength, endurance, and reduced physiologic function that increases an individual's vulnerability for developing increased dependency and/or death." [28] Generally, the frailty phenotype reflects five criteria: shrinking (weight loss), weakness (e.g., decline in grip strength), self-reported fatigue, a decrease in walking speed, and self-reported low activity. In older adults undergoing surgery for nonmetastatic RCC, worse functional health was linked with increased perioperative medical complications and mortality, in addition to higher costs [29].

Reflecting the physiologic reserve of a patient, frailty can be measured via various metrics [30, 31]. Many of these metrics are time- and resource-intensive, making full assessments in routine clinical workflow less feasible. Validated abbreviated tools have been developed to simplify this assessment, such as the Modified Frailty Index of the Canadian Study of Health and Aging (11-CSHA), which derives 11 elements from original 70-variable metric and predicts major complication and readmission after partial nephrectomy [32]. In addition, the FRAIL scale is a five-item assessment tool that can be easily incorporated in routine visits using readily available information from medical records (Table 11.1) which also permits its translation to clinical research relying on administrative data [33].

Nutrition

Malnutrition predicts poor outcomes in RCC and is prevalent among patients with RCC. In surgical patients with localized RCC, 23% met at least one criterion for a composite of hypoalbuminemia, low body mass index (BMI), and weight loss; each of these feature was associated with reduced overall survival [34]. In patients with mRCC, 32% were classified as being at risk for malnutrition according to the Geriatric Nutritional Risk Index (GNRI) [35], which utilizes serum albumin, weight, and ideal body weight [36], and malnutrition was associated with worse overall survival. The GNRI has also been shown to predict postoperative complications in RCC patients [37]. Various other parameters to determine nutritional status have been utilized, including the Mini-Nutritional Assessment Scale-Short Form (MNA-SF), which incorporates BMI, certain comorbidities (dementia, acute illness, or stress), and other patient history (recent weight loss, homebound status, anorexia) [38].

Body Composition

BMI is the most commonly used parameter in the literature and clinical practice to communicate body composition at present. While simple to calculate, this measure is nonspecific, reflecting weight normalized by height alone, rather than more specific factors such as muscle mass [39]. To this end, the data regarding the prognostic benefit of BMI are inconsistent, demonstrating no association between BMI and various perioperative and oncologic outcomes, other studies demonstrating adverse associations with obesity, and still other studies yielding a counterintuitive association between obesity and improved survival [40, 41]. This latter phenomenon has been termed “the obesity paradox” and is thought to result from, at least in part, misclassification bias, related to the lack of specificity of BMI and the differential density of muscle versus adipose mass.

Conversely, granular measurements of body composition, in particular severe deficits in muscle mass, termed *sarcopenia*, have demonstrated prognostic value with respect to overall and cancer-specific survival. Associations between deficits in muscle mass and oncologic outcomes have been demonstrated across the spectrum RCC from localized to metastatic disease, such that low muscle mass is independently associated with death from cancer and death from any cause [42–44]. While sarcopenia has been used to denote a severe deficit of muscle mass [45], contemporary definitions stress the functional decline inherent to this condition such that it is not only an anatomic classification but also encompasses an assessment of strength and physical performance [46]. Detailed body composition analysis may be useful at both single time points and as a dynamic measure that can capture accelerated lean muscle loss prevalent in patients with cancer. Although not yet routinely evaluated in standard clinical practice, muscle mass can be measured using the skeletal muscle index, which reflects the cross-sectional surface of lean muscle at the midpoint of L3 normalized by height in meters squared (cm^2/m^2). The skeletal muscle index is a well-described metric that has been validated against DEXA scans and autopsy studies as a proxy for total body lean muscle mass [47]. Furthermore, these measurements can be derived from axial CT scans or MRI obtained for staging or surveillance purposes in routine clinical practice [44, 48, 49]. Methodology using artificial intelligence and machine-learning platforms are in development to increase access to these measurements in clinical practice.

Immune Profile/Inflammation

Malignancy often results in simultaneously catabolic and inflammatory states, creating a complex interplay between the immune profile and nutritional status. For example, hypoalbuminemia, often utilized as a surrogate for malnutrition, is also an acute-phase reactant, reflecting systematic inflammation. Increased C-reactive protein (CRP), platelet, and erythrocyte sedimentation rate (ESR) have all been associated with decreased survival in RCC [50]. To move beyond individual serum markers though, various scoring systems have been derived to synthesize nutritional and inflammatory parameters. For example, the Onodera Prognostic Nutritional Index (OPNI) score, incorporating serum albumin and total lymphocyte count, has been validated as an independent prognostic factor for overall survival and recurrence-free survival in RCC patients [51]. Similarly, the Controlling Nutritional Status (CONUT) score, which incorporates serum albumin, lymphocyte count, and total serum cholesterol [52], has demonstrated associations with overall survival in RCC surgical patients [53].

Increased neutrophil-to-lymphocyte ratios were associated with poorer overall survival and progression-free survival in both patients with localized RCC and mRCC [54] and appears to perform similarly to the OPNI score [55]. Conversely, lower platelet-to-white blood cell ratios are associated with greater perioperative infectious complications and need for blood transfusion in patients undergoing radical nephrectomy for RCC, although this parameter has not been validated as extensively [56].

Prognostic Models to Convey Risk in Metastatic Disease

Various risk stratification schemes have been developed in the setting of metastatic RCC. The Motzer criteria, also known as the Memorial Sloan Kettering Cancer Center (MSKCC) Criteria, first presented in 1999 [57], predict overall survival in patients with mRCC based on assessment of the following risk factors: KPS <80%, lactate dehydrogenase >1.5× upper limit of normal, anemia, corrected serum calcium >10 mg/dL, and no prior nephrectomy. With the advent of targeted therapies in addition to interferon-based immunotherapy, contemporary risk prediction models have been developed for cancer-specific survival and overall survival after cytoreductive nephrectomy [58, 59]. These have included the Heng criteria, also known as the International Metastatic RCC Database (IMDC) Criteria, which include the following characteristics: KPS <80%, <1-year time from diagnosis to treatment, anemia, serum calcium above upper limit of normal, neutrophil count above upper limit of normal, and platelet count above upper limit of normal [23]. Such models are used to guide decision-making around selection for upfront cytoreductive nephrectomy [60]. Conversely other recently designed prognostic models have been developed at high volume centers from both contemporary and historic cohorts that include more granular data [59].

Laboratory Evaluations

Labs that should be obtained as part of routine preoperative evaluation include a comprehensive blood count, comprehensive metabolic panel, and urinalysis. These labs can help risk-stratify patients based on previously mentioned parameters such as nutritional status and immune profile. eGFR may also guide the decision as to whether a radical versus partial nephrectomy should be performed. Current American Urological Association (AUA) guidelines recommend proceeding with radical nephrectomy if predicted postoperative eGFR is >45 mL/min/1.73 m^2, among other factors [61]. To this end, multiple nomograms have been developed to predict the probability of postoperative eGFR ≤45 mL/min/1.73 m^2 with readily available patient characteristics and preoperative renal function [62, 63]. In addition, CBC may reveal anemia, which has been shown to be associated with decreased survival and earlier recurrence in patients undergoing radical or partial nephrectomy [64]. In the setting of metastatic disease, the aforementioned tests are sufficient for calculating Heng criteria, while lactate dehydrogenase is necessary to ascertain the Motzer/MSKCC criteria.

Comprehensive Geriatric Assessment

A comprehensive geriatric assessment (CGA) represents a multidimensional approach that incorporates many of the above parameters into a more holistic assessment compared to unidimensional or simplistic assessments such as chronologic age or comorbidity scores. CGAs characterize a patient across seven domains, including a patient's functional status, comorbidity, polypharmacy, cognition, psychologic status, social supports, and nutrition [65]. While complex, CGA may better capture functional impairment. Studies in hospitalized older adults have shown that CGA is abnormal in 65% of patients with a "normal" ASA and that an abridged geriatric assessment outperforms KPS in predicting mortality [21, 66]. A recent study of patients who underwent a geriatric assessment prior to partial nephrectomy also found that increased frailty was associated with major postoperative complications [67].

Currently, CGAs are recommended in National Comprehensive Cancer Network (NCCN) guidelines for any older adult who may have difficulty tolerating therapy, although identifying such patients is not straightforward [68]. Full CGAs are time-intensive and best performed by geriatricians or physicians who are specially trained in these assessments. However, abbreviated screening tools focused on functional status, comorbidities, cognition (such as the Mini-Cog), weight loss, and social supports can be more easily incorporated into routine clinical practice [69], which can determine whether referral for complete CGA by specialists is warranted.

Medical/Other Consultation

Appropriate consults should be placed to further evaluate and manage discrete vulnerabilities detected by previously mentioned assessments. These may include formal assessment by a nutritionist for malnutrition, as well as evaluations by specialists in physical therapy, occupational therapy, or physical medicine and rehabilitation (PM&R) in the setting of frailty/poor functional status. These referrals may be particularly useful in patients slated to receive systemic therapy, such as in patients with mRCC planned for upfront systemic therapy and subsequent consideration for deferred cytoreductive nephrectomy. Social work should also be considered to address issues including, but not limited to: food insecurity, housing and utility needs, finances, transport, and social supports at home [26].

Cardiology referrals should be considered for patients at high risk for a major adverse cardiac event, as well as for patients having symptoms such as worsening dyspnea, angina, concerning electrocardiogram findings, those with significant risk factors for coronary artery disease, or those with a history of prior cardiac interventions for severe disease. In patients with a history of poorly controlled diabetes, referral to endocrinology may warrant given associations with elevated hemoglobin A1c with increased length of stay and increased perioperative mortality [70, 71].

In addition, nephrology referral can be considered in those with a high risk of new chronic kidney disease (CKD) or progression of existing disease, particularly in those in whom severe postoperative renal dysfunction is anticipated. It should be noted that the data suggest that patients with surgically induced CKD have slower rates of eGFR decline and mortality compared to those with primarily medically driven CKD [72]. However, there is not a clean divide between these different etiologies of CKD, as patients with RCC often have medical comorbidities linked with preexisting CKD. AUA guidelines account for these differing risk factors and give examples of appropriate patients for nephrology referral as including those with a preoperative eGFR <45 mL/min/1.73 m^2, proteinuria, diabetes with underlying CKD, and those with expected postoperative eGFR <30 mL/min/1.73 m^2 [61].

Previously mentioned nomograms developed by McIntosh and colleagues and Ellis and colleagues may be useful in estimating postoperative eGFR and potential risks of end-stage renal dysfunction and future need for renal replacement therapy [62, 63].

Genetic counseling should be considered in select patients presenting with significant family histories, syndromic presentations, and patients 46 years of age and younger presenting with renal masses [61].

For patients where venous tumor thrombectomy and potential bypass is anticipated, cardiac anesthesiology should be involved in preoperative planning as well as colleagues from vascular surgery, hepatobiliary surgery, and/or cardiothoracic surgery as appropriate to the extent of the tumor and anticipated need for complex vascular reconstruction [73, 74].

Perioperative Optimization

Many of the principles described in the following section fall under the guise of broader Enhanced Recovery After Surgery (ERAS) protocols, which are multidisciplinary data-driven care pathways that aim to improve the consistency of perioperative care using detailed checklists. ERAS protocol has demonstrated improvement in outcomes such as length in stay, readmission rates, and perioperative morbidity across surgical fields. Prospective randomized trials in patients undergoing partial or radical nephrectomy found that ERAS groups had shorter length of stay, as well as reduced or comparable rates of complications [75, 76]. While there is considerable heterogeneity in ERAS protocols, there are often common elements that fall within preoperative, intraoperative, and postoperative considerations, which we will highlight where pertinent.

Counseling/Expectation Setting

Patients should participate in shared decision-making and preoperative education as they consider treatment selection. Frank but compassionate discussions that incorporate patient preferences and concerns should be undertaken, as well as appropriate counseling regarding potential outcomes and potential complications or risks associated with surgery both in general and as related to an individual's unique risk profile. This discussion should also include details regarding perioperative expectations regarding hospital stay, recovery/convalescence, and timing of return to normal activities, in addition to expectations around postoperative disposition and the potential need for discharge to settings other than home, such as a skilled nursing facility. Patient should be given the opportunity to ask questions. Visual aids and techniques such as the "repeat back" may be helpful for improving patient understanding [77]. These conversations also warrant discussion of advance care planning (ACP). While a challenging topic, ACP allows the physician to explore the patient's priorities and preferences in the case of adverse events, as well as ensure that a healthcare proxy is on file.

Laying the groundwork for such patient-centered conversations may aid in more active engagement in perioperative optimization. While traditional risk factors are often static, many of the elements and domains described in the prior sections are potentially modifiable. This represents an exciting area for research on preoperative interventions, termed "prehabilitation," aiming to improve short-term outcomes and potentially to modify treatment strategy or eligibility. Given that expedient surgery is often warranted for RCC patients, instituting interventions with enough time for patients to achieve benefit may be challenging. However, patients on active surveillance and those with advanced or mRCC may have protracted periods of surveillance or nonoperative treatment before surgery is considered, creating potential windows of opportunity for these prehabilitation interventions to be enacted.

Preoperative Nutritional Optimization

Current European Society for Clinical Nutrition and Metabolism (ESPEN) guidelines for nutrition in oncology patients emphasize early screening of nutritional status followed by personalized nutritional support [78]. Gold standard measures would include resting energy expenditure (REE) calculated via indirect calorimetry in these patients. Where REE cannot be measured though, ESPEN guidelines recommend as an initial target 25–30 kcal/kg/day and 1.2–1.5 g of protein/kg/day, although older patients may benefit from even higher protein intake [79].

Although no randomized controlled trials regarding preoperative nutritional supplementation have been undertaken to date for surgical patients with RCC, promising findings have been found in other surgical fields. Perioperative immunonutrition has been found to decrease rates of postoperative complications, particularly infections, and shorten hospital length of stay in the setting of gastrointestinal surgery and other oncologic surgeries [80, 81]. Within urology, limited data are available and preoperative interventions remain largely investigational. A small randomized controlled trial in patients undergoing radical cystectomy demonstrated a reduction in postoperative infectious complications within the group receiving immunonutrition, with concomitant improvement in markers for immune response [82]. Another trial in patients undergoing cystectomy demonstrated that, while enriched oral supplementation prior to surgery did not result in greater hospital-free days compared to multivitamin supplementation, postoperative sarcopenia was less common in the former group [83]. Further randomized controlled trials are in progress at this time [84].

Given the investigational nature of preoperative nutritional efforts, we recommend that physicians consider referrals to nutritionists for patients who are identified to have malnutrition or sarcopenia prior to surgery who are not planned for immediate surgery. For those who are anticipating proceeding to the OR soon, nutritional consultation in the postoperative period can be helpful to optimize nutritional recovery. Regarding the immediate preoperative period, preoperative fasting should not be enforced until 6 hours before surgery and water deprivation enacted only 2 hours before surgery. Glucose supplementation up to this point may also be considered and is included in many ERAS pathways.

Preoperative Exercise Recommendations

Aerobic reserve is an important factor both for tolerating the direct stressors of surgery and participating in postoperative care. Patients should be counseled about the importance to increase their level of physical active preoperatively. Current NCCN guidelines on survivorship prescribe 150–300 minutes of moderate activity or 75 minutes of vigorous activity over the course of a week, as well as two to three strength training sessions per week [85]. While this may not be feasible for all patients, these guidelines should be used to stress the overall importance of physical activity. Referral to PM&R and physical therapy may be considered to assist in optimizing functional status and exercise in the perioperative period.

The feasibility of preoperative conditioning regimens has notably been piloted in the patients with bladder cancer undergoing radical cystectomy. A randomized controlled trial demonstrated improvements in 6-minute walking distance and other measures of fitness, which translated to increased postoperative mobilization after only 2 weeks of home-based training [86]. Translation of these outcomes into improved perioperative outcomes has yet to be demonstrated though. While further trials are ongoing to determine ideal exercise prescriptions, general recommendations at this point include increasing physical activity and weight-bearing activity as much as possible for a patient. These recommendations should be targeted, accounting for an individual's baseline cardiopulmonary fitness and functional status as well as their individual goals and vulnerabilities. For example, while some patients may be able to sustain a high-intensity exercise regimen, others will benefit from increasing the proportion of time they are sitting as opposed to lying in bed or walking short distances with assistive devices.

Smoking Cessation

In addition to detrimental chronic health effects and poorer oncologic outcomes in RCC patients [87], smoking has been associated with increased risk of perioperative complications [88]. A meta-analysis found that while longer periods of smoking cessation are associated with fewer postoperative complications, benefit was still seen for shorter periods [89]. Thus, we recommend cessation as soon as possible and independent of surgery. Although smoking cessation immediately prior to surgery was thought to be potentially detrimental, this has not proven to be the case

[90]. Patients should be provided support for quitting smoking. These resources can involve both nonpharmacologic approaches, such as group counseling sessions, and pharmacologic agents, such as nicotine replacement therapy, bupropion, and varenicline.

Systemic Therapy Hold Parameters

Regarding medication parameters prior to operation, we will focus on several important categories, such as anticoagulants, hypoglycemics, and immunosuppressants. The 2014 American Urological Association (AUA) White Paper summarizes recommendations for antiplatet and anticoagulant agents [91]. This issue is particularly topical for patients with venous tumor thrombus who commonly receive preoperative anticoagulation [73]. Patients with appropriate indications, such as stroke prevention or those with cardiac risk factors, may often be able to continue aspirin perioperatively. While continuation of aspirin is associated with a small risk of increased bleeding, this has not translated to increased transfusion rates. Risk of thrombosis from cessation of anticoagulant agents must be closely weighed against increased risk of bleeding complications and will often warrant multidisciplinary collaboration. Pertinent risk factors for thromboembolic events include history of mechanical heart valves, atrial fibrillation, and deep vein thromboses. In these cases, warfarin and direct oral anticoagulants (DOACs) are typically recommended to be held for 2–5 days before surgery with appropriate bridging depending on risk level.

Regarding hypoglycemic agents, many of these medications can be taken into the morning of surgery, with exceptions for certain classes and modifications for insulin dosing [92, 93]. Patients on chronic steroids may require stress dose steroids at the time of surgery, and referrals to gastroenterology and rheumatology should be placed in the cases where immunomodulatory agents are being used. Otherwise, the merits of discontinuing agents associated with AKI as well as perioperative hypotension, such as ACE inhibitors, nonsteroidal anti-inflammatories, and diuretics, should be considered.

Regarding patients with advanced RCC, there is some evidence that targeted therapies have detrimental effects on wound healing [94]. Given the prolonged half-lives of tyrosine kinase inhibitors (TKIs), such as 24–48 hours for sorafenib, 40–60 hours for sunitinib [95], and 55–99 hours for cabozantinib, these agents are generally held prior to cytoreductive nephrectomy [96]. Per manufacturer recommendations, sorafenib should be held for at least 10 days before surgery and sunitinib and cabozantinib for at least 3 weeks [97–99]. Resumption is recommended no earlier than 2 weeks after surgery, although there are limited data regarding precise timing of cessation and resumption, and practices may vary by clinical institution and surgeon. Notably, bevacizumab has a longer half-life of 21 days [95] and is recommended to be held for 28 days before and after surgery [100]. Conversely, most immunotherapy agents are continued through surgery, including ipilimumab and nivolumab, although a high index of suspicion for uncommon immune-related adverse events unique to these agents should be maintained and holds may be instituted on an individualized basis [101].

Pre-surgical Planning

Key aspects to ensuring that surgical management of RCC progresses in a controlled and optimally safe fashion start with preoperative surgical preparation. In the careful evaluation of available cross-sectional staging imaging, an important factor to assess is hilar anatomy, which includes the number and location of dominant and accessory renal arteries and veins, surrounding and parasitic vasculature, as well as lumbar vessels. It is also important to evaluate the potential involvement of the surrounding viscera and proximity to structures such as the pancreas, liver, intestine, or adrenal gland, which might change the surgical approach or warrant additional caution during certain steps (e.g., Kocherization of the duodenum). Extensive hilar adenopathy should be approached with caution given the potential need for meticulous vascular dissection as well as lymphostasis. Careful preoperative study of available imaging is also necessary to forecast and ensure that appropriate surgical equipment is available (e.g., self-retaining retractors, intraoperative ultrasound). In the case of venous tumor thrombus, understanding the level of the tumor thrombus, involvement of bland thrombus, and extent of venous occlusion is important for planning possible venous reconstruction, substitution, or ligation, as well as early initiation of anticoagulation.

For cases with extensive involvement of surrounding viscera where adjunctive procedures are anticipated (e.g., vascular reconstruction in the form of patch or tube-interposition grafts), it is essential to have vascular surgical support on standby if the primary surgeon is not specifically trained in such reconstructive procedures. For level III or IV venous tumor thrombi, surgeons who do not routinely mobilize the liver and the suprahepatic IVC may consider preoperative consultation of colleagues in hepato-pancreato-biliary surgery. Many high-volume centers of excellence have multidisciplinary Tumor Thrombectomy "Teams" incorporating surgeons from these different disciplines to optimize outcomes in these complex and high-risk cases.

For patients with tumor involving surrounding viscera on preoperative imaging (e.g., the mesentery of the colon, the liver, the tail of the pancreas), involvement of general surgery, colorectal surgery, or hepato-pancreato-biliary surgery may be appropriate if the treating urologic oncologist does not have sufficient expertise to perform relevant adjunctive procedures independently (e.g., partial or subtotal colectomy, partial hepatectomy, distal pancreatectomy). It is preferable and logistically advantageous to alert colleagues who may be needed for an intraoperative consult in advance to ensure that whatever help is needed is available at the time of surgery.

Finally, careful study of the preoperative imaging, understanding of the patient's prior surgical history, and surrounding anatomy with visualization of the case is important to select the optimal surgical approach for a specific patient. For example, a patient with multiple prior abdominal procedures who is anticipated to have significant adhesive disease may benefit from a retroperitoneal/flank approach to avoid the necessity of an extensive adhesiolysis at the time of surgery. Similarly, patients with prior anterior abdominal mesh for hernia repairs around the umbilicus who warrant an intraperitoneal approach may benefit from a subcostal incision vs. a midline incision to avoid the previously placed mesh. Conversely, a patient with extensive common iliac adenopathy may benefit from midline exposure to ensure adequate access to inferior tumor burden. Where possible and if surgeons have appropriate experience and expertise, minimally invasive approaches should be considered given improved perioperative recovery and similar oncologic outcomes with open surgeries [102]. As per AUA guidelines, negative margins should be prioritized in partial nephrectomy, as well as minimization of prolonged warm ischemia [61].

Intraoperative Considerations

In keeping with an AUA White Paper on best practices in the intraoperative setting, effective team communication, such as through use of preoperative huddles and surgical safety checklists, is critical for reduction of medical errors [103]. Regarding antimicrobial prophylaxis, a single administration of intravenous cephalosporin has been shown to significantly reduce rates of infection in patients undergoing radical nephrectomy [104, 105].

Intraoperatively, steps are taken to minimize blood loss. These may include careful ligation of parasitic vessels using ligation, staple ligation, or thermal ligation (e.g., LigaSure®) and ensure that appropriate blood products are proximately available as necessary. In cases with significant potential for intraoperative blood loss such as tumors with extensive venous tumor thrombus involving the inferior vena cava, those with extensive parasitic vessels, as well as tumor or lymphadenopathy encasing the renal hilum or great vessels, additional vascular access, and intraoperative monitoring (e.g., arterial line, central line, large bore IVs) should be considered. Per ERAS protocols, conservative intraoperative fluid administration and maintenance of normothermia should be implemented [76].

Postoperative Optimization

Immediate Postoperative Period

Multimodal analgesic regimens that minimize narcotic use should be used. Such pathways may reduce rates of need for opioids at discharge and reduce adverse effects including hyperalgesia, delirium, somnolence, aspiration, and delayed mobilization as well as ileus [103]. In keeping with ERAS protocols, enteral nutrition is resumed as soon as possible with the objective of having patients resume a normal diet within 2 days of surgery. Early activity is encouraged and is aided by the prompt removal of tethers such as urinary catheters and drains as soon as is appropriate. While there is wide variation in mobilization protocols, these overall appear to shorten length of stay and improve patient quality of life measures [106, 107].

Follow-Up and Cancer Survivorship

Postoperative care for patients should adhere to the principles of survivorship as put forth by NCCN and AUA guidelines (Fig. 11.2) [85, 108]. Regarding surveillance, 2013 AUA guidelines recommend a targeted history and physical and lab testing for renal function during follow-up, as well as chest and abdominal imaging with their frequency based on TNM staging. However, some authors would argue for prolonged and risk-stratified surveillance that incorporates assessments of risk for recurrence as well as life expectancy [109, 110].

In addition to surveillance for new or recurrent tumors, patients should undergo assessment for late effects of cancer treatment, have coordinated care between their primary care providers and specialists, and be counseled regarding healthy practices

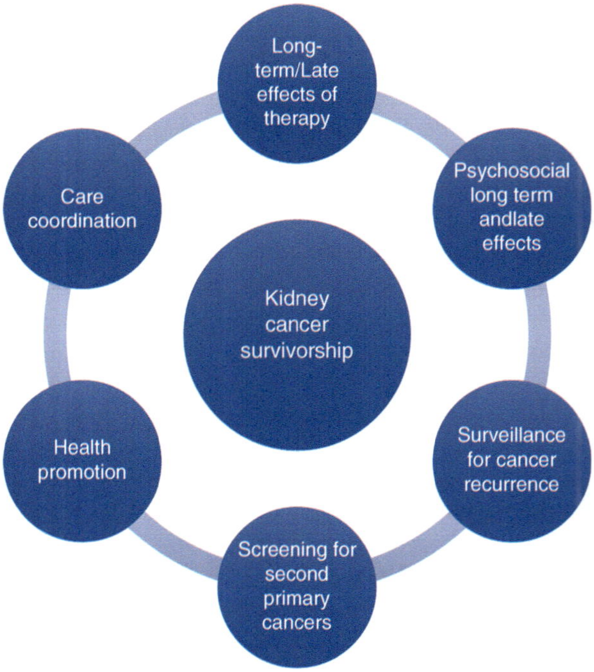

Fig. 11.2 Components of survivorship care, as adapted from NCCN guidelines

[85]. In addition to surveillance through regular physical examinations, laboratory studies, and imaging, patients should also be provided adequate psychosocial support. This may take the form of psychiatric referral, community-based resources such as support groups. Healthy habits such as regular physical activity and smoking cessation are encouraged.

For patients with RCC, control of comorbidities linked with risk of renal insufficiency renal function should be optimized, with referral to nephrology as needed. A systematic review found that >30% of patients who underwent radical nephrectomy and $\geq$ 12% of those who underwent partial nephrectomy for localized RCC had new onset of $\geq$stage 3 CKD [111]. Regarding behavioral modifications, daily salt intake should be limited to <4 g given increasing risk of cardiovascular events and mortality [112]. Low-protein diets are often recommended for those at risk for or with CKD and may reduce progression in those with stage 3 or 4 CKD [113]. However, this should be weighed against the potential of exacerbating preexisting malnutrition and the patient's existing renal function. Pertinent conditions to manage include hypertension and diabetes.

Summary

In this chapter, we have reviewed strategies for perioperative optimization for patients with RCC, for which surgical treatments have substantial morbidity. Detailed and patient-focused preoperative risk stratification can help inform the risks and benefits of a procedure. While routinely evaluated by a host of factors including TNM staging, comorbidity burden, and functional status, refinement of risk through assessment of frailty, nutritional status, and body composition allow for more holistic and personalized evaluation of surgical candidates. Specifically, we recommend incorporating screening questions on patient's ability to perform ADLs and overall functional status as recommended by multiple guideline bodies. The FRAIL scale and MNA-SF provide quick assessment for frailty and nutritional status, respectively. Parameters from routine laboratory evaluation can be used to calculate other prognostic factors such as the OPNI score or the MNA. Together, these tools allow for appropriate consults to be placed where vulnerabilities are identified. Patients should be counseled at the outset when electing a treatment strategy about potential outcomes and complications from intervention and be encouraged to engage in healthy behaviors including smoking cessation and physical activity. The realm of prehabilitation warrants further investigation but represents an exciting frontier in which shorter-term interventions could positively impact perioperative outcomes.

Careful surgical planning is necessary to determine ideal surgical approach and level of support needed from other specialists. ERAS protocols in the perioperative period have been shown to decrease length of stay and complications. Postoperatively, surgeons should engage in principles of survivorship, which not only include cancer surveillance but also assurance of psychosocial support and maintenance of healthy behaviors.

References

1. Padala SA, Barsouk A, Thandra KC, et al. Epidemiology of renal cell carcinoma. World J Oncol. 2020;11(3):79–87.
2. Howlader N, Noone AM, Krapcho M. SEER Cancer Statistics Review 1975–2016. 2019.
3. Abdollah F, Sun M, Thuret R, et al. Mortality and morbidity after cytoreductive nephrectomy for metastatic renal ell carcinoma: a population-based study. Ann Surg Oncol. 2011;18(10):2988–96.
4. Ebbing J, Wiebach T, Kempkensteffen C, et al. Evaluation of perioperative complications in open and laparoscopic surgery for renal cell cancer with tumor thrombus involvement using the Clavien-Dindo classification. Eur J Surg Oncol. 2015;41(7):941–52.
5. Van Poppel H, Da Pozzo L, Albrecht W, et al. A prospective randomized EORTC intergroup phase 3 study comparing the complications of elective nephron-sparing surgery and radical nephrectomy for low-stage renal cell carcinoma. Eur Urol. 2007;51(6):1606–15.
6. Shuch B, Larochelle JC, Onyia T, et al. Intraoperative thrombus embolization during nephrectomy and tumor thrombectomy: critical analysis of the University of California-Los Angeles experience. J Urol. 2009;181(2):492–8; discussion 498–9.
7. Garg T, Young AJ, Kost KA, et al. Burden of multiple chronic conditions among patients with urological cancer. J Urol. 2018;199(2):543–50.
8. ACS NSQIP Surgical Risk Calculator. 2020; https://riskcalculator.facs.org/RiskCalculator/. Accessed 1 Apr 2021.
9. Blair BM, Lehman EB, Jafri SM, Kaag MG, Raman JD. Predicted versus observed 30-day perioperative outcomes using the ACS NSQIP surgical risk calculator in patients undergoing partial nephrectomy for renal cell carcinoma. Int Urol Nephrol. 2018;50(7):1249–56.
10. Winoker JS, Paulucci DJ, Anastos H, et al. Predicting complications following robot-assisted partial nephrectomy with the ACS NSQIP((R)) universal surgical risk calculator. J Urol. 2017;198(4):803–9.
11. Lowrance WT, Yee DS, Savage C, et al. Complications after radical and partial nephrectomy as a function of age. J Urol. 2010;183(5):1725–30.
12. Sirithanaphol W, Pachirat K, Rompsaithong U, Kiatsopit P, Ungareevittaya P, Chindaprasirt J. Perioperative outcomes in elderly patients undergoing nephrectomy for renal cell carcinoma. Res Rep Urol. 2019;11:195–9.
13. Khene ZE, Peyronnet B, Kocher NJ, et al. Predicting morbidity after robotic partial nephrectomy: the effect of tumor, environment, and patient-related factors. Urol Oncol. 2018;36(7):338 e319–26.
14. Lue K, Russell CM, Fisher J, et al. Predictors of postoperative complications in patients who undergo radical nephrectomy and IVC thrombectomy: a large contemporary tertiary center analysis. Clin Genitourin Cancer. 2016;14(1):89–95.
15. Gontero P, Mari A, Marra G, et al. Is partial nephrectomy safe and effective in the setting of frail comorbid patients affected by renal cell carcinoma? Insights from the RECORD 2 multicentre prospective study. Urol Oncol. 2021;39(1):78 e17–26.
16. Charlson ME, Pompei P, Ales KL, MacKenzie CR. A new method of classifying prognostic comorbidity in longitudinal studies: development and validation. J Chronic Dis. 1987;40(5):373–83.
17. Osborn KP IV, Nothelle S, Slaven JE, Montz K, Hui S, Torke AM. Cumulative Illness Rating Scale (CIRS) can be used to predict hospital outcomes in older adults. J Geriatr Med Gerontol. 2017;3(2):030.
18. Oken MM, Creech RH, Tormey DC, et al. Toxicity and response criteria of the Eastern Cooperative Oncology Group. Am J Clin Oncol. 1982;5(6):649–55.
19. Zisman A, Pantuck AJ, Wieder J, et al. Risk group assessment and clinical outcome algorithm to predict the natural history of patients with surgically resected renal cell carcinoma. J Clin Oncol Off J Am Soc Clin Oncol. 2002;20(23):4559–66.

20. Extermann M, Hurria A. Comprehensive geriatric assessment for older patients with cancer. J Clin Oncol Off J Am Soc Clin Oncol. 2007;25(14):1824–31.
21. Ghosn M, Ibrahim T, El Rassy E, Nassani N, Ghanem S, Assi T. Abridged geriatric assessment is a better predictor of overall survival than the Karnofsky performance scale and physical performance test in elderly patients with cancer. J Geriatr Oncol. 2017;8(2):128–32.
22. Bergerot CD, Philip EJ, Bergerot PG, et al. Discrepancies between genitourinary cancer patients' and clinicians' characterization of the eastern cooperative oncology group performance status. Cancer. 2021;127(3):354–8.
23. Heng DY, Xie W, Regan MM, et al. Prognostic factors for overall survival in patients with metastatic renal cell carcinoma treated with vascular endothelial growth factor-targeted agents: results from a large, multicenter study. J Clin Oncol Off J Am Soc Clin Oncol. 2009;27(34):5794–9.
24. Motzer RJ, Bacik J, Murphy BA, Russo P, Mazumdar M. Interferon-alfa as a comparative treatment for clinical trials of new therapies against advanced renal cell carcinoma. J Clin Oncol. 2002;20(1):289–96.
25. Xu Y, Zhang Y, Wang X, Kang J, Liu X. Prognostic value of performance status in metastatic renal cell carcinoma patients receiving tyrosine kinase inhibitors: a systematic review and meta-analysis. BMC Cancer. 2019;19(1):168.
26. Stoffel JT, Montgomery JS, Suskind AM, Tucci C, Vanni AJ. Optimizing outcomes in urologic surgery: pre-operative care for the patient undergoing urologic surgery or procedure. Linthicum Heights: American Urological Association; 2018.
27. Robinson TN, Wu DS, Sauaia A, et al. Slower walking speed forecasts increased postoperative morbidity and 1-year mortality across surgical specialties. Ann Surg. 2013;258(4):582–8; discussion 588–90.
28. Morley JE, Vellas B, van Kan GA, et al. Frailty consensus: a call to action. J Am Med Dir Assoc. 2013;14(6):392–7.
29. Tan HJ, Shirk JD, Chamie K, Litwin MS, Hu JC. Patient function and the value of surgical care for kidney cancer. J Urol. 2017;197(5):1200–7.
30. Fried LP, Tangen CM, Walston J, et al. Frailty in older adults: evidence for a phenotype. J Gerontol A Biol Sci Med Sci. 2001;56(3):M146–56.
31. Searle SD, Mitnitski A, Gahbauer EA, Gill TM, Rockwood K. A standard procedure for creating a frailty index. BMC Geriatr. 2008;8:24-2318-24.
32. Walach MT, Wunderle MF, Haertel N, et al. Frailty predicts outcome of partial nephrectomy and guides treatment decision towards active surveillance and tumor ablation. World J Urol. 2021;39:2843.
33. Abellan van Kan G, Rolland YM, Morley JE, Vellas B. Frailty: toward a clinical definition. J Am Med Dir Assoc. 2008;9(2):71–2.
34. Morgan TM, Tang D, Stratton KL, et al. Preoperative nutritional status is an important predictor of survival in patients undergoing surgery for renal cell carcinoma. Eur Urol. 2011;59(6):923–8.
35. Gu W, Zhang G, Sun L, et al. Nutritional screening is strongly associated with overall survival in patients treated with targeted agents for metastatic renal cell carcinoma. J Cachexia Sarcopenia Muscle. 2015;6(3):222–30.
36. Bouillanne O, Morineau G, Dupont C, et al. Geriatric nutritional risk index: a new index for evaluating at-risk elderly medical patients. Am J Clin Nutr. 2005;82(4):777–83.
37. Watanabe D, Miura K, Yamashita A, et al. A comparison of the predictive role of the geriatric nutritional risk index and immunonutritional parameters for postoperative complications in elderly patients with renal cell carcinoma. J Investig Surg. 2020;34:1072.
38. Rubenstein LZ, Harker JO, Salva A, Guigoz Y, Vellas B. Screening for undernutrition in geriatric practice: developing the short-form mini-nutritional assessment (MNA-SF). J Gerontol A Biol Sci Med Sci. 2001;56(6):M366–72.
39. Psutka SP, Boorjian SA, Moynagh MR, et al. Mortality after radical cystectomy: impact of obesity versus adiposity after adjusting for skeletal muscle wasting. J Urol. 2015;193(5):1507–13.

40. Hakimi AA, Furberg H, Zabor EC, et al. An epidemiologic and genomic investigation into the obesity paradox in renal cell carcinoma. J Natl Cancer Inst. 2013;105(24):1862–70.
41. Steffens S, Ringe KI, Schroeer K, et al. Does overweight influence the prognosis of renal cell carcinoma? Results of a multicenter study. Int J Urol. 2013;20:585–92.
42. Hu X, Liao DW, Yang ZQ, Yang WX, Xiong SC, Li X. Sarcopenia predicts prognosis of patients with renal cell carcinoma: a systematic review and meta-analysis. Int Braz J Urol. 2020;46(5):705–15.
43. Sharma P, Zargar-Shoshtari K, Caracciolo JT, et al. Sarcopenia as a predictor of overall survival after cytoreductive nephrectomy for metastatic renal cell carcinoma. Urol Oncol. 2015;33(8):339 e317–23.
44. Psutka SP, Boorjian SA, Moynagh MR, et al. Decreased skeletal muscle mass is associated with an increased risk of mortality after radical nephrectomy for localized renal cell cancer. J Urol. 2016;195(2):270–6.
45. Fearon K, Strasser F, Anker SD, et al. Definition and classification of cancer cachexia: an international consensus. Lancet Oncol. 2011;12(5):489–95.
46. Bhasin S, Travison TG, Manini TM, et al. Sarcopenia definition: the position statements of the sarcopenia definition and outcomes consortium. J Am Geriatr Soc. 2020;68(7):1410–8.
47. Mourtzakis M, Prado CM, Lieffers JR, Reiman T, McCargar LJ, Baracos VE. A practical and precise approach to quantification of body composition in cancer patients using computed tomography images acquired during routine care. Applied Physiol Nutr Metab. 2008;33(5):997–1006.
48. Khan AI, Reiter DA, Sekhar A, et al. MRI quantitation of abdominal skeletal muscle correlates with CT-based analysis: implications for sarcopenia measurement. Appl Physiol Nutr Metab. 2019;44(8):814–9.
49. Higgins MI, Martini DJ, Patil DH, et al. Quantification of body composition in renal cell carcinoma patients: comparing computed tomography and magnetic resonance imaging measurements. Eur J Radiol. 2020;132:109307.
50. Wu Y, Fu X, Zhu X, et al. Prognostic role of systemic inflammatory response in renal cell carcinoma: a systematic review and meta-analysis. J Cancer Res Clin Oncol. 2011;137(5):887–96.
51. Broggi MS, Patil D, Baum Y, et al. Onodera's prognostic nutritional index as an independent prognostic factor in clear cell renal cell carcinoma. Urology. 2016;96:99–105.
52. Ignacio de Ulibarri J, Gonzalez-Madrono A, de Villar NG, et al. CONUT: a tool for controlling nutritional status. First validation in a hospital population. Nutr Hosp. 2005;20(1):38–45.
53. Elghiaty A, Kim J, Jang WS, et al. Preoperative controlling nutritional status (CONUT) score as a novel immune-nutritional predictor of survival in non-metastatic clear cell renal cell carcinoma of </= 7 cm on preoperative imaging. J Cancer Res Clin Oncol. 2019;145(4):957–65.
54. Nunno VD, Mollica V, Gatto L, et al. Prognostic impact of neutrophil-to-lymphocyte ratio in renal cell carcinoma: a systematic review and meta-analysis. Immunotherapy. 2019;11(7):631–43.
55. Tang Y, Liang J, Liu Z, et al. Clinical significance of prognostic nutritional index in renal cell carcinomas. Medicine (Baltimore). 2021;100(10):e25127.
56. Garbens A, Wallis CJD, Bjarnason G, et al. Platelet to white blood cell ratio predicts 30-day postoperative infectious complications in patients undergoing radical nephrectomy for renal malignancy. Can Urol Assoc J. 2017;11(11):E414–20.
57. Motzer RJ, Mazumdar M, Bacik J, Berg W, Amsterdam A, Ferrara J. Survival and prognostic stratification of 670 patients with advanced renal cell carcinoma. J Clin Oncol Off J Am Soc Clin Oncol. 1999;17(8):2530–40.
58. Lyon TD, Gershman B, Shah PH, et al. Risk prediction models for cancer-specific survival following cytoreductive nephrectomy in the contemporary era. Urol Oncol. 2018;36(11):499 e491–7.
59. McIntosh AG, Umbreit EC, Holland LC, et al. Optimizing patient selection for cytoreductive nephrectomy based on outcomes in the contemporary era of systemic therapy. Cancer. 2020;126(17):3950–60.

60. Network NCC. NCCN clinical practice guidelines in oncology: Kidney cancer version 2.2021 2021.
61. Campbell S, Uzzo RG, Allaf ME, et al. Renal mass and localized renal cancer: AUA guideline. J Urol. 2017;198(3):520–9.
62. McIntosh AG, Parker DC, Egleston BL, et al. Prediction of significant estimated glomerular filtration rate decline after renal unit removal to aid in the clinical choice between radical and partial nephrectomy in patients with a renal mass and normal renal function. BJU Int. 2019;124(6):999–1005.
63. Ellis RJ, Del Vecchio SJ, Gallagher KMJ, et al. A simple clinical tool for stratifying risk of clinically significant CKD after nephrectomy: development and multinational validation. J Am Soc Nephrol. 2020;31(5):1107–17.
64. Xia L, Hu G, Guzzo TJ. Prognostic significance of preoperative anemia in patients undergoing surgery for renal cell carcinoma: a meta-analysis. Anticancer Res. 2017;37(6):3175–81.
65. Hurria A. Geriatric assessment in oncology practice. J Am Geriatr Soc. 2009;57(Suppl 2):S246–9.
66. Ellis G, Whitehead MA, O'Neill D, Langhorne P, Robinson D. Comprehensive geriatric assessment for older adults admitted to hospital. Cochrane Database Syst Rev. 2011;(7):CD006211.
67. Wunderle MF, Hartel N, Wagener N, et al. Prospective geriatric assessment for perioperative risk stratification in partial nephrectomy. Eur J Surg Oncol. 2020;47:913.
68. Network NCC. NCCN clinical practice guidelines in oncology: older adult oncology version 1.2020. National Comprehensive Cancer Network 2020;February 2, 2020.
69. Hernandez Torres C, Hsu T. Comprehensive geriatric assessment in the older adult with cancer: a review. Eur Urol Focus. 2017;3(4–5):330–9.
70. Noordzij PG, Boersma E, Schreiner F, et al. Increased preoperative glucose levels are associated with perioperative mortality in patients undergoing noncardiac, nonvascular surgery. Eur J Endocrinol. 2007;156(1):137–42.
71. Underwood P, Askari R, Hurwitz S, Chamarthi B, Garg R. Preoperative A1C and clinical outcomes in patients with diabetes undergoing major noncardiac surgical procedures. Diabetes Care. 2014;37(3):611–6.
72. Lane BR, Campbell SC, Demirjian S, Fergany AF. Surgically induced chronic kidney disease may be associated with a lower risk of progression and mortality than medical chronic kidney disease. J Urol. 2013;189(5):1649–55.
73. Psutka SP, Leibovich BC. Management of inferior vena cava tumor thrombus in locally advanced renal cell carcinoma. Ther Adv Urol. 2015;7(4):216–29.
74. Psutka SP, Boorjian SA, Thompson RH, et al. Clinical and radiographic predictors of the need for inferior vena cava resection during nephrectomy for patients with renal cell carcinoma and caval tumour thrombus. BJU Int. 2015;116(3):388–96.
75. Recart A, Duchene D, White PF, Thomas T, Johnson DB, Cadeddu JA. Efficacy and safety of fast-track recovery strategy for patients undergoing laparoscopic nephrectomy. J Endourol. 2005;19(10):1165–9.
76. Miao C, Yu A, Yuan H, Gu M, Wang Z. Effect of enhanced recovery after surgery on postoperative recovery and quality of life in patients undergoing laparoscopic partial nephrectomy. Front Oncol. 2020;10:513874.
77. Fink AS, Prochazka AV, Henderson WG, et al. Enhancement of surgical informed consent by addition of repeat back: a multicenter, randomized controlled clinical trial. Ann Surg. 2010;252(1):27–36.
78. Arends J, Baracos V, Bertz H, et al. ESPEN expert group recommendations for action against cancer-related malnutrition. Clin Nutr (Edinburgh, Scotland). 2017;36(5):1187–96.
79. Bozzetti F. Tailoring the nutritional regimen in the elderly cancer patient. Nutrition. 2015;31(4):612–4.
80. Gao B, Luo J, Liu Y, et al. Clinical efficacy of perioperative immunonutrition containing omega-3-fatty acids in patients undergoing hepatectomy: a systematic review and meta-analysis of randomized controlled trials. Ann Nutr Metab. 2020;76:375.

81. Yang FA, Chen YC, Tiong C. Immunonutrition in patients with pancreatic cancer undergoing surgical intervention: a systematic review and meta-analysis of randomized controlled trials. Nutrients. 2020;12(9):2798.
82. Hamilton-Reeves JM, Bechtel MD, Hand LK, et al. Effects of immunonutrition for cystectomy on immune response and infection rates: a pilot randomized controlled clinical trial. Eur Urol. 2016;69(3):389–92.
83. Ritch CR, Cookson MS, Clark PE, et al. Perioperative oral nutrition supplementation reduces prevalence of sarcopenia following radical cystectomy: results of a prospective randomized controlled trial. J Urol. 2019;201(3):470–7.
84. A randomized phase III double-blind clinical trial evaluating the effect of immune-enhancing nutrition on radical cystectomy outcomes. 2019; https://www.swog.org/clinical-trials/s1600. Accessed 1 Apr 2021.
85. Denlinger CS, Sanft T, Moslehi JJ, et al. NCCN guidelines insights: survivorship, version 2.2020. J Natl Compr Cancer Netw. 2020;18(8):1016–23.
86. Jensen BT, Petersen AK, Jensen JB, Laustsen S, Borre M. Efficacy of a multiprofessional rehabilitation programme in radical cystectomy pathways: a prospective randomized controlled trial. Scand J Urol. 2015;49(2):133–41.
87. Ehdaie B, Furberg H, Zabor EC, Hakimi AA, Russo P. Comprehensive assessment of the impact of cigarette smoking on survival of clear cell kidney cancer. J Urol. 2014;191(3):597–602.
88. Yoong SL, d'Espaignet ET, Wiggers J, et al. Tobacco and postsurgical outcomes: WHO tobacco knowledge summaries. Geneva: World Health Organization; 2020.
89. Mills E, Eyawo O, Lockhart I, Kelly S, Wu P, Ebbert JO. Smoking cessation reduces postoperative complications: a systematic review and meta-analysis. Am J Med. 2011;124(2):144–154 e148.
90. Myers K, Hajek P, Hinds C, McRobbie H. Stopping smoking shortly before surgery and postoperative complications: a systematic review and meta-analysis. Arch Intern Med. 2011;171(11):983–9.
91. Culkin DJ, Exaire EJ, Green D, et al. Anticoagulation and antiplatelet therapy in urological practice: ICUD/AUA review paper. J Urol. 2014;192(4):1026–34.
92. Membership of the Working P, Barker P, Creasey PE, et al. Peri-operative management of the surgical patient with diabetes 2015: Association of Anaesthetists of Great Britain and Ireland. Anaesthesia. 2015;70(12):1427–40.
93. Duggan EW, Carlson K, Umpierrez GE. Perioperative hyperglycemia management: an update. Anesthesiology. 2017;126(3):547–60.
94. McCormick B, Meissner MA, Karam JA, Wood CG. Surgical complications of presurgical systemic therapy for renal cell carcinoma: a systematic review. Kidney Cancer. 2017;1(2):115–21.
95. Harshman LC, Yu RJ, Allen GI, Srinivas S, Gill HS, Chung BI. Surgical outcomes and complications associated with presurgical tyrosine kinase inhibition for advanced renal cell carcinoma (RCC). Urol Oncol. 2013;31(3):379–85.
96. Cabozantinib. 2018.
97. SUTENT((R)) (sunitinib malate) capsules. 2021; https://www.pfizerpro.com/product/sutent?gclid=2ab2986bab6817418a0ff80d82cac04e&gclsrc=3p.ds&. Accessed 1 Apr 2021.
98. Prescribing NEXAVAR((R)) (sorafenib). 2021; https://www.hcp.nexavar-us.com/prescribing-nexavar/dosage-administration/?utm_source=bing&utm_medium=cpc&utm_campaign=NEX_X_HCP_BR_SEM_X_X_Al_BNG_BRN_X_X_X_TRA_X_X_X_X_X_209&utm_content=Prescribing+++%7C+Exact&utm_term=sorafenib+package+insert&matchtype=e&device=c&adposition=&loc=103605&gclid=28fc818f4c40110e9577e1e960591d30&gclsrc=3p.ds&msclkid=28fc818f4c40110e9577e1e960591d30. Accessed 1 Apr 2021.
99. Cabometyx((R)) (cabozantinib) tablets. 2021; https://www.cabometyxhcp.com/?gclid=4cb1096d32221cb4c44a690b1881027f&gclsrc=3p.ds&utm_source=bing&utm_medium=cpc&utm_campaign=BS%20-%202021%209er%20Refresh%20-%20BR%20-

%20RCC%20-%20Generic&utm_term=cabozantinib&utm_content=BS%20-%20Generic%20Alone_EX. Accessed 1 Apr 2021.
100. MVASI((R)) (bevacizumab-awwb) injection 100 mg/vial & 400mg/vial. 2021; https://www.mvasi.com/hcp/totality-of-evidence/avastin-bioequivalence?gclid=bd1bf5f871e0161b09d2959e5a8f1332&gclsrc=3p.ds&msclkid=bd1bf5f871e0161b09d2959e5a8f1332&utm_source=bing&utm_medium=cpc&utm_campaign=BND_MVS_HCP_Competitor_2019_PHM&utm_term=avastin%20package%20insert&utm_content=Avastin_Phrase. Accessed 1 Apr 2021.
101. Helmink BA, Roland CL, Kiernan CM, Wargo JA. Toxicity of immune checkpoint inhibitors: considerations for the surgeon. Ann Surg Oncol. 2020;27(5):1533–45.
102. Becher E, Jericevic D, Huang WC. Minimally invasive surgery for patients with locally advanced and/or metastatic renal cell carcinoma. Urol Clin North Am. 2020;47(3):389–97.
103. Chrouser K, Foley F, Goldenberg M, et al. Optimizing outcomes in urologic surgery: intraoperative considerations 2018. American Urological Association, Linthicum Heights, MD.
104. Wolf JS Jr, Bennett CJ, Dmochowski RR, et al. Best practice policy statement on urologic surgery antimicrobial prophylaxis. J Urol. 2008;179(4):1379–90.
105. Steiner T, Traue C, Schubert J. Perioperative antibiotic prophylaxis in transperitoneal tumor nephrectomy: does it lower the rate of clinically significant postoperative infections? Urologe A. 2003;42(1):34–7.
106. Kalisch BJ, Lee S, Dabney BW. Outcomes of inpatient mobilization: a literature review. J Clin Nurs. 2014;23(11–12):1486–501.
107. Castelino T, Fiore JF Jr, Niculiseanu P, Landry T, Augustin B, Feldman LS. The effect of early mobilization protocols on postoperative outcomes following abdominal and thoracic surgery: a systematic review. Surgery. 2016;159(4):991–1003.
108. Donat SM, Diaz M, Bishoff JT, et al. Follow-up for clinically localized renal neoplasms: AUA guideline. J Urol. 2013;190(2):407–16.
109. Stewart SB, Thompson RH, Psutka SP, et al. Evaluation of the National Comprehensive Cancer Network and American Urological Association renal cell carcinoma surveillance guidelines. Clin Oncol. 2014;32:4056.
110. Stewart-Merrill SB, Thompson RH, Boorjian SA, et al. Oncologic surveillance after surgical resection for renal cell carcinoma: a novel risk-based approach. J Clin Oncol Off J Am Soc Clin Oncol. 2015;33(35):4151–7.
111. Patel HD, Pierorazio PM, Johnson MH, et al. Renal functional outcomes after surgery, ablation, and active surveillance of localized renal tumors: a systematic review and meta-analysis. Clin J Am Soc Nephrol. 2017;12(7):1057–69.
112. Kalantar-Zadeh K, Fouque D. Nutritional management of chronic kidney disease. N Engl J Med. 2017;377(18):1765–76.
113. Hahn D, Hodson EM, Fouque D. Low protein diets for non-diabetic adults with chronic kidney disease. Cochrane Database Syst Rev. 2020;10:CD001892.
114. van Walraven C, Austin PC, Jennings A, Quan H, Forster AJ. A modification of the Elixhauser comorbidity measures into a point system for hospital death using administrative data. Med Care. 2009;47(6):626–33.
115. ASA Physical Status Classification. 2020.
116. Karnofsky DA, Burchenal JH. Evaluation of chemotherapeutic agents. New York: Columbia University Press; 1949.
117. Rockwood K, Song X, MacKnight C, et al. A global clinical measure of fitness and frailty in elderly people. CMAJ. 2005;173(5):489–95.
118. Obeid NM, Azuh O, Reddy S, et al. Predictors of critical care-related complications in colectomy patients using the National Surgical Quality Improvement Program: exploring frailty and aggressive laparoscopic approaches. J Trauma Acute Care Surg. 2012;72(4):878–83.
119. Sathianathen NJ, Jarosek S, Lawrentschuk N, Bolton D, Konety BR. A simplified frailty index to predict outcomes after radical cystectomy. Eur Urol Focus. 2018;5:658.

Chapter 12
Surgical Treatment for Metastatic Kidney Cancer

Roy Mano and A. Ari Hakimi

Introduction

Metastatic disease is present in approximately 15% of patients diagnosed with renal cell carcinoma (RCC) [1]. In addition, 20–30% of patients treated for localized RCC will develop distant or local recurrences within 5 years [2]. Common sites for RCC metastases include lung (45%), bone (30%), lymph nodes (22%), liver (20%), adrenal (9%), and brain (8%); 39% of patients have metastases at two or more sites [3]. The approval of sunitinib for treating metastatic RCC (mRCC) in 2005 marked a significant change in the treatment and outcome of patients. Since then, major advancements have been made in the management of metastatic disease including the addition of newer targeted therapies and immunotherapy as first-line treatment options [4]. Surgery for the treatment of mRCC may include the resection of the primary tumor and the kidney (cytoreductive nephrectomy) or the resection of metastases in well-selected patients. Historically, surgery had a central role in the treatment of metastatic RCC; however, its role is currently under question with the advent of new, improved, systemic therapies. In the following chapter, we will review the role of surgery as part of the multidisciplinary treatment for mRCC in the different treatment eras.

R. Mano
Department of Urology, Tel-Aviv Sourasky Medical Center, Sackler School of Medicine, Tel-Aviv University, Tel Aviv-Yafo, Israel

A. Ari Hakimi (✉)
Urology Service, Department of Surgery, Memorial Sloan Kettering Cancer Center, New York, NY, USA
e-mail: hakimia@mskcc.org

K. L. Stratton, A. K. Morgans (eds.), *Urologic Oncology*,
https://doi.org/10.1007/978-3-030-89891-5_12

Cytoreductive Nephrectomy: Historical Perspectives

Cytoreductive nephrectomy (CN) was initially shown to improve overall survival in patients treated with interferon alpha-2b [5–7]. Flanigan et al. performed a randomized controlled trial comparing nephrectomy followed by interferon alpha-2b to interferon alpha-2b alone. The median survival of patients who received surgery ($n = 120$) was 11 months compared to 8 months for patients who did not receive surgery ($n = 121$, $p = 0.05$). This finding remained significant when controlling for performance status, metastatic site, and the presence or absence of a measurable metastatic lesion [5]. In a similar randomized trial, Mickisch et al. compared the outcome of 42 patients receiving combined treatment and 43 patients who received interferon alpha-2b alone. Time to progression (5 vs. 3 months, HR – 0.6, 95% CI 0.36–0.97) and median duration of survival (17 vs. 7 months, HR – 0.54, 95% CI 0.31–0.94) were both significantly longer in patients receiving CN [6]. In an analysis combining both trials, a significant median OS improvement of 6 months was observed when combining CN with interferon compared to interferon alone [7].

Following the publication of these studies, CN became the standard of care for treating patients with mRCC. Consistent with this recommendation, a Surveillance, Epidemiology, and Ends Results (SEER) registry study which examined the temporal trends in the utilization of CN among patients with mRCC treated between the years 1993 and 2010 reported that the proportion of patients undergoing CN increased between the years 1993 and 2004 from 29% to 39% with a decrease in the utilization of CN since 2005 consistent with the approval of targeted therapies for mRCC [8].

Cytoreductive Nephrectomy in the Era of Targeted Therapy

Multiple retrospective studies, based on single- and multicenter cohorts as well as cancer registries, supported the role of CN in patients treated with targeted therapy. Two meta-analyses of studies published by the year 2018 showed that among published nonrandomized studies, nephrectomy followed by targeted therapy was associated with an improved overall survival (OS) compared to targeted therapy alone [9, 10]. Hanna et al. evaluated a group of over 15,000 mRCC patients from the National Cancer Database (NCDB) who were treated with targeted therapies between 2006 and 2013. Approximately a third of these patients underwent CN, a rate that remained stable throughout the years of the study. Patients who were younger, had private insurance, were treated at an academic center, and had lower tumor stage and cN0 were more likely to undergo CN. The median OS was significantly longer among patients who underwent CN (17 vs. 8 months, $p < 0.001$), and CN patients had a lower risk of any death on multivariable Cox-regression analysis after adjusting for all available covariates. This survival benefit remained unchanged even after performing propensity score adjustment [11]. In a retrospective single-center cohort study, the outcomes of CN prior to treatment with TKI were compared to the use of TKI alone in the real-world setting. Multiple imputations and inverse probability of treatment weighting were used to account for missing values and differences between the two groups. Contrary to previously described retrospective studies, no differences were observed in progression-free, overall, and cancer-specific survivals. In subgroup analyses, cancer-related outcomes were improved in patients with sarcomatoid features and clear cell histology who underwent CN [12]. Despite these findings from retrospective studies, level 1 evidence to support the use of nephrectomy prior to targeted therapy was lacking.

The CARMENA trial is a prospective, multicenter, open-label randomized, phase 3 trial which compared nephrectomy followed by sunitinib to sunitinib alone for the treatment of patients diagnosed with metastatic clear cell RCC with a primary endpoint of OS. A total of 450 patients classified as having intermediate- or poor-risk disease according to the Memorial Sloan Kettering Cancer Center (MSKCC) prognostic model were randomized to the study. At a median follow-up of 51 months, the results in the sunitinib-alone group were non-inferior to those in the nephrectomy-sunitinib group with a median overall survival of 18 months and 14 months, respectively (HR = 0.89, 95% CI 0.71–1.1). These findings were consistent when analyzed separately in patients with intermediate-risk and poor-risk disease. Furthermore, no significant differences were noted in the response rates or progression-free survival rates. Major adverse events in sunitinib-treated patients were slightly lower in the nephrectomy-sunitinib group (33% vs. 43%, $p = 0.04$) [13].

A major limitation of the CARMENA trial is the inclusion of patients with intermediate- and high-risk disease, as apparent by the low overall survival of the study group when compared to randomized, controlled trials evaluating sunitinib. Patients with good-risk disease may therefore be more suitable for CN especially when considering the fact that patients with slow-growing disease after nephrectomy may be suitable for prolonged surveillance-only periods limiting the side effects associated with systemic therapy [14, 15]. Additional limitations of the CARMENA trial include the slow and incomplete accrual and the small number of patients enrolled in each one of the 79 trial centers (0.7 patients per year) suggesting not all patients with stage IV disease were enrolled to the trial. Furthermore, the nephrectomy-sunitinib group had a higher percentage of locally advanced tumors (stage T3 or T4) than the sunitinib group (70.1% vs. 51.0%), which could have affected surgical outcomes. Finally, more patients in the nephrectomy group did not receive the assigned treatment (18% did not receive sunitinib and 7% did not undergo nephrectomy), while more patients in the sunitinib-only group received additional nephrectomy (17%) and only 5% did not receive sunitinib, thus complicating the interpretation of the results [14].

Risk Stratification of Patients Planned to Undergo Cytoreductive Nephrectomy

Several studies aimed to identify pretreatment prognostic factors to help select patients who are likely to benefit from CN. Investigators from the MD Anderson Cancer Center evaluated a group of patients who underwent CN, a large part of whom were treated prior to the targeted therapy era, with the aim of identifying preoperative factors that were prognostic for outcomes. On multivariable analysis independent predictors of poor outcome included lactate dehydrogenase level greater than the upper limit of normal, an albumin level less than the lower limit of normal, symptoms at presentation caused by a metastatic site, liver metastasis, retroperitoneal adenopathy, supradiaphragmatic adenopathy, and clinical tumor stage ≥T3. Moreover, inferior OS was positively correlated with the number of risk factors, and patients with ≥4 risk factors did not seem to benefit from CN when compared to a referent group of patients who received medical therapy alone [16]. Margulis et al. expanded the study cohort to include more recently treated patients and developed preoperative and postoperative nomograms to predict cancer-specific survival at 6 and 12 months after CN. The preoperative model included serum albumin and serum lactate dehydrogenase, and the postoperative model included the preoperative predictors as well as pathologic tumor stage, nodal stage, and receipt of blood transfusion. Both models showed good discrimination and calibration when evaluated on a validation dataset [17]. The clinical utility of both preoperative models was validated in an independent cohort of patients treated at MSKCC. Five of the seven risk factors described by Culp et al. (excluding ≥cT3 disease and metastatic symptoms at presentation) were significantly associated with OS, and there was a decreasing rate of OS with the increase in the number of risk factors. The preoperative model suggested by Margulis et al. had a lower AUC than previously published and added little clinical utility for patient management [18]. In a study evaluating preoperative predictors of outcome in a more contemporary cohort of mRCC patients undergoing CN in the targeted therapy era, preoperative predictors included systemic symptoms at diagnosis, retroperitoneal and supradiaphragmatic lymphadenopathy, bone metastasis, clinical T4 disease, a hemoglobin level less than the lower limit of normal, a low serum albumin level, a serum lactate dehydrogenase level greater than the upper limit of normal, and a neutrophil/lymphocyte ratio greater than or equal to 4. Patients were stratified into risk groups based on the number of risk factors present, and high-risk patients (>3 risk factors) did not seem to benefit from CN. Importantly, the median OS of the highest-risk group was longer than that reported for patients in the nephrectomy-sunitinib arm of the CARMENA trial (19.2 months vs. 13.9 months) [19]. A meta-analysis of studies published until 2018 found that good performance status and good/intermediate International Metastatic renal cell carcinoma Database Consortium (IMDC)/ MSKCC risk classification were identified as predictors of an OS benefit associated with the use of CN. Conversely, progression on presurgical systemic treatment, high C-reactive protein, high neutrophil-lymphocyte ratio, poor IMDC/ MSKCC risk classification, sarcomatoid dedifferentiation, and poor performance status were all prognostic for a decrease in OS [10].

Tumor size is an additional prognostic factor among patients with metastatic clear cell RCC. Clear cell tumors ≤4 cm were associated with a lower number of metastatic sites and improved OS which remained longer in smaller tumors even after adjusting for known predictors of outcome. The association between primary tumor size and outcome was not found in patients with non-clear cell RCC [20].

Among patients treated with CN whose tumors were sequenced for genes commonly mutated in RCC, somatic mutations in *SETD2* [HR = 0.58, 95% CI 0.35–0.94, $p = 0.027$] and *KDM5C* (HR = 0.43, 95% CI 0.22–0.85, $p = 0.019$) were associated with a reduced risk of death, whereas *BAP1* mutations were associated with an increased risk of death (HR = 1.81, 95% CI 1.16–2.83, $p = 0.008$). However, the use of genetic findings may be limited by intratumoral heterogeneity present especially in large tumors [21, 22].

Most patients included in previously reported studies evaluating predictors of outcome had clear cell RCC. In a study evaluating a group of patients with non-clear cell RCC who underwent CN, the median OS was 14 months (11–27), and estimated 2- and 5-year survivals were 40% and 12%, respectively. On multivariable analysis, increasing NLR and sarcomatoid features were associated with a worse outcome, while the presence of papillary features was associated with a favorable outcome [23]. In a cohort of patients with metastatic sarcomatoid RCC, estimated 2- and 5-year overall survivals after CN were low (34% and 15%, respectively). On multivariable analysis, metastases to liver, lung, and retroperitoneal nodes and non-clear cell histology were associated with a worse outcome. Notably, median OS increased across each of the therapeutic eras, from 11 months pre-2006 to 21 months in patients treated from 2015 to 2018 [24].

Silagy et al. evaluated reasons physicians were unwilling to perform surgery in a cohort of patients with mRCC referred to CN. When compared to patients who underwent CN, non-operative patients were older, had a reduced performance status, and had a greater metastatic burden and non-clear cell histology. Reasons for avoiding CN included oncologic factors (metastatic burden, unresectable primary tumor, rapidly progressing disease, tumor-driven frailty, and oncologic prioritization) and patient-fitness factors (pre-existing comorbidities and poor renal function). Interestingly, these considerations were associated with decreased OS with four of the oncological factors conferring a median OS of less than 12 months ($p < 0.001$) [25].

The Timing of Cytoreductive Nephrectomy

Concerns associated with performing surgery prior to systemic therapy include delaying the initiation of systemic therapies which have proven efficacy in treating metastatic disease. In a study evaluating complications after CN and the time to receival of systemic therapy, only 5% had a Clavien grade ≥ 3 early complication. Over 60% of patients who were candidates for systemic therapy did not receive the treatment within 60 days; however, the delay was related to the CN in only 11% of patients. On multivariable analysis of preoperative factors, the presence of liver metastases was associated with a higher rate of complications and prolonged length of stay, while the use of a laparoscopic approach for CN was associated with earlier administration of systemic therapy [26]. In a meta-analysis of studies published until 2018, the risk for perioperative mortality was 0–10%, and the risk for Clavien grade ≥ 3 complications was 3–29%. In this meta-analysis 13–30% of patients did not receive systemic therapy after CN [10].

To evaluate the optimal sequence of cytoreductive nephrectomy and targeted therapy, Bhindi et al. used a cohort of patients from the NCDB and compared patients treated initially with CN and those treated initially with targeted therapy while using inverse probability of treatment weighting to account for treatment selection bias. In this study, initial CN was associated with improved overall survival compared to initial targeted therapy. The benefit obtained appeared to be in large part due to the greater likelihood of receiving multimodal therapy among patients treated initially with CN [27]. Using the same cohort of patients, Hanna et al. found a statistically significant survival benefit for patients who underwent CN after receiving targeted therapy. However, the study included only patients who received both CN and targeted therapy; therefore, the group of patients who received initial targeted therapy may be enriched in patients who responded well to systemic therapy and therefore underwent CN [11].

The SURTIME trial is a multicenter, randomized, phase 3 trial which compared immediate CN followed by sunitinib treatment and three cycles of sunitinib followed by CN in the absence of disease progression for the treatment of patients with metastatic clear cell RCC who are surgical candidates. Due to poor accrual, the study was closed prematurely and included a total of 99 patients. The 28-week progression-free survival did not differ significantly between the immediate CN group ($n = 50$, 42%) and the deferred CN group ($n = 49$, 43%). The median OS was significantly longer in the deferred CN arm (32 months) compared to the immediate CN arm (15 months, HR = 0.57, 95% CI 0.34–0.95, $p = 0.03$). Importantly, in the deferred CN arm, systemic progression before CN occurred in 14 patients (29%) who did not undergo nephrectomy, while in the immediate CN arm, 10 patients did not receive sunitinib treatment. The authors concluded that with the deferred approach, more patients received sunitinib and OS was higher [28]. Critics of this study mention that the premature closure of the study due to the poor accrual rendered it underpowered for evaluating the main aims of the study; thus, the results should be regarded as exploratory.

Cytoreductive Nephrectomy in the Era of Checkpoint Inhibitors

After the publication of the CheckMate 214 and the Keynote 426 trials, combination checkpoint blockade immunotherapy with ipilimumab-nivolumab and combination treatment with pembrolizumab-axitinib, respectively, were approved by the FDA for the treatment of newly diagnosed metastatic RCC. Subsequently, multiple guidelines have endorsed these treatment combinations as the preferred first-line regimens for the treatment of metastatic RCC [29, 30].

The benefit of CN in the advent of systemic immunotherapy has been questioned. Initial case series and cancer database studies support the feasibility and safety of CN for mRCC patients treated with immune checkpoint inhibitors (ICI). A study evaluating radical ($n = 10$) and partial ($n = 1$) nephrectomy for ten patients who received initial immunotherapy with nivolumab or combination ipilimumab/nivolumab showed the safety and efficacy of the procedure in this setting. The median time between ICI and surgery was 21 days, and the timing of nephrectomy relative to ICI dosing did not seem to impact outcome. None of the patients developed major intraoperative complications and 4/10 patients developed a Clavien-Dindo grade ≥ 3 complication within 90 days after surgery. Surgical margins were negative for all patients; however, only 1/10 patients exhibited complete response to immunotherapy in the primary tissue, highlighting the possible benefit from CN in ICI-treated patients. Interestingly 3/5 (60%) patients who underwent lymphadenectomy and 3/4 (75%) patients who underwent metastasectomy did not have detectable malignancy in their lymph nodes and metastatic sites, respectively [31]. A recently published case series of five patients further supported the feasibility and safety of CN for mRCC patients who underwent treatment with combination ICI (ipilimumab-nivolumab with or without pembrolizumab-axitinib) for tumors initially deemed as unresectable [32]. In a study based on the NCDB, 391 surgical candidates diagnosed with clear cell mRCC between the years 2015 and 2016 and treated with immunotherapy with or without CN and no other systemic therapies were identified. At a median follow-up of 15 months, patients treated with CN and immunotherapy had superior OS (median not reached (NR) vs. 12 months; hazard ratio 0.23, $p < 0.001$) which remained significant on multivariable analysis. The 20 patients who received immunotherapy prior to cytoreductive nephrectomy had lower stage and grade disease, smaller tumor size, and a lower rate of lymphovascular invasion. Two patients in the delayed CN group had no evidence of disease on pathology, and none of the patients in the group had positive surgical margins. These findings support the role of CN for patients treated with ICI. Moreover, it provides preliminary evidence regarding the timing and safety of CN relative to ICI administration [33].

Two trials are currently underway to provide level 1 evidence for the use of CN in mRCC patients treated with ICI. The phase 2 NORDIC-SUN trial (NCT03977571) will randomize participants to ipilimumab-nivolumab with or without nephrectomy. The primary outcome is overall survival, stratified by IMDC intermediate- and poor-risk disease. The phase 3 PROBE trial (NCT04510597) by the SWOG cancer research network will treat mRCC patients with ipilimumab + nivolumab, pembrolizumab + axitinib, or avelumab + axitinib, after which they will be randomized to either receive or not receive subsequent cytoreductive nephrectomy (Table 12.1) [34].

The Role of CN According to Current Guidelines

The 2021 European Association of Urology (EAU) guidelines recommend performing immediate CN in patients with a good performance status who do not require systemic therapy. CN should be avoided in MSKCC poor-risk patients. Systemic therapy without CN should initially be given to intermediate-risk patients who have an asymptomatic synchronous primary tumor and require treatment, and delayed

Table 12.1 Summary of published and planned randomized controlled trials evaluating the role of cytoreductive nephrectomy in patients with metastatic renal cell carcinoma

Reference (publication year)	Study years	Treatment groups	Performance status/ MSKCC risk group	Median follow-up	Outcomes	Conclusions/ Comments
Flanigan et al. 2001 [5]	1991–1998	Nephrectomy + interferon alpha-2b ($n = 120$) vs. interferon alpha-2b alone ($n = 121$)	Decreased performance status (SWOG PS 1) was found in 45% of the combined treatment group and 58% of the interferon only group	12 months for survivors	Median OS was 11 months in patients assigned to surgery + interferon and 8 months for patients treated with interferon alone ($p = 0.05$)	Nephrectomy followed by interferon therapy results in longer survival among patients with metastatic RCC than does interferon therapy alone
Mickisch et al. 2001 [6]	1995–1998	Nephrectomy + interferon alpha-2b ($n = 42$) vs. interferon alpha-2b alone ($n = 43$)	Decreased performance status (WHO PS 1) was found in 52% of the combined treatment group and 60% of the interferon only group	NA	Time to progression (median 5 vs. 3 months, HR = 0.6, 95% CI 0.36–0.97) and duration of survival (median 17 vs. 7 months, HR = 0.54, 95% CI 0.31–0.94) were significantly better in patients receiving surgery and interferon	Radical nephrectomy before interferon-based immunotherapy might substantially delay time to progression and improve survival of patients with metastatic RCC who present with good performance status

Mejean et al. 2018 [13] (CARMENA)	2009–2017	Nephrectomy + sunitinib ($n = 226$) vs. sunitinib alone ($n = 224$)	In the nephrectomy-sunitinib group, 56% of patients were MSKCC intermediate-risk and 44% were poor-risk; in the sunitinib-alone group, corresponding values were 58.5% and 41.5%	51 months overall	Median OS was 18 months in the sunitinib-alone group and 14 months in the nephrectomy-sunitinib group (HR = 0.89, 95% CI 0.71–1.10) There were no significant differences in response rate or PFS	Sunitinib alone was not inferior to nephrectomy followed by sunitinib in patients with intermediate–/poor-risk metastatic RCC
Bex et al. 2019 [28] (SURTIME)	2010–2016	Immediate CN followed by sunitinib ($n = 50$) vs. treatment with 3 cycles of sunitinib followed by CN and sunitinib ($n = 49$)	In the immediate CN group, 86% of patients were MSKCC intermediate-risk and 14% were poor-risk; in the deferred CN group, corresponding values were 90% and 10%	3.3 years overall	The 28-week PFS was 42% in the immediate CN arm and 43% in the deferred CN arm ($p = 0.61$) Median OS was 32 months in the deferred CN arm and 15 months in the immediate CN arm (HR = 0.57, 95% CI 0.34–0.95, $p = 0.03$)	Deferred CN did not improve the 28-week PFR; however, with the deferred approach, more patients received sunitinib and OS rates were higher

(continued)

Table 12.1 (continued)

Reference (publication year)	Study years	Treatment groups	Performance status/ MSKCC risk group	Median follow-up	Outcomes	Conclusions/ Comments
NORDIC-SUN[a] (NCT03977571)	2020–2025 (estimated)	Deferred CN (induction nivolumab + ipilimumab followed by CN and maintenance nivolumab) vs. no CN with similar systemic therapy	Patients with ≤3 IMDC risk factors deemed suitable for CN will undergo randomization	Patients will be followed for 3 years	Primary outcome will be OS; secondary outcomes will include PFS, time to subsequent systemic treatment, objective response rate, and treatment-related adverse events	Study will include biomarker analyses of TIL, immune cell subsets in blood, genetic profile of circulating tumor DNA and primary tumor tissue and gut microbiome
PROBE[a] (NCT04510597)	2020–2033 (estimated)	Study will compare treatment with standard of care immunotherapy-based drug combination (ipilimumab + nivolumab, pembrolizumab + axitinib or avelumab + axitinib) with or without subsequent CN	Participants must have a WHO PS of 0–1 within 28 days prior to randomization	Patients will be followed for 7 years	Primary outcome will be OS; secondary outcomes will include PFS, objective response, change in maximal tumor diameter, and complications after surgery	NA

[a]Data obtained from https://clinicaltrials.gov/

MSKCC Memorial Sloan Kettering Cancer Center, *SWOG* Southwestern Oncology Group, *PS* performance status, *OS* overall survival, *RCC* renal cell carcinoma, WHO = World Health Organization, *NA* not available, *HR* hazards ratio, *CI* confidence interval, *PFS* progression-free survival, *CN* cytoreductive nephrectomy, *IMDC* International Metastatic RCC Database Consortium, *TIL* tumor-infiltrating lymphocytes

CN should be discussed with patients who derive clinical benefit from systemic therapy. Finally, CN should be performed together with metastasectomy in oligometastatic patients when complete resection of the local tumor and metastases can be achieved [29].

According to the 2021 National Comprehensive Cancer Network (NCCN) guidelines, patients with excellent performance status (ECOG PS <2) and no brain metastases are candidates for cytoreductive therapy prior to systemic treatment if their tumor can be completely resected. In addition, patients with metastatic disease who present with local symptoms related to their primary tumor, such as hematuria, may be offered palliative nephrectomy if they are surgical candidates [30].

Metastasectomy for Renal Cell Carcinoma

The resection of metastatic sites may be used in selected mRCC patients with the aim of achieving a disease-free state. In an NCDB-based study evaluating utilization trends of metastasectomy among patient with mRCC, overall utilization rates increased significantly from 25% in 2006 to 31% in 2013. Patients treated at academic centers and those treated in recent years had higher odds of undergoing metastasectomy. In contrast, patients with increasing age, black and other races, stage pT2 and pT3 tumors, non-clear cell histology, and receipt of targeted therapy had lower odds of undergoing metastasectomy. After propensity score matching, median OS was 24 months for metastasectomy patients compared to 19 months for no metastasectomy ($p < 0.001$). In subgroup analyses, metastasectomy was associated with improved survival both in patients receiving targeted therapy and those who did not receive targeted therapy. In an exploratory analysis evaluating outcome based on site of metastases, metastasectomy was associated with a statistically significant lower risk of death only for lung metastases [35]. A study from Germany evaluating patients with mRCC who underwent metastasectomy during the targeted therapy era showed a significant surge in metastasis-directed therapy, especially surgical resection, during the time of the study, similar to the trend seen in the NCDB-based study. A significant increasing trend for resection of lung, bone, and adrenal metastases was observed, while rates of lymph node resection did not change and those of central nervous system metastases decreased over time. Radiation was used to treat most bone and central nervous system metastases. There was no significant change in the use of radiation for treating metastases throughout the study period [36].

The survival benefit of metastasectomy was shown in a systematic review and meta-analysis of eight comparative studies published until January 2016 which compared survival in patients who underwent complete surgical metastasectomy vs. incomplete or no metastasectomy while adjusting for different baseline characteristics. In the studies included, most patients had clear cell RCC, 12–81% of patients received systemic therapy, and most patients had metastases to multiple organ sites (36–56% of patients). Median overall survival ranged from 37 to 142 months for patient who underwent complete metastasectomy compared to 8–27 months for patients who did not undergo complete metastasectomy. Lack of complete metastasectomy was associated with an increased risk of overall mortality (adjusted HR = 2.37, 95% CI 2.03–2.87; $p < 0.001$) with low heterogeneity between studies [37]. A more recent meta-analysis was published in the year 2021 and included 17 retrospective comparative studies. Consistent with previous findings, patients who did not undergo metastasectomy had a worse OS than those who underwent resection of metastases (HR = 2.15, 95% CI 1.59–2.92, $p < 0.001$). This increased risk of death was observed in patients treated with traditional cytokine therapy (HR = 2.64, 95% CI 1.86–3.74, $p < 0.001$) as well as patients treated with novel targeted therapies and immune checkpoint inhibitors (HR = 1.82, 95% CI 1.23–2.7, $p = 0.003$) [38]. A similar benefit was observed in contemporary comparative studies of single- and multicenter cohorts published since the year 2016 which are reported in Table 12.2 [39–45].

Despite the apparent benefit in metastasectomy according to published studies, it is important to consider the fact they are all retrospective study limited by an apparent selection bias [46]. In addition, these procedures are associated with a high rate of complications which should be discussed with the patients prior to the procedure [47].

Predicting Outcomes After Metastasectomy

Nomograms and risk categories were created to identify which patients may benefit the most from metastasectomy. Predictive variables incorporated in these risk classifiers included high stage and grade of the primary tumor, sarcomatoid dedifferentiation, non-pulmonary metastases (especially brain metastases), multiorgan metastases, incomplete metastasectomy, C-reactive protein levels >1 mg/dL, and disease-free interval ≤ 12 months [48–51]. Reported area under the curve for published nomograms ranged from 0.71 to 0.88 demonstrating the accuracy of these models [48, 51]. In a meta-analysis published in 2021, prognostic factors associated with an improved OS in patient undergoing metastasectomy included lung only metastasis, asynchronous metastasis, fewer metastatic sites, clear cell histology, and prior nephrectomy. Importantly, despite differences among studies in the treatment and patients included, there was little heterogeneity regarding the prognostic factors identified [38].

Molecular subtyping may also assist in identifying which patients will benefit from metastasectomy. Outcomes after complete metastasectomy without systemic treatment were compared between 4 groups of ccRCC patients defined by a 35-gene expression classifier in a small cohort of 43 patients. Patients classified as good prognosis (ccRCC groups 2 and 3) had improved disease-free survival (median of 23 months vs. 9 months, $p = 0.011$), longer time to systemic therapy (92 months vs. 28 months, $p = 0.003$), improved cancer-specific survival (133 months vs. 50 months, $p < 0.001$), and improved overall survival (127 months vs. 50 months, $p = 0.011$);

Table 12.2 Summary of comparative studies, from single or multi-institutional cohorts, published since 2016 evaluating the role of metastasectomy for patient with metastatic renal cell carcinoma

Reference	Study years	MS groups (n)	Histology	Metastatic status	IMDC/ MSKCC risk groups	Systemic treatment type	Median follow-up (IQR)	Median OS (IQR)	OS difference (HR, 95% CI, p-value)
You 2016 [39]	2006–2013	Complete MS (33), incomplete MS (29), no MS (263)	ccRCC in 293 (90%) patients	Synchronous metastases in 180 patients (55%); single metastasis in 121 patients (37%)	81 (25%) favorable, 179 (55%) intermediate, 65 (20%) poor (IMDC)	All patients received TT including tyrosine kinase inhibitors in 302 (93%) and mTOR inhibitor in 23 (7%)	NA	93 months (95% CI 63, 122) for complete MS, 30 months (15, 44) for incomplete MS, and 24 months (19–28) for the no MS ($p < 0.001$)	On multivariable analyses, compared to no-MS, complete MS was associated with improved OS (0.43; 0.26–0.72, $p = 0.001$), but incomplete MS was not (0.86; 0.53–1.4, $p = 0.55$)
Li 2018 [40]	2006–2016	Complete MS (26), incomplete MS (23), no MS (75)	ccRCC in 101 (82%) patients	Single metastasis in 30 patients (24%)	106 (85.5%) favorable-intermediate and 18 (14.5%) poor (MSKCC)	All patients received at least one line of TT including TKIs in 108 (87%)	21 months (10–45)	5.05 years for complete MS, 3.5 years for incomplete MS, and 2.4 years for the non-MS group ($p < 0.024$)	On multivariable analysis, complete MS was associated with increased survival rates (0.5, 0.25–0.98, $p < 0.045$)

(continued)

Table 12.2 (continued)

Reference	Study years	MS groups (n)	Histology	Metastatic status	IMDC/MSKCC risk groups	Systemic treatment type	Median follow-up (IQR)	Median OS (IQR)	OS difference (HR, 95% CI, p-value)
Tornberg 2018 [41]	2006–2017	Complete MS (46), incomplete MS (51)	ccRCC in 86 (89%) patients	Synchronous metastases in 60 patients (62%); single metastasis in 46 patients (55%)	NA	Systemic treatment was given to 55 (57%) patients	46 months (24–74)	5-year OS was 59% for complete MS and 45% for non-complete MS ($p = 0.03$)	On multivariable analysis, non complete MS was associated with an increased likelihood of death (1.92; 1.01–3.64; $p = 0.045$)
Fares 2019 [42]	2007–2016	Complete MS (37), no complete MS (37) in matched cohort	All patients had ccRCC	Synchronous metastases in 21 patients (28%)	21 (28%) favorable, 49 (66%) intermediate, 4 (5%) poor (IMDC)	63 (85%) patients received TT; first-line treatment included sunitinib in 43 (58%) and pazopanib in 17 (23%); and 3 (4%) received temsirolimus	70 months	98 months for the complete MS group vs. 41 months for the non-complete MS group ($p < 0.001$)	On multivariable analysis, complete MS was associated with an improved OS (0.21, 0.09–0.49, $p < 0.001$)
Lyon 2020 [43]	2006–2017	Complete MS (158), no complete MS (428)	ccRCC in 483 (82%) patients	Synchronous metastases in 178 patients (30%); single metastasis in 375 patients (64%)	NA	277 (47%) patients received systemic therapy; most received TT and 45 (8%) received ICI either alone or combined	3.9 years (2.3–6.7)	7.2 years in patients who underwent complete MS	On multivariable analysis, complete MS was associated with an improved OS (0.47, 0.34–0.65, $p < 0.001$)

Dragomir 2020 [44]	2011–2019	Complete MS (229), no MS (803) in matched cohort	ccRCC (85% in both no-MS and MS)	Synchronous metastases in 30% of no-MS patients and 29% in MS patients; single metastasis in 83% in no-MS patients and 88% in MS patients	NA	First-line TT (59% no-MS, 48% MS), second-line TT (31% no-MS, 27% MS)	38 months (20–59) for complete MS and 29 months (16–43) for no-MS	81 months (58–NR) for complete MS and 61 months (26 – NR) for no-MS, ($p < 0.001$)	On multivariable analysis, complete MS was associated with a decreased risk of mortality compared to no-MS (0.41, 0.27–0.63)
Ishihara 2021 [45]	2008–2018	Complete MS (45), incomplete MS (53), no MS (216)	ccRCC in 232 patients (74%)	Synchronous metastases in 161 patients (51%)	41 (13%) favorable, 144 (46%) intermediate, 58 (18%) poor, 71 (23%) unknown (IMDC)	250 patients (80%) received systemic therapy; early TT era ($n = 109$, 35%), late TT era ($n = 139$, 44%), ICI era ($n = 66$, 21%)	25 months (11–52) for the whole cohort	OS was NR (95% CI 122–NR) in the complete-MS group, 82 (45–NR) in the incomplete-MS group ($p = 0.004$), and 28 (23–42) in the no-MS group ($p < 0.001$)	On multivariable analysis, compared to no-MS, incomplete MS (0.56, 0.35–0.90, $p = 0.018$) and complete MS (0.25, 0.12–0.54, $= < 0.001$) were associated with increased OS

MS metastasectomy, *ccRCC* clear cell renal cell carcinoma, *IMDC* International Metastatic RCC Database Consortium, *MSKCC* Memorial Sloan Kettering Cancer Center, *IQR* interquartile range, *OS* overall survival, *HR* hazards ratio, *CI* confidence interval, *TT* targeted therapy, *TKI* tyrosine kinase inhibitors, *ICI* immune checkpoint inhibitor, *NA* not available, *NR* not reached these findings remained significant in multivariable analysis. Pending validation in larger cohorts, the ccRCC classifier may assist in selecting patients for metastasectomy [52].

The role of metastasectomy was evaluated in a matched cohort of patients with metastatic sarcomatoid RCC who received metastasectomy ($n = 40$) and no metastasectomy ($n = 40$). Metastasectomy did not appear to provide a statistically significant survival benefit in patients with sarcomatoid RCC who presented with synchronous metastases (HR = 0.9, 95% CI 0.5, 1.5, $p = 0.62$) or asynchronous metastases (HR = 0.5, 95% CI 0.2, 1.4, $p = 0.17$) at nephrectomy. Pathological LN involvement at nephrectomy conferred a much worse prognosis in patients who undergo metastasectomy for sarcomatoid RCC. Therefore, the authors concluded that metastasectomy should be considered in patients with sarcomatoid RCC if clinically indicated, especially for palliative purposes [53].

Systemic Therapy After Metastasectomy

After metastasectomy, patients have a high risk of recurrence, but to date no postoperative medical treatment has been proven to be beneficial [54, 55]. The use of targeted therapy after complete metastasectomy was evaluated by the RESORT trial, a multicenter, randomized, open-label phase 2 trial. Patients with clear cell mRCC who underwent CN and radical metastasectomy of ≤3 metastatic sites were randomized to receive either sorafenib for a maximum of 52 weeks or observation with a primary endpoint of recurrence-free survival. Most patients had one metastatic site (≥80% in both arms). The trial was prematurely terminated due to the long accrual time and the availability of newer treatments during the time of the study. The median follow-up of the study was 38 months. Patients treated with sorafenib showed a nonsignificant shorter median recurrence-free survival (21 vs. 37 months, $p = 0.4$). Three-year recurrence-free survival rates were 50% for patients in the observation arm compared to 41% for patients receiving sorafenib. Grade ≥ 3 adverse events were more common in the sorafenib arm (22% vs. 3%). While the study did not show a benefit in the use of sorafenib after complete metastasectomy, it did show encouraging recurrence-free survival rates in well-selected patients with mRCC undergoing metastasectomy [56]. A randomized, double blind, placebo-controlled, phase 3 trial conducted by the ECOG-ACRIN cancer research group (E2810, NCT01575548) compared the use of pazopanib for 52 weeks and placebo for mRCC patients who were without evidence of disease after metastasectomy. The study was recently presented in an abstract form after enrolling 129 patients. The median follow-up was 30 months. The use of pazopanib after metastasectomy was associated with a nonsignificant improvement in disease-free survival (HR = 0.85, 95% CI 0.55, 1.31, $p = 0.47$) and a worse overall survival (HR = 2.65, 95% CI 1.02, 6.9, $p = 0.05$). Like the RESORT trial evaluating the use of sorafenib, this study did not show a benefit in using newer targeted agents after complete metastasectomy [57].

The Role of Metastasectomy According to Current Guidelines

The EAU mention in their guidelines that except for brain and bone metastases which may be treated with stereotactic radiotherapy, metastasectomy remains by default the only local treatment for most metastatic sites. They further recommend performing metastasectomy to control local symptoms for patients with favorable disease factors in whom complete resection may be obtained [29]. According to the NCCN guidelines, patients who present with a potentially resectable primary tumor and oligometastatic disease may undergo CN and metastasectomy. In addition, patients who develop oligometastatic disease after a prolonged disease-free state following nephrectomy may also undergo metastasectomy [30].

Conclusions

The role of surgery for the treatment of patients with mRCC is evolving with the ongoing advancements in systemic therapies. Level 1 evidence supported the use of CN in the cytokine era; however, a similar benefit was not observed in the era of targeted therapy, highlighting the importance of proper patient selection. Ongoing trials will shed more light on the role of CN with the recent advancement of ICI to first-line therapy.

Well-selected patients undergoing metastasectomy consistently show longer OS when complete metastasectomy is performed; however, current data stems from retrospective studies prone to selection bias. Additionally, data does not support the use of adjuvant systemic therapy after complete metastasectomy. Future studies may shed further light on the importance of metastasectomy in mRCC.

Funding Information
The Sidney Kimmel Center for Prostate and Urologic Cancers
NIH/NCI Cancer Center Support Grant P30 CA008748

References

1. Siegel RL, Miller KD, Fuchs HE, Jemal A. Cancer statistics, 2021. CA Cancer J Clin. 2021;71(1):7–33.
2. Dabestani S, Beisland C, Stewart GD, Bensalah K, Gudmundsson E, Lam TB, et al. Long-term outcomes of follow-up for initially localised clear cell renal cell carcinoma: RECUR database analysis. Eur Urol Focus. 2019;5(5):857–66.
3. Bianchi M, Sun M, Jeldres C, Shariat SF, Trinh QD, Briganti A, et al. Distribution of metastatic sites in renal cell carcinoma: a population-based analysis. Ann Oncol. 2012;23(4):973–80.
4. Choueiri TK, Motzer RJ. Systemic therapy for metastatic renal-cell carcinoma. N Engl J Med. 2017;376(4):354–66.
5. Flanigan RC, Salmon SE, Blumenstein BA, Bearman SI, Roy V, McGrath PC, et al. Nephrectomy followed by interferon alfa-2b compared with interferon alfa-2b alone for metastatic renal-cell cancer. N Engl J Med. 2001;345(23):1655–9.

6. Mickisch GH, Garin A, van Poppel H, de Prijck L, Sylvester R, European Organisation for R, et al. Radical nephrectomy plus interferon-alfa-based immunotherapy compared with interferon alfa alone in metastatic renal-cell carcinoma: a randomised trial. Lancet. 2001;358(9286):966–70.
7. Flanigan RC, Mickisch G, Sylvester R, Tangen C, Van Poppel H, Crawford ED. Cytoreductive nephrectomy in patients with metastatic renal cancer: a combined analysis. J Urol. 2004;171(3):1071–6.
8. Conti SL, Thomas IC, Hagedorn JC, Chung BI, Chertow GM, Wagner TH, et al. Utilization of cytoreductive nephrectomy and patient survival in the targeted therapy era. Int J Cancer. 2014;134(9):2245–52.
9. Garcia-Perdomo HA, Zapata-Copete JA, Castillo-Cobaleda DF. Role of cytoreductive nephrectomy in the targeted therapy era: a systematic review and meta-analysis. Invest Clin Urol. 2018;59(1):2–9.
10. Bhindi B, Abel EJ, Albiges L, Bensalah K, Boorjian SA, Daneshmand S, et al. Systematic review of the role of cytoreductive nephrectomy in the targeted therapy era and beyond: an individualized approach to metastatic renal cell carcinoma. Eur Urol. 2019;75(1):111–28.
11. Hanna N, Sun M, Meyer CP, Nguyen PL, Pal SK, Chang SL, et al. Survival analyses of patients with metastatic renal cancer treated with targeted therapy with or without cytoreductive nephrectomy: a National Cancer Data Base Study. J Clin Oncol. 2016;34(27):3267–75.
12. Janisch F, Hillemacher T, Fuehner C, D'Andrea D, Meyer CP, Klotzbucher T, et al. The impact of cytoreductive nephrectomy on survival outcomes in patients treated with tyrosine kinase inhibitors for metastatic renal cell carcinoma in a real-world cohort. Urol Oncol. 2020;38(9):739 e9–e15.
13. Mejean A, Ravaud A, Thezenas S, Colas S, Beauval JB, Bensalah K, et al. Sunitinib alone or after nephrectomy in metastatic renal-cell carcinoma. N Engl J Med. 2018;379(5):417–27.
14. Motzer RJ, Russo P. Cytoreductive nephrectomy – patient selection is key. N Engl J Med. 2018;379(5):481–2.
15. Rini BI, Dorff TB, Elson P, Rodriguez CS, Shepard D, Wood L, et al. Active surveillance in metastatic renal-cell carcinoma: a prospective, phase 2 trial. Lancet Oncol. 2016;17(9):1317–24.
16. Culp SH, Tannir NM, Abel EJ, Margulis V, Tamboli P, Matin SF, et al. Can we better select patients with metastatic renal cell carcinoma for cytoreductive nephrectomy? Cancer. 2010;116(14):3378–88.
17. Margulis V, Shariat SF, Rapoport Y, Rink M, Sjoberg DD, Tannir NM, et al. Development of accurate models for individualized prediction of survival after cytoreductive nephrectomy for metastatic renal cell carcinoma. Eur Urol. 2013;63(5):947–52.
18. Manley BJ, Tennenbaum DM, Vertosick EA, Hsieh JJ, Sjoberg DD, Assel M, et al. The difficulty in selecting patients for cytoreductive nephrectomy: an evaluation of previously described predictive models. Urol Oncol. 2017;35(1):35 e1–5.
19. McIntosh AG, Umbreit EC, Holland LC, Gu C, Tannir NM, Matin SF, et al. Optimizing patient selection for cytoreductive nephrectomy based on outcomes in the contemporary era of systemic therapy. Cancer. 2020;126(17):3950–60.
20. DiNatale RG, Xie W, Becerra MF, Silagy AW, Attalla K, Sanchez A, et al. The association between small primary tumor size and prognosis in metastatic renal cell carcinoma: insights from two independent cohorts of patients who underwent cytoreductive nephrectomy. Eur Urol Oncol. 2020;3(1):47–56.
21. Mano R, Gopal N, Hakimi AA. The evolving role of cytoreductive nephrectomy: incorporating genomics of metastatic renal cell carcinoma into treatment decisions. Curr Opin Urol. 2019;29(5):531–9.
22. Tennenbaum DM, Manley BJ, Zabor E, Becerra MF, Carlo MI, Casuscelli J, et al. Genomic alterations as predictors of survival among patients within a combined cohort with clear cell renal cell carcinoma undergoing cytoreductive nephrectomy. Urol Oncol. 2017;35(8):532 e7–e13.

23. Silagy AW, Flynn J, Mano R, Blum KA, Marcon J, DiNatale RG, et al. Clinicopathologic features associated with survival after cytoreductive nephrectomy for nonclear cell renal cell carcinoma. Urol Oncol. 2019;37(11):811 e9–e16.
24. Silagy AW, Mano R, Blum KA, DiNatale RG, Marcon J, Tickoo SK, et al. The role of cytoreductive nephrectomy for sarcomatoid renal cell carcinoma: a 29-year institutional experience. Urology. 2020;136:169–75.
25. Silagy AW, Attalla K, Dinatale RG, Weiss KL, Weng S, Mano R, et al. A qualitative framework of non-selection factors for cytoreductive nephrectomy. World J Urol. 2021;39:3359.
26. Gershman B, Moreira DM, Boorjian SA, Lohse CM, Cheville JC, Costello BA, et al. Comprehensive characterization of the perioperative morbidity of cytoreductive nephrectomy. Eur Urol. 2016;69(1):84–91.
27. Bhindi B, Habermann EB, Mason RJ, Costello BA, Pagliaro LC, Thompson RH, et al. Comparative survival following initial cytoreductive nephrectomy versus initial targeted therapy for metastatic renal cell carcinoma. J Urol. 2018;200(3):528–34.
28. Bex A, Mulders P, Jewett M, Wagstaff J, van Thienen JV, Blank CU, et al. Comparison of immediate vs deferred cytoreductive nephrectomy in patients with synchronous metastatic renal cell carcinoma receiving sunitinib: the SURTIME randomized clinical trial. JAMA Oncol. 2019;5(2):164–70.
29. Ljungberg BLA, Bedke J, Bex A, Capitanio U, Giles RH, Hora M, Klatte T, Lam T, Marconi L, Powles T, Volpe A, Abu-Ghanem Y, Dabestani S, Fernández-Pello MS, Hofmann F, Kuusk T, Tahbaz R. EAU Guidelines on Renal Cell Carcinoma 2021 [June 10,2021]. Available from: https://uroweb.org/guideline/renal-cell-carcinoma/.
30. Network NCC. Kidney Cancer (Version 4.2021) 2021 [June 10, 2021]. Available from: https://www.nccn.org/professionals/physician_gls/pdf/kidney.pdf.
31. Singla N, Elias R, Ghandour RA, Freifeld Y, Bowman IA, Rapoport L, et al. Pathologic response and surgical outcomes in patients undergoing nephrectomy following receipt of immune checkpoint inhibitors for renal cell carcinoma. Urol Oncol. 2019;37(12):924–31.
32. Reimers MA, Figenshau RS, Kim EH, Tucker J, Kasten N, Khan AS, et al. Elective cytoreductive nephrectomy after checkpoint inhibitor immunotherapy in patients with initially unresectable metastatic clear cell renal cell carcinoma. Clin Genitourin Cancer. 2020;18(5):361–6.
33. Singla N, Hutchinson RC, Ghandour RA, Freifeld Y, Fang D, Sagalowsky AI, et al. Improved survival after cytoreductive nephrectomy for metastatic renal cell carcinoma in the contemporary immunotherapy era: an analysis of the National Cancer Database. Urol Oncol. 2020;38(6):604 e9–e17.
34. Zhang T, Hwang JK, George DJ, Pal SK. The landscape of contemporary clinical trials for untreated metastatic clear cell renal cell carcinoma. Cancer Treat Res Commun. 2020;24:100183.
35. Sun M, Meyer CP, Karam JA, de Velasco G, Chang SL, Pal SK, et al. Predictors, utilization patterns, and overall survival of patients undergoing metastasectomy for metastatic renal cell carcinoma in the era of targeted therapy. Eur J Surg Oncol. 2018;44(9):1439–45.
36. Meyer CP, Groeben C, Marks P, Koch R, Huber J. Trends of metastasis-directed treatments in patients with renal cell carcinoma: a total population-based analysis in Germany in the era of targeted therapies. Oncol Res Treat. 2020;43(12):679–85.
37. Zaid HB, Parker WP, Safdar NS, Gershman B, Erwin PJ, Murad MH, et al. Outcomes following complete surgical metastasectomy for patients with metastatic renal cell carcinoma: a systematic review and meta-analysis. J Urol. 2017;197(1):44–9.
38. Hsieh PY, Hung SC, Li JR, Wang SS, Yang CK, Chen CS, et al. The effect of metastasectomy on overall survival in metastatic renal cell carcinoma: a systematic review and meta-analysis. Urol Oncol. 2021;39:422.
39. You D, Lee C, Jeong IG, Song C, Lee JL, Hong B, et al. Impact of metastasectomy on prognosis in patients treated with targeted therapy for metastatic renal cell carcinoma. J Cancer Res Clin Oncol. 2016;142(11):2331–8.

40. Li JR, Ou YC, Yang CK, Wang SS, Chen CS, Ho HC, et al. The impact of local intervention combined with targeted therapy on metastatic renal cell carcinoma. Anticancer Res. 2018;38(9):5339–45.
41. Tornberg SV, Visapaa H, Kilpelainen TP, Taari K, Jarvinen R, Erkkila K, et al. Surgery for metastases of renal cell carcinoma: outcome of treatments and preliminary assessment of Leuven-Udine prognostic groups in the targeted therapy era. Scand J Urol. 2018;52(5–6):419–26.
42. Fares AF, Araujo DV, Calsavara V, Saito AO, Formiga MN, Dettino AA, et al. Complete metastasectomy in renal cell carcinoma: a propensity-score matched by the International Metastatic RCC Database Consortium prognostic model. Ecancermedicalscience. 2019;13:967.
43. Lyon TD, Thompson RH, Shah PH, Lohse CM, Boorjian SA, Costello BA, et al. Complete surgical metastasectomy of renal cell carcinoma in the post-cytokine era. J Urol. 2020;203(2):275–82.
44. Dragomir A, Nazha S, Wood LA, Rendon RA, Finelli A, Hansen A, et al. Outcomes of complete metastasectomy in metastatic renal cell carcinoma patients: the Canadian Kidney Cancer information system experience. Urol Oncol. 2020;38(10):799 e1–e10.
45. Ishihara H, Takagi T, Kondo T, Fukuda H, Tachibana H, Yoshida K, et al. Prognostic impact of metastasectomy in renal cell carcinoma in the postcytokine therapy era. Urol Oncol. 2021;39(1):77 e17–25.
46. Russo P. Kidney cancer and surgical metastasectomy: effective therapy or part of disease natural history? Eur Urol Oncol. 2019;2(2):150–1.
47. Meyer CP, Sun M, Karam JA, Leow JJ, de Velasco G, Pal SK, et al. Complications after metastasectomy for renal cell carcinoma-a population-based assessment. Eur Urol. 2017;72(2):171–4.
48. Tosco L, Van Poppel H, Frea B, Gregoraci G, Joniau S. Survival and impact of clinical prognostic factors in surgically treated metastatic renal cell carcinoma. Eur Urol. 2013;63(4):646–52.
49. Naito S, Kinoshita H, Kondo T, Shinohara N, Kasahara T, Saito K, et al. Prognostic factors of patients with metastatic renal cell carcinoma with removed metastases: a multicenter study of 556 patients. Urology. 2013;82(4):846–51.
50. Takagi T, Fukuda H, Ishihara H, Yoshida K, Kondo T, Kobayashi H, et al. Predictive factors for recurrence after complete metastasectomy in patients with metastatic renal cell carcinoma in the targeted therapy era. Urol Oncol. 2020;38(5):515–20.
51. Wu K, Liu Z, Shao Y, Li X. Nomogram predicting survival to assist decision-making of metastasectomy in patients with metastatic renal cell carcinoma. Front Oncol. 2020;10:592243.
52. Verbiest A, Couchy G, Job S, Caruana L, Lerut E, Oyen R, et al. Molecular subtypes of clear-cell renal cell carcinoma are prognostic for outcome after complete metastasectomy. Eur Urol. 2018;74(4):474–80.
53. Thomas AZ, Adibi M, Slack RS, Borregales LD, Merrill MM, Tamboli P, et al. The role of metastasectomy in patients with renal cell carcinoma with sarcomatoid dedifferentiation: a matched controlled analysis. J Urol. 2016;196(3):678–84.
54. Appleman LJ, Maranchie JK. Systemic therapy following metastasectomy for renal cell carcinoma: using insights from other clinical settings to address unanswered questions. Urol Oncol. 2018;36(1):17–22.
55. Kwak C, Park YH, Jeong CW, Lee SE, Ku JH. No role of adjuvant systemic therapy after complete metastasectomy in metastatic renal cell carcinoma? Urol Oncol. 2007;25(4):310–6.
56. Procopio G, Apollonio G, Cognetti F, Miceli R, Milella M, Mosca A, et al. Sorafenib versus observation following radical metastasectomy for clear-cell renal cell carcinoma: results from the phase 2 randomized open-label RESORT study. Eur Urol Oncol. 2019;2(6):699–707.
57. Appleman LJ, Puligandla M, Pal SK, Harris W, Agarwal N, Costello BA, et al. Randomized, double-blind phase III study of pazopanib versus placebo in patients with metastatic renal cell carcinoma who have no evidence of disease following metastasectomy: a trial of the ECOG-ACRIN cancer research group (E2810). Am Soc Clin Oncol. 2019;49:1287.

Chapter 13
Targeted Therapy for Renal Cell Carcinoma

Juan Javier-DesLoges, Ithaar Derweesh, and Rana R. McKay

Introduction

The 2019 Nobel Prize winning discovery that the von Hippel–Lindau (VHL) tumor suppressor protein regulates hypoxia-inducible factor (HIF) and sensitizes VHL-mutated tumors to vascular endothelial growth factor (VEGF) inhibition revolutionized the management of advanced renal cell carcinoma (RCC) [1] [2]. Since the approval of sunitinib, a VEGF tyrosine kinase inhibitor (TKI), in 2006, VEGF targeting agents have been the mainstay of therapy for advanced RCC [3]. For over a decade, single-agent VEGF TKIs remained the unchallenged first-line treatment for patients with newly diagnosed RCC. The 2018 Nobel Prize winning discovery of the beneficial impact of immune checkpoint blockade ignited a revolution in oncology treatment [4]. In 2015, nivolumab, a programmed death receptor 1 (PD-1) inhibitor, demonstrated improved overall survival in patients previously treated with VEGF blockade and ushered checkpoint inhibitors into the treatment armamentarium for advanced RCC [5]. Now, several regimens of immune checkpoint inhibitors combined with VEGF blockade have demonstrated efficacy for patients with advanced RCC. In this chapter, we aim to summarize the existing literature and concepts on targeted therapy and the role of targeted therapy in the contemporary era.

J. Javier-DesLoges · I. Derweesh
Department of Urology, University of California San Diego, La Jolla, CA, USA

R. R. McKay (✉)
Department of Medicine/Division of Hematology-Oncology,
University of California San Diego, La Jolla, CA, USA

Department of Medical Oncology, Moores UCSD Cancer Center, La Jolla, CA, USA
e-mail: RMcKay@health.ucsd.edu

K. L. Stratton, A. K. Morgans (eds.), *Urologic Oncology*,
https://doi.org/10.1007/978-3-030-89891-5_13

Pathophysiology

An improved understanding of the pathophysiology of RCC has led to the expansion of treatment options for patients with advanced disease, including a broad spectrum of targeted therapies [1]. The Von Hippel–Lindau (*VHL*) gene is a tumor suppressor gene that plays a critical role in the development of clear cell RCC. It is altered in upwards to 90% of clear cell RCC and is a dominant driver of disease pathogenesis [6]. The *VHL* gene, located on chromosome 3p, produces a ubiquitin-mediated degradation protein complex. Under normoxic conditions, the VHL protein complex degrades the HIF protein complex; however, in hypoxic or altered states, the degradation complex is inactive; therefore, HIF will translocate to the cell nucleus where it acts as a transcription factor leading to downstream angiogenesis, proliferation, and cell growth. One of the primary ways that HIF induces angiogenesis is through activation of the VEGF tyrosine kinase receptor. The backbone of systemic therapy for RCC has been drugs that target VEGF [2, 3].

VEGF receptors represent a family of three main receptors: VEGF receptor 1, 2, and 3, the most important of which is VEGF receptor 2 [7]. Each receptor has a similar structure consisting of an extracellular immunoglobulin-like domain, a transmembrane domain, and the intracellular tyrosine kinase domain. The receptors bind VEGF ligands, which leads to VEGF receptor dimerization followed by phosphorylation of the tyrosine protein residues with ATP. This interaction ultimately leads to the activation of the tyrosine kinase domain with initiation of intracellular signaling. While not completely defined, two of the major intracellular signaling pathways are the PI3K-AKT-mTOR and phospholipase Cγ (PLCγ) pathways [8].

Once VEGF receptor is activated, it directly phosphorylates PLCγ, which has a phosphatidylinositol bisphosphate (PIP2) substrate. PIP2 is then transformed into inositol triphosphate (IP3) and diacylglycerol (DAG) subsequently leading to activation of signaling cascades that regulate cell proliferation and survival processes [9]. Additionally, VEGF receptors cross activate the Src kinase family. Src phosphorylates the phosphatidylinositol triphosphate (PIP3). PIP3 then activates the AKT complex, which then activates mTOR. mTOR is a critical serine/threonine protein kinase in RCC pathogenesis that is involved with transcription, cell proliferation, and cell growth [10].

The VEGF TKIs including sunitinib, pazopanib, and axitinib competitively inhibit ATP binding to the intracellular domain of VEGF receptor and consequently inhibit signal transduction. mTOR is primarily inhibited by a class of drugs known as mTOR inhibitors, such as everolimus and temsirolimus, which are now less commonly used as single agents in the treatment of advanced RCC [11].

As described above, VEGF is primarily known for its involvement in cell growth and angiogenesis. However, recent studies on VEGF demonstrate that it also has an important role in immune system modulation [12]. It has been demonstrated that VEGF can block antigen-presenting cell maturation and function resulting in immune suppression [13]. Additionally, VEGFs can inhibit effector T cells, which in turn decrease its proliferation and cytotoxic effects. They can further cause T cell exhaustion by increasing PD-L1 expression [14]. Additionally, VEGFs lead to an increase in suppressive immune cells such as regulatory T cells and myeloid-derived suppressor cells [15]. Lastly, VEGFs can increase the infiltration of tumor-associated macrophages at tumor sites [16]. The sum of these interactions ultimately leads to an immunosuppressive tumor microenvironment that can impede an antitumor response. These findings provide the rationale for a potential synergistic effect of combination VEGF blockade with checkpoint inhibition [17].

Metastatic Renal Cell Carcinoma

Frontline Therapy: Combination Therapy

In 2018, there was a significant change in the frontline treatment paradigm for patients with advanced and metastatic RCC with the reporting of data from the CheckMate 214 phase III trial [18]. CheckMate 214 was a multicenter, international, open-label, randomized phase III trial testing the combination of nivolumab, a PD-1 inhibitor, plus ipilimumab, a checkpoint T-lymphocyte-associated protein-4 inhibitor, compared to sunitinib, the long-standing gold standard frontline treatment in patients with RCC. The primary endpoint of the trial was overall survival (OS) and progression-free survival (PFS) by independent review in International Metastatic RCC Database (IMDC) intermediate- and poor-risk patients. The combination demonstrated improved objective response rate (ORR), PFS, and OS in the intermediate- and poor-risk patients and also in the intention to treat (ITT) population [3] [18]. This led to the FDA approval of nivolumab/ipilimumab as first-line therapy for metastatic RCC.

Additionally, immune checkpoint blockade combined with a VEGF inhibition has been investigated in a series of phase III studies and demonstrated benefit in patients with advanced RCC. These include the IMmotion 151 trial of atezolizumab/bevacizumab, Javelin Renal 101 of avelumab/axitinib, Keynote 426 of pembrolizumab/axitinib, CheckMate 9ER of nivolumab/cabozantinib, and more recently CLEAR Trial of pembrolizumab/lenvatinib. Of these studies, the combination of pembrolizumab/axitinib, nivolumab/cabozantinib, and pembrolizumab/lenvatinib have demonstrated improvements in OS.

The Keynote 426 trial was a phase III randomized control trial of 861 patients with treatment-naïve advanced RCC. The trial compared the combination of immunotherapy (IO) pembrolizumab and TKI axitinib to sunitinib in patients with advanced clear cell RCC. Axitinib is a TKI whose mechanism of action is the inhibition of VEGF receptors 1–3, c-KIT, and platelet-derived growth factor (PDGF) receptor [19]. At the first study analysis conducted at a median follow-up of 12.8 months, the combination of pembrolizumab/axitinib demonstrated superior OS compared to sunitinib, 89.9% compared to 78.3% in the sunitinib group at 12 months (hazard ratio (HR) 0.53; 95% confidence interval (CI), 0.38–0.74; $P < 0.01$). The combination of pembrolizumab and axitinib also had superior PFS (HR, 0.69; 95% CI, 0.57–0.84; $p < 0.01$) and ORR ($p < 0.01$). Lastly, pembrolizumab/axitinib benefited all three risk groups irrespective of PD-L1 expression [19]. In an updated analysis at 23-month minimum follow-up, the benefit of pembrolizumab/axitinib across all three efficacy parameters persisted. The HR for OS in the favorable risk group was 1.06 (95% CI, 0.60–1.86). For intermediate and poor, the HR for OS was 0.63 (95% CI, 0.50–0.81) and for PFS, it was 0.69 (95% CI, 0.56–0.84). The degree of benefit was most pronounced for intermediate- and poor-risk patients and less profound for patients with favorable risk disease [20].

Javelin Renal 101 was another study testing IO/TKI therapy in frontline advanced RCC. This was a phase III trial of 886 patients comparing an IO, avelumab, and TKI, axitinib, to sunitinib in patients with treatment-naïve advanced clear cell RCC in all risk groups. The co-primary endpoints of the study were PFS and OS in PD-L1-positive patients. After a minimum follow-up of 13 months, the combination demonstrated superior PFS, median 13.8 months vs. 7.0 months for avelumab/axitinib compared to sunitinib patients with PD-L1-positive tumors (HR 0.62; 95% CI, 0.49–0.77 $P < 0.01$), median 13.8 months vs. 7.0 months, and also in the overall population (HR, 0.69; 95% CI, 0.57–0.82; $P < 0.01$), median 13.3 months vs. 8.0 months. Furthermore, the ORR was superior compared to sunitinib (52.5% versus 27.3%, respectively) [21]. OS data are still immature at the time of last analysis. Based on the results of this study, the combination was approved by the FDA for treatment in patients with advanced RCC.

Recently, the results from the CheckMate 9ER trial were presented at 2020 European Society for Medical Oncology Virtual Congress. In this trial, 651 patients with treatment-naïve advanced clear cell RCC were randomized to either the combination of cabozantinib (40 mg daily)/nivolumab or sunitinib. Cabozantinib has dual activity as both cMET and VEGF tyrosine kinase receptor inhibitor. At a median follow-up of 18.1 months, the combination of cabozantinib/nivolumab showed significantly improved PFS compared to sunitinib, 16.6 months versus 8.3 months (HR 0.51, 95% CI 0.41–0.64, $p < 0.01$). There was also a 40% decreased risk of death (medians not reached HR 0.60 95% CI 0.40–0.89, $p < 0.01$). Additionally, ORR was higher in patients who received nivolumab/cabozantinib, 55.7%, in contrast to individuals receiving sunitinib, 27.1%, ($p < 0.01$). Finally the, complete response rates were doubled among those receiving nivolumab/cabozantinib (8.0% vs. 4.6%) [22].

In another phase III trial, IMmotion 151 evaluated atezolizumab/bevacizumab against sunitinib in patients with metastatic RCC. Bevacizumab is a monoclonal antibody to VEGF which has shown improved PFS compared to interferon-alfa [23]; atezolizumab is a PD-L1 monoclonal antibody. The trial enrolled 915 patients, who were randomly assigned to atezolizumab/bevacizumab versus sunitinib. Median follow-up was 15 months for PFS analysis and 24 months at the OS interim analysis. Investigator-assessed PFS was prolonged in patients with PD-L1-positive tumors (11.2 months versus 7.7 months, HR 0.74 [95% CI 0·57–0·96]; $p = 0.02$). However, in the ITT population, PFS was not significant (HR 0.93 95% CI 0.76–1.14). Additionally, there was no difference in PFS as assessed by independent radiology review in the PD-L1-positive (HR 0.88 95% CI 0.74–1.04) and ITT population (HR 0.93 95% CI 0.72–1.21). Furthermore, there was no difference in OS with the combination in PD-L1-positive patients or the ITT. Given these results, this regimen is not currently approved for use in the frontline setting in RCC.

More recently, data presented in a press release of the CLEAR trial demonstrated that the combination of lenvatinib and pembrolizumab demonstrated statistically significant improvements in PFS, OS, and ORR versus sunitinib as first-line treatment for patients with advanced RCC. Lenvatinib is a tyrosine kinase inhibitor that blocks VEGF 1–3 receptors and also inhibitors fibroblast growth factor receptors 1–4, PDGFR-alpha, KIT, and RET. We eagerly await complete data regarding the trial's efficacy and safety outcomes at an upcoming future meeting [24].

Taken together, the role for TKI/IO combination therapy continues to grow; however, data to guide choice of regimen in the frontline are lacking, and the optimal sequencing of therapies in the modern era has yet to be defined. While direct comparison across the frontline studies is limited given differing patient populations and study design of the contemporary combinatorial studies, currently clinical parameters are the key determinants that help guide therapy selection in the frontline given lack of biomarkers to optimize therapy selection. There were differences across these trials in CR rates, PD rates, durability of response, PFS, and quality of life which are used to guide therapy selection in the clinical real world (Table 13.1).

Frontline Therapy: Single-Agent Therapy

One of the most widely used targeted therapy drugs in metastatic RCC is sunitinib, a tyrosine kinase inhibitor (TKI) that inhibits the VEGF receptor. The landmark trial that led to sunitinib being approved as frontline therapy for metastatic RCC was SU11248. This trial enrolled 750 patients with metastatic RCC, and patients were randomized to receive sunitinib versus interferon alfa. Sunitinib showed superior ORR 47% versus 12%, $p < 0.0001$ and prolonged PFS, median 11 months versus 5 months HR 0.42 95% CI 0.32–0.54, $p < 0.001$. There was also improved OS, 26.4 months vs. 21.8 months (HR 0.821 95% CI 0.67–1.00 $p = 0.051$) [25].

The second major landmark trial was the COMPARZ trial. In this trial, 1110 patients with clear cell metastatic RCC were randomized to receive pazopanib or sunitinib. This trial demonstrated that PFS with pazopanib was non-inferior compared to sunitinib (HR 1.05 95% CI, 0.90–1.22). Overall, single-agent TKI is being used less frequently in the frontline treatment of advanced RCC given the introduction of IO combinatorial therapy [26].

Despite the evolving data, frontline TKI alone may have a role in the frontline space for a subset of patients with advanced RCC [13]. Despite limitations of subgroup analyses, in patients with IMDC favorable risk disease, CheckMate 214, Keynote 426, and Checkmate 9ER demonstrated no statistical improvement in OS in patients with favorable risk groups [18] [20] [22]. Interestingly, with longer follow-up from CheckMate 214, we see the HR for OS improve in the favorable risk

Table 13.1 Landmark frontline metastatic renal cell carcinoma clinical trials

Trial	CheckMate 214	JAVELIN Renal 101	KEYNOTE 426	IMmotion 151	CheckMate 9ER
Status	Complete	Complete	Complete	Complete	Complete
Study population	*N* = 1096	*N* = 886	*N* = 861	*N* = 915	*N* = 651
Agents	Nivolumab + Ipilimumab vs. Sunitinib	Avelumab + Axitinib vs. Sunitinib	Pembrolizumab/Axitinib vs. Sunitinib	Atezolizumab/ bevacizumab vs. Sunitinib	Cabozantinib and Nivolumab vs. Sunitinib
IMDC risk group	Favorable:23% Intermediate: 61% Poor: 17%	Favorable: 21% Intermediate: 62% Poor: 16%	Favorable: 31% Intermediate: 56% Poor: 13%	Favorable: 20% Intermediate: 69% Poor: 54%	Favorable: 22.9% Intermediate: 58.5% Poor: 25.1%
PD-L1 expression $\geq$ 1%	24%	63%	60%	39.5%	25.1%
Prior nephrectomy %	80%	80%	82.6%	74%	68.7%
Primary endpoint	ORR, PFS, OS in Int/ Poor (IRC)	OS, PFS in PD-L1+ (IRC)	OS, PFS (IRC)	PFS in PD-L1 positive population OS in ITT	PFS
Median follow-up	48 months	12 months	23 months	15 months	18.1 months
ORR	39%	51.4%	60.2%	43%	43%
CR	11%	3.4%	8.8%	9%	8%

PFS (months)	Combination: 12.2 Sunitinib: 12.3 HR 0.89 (95% CI 0.76–1.05) Favorable: Combination: 12.4 months Sunitinib: 28.9 months HR 1.84 (1.29–2.62) Intermediate/poor: Combination: 11.2 months Sunitinib: 8.3 months HR 0.74 (95% CI 0.62–0.88)	Combination: 13.8 Sunitinib: 8.4 Overall: HR 0.69 (95% CI 0.56–0.84) Favorable HR 0.62 (95% CI 0.39–0.98) Intermediate: HR 0.75 (95% CI 0.60–0.94) Poor: 0.51 (95% CI 0.34–0.77)	Combination: 15.4 Sunitinib: 11.1 HR 0.71 (95% CI 0.60–0.84) Favorable HR 0.79 (95% CI 0.57–1.09) Intermediate/poor: HR 0.69 (95% CI 0.56–0.84)	Combination: 11.2 Sunitinib: 8.4 HR 0.83 95% CI 0.70–0.97 Favorable HR 0.62 (95% CI 0.38–0.1.01) Intermediate: HR 0.54 (95% CI 0.40–0.72) Poor: 0.37 (95% CI 0.23–0.58)	Combination: 16.6 Sunitinib: 8.3 HR 0.51 (95%CI 0.41–0.64)
OS	Overall: HR 0.69 (95% CI 0.59–0.81) Favorable: HR 0.93 (95% CI 0.62–1.40) Intermediate/poor: Combination: 48.1 months Sunitinib: 26.6 months HR 0.69 (95% CI 0.59–0.81)	Overall: HR 0.78 (95% CI 0.55–1.08) Favorable: 0.81 (95% CI 0.33–1.96) Intermediate: 0.86 (95% CI 0.61–1.20) Poor: 0.57 (95% CI 0.36–0.89)	HR 0.68 (95% CI 0.55–0.85) Favorable: HR 1.06 (95% CI 0.60–1.86) Intermediate/poor: HR 0.63 (95% CI 0.50–0.81)	HR 0.93 (95% CI 0.76–1.14) Favorable HR 0.84 (95% CI 0.35–1.97) Intermediate: HR 0.70 (95% CI 0.46–1.07) Poor: 0.37 (95% CI 0.21–0.66)	HR 0.59 (0.45–0.78)

patients from 1.45 (95% CI 0.51–4.12) at a minimum follow-up of 17.5 months, 1.22 (0.73–2.04) at a minimum follow-up of 30 months, 1.19 (95% CI 0.77–1.85) at a minimum follow-up of 42 months, and more recently 0.93 (95% CI 0.62–1.40) at a minimum follow-up of 48 months; for Keynote 426 for the favorable risk group, HR 1.06 (95% CI 0.60–1.86) at a median follow-up of 30.6 months; and lastly for Checkmate 9ER for the favorable risk group, HR 0.84 (95% CI 0.35–1.97) [22].

It is hypothesized that differences in underlying disease biology are likely driving this differential response to IO therapy in favorable risk patients. Biological subgroup analyses from the phase II IMmotion 150 study of atezolizumab/bevacizumab demonstrated that the angiogenesis gene expression, which is associated with response to VEGF inhibition, is higher in patients with favorable risk disease compared to intermediate- and poor-risk patients [27]. Furthermore, a recent review demonstrated that angiogenesis, T-effector/IFN-γ response, and myeloid inflammatory gene expression signatures were highly correlated with PFS in patients who receive a TKI [28]. Thus, for a subset of patients with favorable risk disease, single-agent TKI is a potential treatment option that can be utilized.

The CABOSUN trial was a phase II trial that compared cabozantinib versus sunitinib for patients with IMDC intermediate- or poor-risk treatment-naïve RCC [29]. The trial, which included a total of 157 patients, demonstrated that median PFS was higher for cabozantinib 8.6 months (95% CI 6.8–14.0) versus 5.3 months (95% CI 3.0–8.2) (HR 0.48 [95% CI 0.31–0.74]; $p < 0.01$). The ORR was 20% (95% CI 12.0–30.8) versus 9% (95% CI 3.7–17.6), respectively [29]. There was a similar rate of grade 3/4 adverse events, 67% and 68%, respectively. Furthermore, the benefit of cabozantinib was independent of underlying MET status, as determined by immunohistochemistry. The findings of this trial led to the expanded use of cabozantinib to the frontline setting [30]. Cabozantinib remains an option for certain subsets of patients and particularly those who have contraindications to IO, which include patients with active autoimmune disease or rheumatologic conditions [31].

Second-Line Agents: Post-IO Therapy

As the treatment options in the frontline space are rapidly evolving and largely include IO combination therapy, options for post-IO treatment are still evolving. A series of clinical trials and retrospective studies have provided insights in the management strategies post-IO therapy. These studies support the role of some TKI agents in this setting.

The activity of axitinib post IO was evaluated in a phase II trial of 40 patients with clear cell RCC. All patients received axitinib on an individualized dosing algorithm. At a median follow-up of 8.7 months, the median PFS was 8.8 months (95% CI 5.7–16.6). The most common grade 3 side effects were hypertension ($n = 24$, 60%), and there was one grade 4 event (elevated lipase). This study provides rationale for use of axitinib, which is a currently approved agent for RCC, in the post-IO setting [32].

The Tivo-3 trial was a randomized trial for patients who had previously been treated with at least two prior lines of therapies, one of which was a VEGF inhibitor. The study accrued 350 patients who were then randomized to receive tivozanib or sorafenib. The median follow-up was 19.0 months. The study found that median PFS was significantly longer in the tivozanib group 5.6 months vs. 3.9 months (HR 0.73, 95% CI 0.56–0.94; $p = 0.016$. In this trial, 27% of patients in the tivozanib group and 25% of patients in the sorafenib group had received a prior checkpoint inhibitor. The median PFS was 7.3 months vs. 5.1 months (HR = 0.55, 95% CI = 0.32–0.94). Median OS was 16.4 months vs. 19.7 months (HR = 0.99, $p = 0.95$). The study also found that the rates of grade 3 and 4 adverse events were 20% for tivozanib group and 14% for the sorafenib group. Tivozanib is not currently FDA approved for use in patients [33].

The combination of lenvatinib and pembrolizumab has also demonstrated efficacy in the post-IO setting. Based on the results of a phase II trial which enrolled 104 patients, the median PFS was 11.7 months with 12-month PFS and OS at 45% and 77%, respectively. The ORR was 52% by Response Evaluation Criteria in Solid Tumors (RECIST) version 1.1 criteria and 55% by immune RECIST criteria.

The METEOR trial was a phase III trial of 658 patients who were randomized to receive cabozantinib or everolimus after having progressed on a prior TKI. In a subgroup of the METEOR trial, the authors identified 32 patients who received prior IO therapy followed by cabozantinib and determined that the ORR was 22% and PFS was 4.1 months among those patients.

Lastly, complementing these studies are a series of retrospective studies evaluating VEGF-targeted therapy in patients who have progressed on IO therapy. In aggregate, these studies demonstrated activity of VEGF TKIs post IO with ORR ranging from 13% to 41% and the mean PFS was 8.11 months (range 6.4–13.2 months) [34–38] (Table 13.2).

Second-Line Agents: Post-TKI Therapy.

The role of targeted therapy in the second-line setting post TKI has been extensively studied. As mentioned previously, the METEOR trial was a phase III trial where patients were randomized to receive cabozantinib or everolimus after having progressed on a prior TKI. Treatment with cabozantinib resulted in improved OS, PFS, and ORR compared to sunitinib. The median OS was 21.4 months with cabozantinib and 16.5 months with everolimus (HR 0.66 95%CI 0.53–0.83; $p < 0.01$). Cabozantinib had improved PFS (HR 0.51 95% CI 0.41–0.62, $p < 0.01$), and ORR was 17% with cabozantinib versus 3% with everolimus ($p < 0.01$). There was little difference between grade 3 and 4 events, 39% with cabozantinib and 40% with everolimus [39].

In another phase II trial, of 153 patients who had previously progressed on one prior VEGF targeted therapy, patients were randomized to receive lenvatinib/everolimus, lenvatinib alone, or everolimus alone. The lenvatinib/everolimus

Table 13.2 Landmark second-line metastatic renal cell carcinoma clinical trials

Study	Study	Agents	N	ORR	PFS (months)
Retrospective	Albiges (EJC, 2015)[34]	Axitinib/everolimus	56	13%	6.6
Retrospective	Nadal (Annal Oncol, 2016) [35]	VEGF TKI	70	28%	6.4
Retrospective	Derosa (ESMO, 2017)[60]	Cabozantinib/axitinib	56	33%	8.0
Retrospective	McGregor (EJC, 2020) [36]	Cabozantinib	86	36%	6.5
Retrospective	Auvray (EJC, 2020)[37]	Nivolumab/ipilimumab	33	36%	8.0
Retrospective	Shah (EJC, 2019) [38]	TKI	70	41%	13.2
Prospective	Powles (BJC, 2018) [61]	Cabozantinib/ everolimus	32	22%	4.1
Prospective	Ornstein (Lancet Oncol, 2019)[32]	Axitinib	38	45%	8.8
Prospective	Tivo-3 [33]	Tivozanib	350	18%	5.6
Prospective	LenPem [42]	Lenvatinib/ pembrolizumab	104	52%	11.7

combination prolonged PFS compared to everolimus (median 14.6 months versus 5.5 months; HR 0.40 95% CI 0.24–0.68, $p = 0.0005$), but not compared to lenvatinib alone (7.4 months versus 10.2 months; 95% CI 0.39–1.10, $p = 0.12$). Grade 3 or 4 events occurred in 25 patients (50%) receiving single-agent everolimus, 41 (79%) receiving single-agent lenvatinib, and 36 (71%) of patients receiving both. This ultimately led to the FDA approval of the combination of lenvatinib/everolimus in the second-line setting [40].

Future Trials

There are several ongoing studies that will further influence treatment paradigms for patients with advanced RCC. In the frontline space, several ongoing trials will provide further instruction regarding optimal therapy for patients with treatment-naïve advanced or clear cell RCC. The COSMIC-313 trial is a randomized double-blinded phase III trial that will compare nivolumab/ipilimumab/cabozantinib to nivolumab/ipilimumab/placebo in intermediate−/poor-risk patients by IMDC criteria. The primary endpoint is PFS and the secondary endpoint is OS [41]. This trial is investigating triple therapy with nivolumab/ipilimumab/cabozantinib and uses a modern control arm of nivolumab/ipilimumab. The trial recently met its primary endpoint and demonstrated a statistically significant improvement in PFS, OS, and ORR versus sunitinib in the ITT group. Further results are pending [42]. The A031704 PDIGREE is a phase III randomized trial, which will evaluate sequencing for treatment. In this study, all patients will receive treatment with nivolumab/ipilimumab, and individuals with stable disease or a partial response will be

Table 13.3 Future trials for metastatic renal cell carcinoma

Trial	COSMIC 313	CLEAR	AO31704 PDIGREE	MK-6482	Contact 03
Status	Recruiting	Active, not recruiting	Recruiting	Recruiting	Recruiting
Study population	*N* = 676	*N* = 959	*N* = 1046	*N* = 150	*N* = 500
Agents	Nivolumab + ipilimumab + cabozantinib vs. nivolumab + ipilimumab	Lenvatinib + everolimus vs. lenvatinib vs. pembro vs. sunitinib	Nivolumab + ipilimumab followed by nivolumab, nivolumab + cabozantinib, or cabozantinib	Belzutifan vs. everolimus	Atezolizumab + cabozantinib vs. cabozantinib
IMDC risk group	Intermediate or poor risk	All risk groups	Intermediate or poor risk	All risk groups	All risk groups
Primary endpoint	PFS	PFS	OS	ORR	PFS, OS

randomized to either continue nivolumab maintenance or the combination of nivolumab/cabozantinib [19].

For subsequent therapy, the MK-6482-005 trial is evaluating an oral HIF-2a inhibitor in a phase III trial in patients who previously received prior checkpoint inhibition [43]. This trial follows the success of the single-arm phase II study of MK-6482 which demonstrated an ORR was 24% and PFS was 11 months in patients with heavily pretreated advanced RCC [44]. Lastly, Contact-03 is a phase III trial that will test cabozantinib/atezolizumab compared to cabozantinib in patients with advanced RCC who progressed during or following IO therapy [45]. This trial will enroll patients with clear cell, papillary, and unclassified RCC (Tables 13.3, 13.4, and 13.5).

Localized Renal Cell Carcinoma

Adjuvant Therapy

The role of adjuvant systemic therapy has yet to be completely defined in the setting of localized disease. Adjuvant therapy is intended to treat patients who may harbor micrometastatic disease and are at increased risk of disease recurrence. Several large phase III trials have resulted, and overall no targeted agent has demonstrated improvement in OS in the adjuvant setting.

The first adjuvant trial to be reported was the landmark ASSURE trial (ECOG – ACRIN E2805), a multicenter double-blind randomized control trial comparing sunitinib versus sorafenib versus placebo for 54 weeks. The patient population

Table 13.4 Landmark adjuvant therapy trials of targeted therapy agents for non-metastatic renal cell carcinoma [62]

Trial	ASSURE	ASSURE High Risk Patients	S-TRAC	PROTECT	ATLAS	SORCE
Study population	1943	1069	615	1538	724	1171
Agents	Sunitinib vs. sorafenib vs. placebo	Sunitinib vs. placebo	Sunitinib vs. placebo	Pazopanib vs. placebo	Axitinib vs. placebo	Sorafenib for 1 year vs. sorafenib for 3 years vs. placebo
Inclusion criteria	pT1b grade 3/4 to pT4 N+ (resected)	pT3 or greater or N+(resected)	pT3 or greater or N+ (resected)	pT2 grade 3/4, pT3 any grade, N+ (resected)	pT2 or greater or N+	High-risk RCC
Primary endpoint	DFS 5.8 vs. 6.1 vs. 6.6 years Sunitinib: HR 1.02, 97.5% CI 0.85–1.23, $p = 0.80$ Sorafenib: HR 0.97, 97.5% CI 0.80–1.17, $p = 0.70$)	5-year DFS 47.7% vs. 49.9% vs. 50.0% Sunitinib: HR 0.94, 97.5% CI 0.74–1.19, $p = 0.5$ Sorafenib: HR 0.90, 97.5% CI 0.71–1.14, $p = 0.3$	DFS 6.8 vs. 5.6 years HR 0.76, 95% CI 0.59–1.02, $p = 0.03$	DFS 66% vs. 56% HR 0.94, 95% CI 0.77–1.14, $p = 0.50$	DFS HR 0.87, 95% CI 0.66–1.15, $p = 0.3$	5-year DFS 67% sorafenib vs. 65%placebo 10-year DFS 54% sorafenib vs. 53% placebo
Secondary endpoint	5-year OS 77.9% vs. 80.5% vs. 80.3% Sunitinib: HR 1.17, 97.5% CI 0.90–1.52, $p = 0.2$ Sorafenib: HR 0.98, 97.5% CI 0.75–1.28, $p = 0.9$)	5-year OS 75.2% vs. 80.2% vs. 76.5% Sunitinib: HR 1.06, 97.5% CI 0.78–1.45, $p = 0.7$ Sorafenib: HR 0.80, 97.5% CI 0.58–1.11, $p = 0.1$)	OS 20.7% vs. 20.9% HR 1.01, 95% CI 0.72–1.44, $p = 0.9$	OS HR 0.89, 95% CI 0.54–1.46, $p = 0.6$	High-risk patients DFS (HR 0.64, 95% CI 0.468–0.879, $p = 0.005$) Independent reviewer DFS (HR 0.735 95% CI 0.525–1.208, $p = 0.07$)	3-year sorafenib vs. placebo (HR 1.06 95% CI 0.82–1.38, $p = 0.63$) 1-year sorafenib vs. placebo (HR 0.92 95% CI 0.71–1.20 $p = 0.54$).
Adverse events grade 3 and grade 4	63% vs. 72% vs. 25%	66% vs. 72% vs. 28%	63.4% vs. 21.7%	60% vs. 21%	61.2% vs. 30.1%	Overall not reported yet

Table 13.5 Future neoadjuvant/adjuvant therapy trials of targeted therapy for non-metastatic renal cell carcinoma

Trial	Everest	Padres
Status	Active, not recruiting	Recruiting
Type	Adjuvant	Neoadjuvant
Study population	*N* = 1545	*N* = 50
Agents	Everolimus vs. placebo	Axitinib
Primary endpoint	RFS	Percent reduction, ORR, effect on RENAL score, feasibility of partial nephrectomy

consisted of 1943 patients with pT1b grade 3/grade 4, N0, M0 disease to those with resected node positive disease. Both non-clear cell and clear cell patients were eligible. The primary outcome was disease-free survival (DFS). The study demonstrated no difference in DFS between the groups: median DFS was 5.8 years for sunitinib (HR 1.02, 97.5% CI 0.85–1.23, $p = 0.80$), 6.1 years for sorafenib (HR 0.97, 97.5% CI 0.80–1.17, $p = 0.70$), and 6.6 years for placebo. Additionally, there was no significant improvement OS: 5-year OS was 77.9% (HR 1.17 97.5% CI 0.90–1.52) for sunitinib versus 80.5% (HR 0.98 97.5% CI 0.75–1.28, $p = 0.90$) for sorafenib, versus 80.3% for placebo. There was a high rate of grade 3 and 4 adverse events for both sunitinib (63%) and sorafenib (72%), for which a protocol amendment was implemented decreasing the starting dose of sunitinib and sorafenib. Even with the reduced dose, the proportion of grade 3 events exceeded 55% in both the sunitinib and sorafenib arms [46].

One of the major criticisms of ASSURE was the liberal inclusion criteria, enrollment of stage 1 patients with a lower risk of disease recurrence, and enrollment of patients with non-clear cell disease. A secondary post hoc analysis was conducted of 1069 patients with clear cell RCC who were pT3 or greater or had resected node positive disease. This subset analysis did not demonstrate a difference in 5-year DFS or 5-year OS in this higher-risk group of patients: 5-year DFS was 47.7% for sunitinib (HR 0.94, 97.5% CI 0.74–1.19, $p = 0.5$), 49.9% for sorafenib (HR 0.90, 97.5% CI 0.71–1.14, $p = 0.3$), and 50.0% for the placebo arm and 5-year OS 75.2% (HR 1.06, 97.5% CI 0.78–1.45, $p = 0.70$) versus 80.2% (sorafenib HR 0.80, 97.5% CI 0.58–1.11, $p = 0.10$) versus 76.5% for the placebo [47].

In the S-TRAC trial, 615 patients were randomized to either sunitinib or placebo for 1 year or until disease recurrence, toxicity, or withdrawal. Patients with pT3 disease or higher and any resected node-positive disease were eligible. The study demonstrated an improvement in DFS with sunitinib (median DFS of 6.8 years for sunitinib versus 5.6 years for placebo $p = 0.03$) [48]. In an updated analysis at a median follow-up of 6.6 years in the sunitinib arm and 6.7 years in the placebo arm, there was no difference in OS between the arms (HR 0.92, 95% CI 0.66–1.28; $p = 0.6$) [49]. There were also more grade 3 or 4 adverse events in the sunitinib arm (48.4% for grade 3 events and 12.1% for grade 4 events) compared to the placebo group (15.8% grade 3 and 3.6% grade 4 events). Based on this data, the FDA expanded approval of sunitinib for patients with high-risk clear cell RCC. However, given no OS benefit, utility in clinical practice has been limited.

Other VEGF TKIs including pazopanib, axitinib, and sorafenib have failed to demonstrate improvements in DFS and OS for patients with localized RCC. These agents currently do not have role in the adjuvant setting. The PROTECT trial was a multicenter double-blind trial comparing pazopanib to placebo for 1-year post nephrectomy. In this study of 1538 patients, the inclusion population included pT2 Fuhrman grade 3/4, pT3 any grade, or resected node-positive disease. The primary endpoint was 3-year DFS. Given toxicity observed with the 800 mg starting dose of pazopanib, the protocol was amended to decrease the starting dose of pazopanib to 600 mg daily. The study failed to meet its primary endpoint of 3-year DFS in the pazopanib 600 mg starting dose cohort: 3-year DFS 66% in the intention-to-treat arm and 56% in the placebo arm (HR 0.94, 95% CI 0.77–1.14, $p = 0.50$). Additionally, there was no difference in OS with either pazopanib starting dose, and this treatment is not indicated for adjuvant therapy use.

The ATLAS trial was a randomized control trial of 724 patients with pT2 or greater disease or resected node-positive clear cell RCC. Patients were randomized to receive either axitinib or placebo for up to 3 years with a minimum of 1 year unless there was recurrence. The trial was stopped early due to an interim analysis identifying no statistically significance difference in DFS between the two arms (HR 0.87, 95 CI% 0.66–1.15, $p = 0.30$). In the secondary analysis focusing on high-risk patients defined as pT3 grade 3/4, pT4, or any resected nodal disease, there was a difference in investigator-assessed DFS (HR 0.64, 95% CI 0.468–0.879, $p = 0.005$) but not independent reviewer DFS (HR 0.735 95% CI 0.525–1.208, $p = 0.07$). Furthermore, the adverse event rates for grade 3–4 were higher in the axitinib arm versus placebo (49% versus 12%).

In the SORCE adjuvant trial, 1711 patients with intermediate and high RCC (Leibovich score 3–11) were randomized to receive sorafenib for 1 year, sorafenib for 3 years, or placebo. The primary endpoints were DFS and OS. The study demonstrated no difference in 5-year (67% versus 65%) and 10-year DFS (54% versus 53%) between sorafenib- and placebo-treated patients (HR 1.01, 95% CI 0.82–1.23, $p = 0.946$). Furthermore, there was no difference in OS between the arms: 3-year sorafenib versus placebo, HR 1.06, 95% CI 0.82–1.38, $p = 0.63$, and 1-year sorafenib versus placebo HR 0.92, 95% CI 0.71–1.20, $p = 0.54$.

Lastly the E2810 randomized double-blind phase III trial tested the efficacy of pazopanib versus placebo for 52 weeks in patients with M1 disease status post metastasectomy without measurable disease on imaging. The study was unblinded after 83 DFS events occurred, and median follow-up was 30 months (range 0.4–66.5 months). The study did not reach its primary endpoint of improving DFS (HR 0.85, 95% CI 0.55–131, $p = 0.47$). Overall survival was measured at the time of unblinding, and the HR was 2.65 (95% CI 1.02–6.9, $p = 0.05$) in favor of the placebo. Pazopanib unfortunately did not improve DFS in patients who had metastasectomy, and these results are further consistent with the adjuvant studies demonstrating the limited role of VEGF TKI in the adjuvant setting [50].

Overall, the above studies demonstrate the limited utility to targeted therapy in the adjuvant setting given lack of OS benefit and substantial toxicity associated with treatment.

Neoadjuvant Therapy

Targeted therapy in the neoadjuvant setting remains under exploration. The potential benefits to neoadjuvant therapy include downstaging of local disease to facilitate surgical resection, optimizing nephron-sparing operative planning, and also providing an in vivo assessment of response to treatment. There are currently no phase III trials conducted in this disease setting, and data are limited to single-arm phase II studies and retrospective series.

The most robust data stems from two phase II studies. One single-arm phase study investigated the role of neoadjuvant pazopanib in patients with a median tumor size of 7.3 cm and median RENAL score of 11. Eighty percent of patients had high complexity, and 56% of patients had a solitary kidney. The study enrolled 25 patients who receive pazopanib 800 mg once daily for 8 weeks prior to nephrectomy. The primary endpoint was the percentage of patients who could underwent partial nephrectomy after therapy. Secondary endpoint was reduction of tumor volume, diameter, and investigator-assessed RECIST ORR. The study demonstrated a decrease in RENAL score in 71% of patients, and there was also a decrease in tumor volume in 92% of patients. By RECIST criteria, partial response was observed in 36% of tumors. Moreover, 6 patients of 13 who were initially identified as non-partial nephrectomy candidates were able to be safety processed with partial nephrectomy [51].

In another phase II trial, Karam et al. evaluated neoadjuvant axitinib 5 mg twice daily for up to 12 weeks in 24 patients. The inclusion criteria were patients with clinical stage T2b–T3b without evidence of metastatic disease. The primary endpoint was independent review ORR by RECIST criteria. There was a 28.3% median reduction of the tumor diameter, 11 patients had a partial response by RECIST criteria, and 13 had stable disease. The authors did not consider conversion from radical to partial nephrectomy as an endpoint, and therefore this was not evaluated. The drug was reasonably well tolerated, and there were two grade 3 complications and no grade 4 complications [52].

There has been conflicting data of the role of neoadjuvant therapy on venous tumor thrombi. Several small retrospective studies have investigated this approach. In aggregate the data show that in patients receiving sunitinib, tumors may increase, decrease, or be stable in size [53][54]. In contrast to these findings, Field et al. recently evaluated 19 patients with an IVC tumor thrombus receiving neoadjuvant sunitinib, the largest retrospective series on this topic. The authors found a decrease in thrombus size in eight patients, stable disease in ten patients, and an increase in size in one patient. While limited in sample size, these findings are hypothesis-generating to test the utility of TKI therapy in this context [55]. Overall, the role of systemic therapy with an intravenous thrombus will need to be further explored especially in the era of immunotherapy.

Future Trials

There are currently several ongoing trials evaluating adjuvant targeted therapy in localized RCC patients. One of these trials, the EVEREST trial, will test adjuvant everolimus in intermediate high-risk and very high-risk patients post nephrectomy. The trial is expected to accrue 1545 patients and will evaluate recurrence-free survival in RCC patients who will be randomized to 54 weeks of placebo or everolimus [11]. The PADRES trial is a single-arm phase II trial of axitinib given neoadjuvant to surgery in patients with an imperative indication for partial nephrectomy. The trial will enroll 50 patients and will evaluate percent reduction of the longest diameter of the tumor, ORR by RECIST criteria, effect on tumor on RENAL score, as well as the feasibility of partial nephrectomy [56].

Novel Agents

On the forefront of novel agents, there have been several recent trials testing new TKIs as well as other targeted therapy agents. Sapanisertib (TAK-228) is an investigational drug that competitively inhibits ATP suppressing both mTOR complex 1 and 2. In a recent phase 1 trial of 32 patients with metastatic RCC, sapanisertib demonstrated a reasonable safety profile in patients, 1 patient achieved a complete response, and 9 have a partial response [57]. Sapanisertib was also recently tested in combination with TAK117, which is a P13Kα inhibitor [58]. Carotuximab (TRC105) is a monoclonal antibody to endoglin (CD105), an angiogenic target expressed on tumor vessels. A recent study evaluated carotuximab in combination with axitinib versus axitinib alone in 150 patients who had progressed on prior TKI therapy. Median PFS was 6.7 months, and the combination therapy did not prolong PFS compared to axitinib alone [59]. Further study is requisite for these novel agents and their use in RCC patients.

Summary

In summary, targeted therapy continues to play a significant role for patients with metastatic renal cell carcinoma. Combination therapy with IO + TKI agents has demonstrated efficacy in the frontline space. A subset of patients with favorable risk disease and those not candidates for IO can still derive benefit from single-agent TKIs. Additionally, targeted agents either alone or in combination have demonstrated efficacy in the second-line setting. There is a spectrum of other targeted therapies that are currently under investigation that hold promise for improving outcomes for patients. However, we need to continue to refine selection strategies for patients with metastatic disease and integrate biomarkers into clinical decision-making to optimize therapy selection. Adjuvant and neoadjuvant therapy remain an unmet need, and we need improved strategies for localized disease management.

Ultimately, a multidisciplinary team approach will be critical to refining treatment for patients with renal cell carcinoma. Interdisciplinary care involving medical oncology, urologic oncology, radiation oncology, primary care, and palliative care will lead to improved outcomes. Such interwoven teamwork will define the future of cancer care and be needed to help our patients.

Source of Funding None

References

1. Ricketts CJ, et al. The cancer genome Atlas comprehensive molecular characterization of renal cell carcinoma. Cell Rep. 2018;23(1):313–326.e5. https://doi.org/10.1016/j.celrep.2018.03.075.
2. Moslehi J, Rathmell WK. The 2019 Nobel prize honors fundamental discoveries in hypoxia response. J Clin Invest. 2020;130(1):4–6. https://doi.org/10.1172/JCI134813.
3. Motzer RJ, Escudier B, Gannon A, Figlin RA. Sunitinib: ten years of successful clinical use and study in advanced renal cell carcinoma. Oncologist. 2017;22(1):41–52. https://doi.org/10.1634/theoncologist.2016-0197.
4. Zang X. 2018 Nobel prize in medicine awarded to cancer immunotherapy: immune checkpoint blockade – a personal account. Genes Dis. 2018;5(4):302–3. https://doi.org/10.1016/j.gendis.2018.10.003.
5. Rajan A, Kim C, Heery CR, Guha U, Gulley JL. Nivolumab, anti-programmed death-1 (PD-1) monoclonal antibody immunotherapy: role in advanced cancers. Hum Vaccines Immunother. 2016;12(9):2219–31. https://doi.org/10.1080/21645515.2016.1175694.
6. Sanchez DJ, Simon MC. Genetic and metabolic hallmarks of clear cell renal cell carcinoma. Biochim Biophys Acta Rev Cancer. 2018;1870(1):23–31. https://doi.org/10.1016/j.bbcan.2018.06.003.
7. Alonso-Gordoa T, García-Bermejo ML, Grande E, Garrido P, Carrato A, Molina-Cerrillo J. Targeting tyrosine kinases in renal cell carcinoma: 'new bullets against old guys'. Int J Mol Sci. 2019;20:8. https://doi.org/10.3390/ijms20081901.
8. Simons M, Gordon E, Claesson-Welsh L. Mechanisms and regulation of endothelial VEGF receptor signalling. Nat Rev Mol Cell Biol. 2016;17(10):611–25. https://doi.org/10.1038/nrm.2016.87.
9. Lawson ND, Mugford JW, Diamond BA, Weinstein BM. Phospholipase C gamma-1 is required downstream of vascular endothelial growth factor during arterial development. Genes Dev. 2003;17(11):1346–51. https://doi.org/10.1101/gad.1072203.
10. Chen J, et al. Akt1 regulates pathological angiogenesis, vascular maturation and permeability in vivo. Nat Med. 2005;11(11):1188–96. https://doi.org/10.1038/nm1307.
11. "S0931, everolimus in treating patients with kidney cancer who have undergone surgery – full text view – ClinicalTrials.gov." https://clinicaltrials.gov/ct2/show/NCT01120249. Accessed 26 Oct 2020.
12. Yang J, Yan J, Liu B. Targeting VEGF/VEGFR to modulate antitumor immunity. Front Immunol. 2018;9 https://doi.org/10.3389/fimmu.2018.00978.

13. Li Y-L, Zhao H, Ren X-B. Relationship of VEGF/VEGFR with immune and cancer cells: staggering or forward? Cancer Biol Med. 2016;13(2):206–14. https://doi.org/10.20892/j.issn.2095-3941.2015.0070.
14. Ohm JE, Carbone DP. VEGF as a mediator of tumor-associated immunodeficiency. Immunol Res. 2001;23(2–3):263–72. https://doi.org/10.1385/IR:23:2-3:263.
15. Wada J, et al. The contribution of vascular endothelial growth factor to the induction of regulatory T-cells in malignant effusions. Anticancer Res. 2009;29(3):881–8.
16. Varney ML, Johansson SL, Singh RK. Tumour-associated macrophage infiltration, neovascularization and aggressiveness in malignant melanoma: role of monocyte chemotactic protein-1 and vascular endothelial growth factor-a. Melanoma Res. 2005;15(5):417–25. https://doi.org/10.1097/00008390-200510000-00010.
17. Oe R, Fs H. "The intersection between tumor angiogenesis and immune suppression," *Clinical cancer research : an official journal of the American Association for Cancer Research*, Sep 15, 2019. https://pubmed.ncbi.nlm.nih.gov/30944124/. Accessed 24 Nov 2020.
18. Motzer RJ, et al. Nivolumab plus ipilimumab versus sunitinib in advanced renal-cell carcinoma. N Engl J Med. 2018;378(14):1277–90. https://doi.org/10.1056/NEJMoa1712126.
19. "Pembrolizumab plus axitinib versus sunitinib for advanced renal-cell carcinoma | NEJM." https://www.nejm.org/doi/full/10.1056/NEJMoa1816714. Accessed 15 Sep 2020.
20. "Dr. Plimack on updated findings of the KEYNOTE-426 study in RCC," *OncLive*. https://www.onclive.com/view/dr-plimack-on-updated-findings-of-the-keynote426-study-in-rcc. Accessed 23 Sep 2020.
21. Motzer RJ, et al. Avelumab plus axitinib versus sunitinib for advanced renal-cell carcinoma. N Engl J Med. 2019;380(12):1103–15. https://doi.org/10.1056/NEJMoa1816047.
22. "ESMO Virtual Congress 2020: Nivolumab + Cabozantinib vs Sunitinib in First-line Treatment for Advanced Renal Cell Carcinoma: First Results From The Randomized Phase 3 CheckMate 9ER Trial." https://www.urotoday.com/conference-highlights/esmo-2020/kidney-cancer/124542-esmo-virtual-congress-2020-nivolumab-cabozantinib-vs-sunitinib-in-first-line-treatment-for-advanced-renal-cell-carcinoma-first-results-from-the-randomized-phase-3-checkmate-9er-trial.html. Accessed 21 Sep 2020.
23. Yang JC, et al. A randomized trial of bevacizumab, an anti-vascular endothelial growth factor antibody, for metastatic renal cancer. N Engl J Med. 2003;349(5):427–34. https://doi.org/10.1056/NEJMoa021491.
24. "KEYTRUDA® (pembrolizumab) Plus LENVIMA® (lenvatinib) demonstrated statistically significant improvement in Progression-Free Survival (PFS), Overall Survival (OS) and Objective Response Rate (ORR) versus sunitinib as first-line treatment for patients… – Merck.com." https://www.merck.com/news/keytruda-pembrolizumab-plus-lenvima-lenvatinib-demonstrated-statistically-significant-improvement-in-progression-free-survival-pfs-overall-survival-os-and-objective-response-rate/. Accessed 07 Dec 2020.
25. Motzer RJ, et al. Overall survival and updated results for sunitinib compared with interferon alfa in patients with metastatic renal cell carcinoma. J Clin Oncol. 2009;27(22):3584–90. https://doi.org/10.1200/JCO.2008.20.1293.
26. Motzer RJ, et al. Pazopanib versus sunitinib in metastatic renal-cell carcinoma. N Engl J Med. 2013;369(8):722–31. https://doi.org/10.1056/NEJMoa1303989.
27. Argentiero A, et al. Anti-angiogenesis and Immunotherapy: novel paradigms to envision tailored approaches in renal cell-carcinoma. J Clin Med. 2020;9(5) https://doi.org/10.3390/jcm9051594.
28. McDermott DF, et al. Clinical activity and molecular correlates of response to atezolizumab alone or in combination with bevacizumab versus sunitinib in renal cell carcinoma. Nat Med. 2018;24(6):749–57. https://doi.org/10.1038/s41591-018-0053-3.
29. Choueiri TK, et al. Cabozantinib versus sunitinib as initial therapy for metastatic renal cell carcinoma of intermediate or poor risk (Alliance A031203 CABOSUN randomised trial): Progression-free survival by independent review and overall survival update. Eur J Cancer Oxf Engl 1990. 2018;94:115–25. https://doi.org/10.1016/j.ejca.2018.02.012.

30. C. for D. E. and Research, "FDA grants regular approval to Cabometyx for first-line treatment of advanced renal cell carcinoma," FDA, Feb 2019. Accessed 22 Oct 2020. [Online]. Available: https://www.fda.gov/drugs/resources-information-approved-drugs/fda-grants-regular-approval-cabometyx-first-line-treatment-advanced-renal-cell-carcinoma.
31. Salgia NJ, Dara Y, Bergerot P, Salgia M, Pal SK. The changing landscape of management of metastatic renal cell carcinoma: current treatment options and future directions. Curr Treat Options in Oncol. 2019;20(5):41. https://doi.org/10.1007/s11864-019-0638-1.
32. Ornstein MC, et al. Individualised axitinib regimen for patients with metastatic renal cell carcinoma after treatment with checkpoint inhibitors: a multicentre, single-arm, phase 2 study. Lancet Oncol. 2019;20(10):1386–94. https://doi.org/10.1016/S1470-2045(19)30513-3.
33. Rini BI, et al. Tivozanib versus sorafenib in patients with advanced renal cell carcinoma (TIVO-3): a phase 3, multicentre, randomised, controlled, open-label study. Lancet Oncol. 2020;21(1):95–104. https://doi.org/10.1016/S1470-2045(19)30735-1.
34. Albiges L, et al. Everolimus for patients with metastatic renal cell carcinoma refractory to anti-VEGF therapy: results of a pooled analysis of non-interventional studies. Eur J Cancer. 2015;51(16):2368–74. https://doi.org/10.1016/j.ejca.2015.07.030.
35. Nadal R, et al. Safety and clinical activity of vascular endothelial growth factor receptor (VEGFR)-tyrosine kinase inhibitors after programmed cell death 1 inhibitor treatment in patients with metastatic clear cell renal cell carcinoma. Ann Oncol Off J Eur Soc Med Oncol. 2016;27(7):1304–11. https://doi.org/10.1093/annonc/mdw160.
36. McGregor BA, et al. Activity of cabozantinib after immune checkpoint blockade in metastatic clear-cell renal cell carcinoma. Eur J Cancer Oxf Engl 1990. 2020;135:203–10. https://doi.org/10.1016/j.ejca.2020.05.009.
37. Auvray M, et al. Second-line targeted therapies after nivolumab-ipilimumab failure in metastatic renal cell carcinoma. Eur J Cancer. 2019;108:33–40. https://doi.org/10.1016/j.ejca.2018.11.031.
38. Shah AY, et al. Outcomes of patients with metastatic clear-cell renal cell carcinoma treated with second-line VEGFR-TKI after first-line immune checkpoint inhibitors. Eur J Cancer Oxf Engl 1990. 2019;114:67–75. https://doi.org/10.1016/j.ejca.2019.04.003.
39. "Cabozantinib versus everolimus in advanced renal cell carcinoma (METEOR): final results from a randomised, open-label, phase 3 trial - The Lancet Oncology." https://www.thelancet.com/journals/lanonc/article/PIIS1470-2045(16)30107-3/fulltext. Accessed 27 Oct 2020.
40. Motzer RJ, et al. Lenvatinib, everolimus, and the combination in patients with metastatic renal cell carcinoma: a randomised, phase 2, open-label, multicentre trial. Lancet Oncol. 2015;16(15):1473–82. https://doi.org/10.1016/S1470-2045(15)00290-9.
41. "ASCO 2020: COSMIC-313 phase III study of cabozantinib in combination with nivolumab and ipilimumab in patients with previously untreated advanced renal cell carcinoma of intermediate or poor-risk." https://www.urotoday.com/conference-highlights/asco-2020/asco-2020-kidney-cancer/121877-asco-2020-cosmic-313-phase-iii-study-of-cabozantinib-in-combination-with-nivolumab-and-ipilimumab-in-patients-with-previously-untreated-advanced-renal-cell-carcinoma-of-intermediate-or-poor-risk.html. Accessed 22 Oct 2020.
42. "Lenvatinib in combination with pembrolizumab or everolimus shows promise for advanced RCC," *Cancer Network*. https://www.cancernetwork.com/view/lenvatinib-in-combination-with-pembrolizumab-or-everolimus-shows-promise-for-advanced-rcc. Accessed 30 Nov 2020.
43. Merck Sharp & Dohme Corp., "An open-label, randomized phase 3 study of MK-6482 versus everolimus in participants with advanced renal cell carcinoma that has progressed after prior PD-1/L1 and VEGF-targeted therapies," clinicaltrials.gov, Clinical trial registration NCT04195750, Oct. 2020. Accessed 09 Nov 2020. [Online]. Available: https://clinicaltrials.gov/ct2/show/NCT04195750.
44. "ASCO GU 2020 | MK-6482 safety profile | advanced clear-cell RCC | oncology.medicinematters.com." https://oncology.medicinematters.com/asco-gu-2020/renal-cell-carcinoma/mk-6482-well-tolerated-in-advanced-rcc/17751430. Accessed 10 Nov 2020.

45. Exelixis, "A randomized, double-blind, controlled phase 3 study of cabozantinib in combination with nivolumab and ipilimumab versus nivolumab and ipilimumab in subjects with previously untreated advanced or metastatic renal cell carcinoma of intermediate or poor risk," clinicaltrials.gov, Clinical trial registration NCT03937219, Aug. 2020. Accessed 21 Oct 2020. [Online]. Available: https://clinicaltrials.gov/ct2/show/NCT03937219.
46. Haas NB, et al. Adjuvant sunitinib or sorafenib for high-risk, non-metastatic renal-cell carcinoma (ECOG-ACRIN E2805): a double-blind, placebo-controlled, randomised, phase 3 trial. Lancet. 2016;387(10032):2008–16. https://doi.org/10.1016/S0140-6736(16)00559-6.
47. Haas NB, et al. Adjuvant treatment for high-risk clear cell renal cancer. JAMA Oncol. 2017;3(9):1249–52. https://doi.org/10.1001/jamaoncol.2017.0076.
48. Ravaud A, et al. Adjuvant sunitinib in high-risk renal-cell carcinoma after nephrectomy. N Engl J Med. 2016;375(23):2246–54. https://doi.org/10.1056/NEJMoa1611406.
49. Motzer RJ, et al. Adjuvant aunitinib for high-risk renal cell carcinoma after nephrectomy: subgroup analyses and updated overall survival results. Eur Urol. 2018;73(1):62–8. https://doi.org/10.1016/j.eururo.2017.09.008.
50. "ASCO 2019: randomized, double-blind phase III Study of pazopanib versus placebo in patients with mRCC who have no evidence of disease following metastasectomy: a trial of the ECOG-ACRIN Cancer Research Group." https://www.urotoday.com/conference-highlights/asco-2019-annual-meeting/asco-2019-kidney-cancer/113046-asco-2019-randomized-double-blind-phase-iii-study-of-pazopanib-versus-placebo-in-patients-with-mrcc-who-have-no-evidence-of-disease-following-metastasectomy-a-trial-of-the-ecog-acrin-cancer-research-group.html. Accessed 11 Nov 2020.
51. Rini BI, et al. A phase II study of pazopanib in patients with localized renal cell carcinoma to optimize preservation of renal parenchyma. J Urol. 2015;194(2):297–303. https://doi.org/10.1016/j.juro.2015.03.096.
52. Karam JA, et al. Phase 2 trial of neoadjuvant axitinib in patients with locally advanced nonmetastatic clear cell renal cell carcinoma. Eur Urol. 2014;66(5):874–80. https://doi.org/10.1016/j.eururo.2014.01.035.
53. Cost NG, et al. The impact of targeted molecular therapies on the level of renal cell carcinoma vena caval tumor thrombus. Eur Urol. 2011;59(6):912–8. https://doi.org/10.1016/j.eururo.2011.02.032.
54. "Neoadjuvant targeted molecular therapies in patients undergoing nephrectomy and inferior vena cava thrombectomy: is it useful? SpringerLink." https://link.springer.com/article/10.1007/s00345-013-1088-1. Accessed 26 Oct 2020.
55. Field CA, et al. Neoadjuvant sunitinib decreases inferior vena caval thrombus size and is associated with improved oncologic outcomes: a multicenter comparative analysis. Clin Genitourin Cancer. 2019;17(3):e505–12. https://doi.org/10.1016/j.clgc.2019.01.013.
56. "Prior axitinib as a determinant of outcome of renal surgery – full text view – ClinicalTrials.gov." https://clinicaltrials.gov/ct2/show/NCT03438708. Accessed 26 Oct 2020.
57. Voss MH, et al. Phase 1 study of mTORC1/2 inhibitor sapanisertib (TAK-228) in advanced solid tumours, with an expansion phase in renal, endometrial or bladder cancer. Br J Cancer. 2020;20:1901. https://doi.org/10.1038/s41416-020-01041-x.
58. Randomised phase 2 study of sapanisertib (TAK?228/MLN0128) ± TAK-117 versus everolimus in patients with VEGFtargeted therapy-refractory metastatic clear cell renal cell carcinoma.
59. "ESMO 2019: results of the phase 2 TRAXAR study: a randomized phase 2 trial of axitinib and TRC105 (TRAX) versus axitinib alone in patients with advanced or metastatic renal cell carcinoma." https://www.urotoday.com/conference-highlights/esmo-2019/esmo-2019-kidney-cancer/115374-esmo-2019-results-of-the-phase-2-traxar-study-a-randomized-phase-2-trial-of-axitinib-and-trc105-trax-versus-axitinib-alone-in-patients-with-advanced-or-metastatic-renal-cell-carcinoma.html. Accessed 11 Nov 2020.
60. "Randomized phase III trial of adjuvant pazopanib versus placebo after nephrectomy in patients with localized or locally advanced renal cell carcinoma. Journal of Clinical Oncology." https://

ascopubs.org/doi/10.1200/JCO.2017.73.5324?url_ver=Z39.88-2003&rfr_id=ori:rid:crossref.org&rfr_dat=cr_pub%20%200pubmed. Accessed 26 Oct 2020.

61. Choueiri TK, et al. Cabozantinib versus everolimus in advanced renal cell carcinoma (METEOR): final results from a randomised, open-label, phase 3 trial. Lancet Oncol. 2016;17(7):917–27. https://doi.org/10.1016/S1470-2045(16)30107-3.
62. "Update Series (2019) Lesson 19: Integrating Surgical and Systemic Therapies in the Management of Metastatic and High Risk Non-Metastatic Renal Cell Carcinoma I AUA University." https://auau.auanet.org/content/course-299#group-tabs-node-course-default4. Accessed 08 Dec 2020.

Chapter 14
Hereditary Cancer and Genetics in Renal Cell Carcinoma

Hong Truong and Maria I. Carlo

Introduction

Renal cell carcinoma (RCC) represents a spectrum of kidney cancer classified by distinct histologic subtypes, clinical course, and molecular drivers. Most cases of RCCs are sporadic with risk factors that include smoking, obesity, hypertension, chronic renal insufficiency on dialysis, and environmental exposure. About 5%–8% of RCC cases are associated with hereditary RCC syndromes. To date, nine hereditary RCC syndromes have been characterized that are related to inheritance of monogenic germline alteration (Table 14.1). The histologic subtypes and relative risks of RCC vary in these syndromes. Compared to sporadic RCC, hereditary RCC is more likely to occur at an earlier age [1] and is more likely to be multifocal or bilateral [2, 3]. Studies of patients with hereditary RCC syndromes have yielded clues regarding the natural history and molecular pathogenesis of sporadic RCC. Diagnosis of hereditary RCC syndromes allows for screening, early detection, and timely intervention for patients and cascade testing for at-risk family members. Therefore, it is critical for physicians to recognize clinical phenotypes of patients with hereditary RCC syndromes and refer appropriate patients for genetic counseling and germline testing. In this chapter, we review the genetic and clinical features of well-characterized hereditary RCC syndromes and provide a framework on screening and appropriate workup for patients at risk of hereditary RCC syndromes.

H. Truong
Urology Service, Department of Surgery, Memorial Sloan Kettering Cancer Center, New York, NY, USA
e-mail: truongh1@mskcc.org

M. I. Carlo (✉)
Department of Medicine, Memorial Sloan Kettering Cancer Center, New York, NY, USA
e-mail: carlom@mskcc.org

K. L. Stratton, A. K. Morgans (eds.), *Urologic Oncology*,
https://doi.org/10.1007/978-3-030-89891-5_14

Table 14.1 Hereditary renal cell carcinoma syndromes

Syndrome	Chromosome location	Gene(s)	RCC histology	Common extra-renal clinical manifestations
von Hippel-Lindau	3p25.3	*VHL*	Clear cell	Retinal and CNS hemangioblastomas Retinal angiomas Adrenal or paraganglioma Endolymphatic sac tumors Broad ligament and epididymal cystadenomas Pancreatic cysts and neuroendocrine tumors
Hereditary leiomyomatosis and RCC	1q43	*FH*	FH deficient Papillary type 2 HLRCC-associated RCC	Cutaneous and uterine leiomyomas Leiomyosarcomas Adrenal adenoma
Birt-Hogg-Dubé	17p11.2	*FLCN*	Chromophobe Oncocytoma Clear cell Oncocytic hybrid Mixed histology	Cutaneous fibrofolliculoma Pulmonary cysts Spontaneous pneumothorax
Hereditary papillary RCC	7q31.2	*MET*	Papillary type 1	None
Tuberous sclerosis	9q34.13 16p13.3	*TSC1* *TSC2*	Angiomyolipoma Clear cell Oncocytoma Chromophobe	Cardiac rhabdomyoma Angiofibromas, hypomelanotic macules, and other dermatological lesions Cortical dysplasia Subependymal giant cell astrocytoma Retinal nodular and other nonrenal hamartomas Ungual fibromas Oral mucosal lesions
BAP1 tumor predisposition syndrome	3p21.1	*BAP1*	Clear cell Chromophobe	Uveal and cutaneous melanoma Malignant pleural mesothelioma
Hereditary paraganglioma-pheochromocytoma	5p15.33 1p36.13 1q23.3 11q23.1	*SDHA* *SDHB* *SDHC* *SDHD*	SDH deficient Unclassified/eosinophilic variant	Pheochromocytoma Paraganglioma Gastrointestinal stromal tumor
MITF cancer syndrome	3p13	*MITF*	Undefined	Cutaneous melanoma
Cowden syndrome	10q23.31	*PTEN*	Clear cell Papillary Chromophobe	Macrocephaly Breast cancer Thyroid cancer Endometrial cancer

Germline Genetic Testing in Kidney Cancer Patients

Knowledge of clinical features of patients with hereditary RCC syndromes is critical for determining which patients with kidney cancer should be referred for genetic counseling and germline testing. Assessment of genetic risk factors in patients with kidney cancer includes age of diagnosis of kidney cancer, tumor histology, multifocality, stage at presentation, personal history of extra-renal malignancies, and family history. While the median age of onset of patients with sporadic RCC in SEER-17 was 64 years, the median age at presentation of patients with known hereditary RCC syndromes was 37 years [1]. About 70% of hereditary RCC cases were diagnosed at 46 years or younger. Therefore, early age of presentation of kidney cancer may be a sign of an underlying genetic predisposition and has been adopted as a referral criterion for genetic counseling by both the National Comprehensive Cancer Network (NCCN) and the American Urological Association (AUA) kidney cancer guideline panels [4, 5]. Other indications for genetic counseling for RCC include synchronous or metachronous tumor multifocality, bilaterality, and those with histologic characteristics suggestive of a hereditary RCC syndrome such as FH-/SDH-deficient RCC and angiomyolipomas (AMLs) in patient with additional features of tuberous sclerosis complex (TSC). Traditionally, clinically directed single-gene testing has been done for patients with personal or family history suggestive of an underlying hereditary RCC syndrome or in those with first- or second-degree relatives with a known mutation in a cancer susceptibility gene. More recently, kidney cancer multigene panels, assessing 10–20 genes relevant to kidney cancer development, have been more commonly used to streamline testing for patients who meet referral criteria, such as those with early-onset RCC or multifocal/bilateral renal tumors, who lack distinguish clinical features of a classic hereditary cancer syndrome [6].

Surgical Management of Patients with Localized Hereditary Renal Tumors

The goals of surgical management of patients with bilateral, multifocal, or hereditary renal tumors are to prevent development of metastasis, preserve renal function, and minimize treatment-related morbidities. Longitudinal follow-up of patients with hereditary RCC syndromes has made it possible to tailor surgical management based on the underlying genetic alterations, which impact the natural history and clinical outcomes of renal tumors. Tumor growth rates varied significantly between different genetic subtypes. The growth rates of VHL-deficient (0.37 cm/year, interquartile range [IQR] 0.25–0.57 cm/year), FLCN-deficient (0.10 cm/year, IQR 0.04–0.24 cm/year), and MET-activation (0.15 cm/year, IQR 0.05–0.32 cm/year) tumors tend to be slower than BAP1-deficient tumors (0.6 cm/year, IQR 0.57–0.68 cm/year) [7]. For patients with less biologically aggressive tumors, namely, those associated with von Hippel-Lindau (VHL), Birt-Hogg-Dubé (BHD), and hereditary papillary RCC (HPRC) syndromes, an initial period of active surveillance until the largest tumor reaches 3 cm has been adopted to reduce the numbers of renal surgeries and their associated morbidities [8, 9]. The treatment strategy of choice for these patients is tumor enucleation to balance oncologic control and maximal preservation of normal renal parenchyma. On the opposite end of the genetically driven spectrum, hereditary leiomyomatosis and RCC (HLRCC), hereditary paraganglioma-pheochromocytoma, and BAP1 tumor predisposition syndromes are associated with more aggressive tumors. In particular, FH-deficient RCC associated with HLRCC is highly aggressive, and small tumors have the potential to metastasize [10, 11]. The majority of FH-deficient renal tumors have infiltrative margins and invaded renal sinus fat [11]. Therefore, prompt upfront surgical intervention is recommended. A radical nephrectomy or partial nephrectomy with wide margin, when feasible, should be utilized [12].

Implications of Germline Genetics in Management of Metastatic RCC

There is no standard treatment for metastatic RCC in the context of a hereditary syndrome, and treatment is often based on the histology of the original tumor. That being said, several clinical trials have examined regimens in patients with certain genetic syndromes. For VHL, agents that have been used in the treatment of metastatic clear cell RCC seem to have similar efficacy in tumor response, which is expected given that sporadic clear cell RCC is also mostly driven by *VHL* biallelic loss of function. A phase 2 study of pazopanib for patients with VHL reported objective responses in 13 (42%) of 31 patients and 31 (52%) of 59 VHL-associated RCC tumors [13]. In August 2021, the US Food and Drug Administration (FDA) approved the first-in-class, HIF-2 alpha inhibitor belzutifan for patients with VHL-associated RCC, central nervous system hemangioblastomas, or pancreatic neuroendocrine tumors [14]. In a phase 2 trial, HIF-2 alpha inhibitors achieve an overall response rate (ORR) of 49% of patients with VHL-associated RCC. The median duration of response was not reached with 56% of responders having duration of response over 12 months [15]. Belzutifan is currently being studied in sporadic clear cell RCC, with promising results seen in a phase 1 trial [16].

Other therapeutic studies have prospectively included patients with hereditary RCC. A phase 2 trial conducted by the National Cancer Institute (NCI) investigated the efficacy of erlotinib and bevacizumab in patients with advanced papillary RCC. The ORR was 31 (72%) of 43 patients with HLRCC and 14 (35%) of 40 patients with sporadic papillary RCC [17]. The treatment was well tolerated, with 41 (49%) of 83 patients experiencing grade 3 or higher adverse events. Currently, this regimen is included in the NCCN guidelines with special consideration for patients with HLRCC [4]. Additionally, recent retrospective analyses of other phase 2 trials have shown that other regimens also appear active in patients with FH-deficient RCC. In a report of patients with non-clear cell RCC treated with everolimus and bevacizumab, there were seven patients identified with germline *FH* mutations, of whom 4 (57%) had a response [18]. In a phase 2 study of the combination of cabozantinib and nivolumab in patients with non-clear cell RCC, there were five patients identified with germline *FH* mutations, of whom four had a response [19].

MET is known to be a driver in papillary hereditary RCC (where patients mainly present with type 1 papillary RCC) and in sporadic papillary tumors. A study of the *MET* inhibitor foretinib included 10 patients with germline *MET* mutations; of these, 5 patients had an objective response, compared to 5 of 57 patients without germline *MET* mutations [20]. Finally, although metastatic RCC in TSC is rare, everolimus has been shown to have significant activity in the treatment of localized AMLs associated with germline *TSC1* and *TSC2* mutations. 118 patients with AMLs were treated with everolimus. An ORR of 42% was seen, although once agent was discontinued, the AMLs appeared to grow back [21]. Based on this study, everolimus is approved by the FDA for patients with TSC-associated renal AMLs.

Hereditary Renal Cell Carcinoma Syndromes

Von Hippel-Lindau Syndrome (OMIM 193300)

VHL syndrome, the most well-characterized hereditary RCC syndrome, is a highly penetrant autosomal dominant syndrome that predisposes to malignant and benign tumors in multiple organs. VHL is caused by mutations in the *VHL* tumor suppressor gene located on chromosome 3p25.3 that encodes for the VHL protein, an essential part of a multi-protein complex that includes elongin B/C, cullin-2, and Rbx1 [22–24]. VHL protein functions as the recognition site for hypoxia-inducible factor alpha (HIF-alpha) to target proteins for ubiquitin-mediated degradation. Mutations in *VHL* lead to accumulation of HIF-1 and HIF-2 and upregulation of downstream pathways including vascular endothelial growth factor (VEGF), platelet-derived growth factor, and glucose transporters, leading to angiogenesis and cell proliferation [25]. Over 200 distinct mutations have been identified in the *VHL* gene including missense (52%), frameshift (13%), nonsense (11%), deletions (11%), splice site (7%), and inframe deletion/insertion (6%) mutations [26].

The cardinal features of VHL syndrome include clear cell RCC, cerebellar and spinal hemangioblastomas, pheochromocytomas, and endolymphatic sac tumors [27]. Patients with VHL may also have pancreatic cysts and solid tumors. Specific genotypes are associated with certain syndromic manifestations and can guide surveillance and management of patients with VHL. While nonsense and frameshift mutations are associated with higher susceptibility to clear cell RCC, missense mutations are associated with high risk of pheochromocytomas [26]. The lifetime risk of RCC in patients with VHL syndrome approached 75% with median age of onset of 39 years (range 13–70) [26]. VHL-associated RCC tend to be bilateral, multifocal, and recurrent. Clear cell RCC associated with VHL tends to be less biologically aggressive with a robust pseudocapsule. Patients with VHL-associated kidney tumors are recommended to undergo active surveillance until the largest tumors reach 3 cm in diameter. Tumor enucleation is the preferred surgical approach to preserve renal function without compromising oncologic control.

Hereditary Leiomyomatosis and RCC Syndrome (OMIM 150800)

HLRCC syndrome is an autosomal dominant cancer susceptibility syndrome caused by mutations in the *FH* gene, a tumor suppressor, located on chromosome 1q43, which encodes for the enzyme fumarate hydratase, a critical component of the Krebs cycle [28]. *FH* mutations impair oxidative phosphorylation and lead to the accumulation of oncometabolites. HLRCC is characterized by variable development of three tumors: cutaneous leiomyoma, uterine leiomyomata (fibroids), and rarely leiomyosarcomas, and HLRCC (or FH-deficient)-associated RCC. Cutaneous leiomyomas appear firm, flesh-colored to light red/brown papules and develop in nearly all patients by the age of 40 years, but can be subtle to detect. Cutaneous leiomyomas can cause symptoms of variable severity including pain and pruritus in response to touch or temperature changes [29]. Uterine fibroids occur in most women with HLRCC, often causing pelvic symptoms including menorrhagia and pain necessitating hysterectomy at an early age, in many cases before the age of 30 [29, 30]. In rare instances, cutaneous and uterine leiomyosarcomas have been reported in patients with *FH* germline mutations [31, 32]. The lifetime risk of RCC is estimated to be 10–20% with an early age of onset (median age of onset of 37 years, range 10–77 years) [1]. Although rare, RCCs have been reported in children [33]. Unlike other hereditary RCC syndromes, patients with HLRCC tend to have solitary and unilateral tumors with a more aggressive clinical course.

Since 2016, HLRCC-associated RCC has been added as a new RCC entity in the WHO classification of tumors. HLRCC-associated RCC has mixed architectural features including predominantly papillary pattern with tubular, tubulopapillary, tubulocystic, solid, cystic, and collecting duct carcinoma-like elements. Characteristic histologic findings of HLRCC-associated RCC are large nuclei with very prominent eosinophilic nucleolus surrounded by a clear perinucleolar halo. Immunohistochemical analysis of HLRCC-associated RCC reveals loss of FH expression (hence *FH*-deficient RCC is often used to refer to HLRCC-associated renal tumors) and 2-succino-cysteine (2SC) positive immunoreactivity. On CT and MR imaging, FH-deficient RCC tumors appear infiltrative, without circumscribed margins, and have heterogeneous MRI signal and enhancement. Most FH-deficient RCCs are locally advanced with radiographic evidence of invasion into the renal sinus fat or metastatic, particularly through lymph node chains, at the time of diagnosis [11]. However, there are no specific or unique features that would potentially distinguish FH-deficient RCC from other RCC subtypes [11]. Given the potential early age of renal cancer development, annual abdominal screening beginning at the age of 11 years has been recommended.

Of note, the *FH* c.1431_1433dupAAA (p.Lys477dup) germline variant, which is relatively common in certain populations, has conflicting reports on pathogenicity in the heterozygous state. Although in the homozygous state, it is associated with FH deficiency, in the heterozygous state, it does not appear to be associated with increased risk of RCC. In a study of 7571 patients with cancer who underwent germline genetic testing with a multigene panel, 24 patients had the variant, and none had RCC [34]. In another case report, in two patients with the variant and RCC, further pathologic and immunohistochemical studies showed that the RCCs did not have the morphologic features of FH-deficient RCC and had retained FH and no increase in 2SC [35].

Birt-Hogg-Dube Syndrome (OMIM 135150)

BHD is an autosomal dominant cancer predisposition syndrome caused by germline mutations in the *FLCN* gene, which encodes for folliculin. Folliculin is a GTPase-activating protein for RAGC and is involved in the regulation of mTORC1 and TFEB [36, 37]. Although the mechanism by which loss of function of *FLCN* leads to renal tumors is not completely understood, recent work shows the transcription factor TFEB may be a main driver of kidney abnormalities in BHD and that depletion of TFEB in a BHD mouse model leads to rescue of the disease phenotype [38]. BHD is likely underdiagnosed due to the variability in clinical expression, with some mutation carriers having subtle clinical features [39].

Patients with BHD are predisposed to renal tumors, which can vary in spectrum from oncocytomas, chromophobe tumors, or chromophobe oncocytic hybrid, with eosinophilic cytoplasm [40, 41]. As opposed to frequently seen somatic *VHL* mutations in sporadic clear cell RCC, *FLCN* as a somatic driver of sporadic RCC is rarely seen. Fibrofolliculomas are the hallmark cutaneous feature of BHD. These flesh-colored papules are most common in the face, and their incidence increases with age, but in some cases their appearance can be subtle [42]. Additionally, patients with BHD have a high prevalence of pulmonary cysts, and an estimated third of patients develop spontaneous pneumothorax [41]. There is controversy on whether patients with BHD are at increased risk of colon polyps or colorectal cancer. One recent study found an elevated risk of colorectal cancer in BHD patients vs controls (5.1 vs 1.5%, *p*-value .0068) [43]. However, another report from a Dutch registry with 399 patients with BHD and 382 relatives without BHD noted no increased prevalence of colorectal cancer [44]. In that study the rate of colorectal cancer was 3.6% in BHD patients vs 2.6% in relatives ($p = 0.54$). The rate of polyp removal was higher in BHD (12.2 vs 6.3%, $p = 0.005$), but there was no significant difference between the number of polyps and histology in the two groups.

Although there is no prospective data studying the benefits of screening in BHD, consensus guidelines recommend renal imaging, ideally with MRI, every 3 years [4, 45]. There may be limitations with ultrasound in the identification of tumors. In one retrospective study of BHD patients undergoing renal imaging, of 18 who had renal ultrasounds at time of diagnosis of renal mass, half had the tumors identified by CT or MRI and not seen in ultrasound [46]. In terms of management, BHD-associated renal tumors are thought to be relatively slow growing with a lower malignant potential; in a study by Ball et al., the growth rate of these tumors was 0.10 cm/year (IQR 0.04–0.24 cm/yr) [7].

Hereditary Papillary RCC (OMIM 164860)

Hereditary papillary RCC (HPRC) is an extremely rare autosomal dominant condition caused by heterozygous germline mutation in *MET* protooncogene on chromosome 7q31, which encodes for a receptor tyrosine kinase. *MET* mutations lead to constitutive activation of the MET protein and result in uncontrolled cell growth [47, 48]. Patients with HPRC are predisposed to multifocal and bilateral papillary type 1 RCC. Unlike other hereditary RCC syndromes, patients with HPRC do not harbor extra-renal manifestation, making its diagnosis difficult unless the physicians have a high index of suspicion based on tumor multifocality, histology, and family history of papillary type 1 RCC. Due to its indolent nature, MET-activated renal tumors associated with HPRC syndrome are best observed until the tumors reach 3-cm diameter and are amenable to enucleation to preserve renal function without compromising oncologic control [12].

BAP1 Tumor Predisposition Syndrome (OMIM 614327)

BAP1 tumor predisposition syndrome is an autosomal dominant cancer predisposition syndrome caused by germline loss-of-function mutations in the *BAP1* gene. *BAP1* encodes for a deubiquitinating enzyme and is involved in chromatin regulation among other cellular processes [49, 50]. *BAP1* somatic mutations are common in clear cell RCC and associated with worse prognosis [51, 52]. Individuals with *BAP1* germline mutations are at increased risk of cutaneous and uveal melanoma, mesothelioma (both peritoneal and pleural), RCC, and likely other tumors. Compared to other RCC hereditary conditions, BAP1 tumor predisposition syndrome is relatively recently described, and the full phenotypic syndrome, including its penetrance, is not fully understood [53, 54].

In the largest reported series of *BAP1* carriers to date, the incidence of RCC was between 5% and 10% when including probands and relatives [55]. Although it appears that clear cell RCC is the predominant histology, there are also reports of patients with chromophobe tumors with loss of BAP1 on IHC [56]. As opposed to RCCs in patients with VHL and BHD, RCCs in patients with *BAP1* somatic or germline mutations are thought to be aggressive, and consensus recommendations are to perform renal imaging every 2 years [4].

Hereditary Paraganglioma-Pheochromocytoma Syndromes (OMIM 185470)

Hereditary paraganglioma-pheochromocytoma syndrome is an autosomal dominant cancer predisposition syndrome caused by mutations in genes within the SDH complex (*SDHA, SDHB, SDHC, SDHD, SDHAF2,* collectively SDHx), *MAX*, and *TMEM127*. Germline mutations in these genes have been associated with an increased risk of mainly pheochromocytoma and paraganglioma, but gastrointestinal stromal tumors and RCC have also been reported. The majority of cases of RCC within the context of this syndrome are due to germline *SDHB* mutations, and the presenting RCC subtype has typical characteristic histologic features, with the prominent being the presence of cytoplasmic vacuoles and SDHB deficiency on IHC [57, 58]. In 2016, SDHB-deficient RCC was added as a new histologic subtype to the World Health Organization classification of tumors [59]. If SDH deficiency is identified in a renal tumor, there is a high likelihood that it is due to a germline mutation. SDH-deficient RCCs range from slow growing to aggressive. Although there are reports of patients with RCC and germline mutations in *TMEM127* and *MAX*, the association of these genes and the pathogenesis of the RCC have not yet been well established [60, 61].

The incidence of RCC in patients with SDHx mutations is not well established. In a large retrospective study of individuals referred for genetic testing due to a personal or family history of pheochromocytoma or paraganglioma, 876 individuals with *SDHB/C/D* mutations were identified, of which 16 had RCC, all but one in individuals with *SDHB* mutations [62]. The risk of RCC by age 60 in *SDHB* carriers was estimated at 4–5%. Although there are reports of patients with RCC and *SDHA* mutations, the role of the mutation in the pathogenicity of the tumor has not yet been established [63, 64].

Screening for RCC in SDHx carriers is usually obtained within the context of screening for pheochromocytomas and paragangliomas, for which head and neck, thoracic, abdominal, and pelvic MRIs are recommended every 2–3 years[65, 66]. FDG PET may be very sensitive to detect SDH-related tumors, and patients with advanced SDH-deficient RCC can have very high FDG uptake. To date, there is no particular systemic regimen that has been studied in SDH-deficient metastatic RCC.

Other Hereditary Syndromes with Increased Risk of Renal Cancer

There are several other genetic conditions that can predispose to renal tumors. Patients with tuberous sclerosis complex (TSC, OMIM 191100) are at high risk of AML, a renal lesion composed of smooth-muscle-like cells, adipocyte-like cells, and epithelioid cells [67]. Although rare, RCC can also occur with TSC, and several reports have shown a wide spectrum of morphologies and a propensity for bilateral or multifocal lesions [68, 69]. International consensus guidelines recommend imaging, preferably with MRI, every few years and more often if lesions are identified [4].

Patients with Cowden syndrome (OMIM 158350) caused by germline mutations in *PTEN* are also at risk for several malignancies, including breast, endometrial, and thyroid cancer. They are also at increased risk of RCC, although to a lesser extent. RCCs within the context of Cowden typically have non-clear cell histology, with chromophobe and papillary subtypes predominating, although clear cell RCC is also seen [70, 71]. Current NCCN guideline recommends consideration of renal ultrasound every 1–2 years for patients with Cowden syndrome [72].

A germline missense variant in *MITF* p.E318K has been identified to confer a genetic predisposition to melanoma and RCC. Patients with the *MITF* p.E318K variant had a higher than fivefold increased risk of developing melanoma, RCC, or both cancers compared to controls with *MITF* wild type [73]. Therefore, presence of personal or familial melanoma and RCC should prompt referral for genetic counseling.

Conclusions

Knowledge of inherited genetics of patients with RCC continues to evolve. Twelve RCC predisposition genes, *VHL, MET, FH, TSC1/2, FLCN, SDHA/B/C/D, BAP1*, and *MITF*, leading to nine hereditary RCC syndromes have been identified. Studies of hereditary RCC have led to breakthrough discoveries into the genetic basis of kidney cancer and revolutionized the surgical management and more effective targeted therapies for patients with both hereditary and sporadic forms of RCC. It is critical that physicians managing patients with RCC recognize and refer patients at risk of hereditary RCC syndromes for genetic counseling and germline testing because well-defined RCC management strategies exist for these patients, and early screening, detection, and intervention of at-risk organs minimize cancer-specific morbidity and mortality.

References

1. Shuch B, Vourganti S, Ricketts CJ, Middleton L, Peterson J, Merino MJ, Metwalli AR, Srinivasan R, Linehan WM. Defining early-onset kidney cancer: implications for germline and somatic mutation testing and clinical management. J Clin Oncol. 2013;32:431–7.
2. Klatte T, Patard J-J, Wunderlich H, et al. Metachronous bilateral renal cell carcinoma: risk assessment, prognosis and relevance of the primary-free interval. J Urology. 2007;177:2081–7.
3. Klatte T, Wunderlich H, Patard J, et al. Clinicopathological features and prognosis of synchronous bilateral renal cell carcinoma: an international multicentre experience. BJU Int. 2007;100:21–5.
4. Motzer RJ, Jonasch E, Boyle S, et al. NCCN guidelines insights: kidney cancer, version 1.2021: featured updates to the NCCN guidelines. J Natl Compr Canc Ne. 2020;18:1160–70.

5. Campbell SC, Clark PE, Chang SS, Karam JA, Souter L, Uzzo RG. Renal mass and localized renal cancer: evaluation, management, and follow-up: AUA guideline: part I. J Urology. 2021;206:199–208.
6. Shuch B, Zhang J. Genetic predisposition to renal cell carcinoma: implications for counseling, testing, screening, and management. J Clin Oncol. 2018;36:3560–6.
7. Ball MW, An JY, Gomella PT, et al. Growth rates of genetically defined renal tumors: implications for active surveillance and intervention. J Clin Oncol. 2020;38:1146–53.
8. Walther MM, Choyke PL, Glenn G, Lyne JC, Rayford W, Venzon D, Linehan WM. Renal cancer in families with hereditary renal cancer: prospective analysis of a tumor size threshold for renal parenchymal sparing surgery. J Urology. 1999;161:1475–9.
9. Metwalli AR, Linehan WM. Nephron-sparing surgery for multifocal and hereditary renal tumors. Curr Opin Urol. 2014;24:466–73.
10. Choyke PL, Glenn GM, Walther MM, Zbar B, Linehan WM. Hereditary renal cancers. Radiology. 2003;226:33–46.
11. Nikolovski I, Carlo MI, Chen Y-B, Vargas HA. Imaging features of fumarate hydratase-deficient renal cell carcinomas: a retrospective study. Cancer Imaging. 2021;21:24.
12. Gomella PT, Linehan WM, Ball MW. Precision surgery and kidney cancer: knowledge of genetic alterations influences surgical management. Genes-basel. 2021;12:261.
13. Jonasch E, McCutcheon IE, Gombos DS, et al. Pazopanib in patients with von Hippel-Lindau disease: a single-arm, single-centre, phase 2 trial. Lancet Oncol. 2018;19:1351–9.
14. (n.d.) FDA approves belzutifan for cancers associated with von Hippel-Lindau disease. https://www.fda.gov/drugs/resources-information-approved-drugs/fda-approves-belzutifan-cancers-associated-von-hippel-lindau-disease. Accessed 17 Aug 2021.
15. Srinivasan R, Donskov F, Iliopoulos O, et al. Phase 2 study of belzutifan (MK-6482), an oral hypoxia-inducible factor 2α (HIF-2α) inhibitor, for Von Hippel-Lindau (VHL) disease-associated clear cell renal cell carcinoma (ccRCC). J Clin Oncol. 2021;39:4555.
16. Choueiri TK, Bauer TM, Papadopoulos KP, et al. Inhibition of hypoxia-inducible factor-2α in renal cell carcinoma with belzutifan: a phase 1 trial and biomarker analysis. Nat Med. 2021;27:802–5.
17. Srinivasan R, Gurram S, Harthy MA, et al. Results from a phase II study of bevacizumab and erlotinib in subjects with advanced hereditary leiomyomatosis and renal cell cancer (HLRCC) or sporadic papillary renal cell cancer. J Clin Oncol. 2020;38:5004.
18. Feldman DR, Ged Y, Lee C, et al. Everolimus plus bevacizumab is an effective first-line treatment for patients with advanced papillary variant renal cell carcinoma: final results from a phase II trial. Cancer. 2020;126:5247–55.
19. Lee C-H, Voss MH, Carlo MI, et al. Nivolumab plus cabozantinib in patients with non-clear cell renal cell carcinoma: results of a phase 2 trial. J Clin Oncol. 2021;39:4509.
20. Choueiri TK, Vaishampayan U, Rosenberg JE, et al. Phase II and biomarker study of the dual MET/VEGFR2 inhibitor foretinib in patients with papillary renal cell carcinoma. J Clin Oncol. 2012;31:181–6.
21. Bissler JJ, Kingswood JC, Radzikowska E, et al. Everolimus for angiomyolipoma associated with tuberous sclerosis complex or sporadic lymphangioleiomyomatosis (EXIST-2): a multicentre, randomised, double-blind, placebo-controlled trial. Lancet. 2013;381:817–24.
22. Kibel A, Iliopoulos O, DeCaprio J, Kaelin W. Binding of the von Hippel-Lindau tumor suppressor protein to Elongin B and C. Science. 1995;269:1444–6.
23. Pack SD, Zbar B, Pak E, et al. Constitutional von Hippel-Lindau (VHL) gene deletions detected in VHL families by fluorescence in situ hybridization. Cancer Res. 1999;59:5560–4.
24. Kamura T, Koepp DM, Conrad MN, et al. Rbx1, a component of the VHL tumor suppressor complex and SCF ubiquitin ligase. Science. 1999;284:657–61.
25. Majmundar AJ, Wong WJ, Simon MC. Hypoxia-inducible factors and the response to hypoxic stress. Mol Cell. 2010;40:294–309.
26. Nielsen SM, Rhodes L, Blanco I, Chung WK, Eng C, Maher ER, Richard S, Giles RH. Von Hippel-Lindau disease: genetics and role of genetic counseling in a multiple neoplasia syndrome. J Clin Oncol. 2016;34:2172–81.

27. Hampel H, Bennett RL, Buchanan A, Pearlman R, Wiesner GL, Committee GDG American College of Medical Genetics and Genomics Professional Practice and Guidelines Committee and National Society of Genetic Counselors Practice Guidelines. A practice guideline from the American College of Medical Genetics and Genomics and the National Society of Genetic Counselors: referral indications for cancer predisposition assessment. Genet Med. 2015;17:70–87.
28. Tomlinson IPM, Alam NA, Rowan AJ, et al. Germline mutations in FH predispose to dominantly inherited uterine fibroids, skin leiomyomata and papillary renal cell cancer. Nat Genet. 2002;30:406–10.
29. Smit D, Mensenkamp A, Badeloe S, et al. Hereditary leiomyomatosis and renal cell cancer in families referred for fumarate hydratase germline mutation analysis. Clin Genet. 2011;79:49–59.
30. Lehtonen HJ. Hereditary leiomyomatosis and renal cell cancer: update on clinical and molecular characteristics. Familial Cancer. 2011;10:397–411.
31. Toro JR, Nickerson ML, Wei M-H, et al. Mutations in the fumarate hydratase gene cause hereditary Leiomyomatosis and renal cell cancer in families in North America. Am J Hum Genet. 2003;73:95–106.
32. Wei M-H, Toure O, Glenn GM, et al. Novel mutations in FH and expansion of the spectrum of phenotypes expressed in families with hereditary leiomyomatosis and renal cell cancer. J Med Genet. 2006;43:18.
33. Hol JA, Jongmans MCJ, Littooij AS, et al. Renal cell carcinoma in young FH mutation carriers: case series and review of the literature. Familial Cancer. 2020;19:55–63.
34. Zhang L, Walsh MF, Jairam S, et al. Fumarate hydratase FH c.1431_1433dupAAA (p.Lys477dup) variant is not associated with cancer including renal cell carcinoma. Hum Mutat. 2020;41:103–9.
35. Gupta S, Shen W, Jimenez RE, Cheville JC. Fumarate Hydratase (FH) c.1431_1433dupAAA (p.Lys477dup) variant is not associated with FH protein deficiency and increased 2SC in two separate patients with renal neoplasia. Hum Mutat. 2021; https://doi.org/10.1002/humu.24268.
36. Lawrence RE, Fromm SA, Fu Y, et al. Structural mechanism of a rag GTPase activation checkpoint by the lysosomal folliculin complex. Science. 2019;366:971–7.
37. Alesi N, Akl EW, Khabibullin D, et al. TSC2 regulates lysosome biogenesis via a non-canonical RAGC and TFEB-dependent mechanism. Nat Commun. 2021;12:4245.
38. Napolitano G, Malta CD, Esposito A, et al. A substrate-specific mTORC1 pathway underlies Birt–Hogg–Dubé syndrome. Nature. 2020;585:597–602.
39. Menko FH, van Steensel MA, Giraud S, et al. Birt-Hogg-Dubé syndrome: diagnosis and management. Lancet Oncol. 2009;10:1199–206.
40. Sattler EC, Reithmair M, Steinlein OK. Kidney cancer characteristics and genotype-phenotype-correlations in Birt-Hogg-Dubé syndrome. PLoS One. 2018;13:e0209504.
41. Houweling AC, Gijezen LM, Jonker MA, et al. Renal cancer and pneumothorax risk in Birt–Hogg–Dubé syndrome; an analysis of 115 FLCN mutation carriers from 35 BHD families. Br J Cancer. 2011;105:1912–9.
42. Schmidt LS, Linehan WM. Molecular genetics and clinical features of Birt–Hogg–Dubé syndrome. Nat Rev Urol. 2015;12:558–69.
43. Sattler EC, Syunyaeva Z, Reithmair M, Dempke W, Steinlein OK. Colorectal cancer risk in families with Birt-Hogg-Dubé syndrome increased. Eur J Cancer. 2021;151:168–74.
44. van de Beek I, Glykofridis IE, Wolthuis RMF, Gille HJJP, Johannesma PC, Meijers-Heijboer HEJ, van Moorselaar RJA, Houweling AC. No evidence for increased prevalence of colorectal carcinoma in 399 Dutch patients with Birt-Hogg-Dubé syndrome. Br J Cancer. 2020;122:590–4.
45. Carlo MI, Hakimi AA, Stewart GD, et al. Familial kidney cancer: implications of new syndromes and molecular insights. Eur Urol. 2019;76:754–64.
46. Johannesma PC, van de Beek I, van der Wel TJWT, et al. Renal imaging in 199 Dutch patients with Birt-Hogg-Dubé syndrome: screening compliance and outcome. PLoS One. 2019;14:e0212952.

47. Schmidt LS, Nickerson ML, Angeloni D, et al. Early onset hereditary papillary renal carcinoma. J Urology. 2004;172:1256–61.
48. Schmidt L, Duh F-M, Chen F, et al. Germline and somatic mutations in the tyrosine kinase domain of the MET proto-oncogene in papillary renal carcinomas. Nat Genet. 1997;16:68–73.
49. Ventii KH, Devi NS, Friedrich KL, Chernova TA, Tighiouart M, Meir EGV, Wilkinson KD. BRCA1-associated protein-1 is a tumor suppressor that requires deubiquitinating activity and nuclear localization. Cancer Res. 2008;68:6953–62.
50. Campagne A, Lee M-K, Zielinski D, et al. BAP1 complex promotes transcription by opposing PRC1-mediated H2A ubiquitylation. Nat Commun. 2019;10:348.
51. Voss MH, Reising A, Cheng Y, et al. Genomically annotated risk model for advanced renal-cell carcinoma: a retrospective cohort study. Lancet Oncol. 2018;19:1688–98.
52. Peña-Llopis S, Vega-Rubín-de-Celis S, Liao A, et al. BAP1 loss defines a new class of renal cell carcinoma. Nat Genet. 2012;44:751–9.
53. Testa JR, Cheung M, Pei J, et al. Germline BAP1 mutations predispose to malignant mesothelioma. Nat Genet. 2011;43:1022–5.
54. Abdel-Rahman MH, Pilarski R, Cebulla CM, Massengill JB, Christopher BN, Boru G, Hovland P, Davidorf FH. Germline BAP1 mutation predisposes to uveal melanoma, lung adenocarcinoma, meningioma, and other cancers. J Med Genet. 2011;48:856.
55. Walpole S, Pritchard AL, Cebulla CM, et al. Comprehensive study of the clinical phenotype of germline BAP1 variant-carrying families worldwide. Jnci J Natl Cancer Inst. 2018;110:1328–41.
56. Carlo MI, Mukherjee S, Mandelker D, et al. Prevalence of germline mutations in cancer susceptibility genes in patients with advanced renal cell carcinoma. JAMA Oncol. 2018;4:1228.
57. Williamson SR, Eble JN, Amin MB, Gupta NS, Smith SC, Sholl LM, Montironi R, Hirsch MS, Hornick JL. Succinate dehydrogenase-deficient renal cell carcinoma: detailed characterization of 11 tumors defining a unique subtype of renal cell carcinoma. Modern Pathol. 2015;28:80–94.
58. Gill AJ, Hes O, Papathomas T, et al. Succinate Dehydrogenase (SDH)-deficient renal carcinoma. Am J Surg Pathol. 2014;38:1588–602.
59. Moch H, Cubilla AL, Humphrey PA, Reuter VE, Ulbright TM. The 2016 WHO classification of tumours of the urinary system and male genital organs—part a: renal, penile, and testicular Tumours. Eur Urol. 2016;70:93–105.
60. Hernandez KG, Ezzat S, Morel CF, Swallow C, Otremba M, Dickson BC, Asa SL, Mete O. Familial pheochromocytoma and renal cell carcinoma syndrome: TMEM127 as a novel candidate gene for the association. Virchows Arch. 2015;466:727–32.
61. Casey RT, Warren AY, Martin JE, et al. Clinical and molecular features of Renal and Pheochromocytoma/Paraganglioma Tumor Association Syndrome (RAPTAS): case series and literature review. J Clin Endocrinol Metab. 2017;102:4013–22.
62. Andrews KA, Ascher DB, Pires DEV, et al. Tumour risks and genotype–phenotype correlations associated with germline variants in succinate dehydrogenase subunit genes SDHB, SDHC and SDHD. J Med Genet. 2018;55:384.
63. Wurth R, Jha A, Kamilaris C, Gill AJ, Poplawski N, Xekouki P, Quezado MM, Pacak K, Stratakis CA, Hannah-Shmouni F. A case of carney triad complicated by renal cell carcinoma and a germline SDHA pathogenic variant. Endocr Diabet Metabol Case Rep. 2021; https://doi.org/10.1530/edm-20-0170.
64. Gault MD, Mandelker D, DeLair D, et al. Germline SDHA mutations in children and adults with cancer. Mol Case Stud. 2018;4:a002584.
65. Amar L, Pacak K, Steichen O, et al. International consensus on initial screening and follow-up of asymptomatic SDHx mutation carriers. Nat Rev Endocrinol. 2021;17:435–44.
66. Rednam SP, Erez A, Druker H, et al. Von Hippel–Lindau and hereditary pheochromocytoma/paraganglioma syndromes: clinical features, genetics, and surveillance recommendations in childhood. Clin Cancer Res. 2017;23:e68–75.
67. Henske EP, Jóźwiak S, Kingswood JC, Sampson JR, Thiele EA. Tuberous sclerosis complex. Nat Rev Dis Primers. 2016;2:16035.

68. Guo J, Tretiakova MS, Troxell ML, et al. Tuberous sclerosis–associated renal cell carcinoma. Am J Surg Pathol. 2014;38:1457–67.
69. Bjornsson J, Short MP, Kwiatkowski DJ, Henske EP. Tuberous sclerosis-associated renal cell carcinoma. Clinical, pathological, and genetic features. Am J Pathol. 1996;149:1201–8.
70. Kim RH, Wang X, Evans AJ, Campbell SC, Nguyen JK, Farncombe KM, Eng C. Early-onset renal cell carcinoma in PTEN harmatoma tumour syndrome. Npj Genom Medicine. 2020;5:40.
71. Gupta S, Erickson LA. Renal neoplasia in Cowden syndrome. Mayo Clin Proc. 2020;95:2808–9.
72. Daly MB, Pal T, Berry MP, et al. Genetic/familial high-risk assessment: breast, ovarian, and pancreatic, version 2.2021, NCCN clinical practice guidelines in oncology. J Natl Compr Canc Netw. 2021;19:77–102.
73. Bertolotto C, Lesueur F, Giuliano S, et al. A SUMOylation-defective MITF germline mutation predisposes to melanoma and renal carcinoma. Nature. 2011;480:94–8.

Chapter 15
Immunotherapy

Georgia Sofia Karachaliou, Nathan Hirshman, and Tian Zhang

At initial presentation, approximately 19% of renal cell carcinoma (RCC) patients either have locally advanced disease or distant metastases [1]. While surgical resection of the tumor is typically considered the only curative option for patients with early-stage disease, new treatment options have arisen for both early-stage disease and advanced/metastatic disease. Specifically, systemic immunotherapy is now considered part of the treatment paradigm for individuals with RCC. In metastatic renal cell carcinoma (mRCC), the International Metastatic renal cell carcinoma Database Consortium (IMDC) has implemented risk stratification with six risk factors, hypercalcemia, neutrophilia, anemia, thrombocytosis, less than a year from initial diagnosis to systemic therapy, and poor performance status (Karnofsky Performance Status <70), and is now used for trial stratification and treatment selection [2].

In 1992, high-dose interleukin (IL)-2 was the first approved immunotherapeutic agent for RCC, despite significant toxicities, because of improved clinical outcomes in a subset of mRCC patients [3, 4]. Importantly, durable complete responses (CR) were observed in 5–9% of patients [4, 5]. The most common side effects were capillary leak syndrome, urinary tract and catheter site infections, hypotension,

G. S. Karachaliou
Duke University Hospital, Department of Medicine/Division of Medical Oncology, Durham, NC, USA
e-mail: georgiasofia.karachaliou@duke.edu

N. Hirshman
Duke University Medical Center, Department of Medicine, Durham, NC, USA
e-mail: Nathan.hirshman@duke.edu

T. Zhang (✉)
Division of Hematology and Oncology, Department of Internal Medicine, University of Texas Southwestern Medical Center, Dallas, TX, USA
e-mail: tian.zhang2@duke.edu, zhang@utsouthwestern.edu

K. L. Stratton, A. K. Morgans (eds.), *Urologic Oncology*,
https://doi.org/10.1007/978-3-030-89891-5_15

tachycardia, dyspnea, renal dysfunction, hyperbilirubinemia, transaminase elevations, and neurological changes [6]. Currently, high-dose IL-2 is still possible to be given as first-line treatment for selected patients with favorable risk RCC, excellent performance status, and normal organ function [7]. However, the recent development and approvals of immune checkpoint inhibitors (ICIs) have improved targeted activation of immune surveillance.

Recently, ICIs have been further studied in renal cell carcinoma, given RCC's immunogenicity and increased infiltration of different immune cells such as T cells and NK cells [8]. In addition, regulatory T cells (Tregs), tumor-associated macrophages, and myeloid-derived suppressor cells (MDSCs) have been shown to be responsible for suppression of anti-cancer activity in RCC [8]. Anti-PD-1 and anti-CTLA-4 antibodies improve T-cell responses and allow upregulation of anticancer activity by suppressing Treg activity, thereby increasing IFN-γ and IL-2 production in the tumor microenvironment. Currently, these antibodies targeting PD-1 and CTLA-4 pathways represent new treatment options for RCC.

In this chapter, we will highlight the current immunotherapeutic options, including anti-PD-1 and anti-CTLA-4 antibodies, along with the ongoing clinical trials in metastatic RCC as well as local RCC that are important in informing multidisciplinary care of RCC.

Immunotherapy in Patients with Metastatic RCC

The landscape of systemic treatment regimens for mRCC has expanded dramatically over the past 15 years with the rise of immunotherapy [17]. Specifically, the role of PD-1 inhibitors is growing in treatment of patients with mRCC. Nivolumab, the first-in-class PD-1 inhibitor, was first approved by the US FDA in 2015 in second-line treatment of mRCC, based on the improved overall survival (OS) demonstrated in CheckMate 025, a trial comparing the efficacy of nivolumab to everolimus in patients who were previously treated for mRCC [9]. Subsequently, pembrolizumab, a selective, fully humanized immunoglobulin G4-κ monoclonal antibody against PD-1, was investigated in combination with axitinib in first-line treatment of mRCC. Several clinical trials with combination immunotherapy agents have now improved clinical outcomes in mRCC (Table 15.1).

The CheckMate 214 randomized phase 3 clinical trial randomly assigned 1096 patients to nivolumab plus ipilimumab (a CTLA-4 inhibitor) or sunitinib (a receptor tyrosine kinase inhibitor targeted against vascular endothelial growth factor receptors [VEGFRs]) [10]. With a median follow-up of 55 months, concurrent nivolumab and ipilimumab for four cycles followed by maintenance nivolumab improved median overall survival (OS) versus sunitinib in all patients (median OS not reached versus 38.4 months; HR 0.69, 95%CI 0.59–0.81]) [11]. Specifically, in the subset of patients with IMDC intermediate-poor-risk disease, OS was improved further (median OS 48.1 versus 26.6 months; HR 0.65, 95%CI 0.54–0.78). PFS was noted to be relatively comparable between the two groups (median PFS was 12.2 months versus 12.3 months, HR 0.89 [95%CI 0.76–1.05]), with 4-year PFS better for

Table 15.1 Completed phase 3 clinical trials investigating immunotherapeutic agents in metastatic renal cell carcinoma

Trial					
	CheckMate 214	KeyNote-426	CheckMate 9ER	JAVELIN 101	CLEAR
Clinicaltrial.gov identifier	NCT02231749	NCT02853331	NCT03141177	NCT02684006	**NCT02811861**
Intervention	Ipi + nivo	Pembro+axi	Nivo+cabo	Ave + axi	Pembro+lenva
12-month OS	Ipi + nivo 80% Sun72%	Pembro+axi 90% Sun 78%	Nivo+cabo 86% Sun 75%	Ave + axi 86% Sun 83%	NR NR
HR OS	0.66	0.53	0.60	0.80	N/A
PFS	Ipi + nivo 8.2 m Sun 8.3 m	Pembro+axi 15.1 m Sun 11.1 m	Nivo+cabo 16.6 m Sun 8.3 m	Ave + axi 13.8 m Sun 8.4 m	Pembro+lenva 23.9 m Sun 9.2 m
ORR	42%	59%	56%	51%	71%

OS overall survival, *HR* hazard ratio, *PFS* progression-free survival, *ORR* objective response rate, *Ipi* ipilimumab, *Nivo* nivolumab, *Sun* sunitinib, *Pembro* pembrolizumab, *Axi* axitinib, *Cabo* cabozantinib, *Ave* avelumab, *Lenva* lenvatinib, *NR* not reached, *N/A* not applicable

patients treated with ipilimumab-nivolumab versus sunitinib (31% versus 17%). Furthermore, in the subset of patients with intermediate-poor-risk disease, median PFS was 11.2 months versus 8.3 months for ipilimumab-nivolumab versus sunitinib, respectively. The most common observed grade 3–4 treatment-related adverse events in the combination group were increased lipase levels in 10% (57/547), amylase levels in 6% (31/547), and alanine aminotransferase levels in 5% (28/547). Notably, eight deaths in the nivolumab plus ipilimumab group and four deaths in the sunitinib group were reported as treatment-related [10]. Ultimately, given the improved overall survival, this pivotal trial led to US FDA approval of the nivolumab plus ipilimumab combination for patients with treatment-naïve mRCC and IMDC intermediate- and poor-risk disease.

Given the need to establish more treatment options in mRCC, Keynote 426, an open-label, phase 3 trial [12], investigated the efficacy of the combination of pembrolizumab and axitinib (a VEGFR-targeted TKI) compared with sunitinib. A total of 861 patients with previously untreated advanced RCC were randomly assigned to receive pembrolizumab 200 mg intravenously once every 3 weeks plus axitinib 5 mg orally twice daily or sunitinib 50 mg orally once daily for the first 4 weeks of each 6-week cycle. With a median follow-up for all patients of 30.6 months [13], the combination of pembrolizumab plus axitinib prolonged overall survival when compared to sunitinib (median OS NR versus 35.7 months, HR 0.68, 95%CI 0.55–0.85, $p < 0.001$) [14]. The median PFS for the combination cohort was 15.4 months (95%CI 12.7–18.9) compared to 11.1 months (95%CI 9.1–12.5) for the sunitinib group (HR 0.71, 95%CI 0.60–0.84, $p < 0.0001$). Furthermore, the objective response rate was 60% versus 40% ($p < 0.0001$), and the median duration of response was 23.5 months compared to 15.9 months. It is also important to highlight that the pembrolizumab plus axitinib showed a clinical benefit in all subgroups tested (including

IMDC risk and PD-L1 expression subgroups). Given the results of this trial, the US FDA approved this combination as first-line treatment for metastatic ccRCC.

CheckMate 9ER, an open-label multinational phase 3 trial, has subsequently compared the combination of nivolumab plus cabozantinib, a TKI and VEGF inhibitor, to sunitinib in patients with previously untreated advanced or metastatic RCC [15]. It is proposed that nivolumab's ability to prevent cancer from evading immune detection [16, 17] and cabozantinib's immunomodulatory and antiangiogenic properties [18, 19] may provide a synergistic effect for tumor immunosuppression. The investigators recently announced that the study met its primary endpoint of progression-free survival (PFS) at final analysis, as well as its secondary endpoints of OS and objective response rate at a pre-specified interim analysis. With a median follow-up of 18.1 months, median OS had not been reached in either treatment cohort [20]. The objective response rate was higher (55.7% for cabozantinib-nivolumab-treated patients versus 27.1% for patients treated with sunitinib), and the combination cabozantinib-nivolumab had a PFS benefit (median PFS 16.6 months for cabozantinib-nivolumab versus 8.3 months for sunitinib group, $p < 0.0001$); this benefit was seen across predefined patient populations (i.e., IMDC risk status, tumor PD-L1 expression, and bone metastases). The most common AEs in the nivolumab plus cabozantinib group were diarrhea, fatigue, hepatotoxicity, and palmar-plantar erythrodysesthesia syndrome. The data from the CheckMate 9ER trial supports the combination of nivolumab plus cabozantinib as a first-line treatment option for patients with mRCC which was approved by the US FDA in January 2021.

Another phase 3 trial, JAVELIN Renal 101 [21, 22], has demonstrated significantly prolonged PFS with first-line avelumab (PD-L1 inhibitor) plus axitinib versus sunitinib in advanced RCC. Treatment-naive patients with mRCC were randomly assigned to receive avelumab 10 mg/kg intravenously every 2 weeks plus axitinib 5 mg orally twice daily or sunitinib 50 mg orally once daily for 4 weeks out of each 6-week cycle. Of the total of 886 patients who were enrolled in this study, 442 were randomized to the combination cohort and 444 to the sunitinib cohort. At a follow-up of 13 months, median PFS was 13.8 months (95%CI 10.1–20.7) in the avelumab plus axitinib group compared to 7.0 months (95%CI 5.7–9.6) in the sunitinib group [22]. In the avelumab plus axitinib cohort, objective responses occurred in 30.7% and 51.2% of patients at the 7-week and 13-week landmark, respectively, compared to 7.1% and 20% of patients in the sunitinib cohort, respectively. The mean duration of response was longer in the avelumab plus axitinib cohort than in the sunitinib cohort at the 13-week landmark. Of note, it is important to highlight that neither the expression of PD-L1 nor tumor mutational burden differentiated the PFS in either treatment cohort. Ultimately given the results of the JAVELIN Renal 101, the US FDA approved the combination of avelumab/axitinib for first-line treatment of ccRCC in May 2019 [21].

In addition, the KEYNOTE-581/CLEAR study [23, 24], a multicenter, randomized, open-label phase 3 trial, evaluated the efficacy of the combination of lenvatinib plus everolimus (two targeted therapies) or the combination of lenvatinib plus pembrolizumab compared to the standard first-line therapy with sunitinib as a single agent in patients with advanced or mRCC. In particular, in line with the recently published data of this study, a total of 1069 patients were randomly assigned to receive lenvatinib plus pembrolizumab, lenvatinib plus everolimus, or sunitinib.

Patients in the lenvatinib plus pembrolizumab group achieved a significantly longer PFS of 23.9 months compared to 9.2 months in the sunitinib group (HR 0.39, 95%CI 0.32 to 0.49, $p < 0.001$). Despite the fact that the median OS in the pembrolizumab plus lenvatinib group was longer over sunitinib group (but not reached), this benefit was not observed in the lenvatinib plus everolimus group compared to sunitinib group. Regarding the ORR, 71.0%, 53.5%, and 36.1% were achieved in the lenvatinib plus pembrolizumab, lenvatinib plus everolimus, and sunitinib, respectively. Similar percentages of grade ≥ 3 were reported among the groups, and in at least 10% of the patients in any group, hypertension, diarrhea, and elevated lipase levels were the most common grade ≥ 3. Consequently, this combination adds more to treatment armamentarium for patients with mRCC.

Lastly, the phase 3 trial, IMmotion 151, improved PFS favoring the combination of atezolizumab (a PD-L1 inhibitor) plus bevacizumab (anti-VEGF) group compared to the sunitinib group [25]. Of a total of 915 patients who were enrolled, 454 were randomly assigned to the atezolizumab plus bevacizumab cohort and 461 patients were treated with sunitinib. Forty percent (362/915) of the patients had PD-L1-positive tumors. The PD-L1-positive population achieved a median PFS of 11.2 months in the combination of atezolizumab plus bevacizumab group compared to those in sunitinib group, who achieved a PFS of 7.7 months (HR 0.74, 95%CI 0.57–0.96; $p = 0.0217$). The combination demonstrated a better side effect profile with 40% of patients in the atezolizumab plus bevacizumab group and 54% in the sunitinib group experiencing treatment-related grade 3/4 adverse events (the most common AE reported in both groups was hypertension (14% versus 17%, respectively) followed by proteinuria and diarrhea. Fatigue was also reported as a frequent AE (<5%) in the atezolizumab plus bevacizumab group, while thrombocytopenia (5%) and palmar-plantar erythrodysesthesia (9%) were commonly reported in the sunitinib group). Additionally, only 5% in the atezolizumab plus bevacizumab group compared to 8% in the sunitinib group discontinued treatment because of adverse events.

Interestingly, a subgroup analysis of the IMmotion 151 clinical trial was conducted in previously untreated patients with advanced or mRCC and sarcomatoid features [26]. Patients whose tumor had any component of sarcomatoid features were included and received atezolizumab plus bevacizumab ($n = 68$) or sunitinib ($n = 74$). Median PFS was significantly longer in the group receiving atezolizumab plus bevacizumab overall (8.3 versus 5.3 months; HR 0.52, 95%CI 0.34–0.79) as well as a further subset of patients with PD-L1-positive tumors and sarcomatoid features (8.6 versus 5.6 months; HR 0.45, 95%CI 0.26–0.77). Patients treated with atezolizumab plus bevacizumab achieved an ORR of 49% versus 14% in sunitinib-treated patients, including complete responses of 10% versus 3% of patients treated with sunitinib. While encouraging that this combination can improve PFS, this combination has not received FDA approval, and expanded follow-up is warranted to evaluate for further survival benefits.

Additionally, a subgroup analysis of the CheckMate 214 clinical trial investigated the efficacy of the combination of nivolumab plus ipilimumab compared to sunitinib in a total of 145 patients with sarcomatoid RCC (sRCC) (139 patients with intermediate−/poor-risk disease and 6 with favorable risk) [27]. In the intermediate−/poor-risk disease patients, median OS was not reached in the combination ICI

Table 15.2 NCCN guidelines for first-line treatment of relapsed or metastatic renal cell carcinoma (Version 3.2022)

	Preferred regimens	Other recommended regimens
IMDC favorable risk	Axitinib + pembrolizumab (1) Cabozantinib + nivolumab (1) Lenvatinib + pembrolizumab (1)	Ipilimumab + nivolumab (2A) Cabozantinib (2B) Axitinib+ avelumab (2A) Pazopanib (2A) Sunitinib (2A)
IMDC intermediate/poor risk	Ipilimumab + nivolumab (1) Axitinib + pembrolizumab (1) Nivolumab + cabozantinib (1) Lenvatinib + pembrolizumab (1) Cabozantinib (2A)	Pazopanib (2A) Sunitinib (2A) Axitinib + avelumab (2A)

1 = based on one randomized controlled phase 3 trial
2A = based on at least one randomized controlled phase 2 trial

group compared to 14.5 months in the sunitinib group (HR 0.45, $p = 0.004$). Further, the median PFS was 26.5 months compared to 5.1 months (95%CI 0.33–0.86; $p = 0.0093$), while the ORR was 60.8% versus 23.1%, respectively. These findings are similar to other subgroup analyses that have supported the efficacy of ICI-based therapies in individuals with sRCC. These studies include KEYNOTE-426 which demonstrated improved outcomes with pembrolizumab-axitinib (12-month OS of 83.4%, ORR of 58.8%, and CR of 11.8%), JAVELIN Renal 101 which showed improved outcomes with avelumab-axitinib (12-month OS 8%, ORR of 47%, and CR of 4%), and IMmotion151 which showed improved outcomes with atezolizumab-bevacizumab (12-month OS69%, ORR 49%, CR of 10%). The genetic heterogeneity of sRCC may play a role in determining why certain individuals respond to ICIs, while others do not. Particularly, mutations in *TP53*, *NF2*, and other members of the Hippo pathway, *CDKN2A/2B, PI3K, BAP1,* and enrichment of TGF-β signaling are growing areas of interest for understanding the mechanisms of ICI resistance [28].

Table 15.2 summarizes the current NCCN guidelines for patients with either relapsed or stage IV disease.

In summary, first-line treatment options for mRCC have significantly expanded to pure immunotherapy combinations and to combinations of immunotherapy checkpoint inhibitors with tyrosine kinase inhibitors of the VEGFR pathway. Importantly, patients with mRCC are achieving complete responses and durable responses. Clinical questions that remain for patients achieving responses will include when patients can safely discontinue treatment and when (if a primary is intact) patients can optimally undergo cytoreductive nephrectomy.

Immunotherapy in the Adjuvant Setting in Patients with Local/Locally Advanced RCC

In individuals with localized RCC, the main staple of therapy is surgical resection. Following resection, disease progression usually occurs in distant sites via circulating tumor cells and micrometastases from the primary tumor. Targeting micrometastases by initiating immunotherapy after surgical resection of the primary tumor, when the tumor burden is lowest, is a promising new line of adjuvant treatment. Conducting adjuvant clinical trials provides the opportunity to determine biomarkers associated with recurrence as well as predictive biomarkers for response to treatment [29].

There are multiple trials investigating the administration of immunotherapy in the adjuvant setting in RCC, including at least three purely adjuvant studies. In particular, IMmotion 010 is a phase 3, multicenter, randomized, placebo-controlled, double-blind study aiming to evaluate the efficacy and safety of the administration of atezolizumab versus placebo in patients with RCC who are at high risk of disease recurrence following nephrectomy. The participants in the experimental cohort received atezolizumab 1200 mg IV infusion every 3 weeks for 16 cycles (each cycle = 21 days) or 1 year (whichever occurs first), whereas patients in the control cohort received intravenous placebo for the same time frame. The CheckMate 914 trial (NCT03138512) is an ongoing phase 3 clinical trial with a target enrollment of approximately 1600 randomized patients across 22 countries. Checkmate 914 randomizes patients to nivolumab alone or nivolumab with ipilimumab or placebo and aims to evaluate these treatments for efficacy in delaying recurrence of cancer in patients after partial or full nephrectomy. In the first part of the trial, patients are randomized 1:1 to receive nivolumab plus ipilimumab or placebo infusions. In the second part, patients are randomized 1:1:2 to receive nivolumab plus ipilimumab, placebo infusions, or nivolumab with ipilimumab placebo. All treatments are given for 24 weeks or until evidence of disease recurrence, unacceptable toxicity, or withdrawal of consent [30]. Finally, the Keynote-564 study (NCT03142334) aims to evaluate the safety and efficacy of pembrolizumab in the adjuvant treatment of adult participants who have intermediate-high- or high-risk localized disease and had undergone nephrectomy or who had oligometastatic disease and had undergone metastasectomy, without evidence of residual disease. 496 patients in the experimental cohort received pembrolizumab 200 mg IV infusion every 3 weeks for up to 17 cycles, while 498 patients in the control cohort received placebo IV infusion every 3 weeks [31, 32]. With a median follow-up of 24.1 months, patients treated with pembrolizumab had improved disease-free survival (HR 0.68, 95% CI 0.55–0.87, $p = 0.002$), with neither cohort meeting the median disease-free survival timepoint. Common any-grade adverse events included fatigue, diarrhea, pruritus, arthralgia, hypothyroidism, and rash, without any unexpected AEs. This represents the first positive trial in the adjuvant setting of clear cell RCC, approved for adjuvant treatment of RCC by the US FDA in November 2021. As of August 2021, only CheckMate 914 is currently still enrolling patients.

Lastly, the PROSPER RCC is an unblinded, phase 3 study in the National Clinical Trials Network that includes patients with RCC and clinical stage T2 or higher or any nodal disease planned for radical or partial nephrectomy. PROSPER RCC randomizes patients to either nephrectomy and standard postoperative follow-up or preoperative nivolumab, surgical resection, and then adjuvant nivolumab for up to a year [34]. This study aims to improve clinical outcomes by priming the immune system with neoadjuvant nivolumab prior to surgical resection of the tumor as well as continued immune system engagement with adjuvant nivolumab in patients with high-risk RCC. Only select patients with oligometastatic disease are included in the study, specifically if they undergo metastasectomy and do not have other evidence of disease. Patients will be stratified by clinical T stage, node positivity, and M stage. In order to improve historical 5-year DFS rates of 56% seen in the ASSURE trial to a hypothesized 70%, with 84.2% power, PROSPER RCC is set to enroll up to 807 patients and completed accrual in 2021. This study is also designed to evaluate improvements in OS and critical perioperative therapy considerations such as safety, feasibility, and quality of life metrics. Furthermore, the PROSPER RCC study also promises many translational studies to evaluate the contribution of the baseline immune microenvironment components on clinical outcomes. Ultimately, if positive, PROSPER RCC is poised to transform the current treatment paradigm for patients with localized, high-risk RCC.

Ongoing Clinical Trials in Metastatic RCC

Currently several ongoing clinical trials are investigating the role of immunotherapy treatments in patients with mRCC [33]. The randomized, multicenter phase 3 trial, PDIGREE trial (NCT03793166) [35], is based off of the survival improvements seen in both Checkmate 214 and Checkmate 9ER. PDIGREE investigates the efficacy of the combination of nivolumab plus ipilimumab, followed by either nivolumab with cabozantinib or nivolumab alone in patients with treatment-naïve, IMDC intermediate- or poor-risk mRCC. All patients are first treated with induction ipilimumab 1 mg/kg and nivolumab 3 mg/kg intravenously once every 3 weeks for up to four cycles. Following the initial 3-month radiographic evaluation, treatment is adapted for responses. Patients who achieve complete response continue with nivolumab 480 mg intravenously every 4 weeks as maintenance. Patients who demonstrate progressive disease will subsequently be switched to cabozantinib 60 mg oral daily. For patients without complete response or progressive disease (i.e., those with stable disease or partial responses), they are then randomized to nivolumab 480 mg intravenously every 4 weeks versus nivolumab 480 mg intravenously every 4 weeks with cabozantinib 40 mg oral daily. The participants will be stratified based on the IMDC risk group and presence of bone metastases. The investigators hypothesize that the 3-year OS will be improved to 70% for nivolumab-cabozantinib compared to 60% for nivolumab alone; with a power of 85% and two-sided alpha of 0.05, PDIGREE is set to randomize 696 patients and to potentially enroll up to 1046 patients. While the primary endpoint is 3-year OS, CR at 1 year, PFS, ORR are key secondary endpoints. Consolidative nephrectomy can be considered for those patients who will achieve excellent partial responses resulting in a prospective treatment discontinuation. As per investigators till January 2021, more than 300 patients are already enrolled in this study. Additionally, tissue- and plasma-based biomarkers will be evaluated to associate with treatment response or resistance.

Further building on the combination of cabozantinib and nivolumab, the COSMIC-313 study [36] is a global, randomized, placebo-controlled, double-blind phase 3 trial, with a planned enrollment of 676 patients, investigating the efficacy and safety of the concurrent administration of cabozantinib with nivolumab plus ipilimumab compared to nivolumab plus ipilimumab. Patients randomized to the combination cohort will receive cabozantinib 40 mg orally once daily plus nivolumab 3 mg/kg intravenously plus ipilimumab 1 mg/kg intravenously once every 3 weeks for four doses, followed by cabozantinib 40 mg orally once daily plus nivolumab 480 mg intravenously once every 4 weeks. The control cohort will receive a cabozantinib-matched placebo and the same treatment regimen for nivolumab plus ipilimumab. The main primary endpoint that drives the sample size of 676 patients is improvement of the PFS, while secondary endpoints include OS, objective response rate, duration of responses, and safety. Finally, correlation of biomarkers with clinical outcomes will also be evaluated.

Recently in a phase 1/2 study, the combination of bempegaldesleukin (BEMPEG), first-in-class pegylated interleukin-2, with nivolumab showed a manageable safety profile as well as an encouraging objective response rate of 46% in advanced RCC. Based on these results, the PIVOT 09 study [37], a global, multicenter, randomized, open-label phase 3 study, is also currently open and studying the efficacy and safety of the concurrent administration of BEMPEG plus nivolumab compared to investigator's choice of tyrosine kinase inhibitor (sunitinib or cabozantinib) in patients with previously untreated advanced or mRCC. Patients are randomized to receive either BEMPEG 0.006 mg/kg with 360 mg nivolumab intravenously every 3 weeks or sunitinib 50 mg orally daily 4 weeks on, 2 weeks off schedule or 60 mg cabozantinib orally once daily. Objective response rate, OS, and PFS in the intermediate- and poor-risk population will be evaluated as well as safety, PD-L1 expression as a predictive biomarker, and quality of life [37].

To build on cabozantinib effect in previously treated mRCC, the open-label phase 3 study CONTACT-03 opened in July 2020 and is investigating the administration of atezolizumab plus cabozantinib versus cabozantinib monotherapy following progression on/after prior ICI treatment in patients with advanced/metastatic RCC. Patients enrolled to the CONTACT-03 trial will be randomized in two groups, receiving either atezolizumab intravenously 1200 mg every 3 weeks with cabozantinib 60 mg orally daily or cabozantinib 60 mg daily. The primary endpoints will be PFS and OS in the intent-to-treat (ITT) population. The secondary endpoints will be the investigator-assessed PFS per RECIST 1.1 criteria and the independent review and investigator-assessed ORR and DoR.

Finally, an important trial to note for multimodality care of renal cell carcinoma is the PROBE trial, which opened in the NCTN in November 2020 (NCT04510597). Importantly, for patients with synchronous metastatic RCC and intact primary, the CARMENA trial showed that starting sunitinib upfront is noninferior to cytoreductive nephrectomy followed by sunitinib. The PROBE trial is a phase 3 randomized trial of patients with intact primary and synchronous metastatic RCC. Patients are randomized to receiving any approved immunotherapy combinations or cytoreductive nephrectomy upfront, followed by any of the approved immunotherapy combinations.

Biomarkers for Immunotherapy in Metastatic Renal Cell Carcinoma

With multiple immunotherapy combinations, there is growing need to identify predictive biomarkers for patients with kidney cancer to select optimal treatment combinations and sequential treatments. Based on all first-line phase 3 trials of mRCC (Checkmate 214, Keynote 426, IMmotion 151, and JAVELIN Renal 101), PD-L1 status has not demonstrated a clear predictive response to ICIs. In these trials, the PD-L1 positivity has been shown to be more of a poor prognostic indicator than predictive of treatment effect, and patients with both PD-L1-negative and PD-L1-positive tumors tend to benefit from combination immunotherapy treatments over sunitinib. Tumor mutational burden (TMB) is another biomarker that has been used in other malignancies as a predictor for response to ICIs, notably gaining a tumor-agnostic indication for pembrolizumab in treatment of tumors with TMB greater than 10 mutations per megabase (muts/Mb) [38]. However, the tumor mutational burden for RCC is overall quite low. From the Memorial Sloan Kettering data, the TMB cutoff point for the top 20% of RCC cases was 5.9 muts/Mb, which is quite low compared with other tumor types, and suggests that few RCC tumors have "high TMB" by standard definitions, and the ICI treatment response likely stems from other mechanisms. Therefore, further biomarkers are needed to help guide treatment selection.

Notably, molecular classification by transcriptome gene expression can subtype RCC tumors, with some subsets of RCC tumors showing treatment response to atezolizumab monotherapy or in combination with bevacizumab [39]. Specifically, IMmotion 150, a randomized phase 2 trial studying atezolizumab monotherapy or combination with bevacizumab versus sunitinib in treatment-naïve metastatic RCC, investigated the importance of genes of tumor angiogenesis, pre-existing immunity, and immunosuppressive myeloid inflammation on treatment response. The study determined that high expression of angiogenic genes was associated with improved ORR (46% versus 9%) and PFS (HR 0.31, 95% CI, 0.18–0.55) when compared to low angiogenic gene expression. No difference in PFS was observed in the high angiogenic gene groups between combination or monotherapy groups and sunitinib. Interestingly, the study demonstrated improved PFS in individuals with low angiogenic gene expression when treated with combination ICI versus sunitinib (HR 0.59, 95%CI 0.35–0.98). High pre-existing immune response (High T_{eff}) compared to low T_{eff} was associated with improved ORR (49% versus 16%) and PFS (HR 0.50, 95%CI, 0.30–0.86). When compared across treatment groups, high Teff gene expression was associated with improved PFS in the combination group compared to sunitinib (HR 0.55, 95% CI 0.32–0.95). Further, high myeloid inflammatory gene signature (myeloid high) was associated with reduced PFS in the atezolizumab monotherapy group (HR 2.98, 95% CI 1.68–5.29) and combination group (HR 1.71, 95% CI 1.01–2.088). When compared across groups, myeloid high status was associated with worse PFS with atezolizumab monotherapy versus sunitinib (HR 2.03, 95% CI 1.21–3.40). Although still requiring further investigation, this study suggests that clinical benefit from immunotherapy treatments may be predicted by classifying genetic profiles with specific focus on tumor angiogenesis, pre-existing immunity, and myeloid inflammation.

Subsequently, a recent analysis from the IMmotion 151 trial performed transcriptomic evaluation of 823 tumors from advanced RCC patients and revealed 7 subtypes of RCC with distinct tumor molecular characteristics [40]. Subtypes were characterized by distinct angiogenesis, immune, cell cycle, metabolism, and stromal programs. In particular, clusters 1 (angiogenic/stromal) and 2 (angiogenic) are characterized by high angiogenesis with higher stroma-specific expression in cluster 1 and increased catabolic metabolism in cluster 2. Group 3 (complement/oxidation) demonstrated high expression of the complement cascade as well as high expression of Ω-oxidation-related genes. In clusters 4, 5, and 6, the cell cycle transcriptional programs are enriched. Specifically, in cluster 4 (t-effector/proliferative), there is a strong enrichment in T-effector, JAK/STAT, and interferon-α and interferon-ɣ signature, cluster 5 (proliferative) showed a high expression of the FAS/pentose phosphate pathway-associated genes, and cluster 6 (stromal/proliferative) demonstrated high expression of both the epithelial-mesenchymal transition (EMT) transcriptional module and the collagen-/fibroblast-associated stromal genes. Finally, in cluster 7, high expression of small nucleolar RNA (snoRNA) was identified, which is associated with carcinogenesis [41].

The authors evaluated clinical outcomes to atezolizumab plus bevacizumab and sunitinib in each cluster. Patients with angiogenic clusters (1 and 2) demonstrated longer PFS in both treatment groups, suggesting better outcomes regardless of treatment. Conversely, those in the group 6 (stromal/proliferative) had shorter PFS in both groups. When compared across treatment groups, atezolizumab plus bevacizumab demonstrated improved OR rate (52.0% versus 19.4%, $p < 0.001$) and PFS (HR 0.52, 95%CI 0.33–0.92) versus sunitinib in cluster 4 (t-effector/proliferative). Similar improved outcomes were seen in cluster 5 (proliferative cluster) and cluster 7 (snoRNA cluster) [41]. These findings further suggest that molecularly stratifying patient tumors may help predict patient response to ICI and antiangiogenic therapies.

Germline HLA-I evolutionary divergence (HED) may also represent a promising predictive biomarker for ICI treatment response in mRCC. HED is associated with response to ICIs in patients treated for cancer and with the diversity of tumor, viral, and human immunopeptidomes [42]. Compared with TMB, which can be challenging to accurately estimate due to tumor purity or clonal fraction, HED can be reliably inferred from normal tissue DNA sequencing. It is possible that combining information of HED with TMB may help us identify patients who are most likely to benefit from ICI therapy, but further prospective validation will be needed before clinical use of this biomarker [42].

Another gene which initially seemed promising for predicting ICI response is *PBRM1*. *PBRM1* mutations occur commonly in RCC, and an initial study demonstrated better responses and better survival for patients with *PBRM1* mutations when treated with nivolumab [43]. Specifically, the odds ratio for *PBRM1*-mutated disease among the responders versus the nonresponders was statistically significant [9]. However, there were nonresponders to nivolumab who also had the *PBRM1* mutation, and subsequent analysis did not show that *PBRM1* mutations could predict for treatment response from the combination of atezolizumab and bevacizumab [25]. Therefore, *PBRM1* mutations cannot be used independently to predict for ICI response.

In summary, multiple genomic, transcriptomic, and protein-level biomarkers are being explored in mRCC. Ultimately, prospective validation of promising biomarkers will help oncologists and patients with treatment selection. Identifying and validating predictive biomarkers will be necessary for individualizing immunotherapy selection and sequencing in the era of precision oncology.

Conclusions and Multimodality Care in Renal Cell Carcinoma in the Immunotherapy Era

The standard of care for patients with mRCC is rapidly changing with multiple approvals of immunotherapy agents and combinations. Both first- and second-line treatments centered on immunotherapy are becoming mainstays for mRCC treatment. Ongoing clinical questions pertaining to multimodality care include timing of cytoreductive nephrectomy for patients who have synchronous metastatic RCC, the utility and timing of perioperative immunotherapy treatment, as well as utility and timing of radiation therapy. The identification of new predictive markers will also play an important role to better understand the tumor microenvironment and guide treatment selection. Currently, there is significant investigation into multimodality strategies for patients with both mRCC and local RCC in attempts to identify the optimal treatment plan for each patient. Surgical and radiation treatment modalities will undoubtedly have their roles, and ongoing trials will provide evidence for optimal treatment sequencing.

References

1. Patel HD, Gupta M, Joice GA, et al. Clinical stage migration and survival for renal cell carcinoma in the United States. Eur Urol Oncol. 2019;2(4):343–8.
2. Heng DYC, Xie W, Regan MM, et al. Prognostic factors for overall survival in patients with metastatic renal cell carcinoma treated with vascular endothelial growth factor-targeted agents: results from a large, multicenter study. J Clin Oncol. 2009;27(34):5794–9.
3. Frfrs G. Results of treatment of 255 patients with metastatic renal cell carcinoma who received high-dose recombinant interleukin-2 therapy. J Clin Oncol. 1995;13(3):688–96.
4. Fisher RI, Rosenberg SA, Sznol M, Parkinson DR, Fyfe G. High-dose aldesleukin in renal cell carcinoma: long-term survival update. Cancer J Sci Am. 1997;3(Suppl 1):S70–2.
5. Rosenberg SA, Yang JC, White DE, Steinberg SM. Durability of complete responses in patients with metastatic cancer treated with high-dose interleukin-2: identification of the antigens mediating response. Ann Surg. 1998;228(3):307–19.
6. Schwartz RN, Stover L, Dutcher JP. Managing toxicities of high-dose interleukin-2. Oncology (Williston Park). 2002;16(11 Suppl 13):11–20.

7. NCCN Guidelines for Treatment of Cancer by Site. National Comprehensive Cancer Network. 2019;20:2020.
8. Murphy KA, James BR, Guan Y, Torry DS, Wilber A, Griffith TS. Exploiting natural anti-tumor immunity for metastatic renal cell carcinoma. Hum Vaccin Immunother. 2015;11(7):1612–20.
9. Motzer RJ, Escudier B, McDermott DF, et al. Nivolumab versus everolimus in advanced renal-cell carcinoma. N Engl J Med [Internet] 2015;373(19):1803–13. Available from: http://www.ncbi.nlm.nih.gov/pubmed/26406148.
10. Motzer RJ, Rini BI, McDermott DF, et al. Nivolumab plus ipilimumab versus sunitinib in first-line treatment for advanced renal cell carcinoma: extended follow-up of efficacy and safety results from a randomised, controlled, phase 3 trial. Lancet Oncol. 2019;20(10):1370–85.
11. Albiges L, Tannir NM, Burotto M, et al. Nivolumab plus ipilimumab versus sunitinib for first-line treatment of advanced renal cell carcinoma: extended 4-year follow-up of the phase III CheckMate 214 trial. ESMO open [Internet]. 2020;5(6):e001079. Available from: http://www.ncbi.nlm.nih.gov/pubmed/33246931
12. Rini BI, Plimack ER, Stus V, et al. Pembrolizumab plus axitinib versus sunitinib for advanced renal-cell carcinoma. N Engl J Med. 2019;380(12):1116–27.
13. Powles T, Plimack ER, Soulières D, et al. Pembrolizumab plus axitinib versus sunitinib monotherapy as first-line treatment of advanced renal cell carcinoma (KEYNOTE-426): extended follow-up from a randomised, open-label, phase 3 trial. Lancet Oncol [Internet]. 2020;21(12):1563–73. Available from: http://www.ncbi.nlm.nih.gov/pubmed/33284113.
14. Plimack ER, Rini BI, Viktor Stus V, et al. Pembrolizumab plus axitinib versus sunitinib as first-line therapy for advanced renal cell carcinoma (RCC): updated analysis of KEYNOTE-426. J Clin Oncol. 2020;38:15_suppl.5001.
15. Choueiri TK, Apolo AB, Powles T, et al. A phase 3, randomized, open-label study of nivolumab combined with cabozantinib vs sunitinib in patients with previously untreated advanced or metastatic renal cell carcinoma (RCC; CheckMate 9ER). J Clin Oncol. 2018;36:15_suppl.TPS4598.
16. Wang C, Thudium KB, Han M, et al. In vitro characterization of the anti-PD-1 antibody nivolumab, BMS-936558, and in vivo toxicology in non-human primates. Cancer Immunol Res. 2014;2(9):846–56.
17. Ribas A, Wolchok JD. Cancer immunotherapy using checkpoint blockade. Science. 2018;359(6382):1350–5.
18. Apolo AB, Nadal R, Girardi DM, et al. Phase I study of cabozantinib and nivolumab alone or with Ipilimumab for advanced or metastatic urothelial carcinoma and other genitourinary tumors. J Clin Oncol. 2020;38(31):3672–84.
19. Apolo AB, Nadal R, Tomita Y, et al. Cabozantinib in patients with platinum-refractory metastatic urothelial carcinoma: an open-label, single-centre, phase 2 trial. Lancet Oncol. 2020;21(8):1099–109.
20. Choueiri TK, Powles T, Burotto M, et al. Nivolumab plus cabozantinib versus sunitinib for advanced renal-cell carcinoma. N Engl J Med [Internet] 2021;384(9):829–41. Available from: http://www.ncbi.nlm.nih.gov/pubmed/33657295.
21. Motzer RJ, Penkov K, Haanen J, et al. Avelumab plus axitinib versus sunitinib for advanced renal-cell carcinoma. N Engl J Med. 2019;380(12):1103–15.
22. Choueiri TK, Motzer RJ, Rini BI, et al. Updated efficacy results from the JAVELIN renal 101 trial: first-line avelumab plus axitinib versus sunitinib in patients with advanced renal cell carcinoma. Ann Oncol Off J Eur Soc Med Oncol. 2020;31(8):1030–9.
23. Motzer R, Alekseev B, Rha S-Y, et al. Lenvatinib plus Pembrolizumab or Everolimus for advanced renal cell carcinoma. N Engl J Med [Internet] 2021;Available from: http://www.ncbi.nlm.nih.gov/pubmed/33616314.
24. Grünwald V, Powles T, Choueiri TK, et al. Lenvatinib plus everolimus or pembrolizumab versus sunitinib in advanced renal cell carcinoma: study design and rationale. Future Oncol. 2019;15(9):929–41.
25. Rini BI, Powles T, Atkins MB, et al. Atezolizumab plus bevacizumab versus sunitinib in patients with previously untreated metastatic renal cell carcinoma (IMmotion151): a mul-

ticentre, open-label, phase 3, randomised controlled trial. Lancet (London, England). 2019;393(10189):2404–15.
26. Rini BI, Motzer RJ, Powles T, et al. Atezolizumab plus bevacizumab versus sunitinib for patients with untreated metastatic renal cell carcinoma and sarcomatoid features: a prespecified subgroup analysis of the IMmotion151 clinical trial. Eur Urol. 2020;
27. Tannir NM, Signoretti S, Choueiri TK, et al. Efficacy and safety of nivolumab plus ipilimumab versus sunitinib in first-line treatment of patients with advanced sarcomatoid renal cell carcinoma. Clin Cancer Res. 2021;27(1):78–86.
28. Hwang JK, Agarwal N, Brugarolas J, Zhang T. Checking the hippo in sarcomatoid renal cell carcinoma with immunotherapy. Clin Cancer Res. 2021;27(1):5–7.
29. Chowdhury N, Drake CG. Kidney cancer: an overview of current therapeutic approaches. Urol Clin North Am. 2020;47(4):419–31.
30. Bex A, Russo P, Yoshihiko Tomita Y, et al. A phase III, randomized, placebo-controlled trial of nivolumab or nivolumab plus ipilimumab in patients with localized renal cell carcinoma at high-risk of relapse after radical or partial nephrectomy (CheckMate 914). J Clin Oncol. 2020;38:15_suppl.TPS5099.
31. Choueiri TK, Quinn DI, Zhang T, et al. KEYNOTE-564: a phase 3, randomized, double blind, trial of pembrolizumab in the adjuvant treatment of renal cell carcinoma. J Clin Oncol. 2018;36:15_suppl.TPS4599.
32. Choueiri TK, Tomczak P, Park B, et al. Adjuvant pembrolizumab after nephrectomy in renal cell carcinoma. N Engl J Med. 2021;385:683–94.
33. Zhang T, Hwang JK, George DJ, Pal SK. The landscape of contemporary clinical trials for untreated metastatic clear cell renal cell carcinoma. Cancer Treat Res Commun. 2020;24:100183.
34. Haas NB, Puligandla M, Allaf ME, et al. versus observation in patients with renal cell carcinoma (RCC) undergoing nephrectomy (ECOG-ACRIN EA8143). J Clin Oncol. 2020;38:15_suppl.TPS5101.
35. Zhang T, Ballman KV, Choudhury AD, et al. PDIGREE: an adaptive phase III trial of PD-inhibitor nivolumab and ipilimumab (IPI-NIVO) with VEGF TKI cabozantinib (CABO) in metastatic untreated renal cell cancer (Alliance A031704). J Clin Oncol. 2020;38:15_suppl.TPS5100.
36. Choueiri TK, Albiges L, Powles T, et al. A phase III study (COSMIC-313) of cabozantinib (C) in combination with nivolumab (N) and ipilimumab (I) in patients (pts) with previously untreated advanced renal cell carcinoma (aRCC) of intermediate or poor risk. J Clin Oncol. 2020;38:6_suppl.TPS767.
37. Tannir NM, Agarwal N, Pal SK, et al. PIVOT-09: a phase III randomized open-label study of bempegaldesleukin (NKTR-214) plus nivolumab versus sunitinib or cabozantinib (investigator's choice) in patients with previously untreated advanced renal cell carcinoma (RCC). J Clin Oncol. 2020;38:6_suppl.TPS763.
38. Samstein RM, Lee C-H, Shoushtari AN, et al. Tumor mutational load predicts survival after immunotherapy across multiple cancer types. Nat Genet. 2019;51(2):202–6.
39. McDermott DF, Huseni MA, Atkins MB, et al. Clinical activity and molecular correlates of response to atezolizumab alone or in combination with bevacizumab versus sunitinib in renal cell carcinoma. Nat Med. 2018;24(6):749–57.
40. Motzer RJ, Banchereau R, Hamidi H, et al. Molecular subsets in renal cancer determine outcome to checkpoint and angiogenesis blockade. Cancer Cell. 2020;38(6):803–817.e4.
41. Braicu C, Zimta A-A, Harangus A, et al. The function of non-coding RNAs in lung cancer tumorigenesis. Cancers (Basel). 2019;11(5)
42. Chowell D, Krishna C, Pierini F, et al. Evolutionary divergence of HLA class I genotype impacts efficacy of cancer immunotherapy. Nat Med. 2019;25(11):1715–20.
43. Miao D, Margolis CA, Gao W, et al. Genomic correlates of response to immune checkpoint therapies in clear cell renal cell carcinoma. Science. 2018;359(6377):801–6.

Chapter 16
Evolving Treatment in Non-muscle-Invasive Bladder Cancer

Benjamin M. Eilender, Andrew B. Katims, John L. Pfail, and John Sfakianos

Introduction

Bladder cancer is the fifth most common malignancy in the United States with an estimated 81,400 new cases in 2020. This represents 4.5% of all new cancer cases in the United States. There was an estimated 17,980 deaths in the United States attributed to bladder cancer in 2020, which equates to 3.0% of all cancer-related deaths during this period [1, 2]. Non-muscle-invasive bladder cancer (NMIBC) is defined as malignancy of the bladder without invasion of the detrusor muscle layer of the bladder and possibly the deeper layers. NMIBC accounts for approximately 70–80% of new bladder cancer diagnosis and includes Ta, T1, and carcinoma in situ (CIS) disease stages [3]. NMIBC encompasses a wide range of disease pathology, ranging from low-grade, superficial cancer with a relatively benign disease process to a potentially very aggressive invasive cancer. Overall, the cancer-specific survival (CSS) for NMIBC at 15 years is as high as 85%, which is significantly higher than that of muscle-invasive bladder cancer (MIBC) [4]. The range of treatment options for patients with NMIBC continues to evolve with the improvement in understanding of the disease process. Yet, effective treatment of NMIBC still presents a substantial challenge for clinicians and financial burden on the US healthcare system.

This chapter will first touch upon the tumor genetics, biology, and risk stratification of NMIBC. Then, the focus will shift to the various treatment options for NMIBC, beginning with endoscopic surgical management of NMIBC and surveillance of the disease. Further treatment with intravesical chemotherapies and immunotherapies which are currently being used and trialed will then be discussed. Emerging therapies with the latest areas of focus in treatment for NMIBC including

B. M. Eilender · A. B. Katims · J. L. Pfail · J. Sfakianos (✉)
Department of Urology, Icahn School of Medicine, New York, NY, USA
e-mail: Benjamin.eilender@mountsinai.org; Andrew.katims@mountsinai.org; John.Pfail@icahn.mssm.edu; john.sfakianos@mountsinai.org

K. L. Stratton, A. K. Morgans (eds.), *Urologic Oncology*,
https://doi.org/10.1007/978-3-030-89891-5_16

gene therapy, viral therapy, and enhanced chemotherapies with their relevant studies are included. Finally, the chapter concludes with surveillance protocols and the role for early cystectomy in patients with NMIBC.

Tumor Biology, Genetics, and Risk Stratification

Tumor Biology and Genetics

The understanding of NMIBC tumor genetics, grading, and staging is essential for full comprehension of the disease. The pathologic grading system created by the World Health Organization (WHO) and the International Society of Urologic Pathology (ISUP) in 1998 for urothelial carcinoma (UC) of the bladder is accepted as the gold standard for classification for Ta and T1 UC tumors. This classification system includes the full range of non-muscle-invasive bladder tumors including hyperplastic regions (flat and papillary), flat lesions with atypia (carcinoma in situ (CIS)), dysplasia and reactive atypia, and noninvasive papillary neoplasms (papilloma, papillary carcinoma of varying grades, and papillary neoplasm of low malignant potential (PUNLMP)) [5, 6]. Broadly, NMIBC can be divided into two groups, low-grade or high-grade tumors [7]. Pathological grading, low-grade versus high-grade, continues to be the most significant prognostic factor when evaluating NMIBC. Low-grade versus high-grade NMIBC urothelial carcinoma can be dichotomized into two distinct disease processes, based on different tumor behavior, genetic mutations, tumor development, and treatment options [8]. Low-grade, noninvasive, papillary tumors tend to follow the tumorigenesis cascade of either a loss of heterozygosity of parts of chromosome 9, oncogenic mutations that lead to the overexpression of fibroblast growth factor 3 (FGFR3), or increased expression of the RAS pathway [9]. The tumorigenesis pathway of higher-grade urothelial carcinoma, including disease variants such as CIS, T1, and muscle-invasive bladder cancer (MIBC), often involves chromosomal aneuploidy, especially chromosomes 7, 9, and 17 and/or increased expression of pRb, p53, and/or p21 [10–13]. It is important to understand differences in NMIBC tumor tumorigenesis characteristics and pathways when exploring potential pathways to target for treatment options.

Risk Stratification

Risk stratification for NMIBC holds significant predictive implications for disease characteristics and therefore dictates therapeutic options offered to patients. The European Organization for Research and Treatment of Cancer (EORTC) risk calculator is a frequently used tool to predict Ta/T1 NMIBC disease recurrence and progression at 1 and 5 years. The EORTC nomogram looks at number of tumors, tumor size, Ta vs T1 disease, CIS prevalence, and presence of previously documented disease recurrence with recurrence frequency [14]. Although frequently used, there are limitations to the EORTC tool, including lack of real-life applicability to more recent patient groups who have received intravesical chemotherapy, immunotherapy, or restaging TURBT [15]. The American Urological Association (AUA) and Society of Urologic Oncology (SUO) have developed a risk stratification system to divide patients with NMIBC urothelial carcinoma into low-risk, intermediate-risk, and high-risk disease. Low-risk NMIBC is classified as any low-grade, Ta, solitary urothelial carcinoma growth ≤3 cm, or papillary urothelial neoplasm of low malignant potential. Intermediate-risk disease includes low-grade Ta solitary lesion greater than 3 cm, multifocal low-grade Ta disease, low-grade Ta with recurrence within 1 year, high-grade Ta ≤ 3 cm, or low-grade T1 disease. High-risk NMIBC includes high-grade T1, recurrent high-grade Ta, CIS, variant histology, any BCG failure in a high-grade patient, any presence of lymphovascular invasion or high-grade prostatic urethral involvement, high-grade Ta > 3 cm, and/or multifocal high-grade Ta [15] (Table 16.1).

Summary
- The term NMIBC encompasses any variant of bladder cancer that does not invade into the muscular layer.
- Pathologically, NMIBC can be subdivided into low-grade or high-grade disease.
- Low-grade and high-grade NMIBC follow different tumorigenesis pathways.
- The AUA and SUO risk-stratify NMIBC into low-risk, intermediate-risk, and high-risk disease, which is important when determining treatment options for patients.

Endoscopic/Cystoscopic Treatment and Management

Endoscopic management is the mainstay treatment option for NMIBC. Patients referred to urologists for suspicion of bladder tumor should undergo some form of cystoscopy. Cystoscopy allows for direct visualization of the bladder and allows for identification of potential bladder tumor(s) while concurrently assessing the number, size, and location of tumor(s) prior to attempted surgical resection.

Transurethral Resection of Bladder Tumor (TURBT)

Transurethral resection of bladder tumor (TURBT) is the most important first step in management of bladder cancer, for both NMIBC and muscle-invasive bladder cancer (MIBC). It provides diagnostic, both pathologic and staging, and therapeutic utility to the patient. The goal of original TURBT is to remove all visible tumor if possible, as the presence of residual bladder tumor after original TURBT is associated with higher risk of neoplasm recurrence [16]. Before beginning the resection,

Table 16.1 Risk stratification of NMIBC based on AUA/SUO classification system

NMIBC Risk-stratification based on AUA/SUO Classification

Low-risk	**Intermediate-risk**	**High-risk**
Low-grade solitary Ta ≤3 cm	*Low-grade T1, multifocal low-grade Ta*	*CIS, variant histology, lymphovascular invasion*
Papillary urothelial neoplasm of low malignant potential	*High-grade Ta ≤3 cm*	*High-grade T1*
	Solitary low-grade Ta >3cm	*Recurrent high-grade Ta, high grade Ta >3cm or multifocal*
	Recurrence < 1yr, Low-grade Ta	*BCG failure in high-grade*
		High-grade prostatic urethral involvement

it is imperative to do a bimanual exam to assess for any palpable masses or a fixed bladder to assess clinical staging. While performing a TURBT, it is important to note the number and size of lesions, the gross appearance of the tumor, and involvement of critical structures including the trigone, ureteral orifices, or prostatic urethra [17]. Both bipolar and monopolar electrocautery are acceptable options for TURBT of NMIBC as there is no statistically significant difference between the two in terms of disease recurrence or risk of bladder perforation, although bipolar TURBT is associated with decreased resection time, need for blood transfusion, risk of TUR syndrome, and length of hospital stay postoperatively and is therefore more commonly used in clinical practice today [18, 19].

Achieving a complete resection of all visible bladder tumor on original TURBT can be technically very challenging. There are many surgical techniques that can be used to achieve this. One preferred method is the complete en bloc resection of the bladder tumor(s) (EBR). EBR involves complete resection of the tumor in one continuous resection bite instead of multiple smaller resections to achieve the same end point, compared to a fragmented resection. Ideally, the EBR also involves normal tissue at the ends of the specimen to assess for negative tumor margins when assessing for complete resection of tumor [20]. This approach provides a high-quality specimen with less electrocautery artifact with no difference in recurrence rates compared to non-EBR. But this technique can be limited by factors such as tumor size, location, and surgeon experience [21]. Further, laser EBR is a feasible and safe option and has been funded to be equally effective in terms of tumor excision and recurrence rates compared to resection with electrocautery [21].

Tumor location plays a key role in successful resection, with those located on the anterior bladder wall or dome often presenting more difficulties for the surgeon to reach when resecting. Often, one must apply abdominal pressure while limiting hydrodistension to get these anterior/dome tumors within distance to resect. Tumors in bladder diverticulum can also present challenges to the surgeon with innately no muscular layer present in this area of tissue. If concerned for bladder perforation from extensive resection, the surgeon should terminate the procedure and also stop filling the bladder. If an extraperitoneal perforation, often this can be treated conservatively with a large Foley catheter postoperatively. If an intraperitoneal bladder injury occurs, cystorrhaphy should be performed, in addition to placement of a large catheter. If extensive resection is performed and there is any concern for bladder perforation, no intravesical immunotherapy or chemotherapy should be instilled [22]. Close attention must also be paid while removing tumors on or near the ureteral orifices. Resecting near or at the distal ureter can cause acute obstruction to the renal unit or the potential refluxing of malignant cells into the upper tract. Because of this, one should only use the cutting function rather than coagulation while near a ureteral orifice and may leave a stent postoperatively if concerned for damage [5].

A complete resection should be performed at original TURBT. Regardless if all visible tumor is able to be resected at original TURBT, inclusion of the detrusor muscle layer must be involved during this first resection to ensure proper staging and to determine next steps of management. Often, for original resections where muscle is not present in the specimen, complete surgical resection is not achievable, or in the case of documented NMIBC on original resection that demonstrates high-grade T1 disease, it is necessary to perform repeat TURBT within 4–6 weeks from the primary tumor resection. Repeat TURBT for original resection showing T1 NMIBC within 4–6 weeks can lead to upstaging to MIBC and/or the discovery of new pathologic adverse risk factors in a significant number of patients. In patients with NMIBC with muscle present in original specimen, upstaging to MIBC occurred 2–28% of the time with repeat resection, while upstaging to MIBC from non-muscle-invasive disease can be seen in as high as 49% of repeat TURBTs in patients who have no muscle present in original sample [23, 24]. Other studies have shown that restaging TURBT in patients with high-risk non-muscle-invasive disease provides an improved tumor initial response rate to intravesical BCG therapy when compared to patients who underwent BCG without restaging resection. In one study, in the re-resection plus BCG group, 29% of patients had residual/recurrent tumor and 7% with disease progression at first follow-up surveillance cystoscopy, compared to 57% and 34%, respectively, in the group that did not undergo restaging TURBT [25]. In patients with persistent T1 NMIBC on original and restaging TURBT, the risk of eventual progression to T2 or muscle-invasive disease in the future can be as high to 80% [26].

Bladder biopsy followed by fulguration of suspicious lesions is another method of endoscopic management used in clinical practice for diagnosis and management of NMIBC. Biopsies can be focused, on areas of erythema or irregularity, when concerned for carcinoma in situ (CIS) or other suspicious looking tissue, or dispersed, truly random biopsies across the bladder, in patients deemed high risk for invasive disease, for example, patients with positive cytology but no visible lesions on cystoscopy. Some studies have shown very low yield to finding any additional form of NMIBC in true random biopsies, with only 8% of patients undergoing random biopsies being positive for malignancy. But these random samplings may be more useful in patients with positive high-grade cytology or in the presence of multifocal broad-based papillary tumors [27]. The current AUA guidelines do not recommend performing random bladder biopsies in patients at low risk for developing invasive urothelial carcinoma. There is no consensus if bladder biopsies are warranted in patients at high risk for developing muscle-invasive disease. Prostatic urethral biopsies or tissue sampling can also be considered if concerned for involvement of the prostatic urethra or to ensure negative distal margins of the bladder, especially if eventual orthotopic urinary diversion may be considered. But this must be weighed against the potential harm of seeding bladder tumor into prostatic urethra in patients with no known disease in the prostate and documented malignancy in the bladder [5].

There are several newer enhanced cystoscopy techniques that allow for better detection of intravesical tumors. Blue light cystoscopy (BLC) incorporates cystoscopy in combination with injection of 5-aminolevulenic acid (5-ALA) or hexaminolevulinate into the bladder which selectively enters the cytoplasm of abnormal urothelial cells and appears red under blue fluorescent light [28]. Studies have shown improved detection of CIS, superficial papillary tumors, and dysplasia with blue light technology and therefore decreased residual tumor rates and increased recurrence-free survival, when compared to the use of the regular white light cystoscopy (WLC). One phase 3 controlled study demonstrated 96% overall tumor detection with BLC, in comparison to 77% with standard WLC. In the subgroup analysis, BLC significantly outperformed WLC in detecting CIS (95% versus 68%) and dysplasia of the urothelium (93% versus 48%) [29, 30]. Narrowband imaging (NBI) is another advanced cystoscopic tool that can be offered for better detection of CIS and papillary tumors. NBI uses precise wavelengths of light that are better absorbed by hemoglobin, compared to WLC, and translates into better visualization of vascularity seen with neoplasms in the bladder. There is varying information as to the efficacy of NBI compared to the standard WLC. Many studies have shown increased detection of CIS with a significant decrease in cancer recurrence rates with NBI compared to WLC [31]. However, other literature shows no statistically significant difference in disease recurrence rates after transurethral resection between NBI and WLC groups [32, 33]. Overall, these more sensitive cystoscopy methods should be considered in patients with NMIBC to better detect tumor and allow for more complete resection.

Summary

- TURBT is the first step in management of NMIBC and provides both diagnostic and therapeutic utility to the clinician.
- Complete resection of tumor should be performed at original TURBT. Often there are technical challenges that can make complete resection difficult, based on tumor burden and location of tumor.
- Repeat TURBT showing non-muscle-invasive disease should be performed within 6 weeks of original resection.
- Enhanced cystoscopy techniques may be helpful in identifying tumors hard to see on regular white light cystoscopy.

Surveillance

Surveillance cystoscopy, urine cytology, urinary biomarkers, and upper tract imaging are the key modalities used to monitor disease recurrence and possible progression of NMIBC. Surveillance schedules should be determined based on risk stratification of a given patient. Patients are categorized into low-risk, intermediate-risk, or high-risk NMIBC as determined by AUA/SUO NMIBC guidelines which were previously described in Sect. 14.2 of this chapter [5, 15]. After initial treatment of patient with NMIBC, it is recommended for first surveillance cystoscopy to be within 3–4 months of original treatment. Low-risk patients with a negative first surveillance cystoscopy and in the absence of symptoms should be offered repeat cystoscopy at 6–9 months after first surveillance and annually thereafter for 5 years. At 5 years, if still no evidence of disease, patients and their urologist should undergo a shared decision-making process as to whether to continue forward with surveillance cystoscopies. If a low-risk Ta patient does have a solitary <1 cm papillary lesion seen on cystoscopy, the urologist may offer office fulguration instead of full TURBT. Upper tract imaging and cytology in these low-risk, asymptomatic patients without hematuria are not recommended. For intermediate-risk patients with a first negative surveillance cystoscopy at 3–4 months, urologists should perform repeat cystoscopy and urine cytology every 3–6 months for 2 years, every 6–12 months for years 3 and 4, and then annually every year after that. High-risk patients should undergo cystoscopy, cytology, and possible tumor markers every 3–4 months for years 1 and 2, every 6 months for years 3 and 4, and annually after that. For both intermediate- and high-risk patients, upper tract imaging should be considered every 1–2 years as part of upper tract surveillance [15]. If tumor recurrence does occur during the surveillance schedule described above, there is a restart of the timeline beginning with the latest recurrence as time zero (Table 16.2).

Factors that must be considered when placing a patient on a surveillance schedule for NMIBC in addition to risk category include likelihood for patient to adhere to protocols; patient's life expectancy, including overall medical comorbidities; and overall functional status [34]. One study showed that only about 40% of patients followed standardized surveillance protocols, with patients who were elderly, non-white, and with significant other comorbidities and favorable disease pathology being associated with a decrease in compliance with surveillance scheduling [35]. Adding to this problem is the ongoing poor compliance of physicians to guidelines for NMIBC. Though 82% of physicians would perform surveillance cystoscopy, less than 50% of physicians follow treatment guidelines in terms of intravesical therapy, repeat TURBT, and early cystectomy [36]. Although repeat cystoscopies are considered to be bothersome to many patients, one study shows that unless a less

Table 16.2 Recommended surveillance schedule for NMIBC

Recommended Surveillance NMIBC

Risk-stratifiction	Cystoscopy	Upper Tract Imaging	Cytology
Low-risk	Year 1: 3 months, 9-12 months Years 2-5: annual > Year 5: shared decision making	X	X
Intermediate-risk	Years 1-2: every 3-6 months Years 3-4: every 6-12 months ≥ Year 5: annual	✓ every 1-2 years	✓ Same as cystoscopy timeline
High-risk	Years 1-2: every 3-4 months Years 3-4: every 6 months ≥ Year 5: annual	✓ every 1-2 years	✓ Same as cystoscopy timeline

invasive test was as sensitive for picking up disease recurrence as cystoscopy, patients would not replace regular cystoscopies with a less invasive test such as urinary biomarkers [37].

Microscopic evaluation by a pathologist of urine cytology specimens plays a crucial and noninvasive role as an adjunctive test in surveillance protocols for patients with NMIBC. Urine cytology has a high specificity, in some studies up to 90%, but lower sensitivity, between 15 and 30%, especially in lower-grade UC tumors [5, 38]. Furthermore, there are newer tumor markers developed recently to supplement or replace the conventional urine cytology test. Some of the more frequently used urine tumor markers used include *Immunocyst*, *NMP22 BladderChek*, *UroVysion*, *BTA stat*, and *BTA TRAK*. Although many of the biomarkers listed above have shown promise, many with higher sensitivities compared to standard urine cytology, there is a lack of high-quality evidence, which has prevented many of these from being regularly implemented into practice guidelines [39]. The noninvasive urine monitoring test, Cxbladder Monitor, has shown utility to use in confirmation with a negative cystoscopy to rule out recurrent UC disease. In direct comparison to other noninvasive urinary monitoring tests including UroVysion FISH and NMP22 BladderChek, Cxbladder Monitor outperformed both in terms of sensitivity and negative predictive value [40]. Overall, the AUA guidelines do not recommend using biomarkers in place of cystoscopy and also recommend against using biomarkers, just as with cytology, in patients with low-risk disease and negative cystoscopy. Urinary biomarkers may be used in patients to assess response to intravesical treatment for NMIBC or to assist when urine cytology is indeterminate [15].

Upper tract disease monitoring is the final component of surveillance in NMIBC. Although early literature suggested the prevalence of upper tract urothelial carcinoma (UTUC) after primary bladder malignancy was in the range of 2–7%, other studies have shown the presence of UTUC in this patient population is less than 1%. Factors that independently led to increased occurrence of upper tract tumors include primary bladder tumors that are high grade, have CIS features, or are located in close proximity to the ureteral orifices [41]. As mentioned above, this explains why current AUA guidelines caution against upper tract imaging in low-risk patients without hematuria or other symptoms while recommending upper tract imaging in intermediate-risk and high-risk patients every 1–2 years [15]. Options for upper tract imaging include computed tomography urography (CTU), magnetic resonance urography (MRU), renal bladder ultrasound (RBUS), or retrograde ureteropyelogram. Selective cytology is a strategy implemented by some to monitor for isolated positive urine cytology of the upper tracts in surveillance of NMIBC. Though much of the literature demonstrates that with a history of superficial NMIBC and an absence of upper tract filling defects seen on imaging, it may not be beneficial to obtain selective cytologies [42]. Although uncommon in patients with NMIBC, those who do develop upper tract disease tend to have poor outcomes with high rates of mortality.

Summary

- Cystoscopy, urine cytology, upper tract imaging, and tumor biomarkers can all be used for surveillance of NMIBC.
- Surveillance schedules should be determined based on patient's risk stratification category (low vs intermediate vs high).
- For every disease recurrence, surveillance schedules should be restarted from time zero.
- Following regular, recommended surveillance cystoscopies and imaging can present challenges for both physician and patient.

Intravesical BCG

In addition to surgical resection, immunotherapy, particularly bacillus Calmette-Guerin (BCG), is an important treatment option for those harboring NMIBC [43]. With the advent of BCG, bladder cancer was one of the earliest cancers in which immunotherapy was employed.

Bacillus Calmette-Guerin (BCG)

BCG was first shown to prevent the growth of tumors in animal models by Old et al. in 1959 and was first used in humans in 1976 for treatment of recurrent superficial bladder tumors [44, 45]. Intravesical instillation of BCG remains the gold standard for patients with either intermediate- or high-risk NMIBC [46, 47].

Mechanism of Action

The exact mechanism of action of BCG in its ability to treat bladder cancer is not fully understood. However, the effect of BCG on stimulation of the immune system is well recognized [48]. A tentative model of the mechanism of action of BCG in bladder cancer begins with the attachment of live BCG to the urothelium followed by internalization of BCG by bladder cancer cells. In response to internalization of BCG, bladder cancer cells upregulate expression of MHC class II and ICAM-1 and secrete various cytokines. Th1 cytokines (IL-2, tumor necrosis factor, IL-12, and IFN-γ) and Th2 cytokines (IL-4, IL-5, IL-6, and IL-10) along with IL-8 and IL-17 are all involved. Cytotoxicity to bladder cancer cells proceeds through activation of natural killer cells and secretion of tumor necrosis factor-related apoptosis-inducing ligand (TRAIL) by polymorphonuclear cells and macrophages. Additionally, direct cytotoxicity by BCG might also have a role in recruitment of immune cells [49].

Induction and Maintenance Regimens

Induction with BCG is typically started 2–4 weeks after TURBT to allow for re-epithelialization of the bladder and reduce the potential for systemic absorption. In the absence of an infection or traumatic catheter placement, reconstituted BCG powder in 50 mL of saline is administered through a urethral catheter and held in place for 1 to 2 hours. Limiting fluids and diuretics 2 hours prior to instillation allows for ease of retention. There has been no evidence to support patients turning from side to side to coat the entire urothelium, though some clinicians still advocate for this practice [50, 51].

The optimal treatment schedule for BCG is yet to be established. All patients treated with BCG should undergo a 6-week induction course, though induction alone is likely insufficient to gain an optimal response [22]. Traditional maintenance therapy includes 3 weekly instillations after induction at 3 and 6 months and then every 6 months. However, most patients in the trial developing the aforementioned schedule were unable to complete the goal of 3 years of maintenance due to side effects, and given the benefit in recurrence-free survival, maximum therapeutic effect may be seen at an earlier date [52].

The AUA recommends considering BCG maintenance therapy for up to 1 year for intermediate-risk patients who have complete response to induction and continuation up to 3 years for high-risk patients, as tolerated [22].

Risks/Adverse Reactions

In general, BCG is fairly well tolerated but rarely can be fatal, which must be a consideration to its clinical use [53]. Fatalities from disseminated BCG are most common in immunocompromised patients; therefore, systemic conditions or pharmacotherapies that interfere with the immune system must be considered prior to initiating therapy. However, more commonly, BCG produces irritating lower urinary tract symptoms, such as frequency and dysuria, which are often limited to a few days following treatment. Less common manifestations of BCG toxicity (occurring in less than 5% of cases) include fever, significant hematuria, prostatitis, arthralgia, epididymitis, sepsis, rash, and renal abscess [50].

Side effects, toxicity, and adverse reactions can be divided into three grade categories.

Grade 12 includes moderate symptoms for <48 hours. This includes mild or moderate irritative voiding symptoms, hematuria, or fever <38.5 °C. Clinicians can consider sending a urine culture to rule out bacterial infection. Management should be based on symptom management and can include nonsteroidal anti-inflammatory drugs, anticholinergics, and antispasmodics. If these symptoms last longer than 48 hours, or become severe, patients are upgraded to grade 2 and require more significant intervention. Patients should be worked up with a urine culture, chest X-ray, and liver function tests. Management should include local symptoms management as per grade 1 recommendations, treatment of urine culture if appropriate, and initiation of oral isoniazid and rifampin until symptoms resolve. Vitamin B6 or pyridoxine should be given with these medications.

Grade 3 toxicity includes severe systemic reactions that can be life threatening. The treatment and work-up for grade 1 and 2 reactions should be initiated. These patients should also be assessed for solid organ involvement. Infectious disease consultation is recommended. Prednisone may be added if there are signs of septic shock [5, 54].

BCG Failure

Despite a response seen in more than 60% of patients treated with intravesical BCG, BCG-unresponsive patients are left with limited options [55]. Poor prognostic factors associated with disease progression and/or treatment unresponsiveness after intravesical BCG include female gender, higher-grade tumors, presence of CIS, and increased multiplicity of tumors [56]. BCG unresponsiveness indicates a patient must have either [1] persistent or recurrent CIS alone or with recurrent Ta/T1 disease within 12 months of completion of adequate BCG therapy; [2] recurrent high-grade Ta/T1 disease within 6 months of completion of adequate BCG therapy; or [3] T1 high-grade disease at the first evaluation following an induction BCG course [57]. Current AUA/SUO guidelines recommend these patients undergo radical cystectomy, which will be discussed later in this chapter [58, 59]. Figure 16.1 shows treatment options for patients who fall into the BCG failure category.

Summary
- Intravesical BCG is a mainstay of treatment for NMIBC.
- An induction course of BCG is usually started within weeks following TURBT and should last for 6 weeks.
- Maintenance intravesical BCG entails 3 weekly instillations starting 3 months after induction BCG and then goes to every 6 months, with 3 weekly instillations, after that.
- BCG adverse side effects can be divided into grade 1, grade 2, and grade 3.
- Although intravesical BCG works for many patients with NMIBC, BCG failure does occur. Treatment options after BCG failure are listed in Fig. 16.1.

Intravesical Chemotherapy

Chemotherapy Post-TURBT

Instillation of intravesical chemotherapy after resection of NMIBC has been well established to reduce the rate of recurrence. As early as 1981, a trial of Adriamycin after TURBT showed a significant decrease in recurrence, with 72% of patients

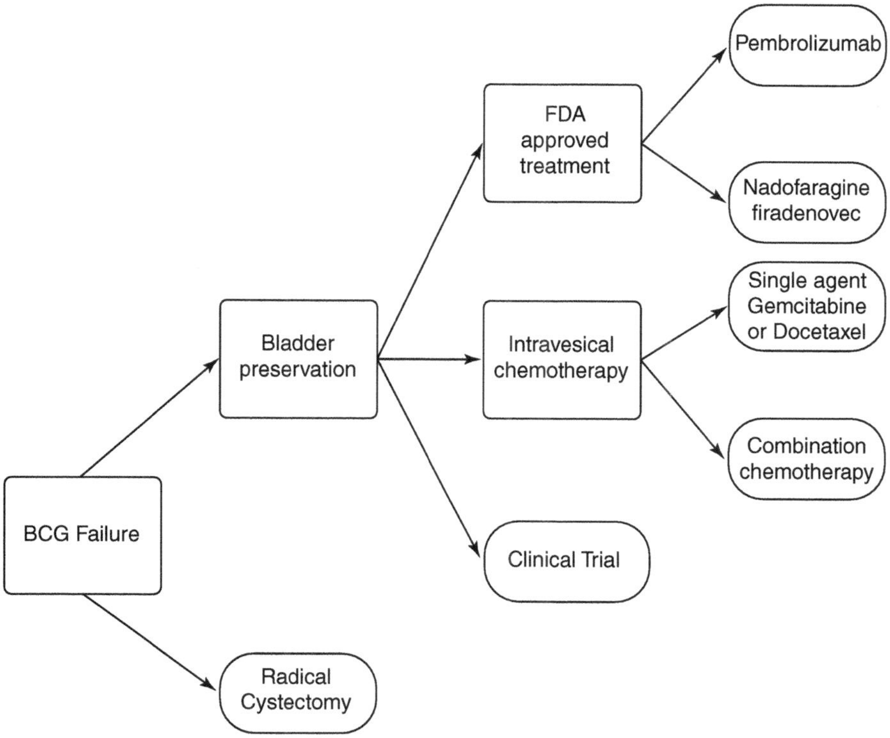

Fig. 16.1 NMIBC BCG failure decision-making

having a reduction in the number of recurrent papillomas after a single instillation compared to 39% in the control group for Ta or T1 disease [60]. Immediate instillation, within 24 hours of resection, is thought to prevent recurrence by destruction of free-circulating tumor cells after resection prior to implantation, or by destruction of small tumors at the resection site [61, 62]. There can be adherence of free tumor cells to the bladder wall within 1 hour of resection with a maximum time of 24 hours [63].

A single instillation of intravesical chemotherapy within 24 hours of TURBT is recommended by the AUA, European Association of Urology (EAU), and National Comprehensive Cancer Network (NCCN) [22, 46, 64]. Gemcitabine, mitomycin C (MMC), epirubicin, and pirarubicin have all been shown to be efficacious in placebo-controlled trials to significantly reduce the risk of recurrence and prolong recurrence-free survival, particularly for low-grade tumors [65–67]. Yet, there is a lack of efficacy in patients at high-risk for recurrence, for example, patients with more than one recurrence per year [68]. There are no head-to-head trials comparing these agents.

A meta-analysis among all intravesical agents found that instillation within 24 hours of TURBT prolonged recurrence-free survival by 38% [69]. Intravesical chemotherapy after TURBT is generally well tolerated, with the most common side effect being temporary irritative voiding symptoms. However, in the event of a perforation, extensive tumor resection, ongoing significant bleeding, or gross evidence of muscle-invasive disease, intravesical chemotherapy should be avoided due to the risk for systemic absorption with potential significant adverse reactions [70].

Adjuvant Intravesical Chemotherapy

The use of adjuvant intravesical therapy has gained traction, particularly in the era of a BCG shortage. Intravesical chemotherapy should be tailored based on risk stratification.

Low-Risk NMIBC

The standard therapy for low-risk NMIBC is a single instillation of intravesical chemotherapy post TURBT. Multiple trials utilizing MMC, epirubicin, or pirarubicin have shown no benefit to additional intravesical therapy beyond a single post-resection dose for this group of patients [67, 71–73]. For example, Tolley et al. compared recurrence-free interval for post-resection MMC in either a single instillation, instillation after resection followed by four more doses at each cystoscopy for the first year, and no MMC. Both the single-instillation and multiple-instillation group outperformed the control group for recurrence-free survival ([HR 0.66; CI 0.48–0.91] and [HR 0.50; CI 0.36–0.70], respectively). There was no significant difference between the two groups receiving MMC [68]. As such, the EAU, AUA, and NCCN recommend no adjuvant intravesical chemotherapy beyond a single post-resection instillation for low-risk NMIBC [22, 46, 64].

Intermediate-Risk NMIBC

While a single post-resection chemotherapy instillation decreases the rate of recurrence, it is insufficient treatment for patients with intermediate-risk NMIBC [74, 75]. The AUA and EAU recommend induction and maintenance therapy for up to 1 year with either intravesical BCG or chemotherapy [22, 46]. Multiple trials have evaluated BCG, MMC, doxorubicin, and epirubicin compared to no intravesical therapy, and all have been found to reduce the risk of recurrence. Further, a meta-analysis analyzed benefits of intravesical therapies as compared to no intravesical therapy and found three trials with BCG (RR 0.56; CI 0.43–0.71), eight trials with MMC (RR 0.71; CI 0.57–0.89), ten trials with doxorubicin (RR 0.80; CI 0.72–0.88), and nine trials with epirubicin (RR 0.63; CI 0.53–0.75). BCG had similar rates of recurrence prevention to MMC, and both outperformed doxorubicin or epirubicin [76]. Meta-analyses directly compared MMC to BCG and found overall results with no significant difference for development of tumor progression after induction therapy (9.44% vs 7.2%). However, BCG did outperform MMC when BCG maintenance therapy was given [77, 78]. This included a meta-analysis with 74% of patients having intermediate-risk disease which found a 32% risk reduction for BCG maintenance versus MMC maintenance therapy [79]. Importantly, intravesical chemotherapy has a much better safety and tolerability profile compared to BCG, and given the similarity in efficacy and BCG shortage, intravesical MMC is gaining popularity [76].

Mitomycin C (MMC)

Mechanism of Action

Mitomycin C is a chemotherapeutic agent which acts primarily through alkylation and crosslinking of DNA strands, resulting in cellular apoptosis. It is particularly useful for intravesical therapy due to its large molecular weight (334 kDa), which prevents physiologic uptake and limits effects to a local area [80]. Induction therapy consists of 6 weekly instillations of 40 mg of MMC in 20 cc of sterile water.

Optimizing Response to MMC

Efficacy of MMC can be optimized by performing the following prior to instillation [81]:

1. Dehydration – no fluids for 8 hours prior to treatment.
2. Urinary alkalinization – 1.3 g of oral NaHCO3 the night prior to, morning of, and 30 minutes prior to therapy.
3. Complete bladder emptying prior to instillation – post-void residual <10 cc upon bladder scan.
4. High MMC concentration – 40 mg in 20 cc of sterile water.

These recommendations are based on a computational model which simulated treatment parameters, creating the most efficacious therapy, and proven in a clinical study [82]. A phase 3 RCT found that patients in the MMC optimized group had a longer median time to recurrence versus the standard group (20-mg dose with no pharmacokinetic manipulations or urinary alkalinization), with median recurrence at 29.1 months for the optimized group versus 11.8 months for the standard group. Further, 5-year recurrence-free survival was 41.0% versus 24.6% in the optimized versus standard MMC groups, respectively [83]. Other methods at optimizing MMC efficacy, such as chemohyperthermia and electromotive drug administration, have been successful and are detailed later in this chapter.

Maintenance MMC

Fewer studies have looked at maintenance therapy with MMC. One promising multicenter trial randomized 495 patients to BCG induction, MMC induction, or MMC induction with 3 years of maintenance therapy. Three-year recurrence-free rates were similar for the BCG and MMC induction groups, 65.5% and 68.6%, respectively. The MMC maintenance group vastly outperformed either group, with a 3-year recurrence-free rate of 86.1% [84]. Further studies are needed to validate these results. The optimal duration of maintenance therapy has not yet been determined. There is some evidence to support that a shorter duration of high-density therapy is as effective as longer courses of lower-density solution. Additionally, long-term MMC therapy (>1 year) seems only beneficial when no immediate post-resection dose is given [85].

Epirubicin

Mechanism of Action and Side Effects

Epirubicin is an anthracycline antineoplastic agent that inhibits DNA replication, transcription, and repair by binding to nucleic acid. There can be systemic absorption of this drug, with studies showing 58–84% of each dose recovered from the bladder after treatment. However, tumors absorb 2–10x more epirubicin compared to normal urothelium, making it an attractive option [86]. Further, epirubicin is generally well tolerated, more so than BCG, with the most common side effect being chemical cystitis [87].

Epirubicin Versus Other Agents

Overall, BCG outperforms epirubicin in regard to time to recurrence. The largest, phase 3 randomized trial compared time to first recurrence among patients treated with BCG, BCG plus isoniazid, and epirubicin. Patients treated with epirubicin had a significantly shorter time to recurrence compared to the other two groups. At 3 years, 49% of patients in the epirubicin group were recurrence-free compared to 65% in the BCG group and 64% in the BCG plus isoniazid group. A relatively small number of patients (n – 43, 5%) in the entire cohort progressed to muscle-invasive disease. Progression to muscle-invasive disease did not differ between any of the three groups, including patients with high-risk disease. Of note, patients in the BCG plus isoniazid group did not experience fewer side effects compared to BCG alone [87]. One study comparing three different treatment schemes with epirubicin, two maintenance therapies, and one group with immediate post-TURBT instillation followed by an extra instillation within 48 hours found no difference in recurrence-free survival between the three groups. On average, 44% of patients were recurrence-free at 5 years out [88].

Indeed, the performance data for epirubicin is generally weaker than BCG or MMC. A recent randomized trial found that a single instillation of epirubicin after TURBT was ineffective for preventing recurrence for intermediate- and high-risk disease [89]. Further, a randomized trial demonstrated long-term superiority of BCG over epirubicin in terms of disease-free survival, distant metastasis, and overall and disease-specific survival for intermediate- and high-risk patients [90]. There is no standardized maintenance schedule or dosage of epirubicin. Some studies have reported 30–80 mg of epirubicin, with weekly induction from 4 to 8 weeks, with or without maintenance once every 1–4 months, for 10–24 months [86].

High-Risk NMIBC and BCG Failure

BCG induction plus maintenance for 1–3 years remains the standard of care for high-risk NMIBC [22, 46]. No study to date has shown neither superiority nor non-inferiority of intravesical chemotherapy compared to BCG for high-risk NMIBC. However, BCG failure, which is described in more detail in Sect. 14.5, necessitates ongoing trials for bladder-preserving therapy. Currently, the only FDA-approved intravesical chemotherapy for BCG-refractory CIS is valrubicin, for which a long-term follow-up study found only 4% complete response rate at 24 months [91]. As such, valrubicin is rarely used and not regularly recommended (Fig. 16.2).

Gemcitabine

Mechanism of Action, Comparison to Other Agents, and Side Effects

Gemcitabine is a deoxycytidine analogue that is transported into cells, phosphorylated, and then incorporated into DNA and RNA, which inhibits growth activity and leads to apoptosis [92]. Several trials have validated the efficacy of single-agent gemcitabine for BCG failure NMIBC patients. Two randomized controlled trials compared patients with recurrence after BCG treated with either re-induction BCG, MMC, or gemcitabine. Gemcitabine outperformed BCG in regard to disease

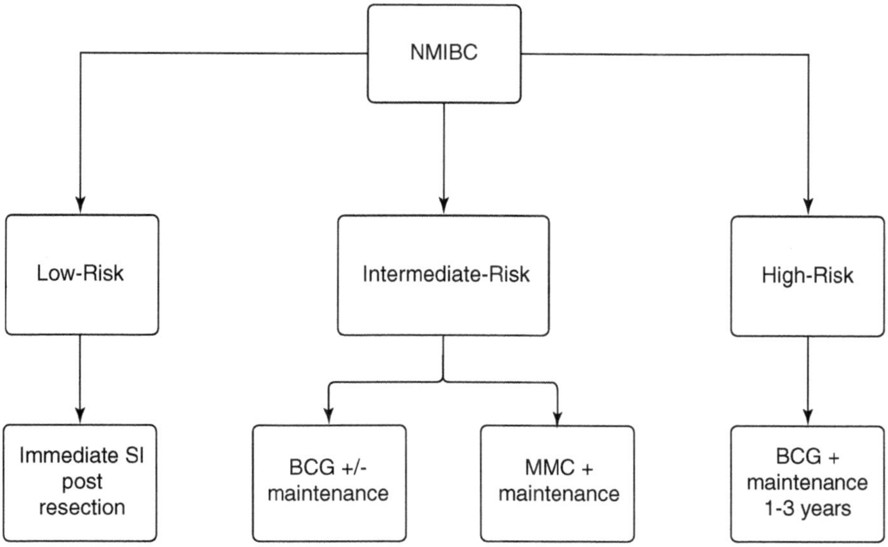

Fig. 16.2 NMIBC post-resection TURBT treatment options based on risk stratification

recurrence, with 52% of patients treated with gemcitabine having recurrence vs 88% treated with BCG [93]. Gemcitabine also outperformed MMC, with 72% versus 61% of patients being recurrence-free after 36 months, respectively. Gemcitabine had a favorable side effect profile compared to MMC, with less patients experiencing chemical cystitis [94]. However, a more recent phase 2 study, utilizing more detailed understanding of BCG-refractory disease, found gemcitabine to have a durable response in less than 30% of patients after 12 months [95].

Of note, a Cochrane review found gemcitabine to be similarly efficacious to BCG for intermediate-risk NMIBC, offering a potential additional option for intravesical chemotherapy aside from MMC [96].

Docetaxel

Mechanism of Action and Usage

Docetaxel is a taxane cytotoxic agent which binds to and stabilizes microtubules. This disrupts cellular division and normal cellular activity which ultimately leads to apoptosis [97]. In vitro, docetaxel has been shown to be one of the most effective agents at inhibiting growth in urothelial carcinoma [98]. In a small cohort of patients, intravesical docetaxel has shown long-term efficacy in BCG failure NMIBC disease. The initial study had a complete response rate of 56% and 4-year durable response of 22% [99]. Two follow-up studies have shown that maintenance intravesical docetaxel after induction may prolong the complete response rate and reduce the need for radical cystectomy [100, 101].

Combination Therapy

Multiple different combinations of intravesical chemotherapy have been studied to improve response rates over single-agent therapy. Early trials assessed combinations of doxorubicin and MMC for CIS and epirubicin and IFN-α for high-risk recurrence. The first study had a relatively poor long-term disease-free survival (<50%) and significant side effects [102]. The later study was stopped early due to poor accrual, but BCG was significantly superior compared to epirubicin and IFN-α [103].

More promising results were seen with combination therapy of gemcitabine and MMC in BCG-refractory patients. Patients were treated with intravesical gemcitabine for 90 minutes followed by intravesical MMC for 90 minutes, followed by monthly maintenance treatment. Disease-free survival was found to be 48% at 1 year and 38% at 2 years [104]. Another study evaluated gemcitabine and docetaxel in BCG-refractory NMIBC. Gemcitabine was instilled for 90 minutes followed by docetaxel for 2 hours. Patients who had complete response were continued on maintenance therapy. At 1 year, disease-free survival was 54% and 34% at 2 years [105].

One ongoing phase 1 trial is evaluating intravesical therapy with cabazitaxel, gemcitabine, and cisplatin in a cohort of patients with BCG failure. Initial complete response rate was 89%, and recurrence-free survival at 1 year was 83% [106].

Summary

- Most patients with NMIBC should have a single instillation of intravesical chemotherapy within 24 hours of transurethral resection unless a specific contraindication exists.
- Patients with low-risk NMIBC do not have a further cancer-specific benefit for intravesical chemotherapy beyond the single post-resection dose.
- BCG with maintenance therapy has the best outcomes for intermediate-risk NMIBC.
- Intermediate-risk NMIBC appears to be equally responsive to maintenance mitomycin C compared to induction BCG and has fewer side effects.
- BCG remains the standard of care for high-risk NMIBC.
- Patients with BCG failure who do not undergo early cystectomy may undergo a trial of single or combination intravesical therapy or can consider enhanced chemotherapy or photodynamic therapy (see Sect. 14.8).

Non-BCG Immunotherapy

Programmed Cell Death Protein (PD1) and PD1 Ligand (PDL1) Inhibitors

The successful use of inhibitors of programmed cell death protein (PD1) and PD1 ligand (PDL1) in metastatic bladder cancer [107] has led to increased interest in using checkpoint immunotherapy in BCG-unresponsive patients. Inhibitors of PD1 and PDL1 act by interrupting the suppressive effect on T-cell activation, thereby initiating an immune response.

Pembrolizumab

One such agent is pembrolizumab, which was granted FDA approval in January 2020 for BCG-unresponsive CIS based on the results of the KEYNOTE-057 trial. This multicenter trial included 102 patients with BCG-unresponsive CIS or high-grade Ta/T1 disease who were then treated with 200 mg of pembrolizumab intravenously every 3 weeks for up to 24 months. Overall, 40.6% of patients experienced complete response for a median duration of response lasting for 16.2 months [108]. KEYNOTE-676 is an open-label phase 3 two parallel-arm study on the safety and antitumor activity of combination treatment with pembrolizumab and BCG, as compared to BCG alone in patients with high-risk NMIBC (NCT03711032). Similarly, a phase 1, single-arm, open-label study is currently being conducted on the tolerability and efficacy of combination therapy with pembrolizumab and BCG in high-risk or BCG-refractory patients. This study is also investigating tumor characteristics that correlate with greater pembrolizumab efficacy (NCT02808143).

Risk/Adverse Effects

The most common adverse events observed in patients receiving pembrolizumab as a single agent in clinical trials have been fatigue, musculoskeletal pain, decreased appetite, pruritus, diarrhea, nausea, rash, pyrexia, cough, dyspnea, constipation, pain, and abdominal pain. Serious adverse events include pneumonia, cardiac ischemia, colitis, pulmonary embolism, sepsis, and urinary tract infection. In addition, pembrolizumab carries precautions for immune-mediated pneumonitis, immune-mediated colitis, immune-mediated hepatitis, immune-mediated endocrinopathies, immune-mediated nephritis, immune-mediated skin adverse reactions, infusion-related reactions, complications of allogeneic hematopoietic stem cell transplantation before and after pembrolizumab treatment, and embryofetal toxicity.

Atezolizumab

In the SWOG S1605 trial, atezolizumab, another inhibitor of the PD1/PDL1 axis, has shown promising results for the treatment of patients with BCG-unresponsive NMIBC. This trial is a single-arm phase 2 trial in which patients are treated with 1200 mg of atezolizumab every 3 weeks for 1 year. Recent results have shown 41.1% and 20.5% complete response at 3 and 6 months, respectively [109]. A phase 1, open-label, non-randomized, dose de-escalation, single-arm trial (BladderGATE) is being conducted to study dose-limiting toxicity and recurrence-free survival in BCG-naïve, high-risk, NMIBC patients receiving one installation of intravesical BCG per week and 1200 mg of intravenous atezolizumab every 3 weeks (NCT04134000). Additionally, the multicenter ALBAN study is a phase 3, open-label, randomized, two parallel-arm trial of combination therapy with BCG and atezolizumab compared with BCG alone in BCG-naïve patients with high-risk NMIBC (NCT03799835).

Risks/Adverse Effects

Generally, atezolizumab has been well tolerated across bladder cancer studies with most adverse events being mild to moderate in grade. Most common adverse events include fatigue, nausea, decreased appetite, pyrexia, diarrhea, anemia, dyspnea, nausea, vomiting, and hypertension. Similar to pembrolizumab, atezolizumab may result in immune-related adverse events, such as immune-mediated pneumonitis, colitis, and hepatitis.

Summary

- There has been an increase interest in PD1 and PDL1 inhibitors such as pembrolizumab and atezolizumab in patients not responding to BCG immunotherapy treatment.
- Pembrolizumab is the only PD1/PDL1 inhibitor that is currently approved for patients with NMIBC outside of clinical trials.

Emerging Therapies

Nadofaragene Firadenovec (rAD-IFN/Syn-3)

In addition to inhibitors targeting the PD1/PDL1 axis, other novel immunotherapy approaches such as nadofaragene firadenovec (rAD-IFN/Syn-3) are being explored. RAD-IFN/Syn-3 is a viral gene therapy and the first of its kind to be used in the treatment of bladder cancer. This therapy consists of rAd-IFN alpha, a non-replicating recombinant adenovirus vector-based gene therapy that delivers a copy of the human interferon alfa-2b gene to urothelial cells, and Syn3, a polyamide surfactant that enhances the viral transduction of the urothelium [110]. Once the virus enters the urothelial tumor cells, it is transported to the nucleus, and endogenous IFN alpha 2b is produced by the cell leading to tumor cell cytotoxicity. It has been shown in preclinical studies that recombinant interferon alfa gene therapy results in local rather than systemic interferon alfa-2b production and therefore results in a local response [111, 112].

RAD-IFN/Syn-3 has been shown in a randomized phase 2 study to be well tolerated and demonstrate promising efficacy in patients with high-grade (HG) BCG-refractory or relapsed NMIBC. This trial included 40 patients who received rAD-IFN/Syn-3, 35% of which remained free of HG recurrence 12 months after initial treatment [113]. Recently, a multicenter, open-label phase 3 study investigated rAD-IFN/Syn-3 for HG NMIBC (CIS ± Ta/T1, or Ta/T1 alone) unresponsive to BCG. This trial included 151 patients, of which 103 had CIS and 48 had HG Ta/T1 disease. Of the patients with CIS, 53.4% achieved a complete response within 3 months and 24.3% remained disease-free at 12 months. Of the patients with HG Ta/T1 disease, 72.9% and 43.8% were free from recurrence at 3 and 12 months, respectively.

Overall, 66% and 4% of patients experienced grade 1–2 and grade 3 drug-related adverse events, respectively. These events included discharge around the catheter during instillation, fatigue, bladder spasm, micturition urgency, chills, dysuria, pyrexia, syncope, hypertension, and urinary incontinence [114].

ALT-801 and ALT-803

Cytokine therapy focusing on interleukin-2 (IL-2), interleukin-15 (IL-15), and interleukin-2R beta-gamma pathways in lymphocytes has been studied for several decades in the management of several cancers including renal cell carcinoma [115] [116]. Intravesical ALT-801 is a recombinant fusion protein of IL-2 and a soluble T-cell receptor against p53-derived antigen that is being studied in patients with NMIBC. A phase 1 study of ALT-801 plus gemcitabine showed a good safety profile with immune responses in a cohort of BCG-unresponsive patients (NCT01625260) [117]. Adverse events in this trial included hepatotoxicity, anorexia, pruritus, rash, edema, fatigue, and chills.

Similarly, ALT-803, an IL-15 superagonist that promotes proliferation and activation of natural killer (NK) cells and CD8+ T cells, is being investigated in two clinical trials. The first of which is a phase 2 trial in combination with BCG in BCG-unresponsive CIS with or without Ta or T1 disease (QUILT-3.032, NCT03022825). Preliminary results show that 82% of patients with CIS have achieved a complete response and 78% remained disease-free at 3 months. Similarly, 77% of patients with papillary disease remained disease-free at 6 months. Serious adverse events reported were *E. coli* infection, anemia, and bacteremia, with no immune-related adverse events [118]. The safety profile of ALT-803 in combination with BCG is also under investigation in a phase 1b/2 study in patients with high-grade BCG-naïve NMIBC (QUILT-2.005, NCT02138734). Of the nine patients enrolled, all were disease-free at 24 months, and zero patients experienced disease recurrence or progression. ALT-803 was well tolerated with adverse events being hematuria, urinary tract pain, and hypertension [119].

Vicinium (VB4–845)

Vicinium contains the active pharmaceutical ingredient VB4–845, which is a recombinant fusion protein that expresses a humanized single-chain antibody fragment specific for the epithelial cell adhesion molecule (EpCAM) antigen linked to ETA (252–608). Once bound to the EpCAM antigen on the surface of carcinoma cells, Vicinium is internalized through an endolytic pathway. The ETA (252–608) is cleaved off and induces cell death by irreversibly blocking protein synthesis [120]. A phase 2 study evaluated once-weekly instillations of Vicinium 30 mg over 6 or 12 weeks, followed by up to 3 maintenance cycles in 45 subjects with bladder cancer and residual CIS with or without concurrent Ta or T1 disease who were refractory or intolerant to BCG. A complete response was achieved by 44% of patients, and 16% remained disease-free at 1 year. The median time to recurrence was 134 days longer in subjects who received 12 weeks of induction therapy compared to 6 weeks (NCT00462488) [121]. In this trial, 65.2% of patients experienced at least one adverse event with the most common being renal and urinary disorders, bladder pain, urinary tract infections, urgency, and hematuria. There is also a phase 1 trial that is investigating the efficacy and safety of combination durvalumab and Vicinium for BCG unresponsive NMIBC patients. This study is currently enrolling patients with an estimated primary completion date of August 30, 2022 (NCT03258593).

VPM1002BC

VPM1002BC is a modified mycobacterium BCG for the treatment of NMIBC. The genetic modifications are expected to result in better immunogenicity and less side effects. A phase 1 trial including six patients with BCG failure investigated the safety and immunology of VPM1002BC treatment. This trial reported the first intravesical application of VPM1002BC for the treatment of NMIBC. In the trial, no dose-limiting toxicity and no grade ≥ 3 adverse events occurred. Plasma levels of TNF alpha significantly increased after treatment, and blood-derived CD4+ T cells significantly increased intracellular IFN expression. Grade 1 or 2 adverse events experienced in this trial included anemia, abdominal pain, bladder infection, prostate infection, urinary tract infection, headache, hematuria, increased creatinine, and hematoma [122]. The efficacy of this treatment for BCG-unresponsive patients was recently presented and demonstrated a recurrence-free survival of 49% at 60 months, with only 5% of patients unable to tolerate adequate induction therapy [123]. The estimated completion of this study is December 21, 2022 (NCT02371447).

Enhanced Chemotherapy

Device-assisted drug delivery, such as chemohyperthermia (CHT) via microwave/radiofrequency induction and electromotive drug administration (EMDA), is an active area of research.

Chemohyperthermia (CHT)

Hyperthermia is thought to increase drug penetration by increased urothelial cellular membrane permeability and modified blood perfusion. Further, hyperthermia can be directly cytotoxic and increase tumor cell apoptosis [124]. Synergo® (Medical Enterprises, Amsterdam, Netherlands) is an FDA-approved device which induces bladder wall hyperthermia utilizing a three-way catheter with a microwave applicator at the tip [125]. In a multicenter study of 83 patients, MMC delivered with the Synergo® system had a significant decrease in recurrence rate after 24 months, 17.1% versus 57.5%, when compared to standard intravesical MMC. There were significantly more side effects in the CHT group, though all localized and transient [126]. A 90-month follow-up had recurrence rates of 40% in the CHT group and 80% in the traditional MMC group [127]. Another promising trial evaluated 51 patients with BCG-refractory CIS and found an initial complete response rate of 92% after treatment with hyperthermic MMC. Fifty percent of patients had ongoing response at 2 years [128]. In intermediate- and high-risk groups treated with CHT, recurrence rates were found to be 14.3% at 1 year and 24.6% at 2 years [129]. While these results are promising, most trials have relatively short follow-up with small sample sizes.

Electromotive Drug Administration (EMDA)

EMDA applies an electric field into the bladder mucosa, which may increase penetration of MMC through iontophoresis, electroosmosis, or electrophoresis and electroporation. The patient is grounded, and an active electrode on a catheter tip is placed into the bladder. MMC delivery with EMDA can reduce dwell time to 30 minutes instead of 2 hours [130]. One study compared treatment of patients with low-intermediate NMIBC treated with CHT, EMDA, or MMC alone and found complete response rates of 66%, 40%, and 27.7%, respectively [131]. Another study randomized high-risk NMIBC patients to treatment with MMC alone, EMDA, or BCG and found similar complete response rates in the EMDA and BCG groups, both of which were superior to MMC alone [132]. Further, a randomized trial compared patients with BCG induction for 6 weeks plus maintenance therapy versus BCG induction for 2 weeks followed by EMDA/MMC induction and maintenance therapy for pT1 disease. The BCG + EMDA/MMC group significantly outperformed BCG alone in terms of recurrence rate (41.9% vs 57.9%), disease-free survival (69 months vs 21 months), progression rate (9.3% vs 21.9%), and disease-specific mortality rate (5.6% vs 16.2%) [133, 134]. Finally, one randomized study found that EMDA/MMC given immediately prior to TURBT had a lower recurrence rate (38%) compared to those that received an immediate post-TURBT, traditional MMC dose (59%) and to those who had TURBT alone (64%). Further, there was a significantly longer disease-free survival in the EMDA/MMC group compared to MMC or TURBT alone (52 months vs 16 months and 12 months, respectively) [135]. Despite the above results, EMDA has not yet reached FDA approval.

Photodynamic Therapy

Photodynamic therapy (PDT) involves the administration, either oral, intravenous, or intravesical, of a photosensitizing agent, followed by activation with light. A photochemical reaction occurs creating reactive oxygen species that are lethal to cells [136]. There is preferential uptake in tumor cells of photosensitizing agents; however, the exact mechanism has not yet clearly been elucidated [137]. The most studied and utilized agent for NMIBC is 5-aminolevulinic acid (5-ALA), which is an endogenous substance of heme biosynthesis. 5-ALA is metabolized to protoporphyrin IX (PP IX), which, when irradiated with visible light, produces reactive oxygen species causing cell destruction [138]. This agent can be given orally or intravesically, though there are significantly more adverse effects when given orally, such as hypotension and tachycardia [139]. A small, single-center study found that 5-ALA given intravesically to a mixed cohort of patients with superficial tumors was effective. Of the patients that received PDT as primary treatment after TURBT, 83% (n = 5) were disease-free, and 57% had complete response. There was an initial complete response of 40% in BCG-refractory CIS. Importantly, side effects were local and mild for all patients [140]. More recently, a prospective, multicenter trial evaluated patients undergoing TURBT who had not previously had BCG therapy and found an overall recurrence-free rate of 78% after 12 months of PDT [141]. A newer agent, Radachlorin, shows promise against BCG-refractory CIS. One study found high recurrence-free rates after administering Radachlorin to patients with BCG-refractory CIS: 90.9% at 12 months, 64.4% at 24 months, and 60.1% at 30 months with no significant adverse events [142] (Table 16.3).

Summary

- There are a number of emerging therapies being studied for treatment of NMIBC.
- Areas of focus include gene therapy, cytokine therapy, and advanced chemotherapies, among others.

Role for Radical Cystectomy

There is a role for surgical, non-endoscopic management in the treatment of NMIBC in certain patient populations. Patients found to have high-grade superficial bladder cancer, especially those with deep lamina propria invasion, both have an increased risk of local disease progression and present with increased risk of developing subsequent upper tract malignancies. Studies have shown that approximately one-half of patients with high-grade NMIBC will eventually have disease progression and approximately one-third of these patients will die from bladder cancer over a 15-year follow-up [4]. In these patients with high-risk superficial disease who are at risk of progression, there is literature that supports early radical cystectomy, especially since many of patients may have unknown muscle involvement at the time

Table 16.3 NMIBC non-surgical evolving therapies

Immunotherapy	Chemotherapy	Viral gene therapy	Cytokine therapy	Other emerging therapies
BCG	Mitomycin C	Nadofaragene	ALT-801	Vicinium (VB4–845)
Pembrolizumab	Epirubicin		ALT-803	VPM1002BC
Atezolizumab	Gemcitabine			Chemohyperthermia
	Docetaxel			EDMA
				Photodynamic therapy

which results in pathologic upstaging at the time of surgery. Studies have shown that for patients with high-grade clinical T1 tumors, early radical cystectomy increased life expectancy and disease-free survival at 10 years for those that underwent the procedure earlier compared to those that waited for documented muscle invasion [143].

According to AUA guidelines, clinicians should not offer radical cystectomy in patients with low-risk or intermediate-risk Ta disease until all feasible bladder-sparing therapies have been unsuccessful. In select high-risk patients who present with T1 disease on both original and re-staging TURBT or those who have T1 disease on original staging TURBT in association with adverse pathological features, such as CIS, variant histology, or lymphovascular invasion, these patients should be offered up-front radical cystectomy due to increased risk of developing muscle-invasive disease. Those high-risk patients who fail two induction cycles of intravesical BCG or maintenance BCG within 1 year with notable disease persistence should also be offered radical cystectomy [15]. In general, patients with high-grade T1 disease and poor pathologic features such as CIS and lymphovascular invasion, involvement of prostatic urethra or ureteral orifices, or tumors too large for complete endoscopic resection should also be considered for early cystectomy before documented T2 disease [144].

However, it is important to consider that many of these patients who may undergo radical cystectomy with high-risk NMIBC may end up being overtreated. This is important because radical cystectomy with or without continent diversion is a life-altering procedure, associated with a high risk of perioperative morbidity. A recent meta-analysis reported that 59% of patients undergoing radical cystectomy with either extracorporeal or intracorporeal conduit diversion experience complications in the 90-day postoperative period. Likewise, in patients undergoing radical cystectomy with intracorporeal continent diversion, the overall 30-day complication rate was 45.7%. Furthermore, mean in-hospital stay was 9 days for all diversion types, and 90-day mortality was 3% [58].

Many patients undergoing this procedure require lifelong ostomies which have a significant effect on a patient's quality of life and overall psychological well-being. In a recent study, both patients and caregivers reported having insufficient psychological preparation for ostomy surgeries and very limited hands-on training with stoma care and utility of stomal appliances. Patients reported depression, anxiety, and distress caused by changes in body image and sexual, urinary, and bowel function. Patients and caregivers also reported significant patient medical needs in the postoperative period including pain, fatigue, sleep disturbance, inflammation, and complications resulting in hospital readmissions [145].

The 5- and 10-year recurrence-free survival for patients with organ-confined, lymph node-negative Pis, Pa, and P1 disease who underwent radical cystectomy range from 79% to 91% and 74% to 89%, respectively [146]. Granted, radical cystectomy is curative for these patients early in their disease course; many patients may seek bladder-sparing treatments or may harbor too many comorbidities and are therefore ineligible for cystectomy. There continues to be clear and urgent need for alternative therapies for these patients (Table 16.4).

Table 16.4 Summary of NMIBC treatment options

Surgery	Intravesical chemotherapies	Immunotherapies	Emerging therapies	Device-assisted drug delivery
TURBT	Mitomycin C	BCG	Nadofaragene firadenovec (rAD-IFN/Syn-3)	Chemohyperthermia
Radical cystectomy	Epirubicin	Pembrolizumab	ALT-801, ALT-803	Electromotive drug administration
	Doxorubicin	Atezolizumab	Vicinium (VB4–845)	Photodynamic therapy
	Gemcitabine		VPM1002BC	
	Docetaxel			

Summary

- There is a role for radical cystectomy in specific patients with NMIBC who are at high risk for disease progression and may be curative in some of these patients.
- Conversely, there are patients with NMIBC who undergo radical cystectomy that end up being overtreated and have to live with the sequelae of a life-changing surgery.
- Because of this, there is still a need for alternative therapies for these patients.

References

1. SEER*Explorer Application [Internet]. [cited 2021 Jan 2]. Available from: https://seer.cancer.gov/explorer/application.html?site=71&data_type=1&graph_type=2&compareBy=stage&chk_stage_104=104&chk_stage_105=105&chk_stage_106=106&chk_stage_107=107&sex=1&race=1&age_range=1&hdn_rate_type=1&advopt_precision=1&advopt_display=2.
2. Bladder Cancer — Cancer Stat Facts [Internet]. [cited 2021 Jane 4]. Available from: https://seer.cancer.gov/statfacts/html/urinb.html.
3. Heney NM. Natural history of superficial bladder cancer: prognostic features and long-term disease course. Urol Clin N Am. 1992;93:249.
4. Cookson MS, Herr HW, Zhang ZF, Soloway S, Sogani PC, Fair WR. The treated natural history of high risk superficial bladder cancer: 15- year outcome. J Urol. 1997;158:62.
5. Partin AW, Dmochowski RR, Louis R, Kavoussi CAP. Campbell-Walsh-Wein Urology. In: Campbell-Walsh-Wein Urology. 2020.
6. Epstein JI. The new World Health Organization/International Society of Urological Pathology (WHO/ISUP) classification for TA, T1 bladder tumors: is it an improvement? Crit Rev Oncol/Hematol. 2003;47:83–9.
7. Humphrey PA, Moch H, Cubilla AL, Ulbright TM, Reuter VE. The 2016 WHO classification of tumours of the urinary system and male genital organs—part B: prostate and bladder tumours. Eur Urol. 2016;
8. Droller MJ. Biological considerations in the assessment of urothelial cancer: A retrospective. Urology [Internet]. 2005 Nov [cited 2021 Jan 2];66(5 SUPPL.):66–75. Available from: https://pubmed.ncbi.nlm.nih.gov/16194710/.
9. Wolff EM, Liang G, Jones PA. Mechanisms of disease: genetic and epigenetic alterations that drive bladder cancer [Internet]. Vol. 2, Nature Clinical Practice Urology. Nature

Publishing Group; 2005 [cited 2021 Jan 2]. p. 502–10. Available from: www.nature.com/clinicalpractice/uro
10. Olumi AF, Tsai YC, Nichols PW, Skinner DG, Cain DR, Bender LI, et al. Allelic loss of chromosome 17p distinguishes high grade from low grade transitional cell carcinomas of the bladder. Cancer Res. 1990;
11. Cohen MB, Carroll PR, Kerschmann R, Cohen MB, Field FG, Mayall BH. Centromeric copy number of chromosome 7 is strongly correlated with tumor grade and labeling index in human bladder cancer. Cancer Res. 1991;
12. Degtyar P, Neulander E, Zirkin H, Yusim I, Douvdevani A, Mermershtain W, et al. Fluorescence in situ hybridization performed on exfoliated urothelial cells in patients with transitional cell carcinoma of the bladder. Urology [Internet]. 2004 [cited 2021 Jan 2];63(2):398–401. Available from: https://pubmed.ncbi.nlm.nih.gov/14972510/
13. Chatterjee SJ, Datar R, Youssefzadeh D, George B, Goebell PJ, Stein JP, et al. Combined effects of p53, p21, and pRb expression in the progression of bladder transitional cell carcinoma. J Clin Oncol [Internet]. 2004 [cited 2021 Jan 2];22(6):1007–13. Available from: https://pubmed.ncbi.nlm.nih.gov/14981105/
14. EORTC risk tables: predicting recurrence and progression in stage Ta T1 bla – Evidencio [Internet]. [cited 2021 Jan 10]. Available from: https://www.evidencio.com/models/show/1025.
15. Bladder Cancer: Non-Muscle Invasive Guideline – American Urological Association [Internet]. [cited 2021 Jan 10]. Available from: https://www.auanet.org/guidelines/bladder-cancer-non-muscle-invasive-guideline.
16. Mariappan P, Zachou A, Grigor KM. Detrusor muscle in the first, apparently complete transurethral resection of bladder tumour specimen is a surrogate marker of resection quality, predicts risk of early recurrence, and is dependent on operator experience. Eur Urol [Internet]. 2010 May [cited 2021 Jan 2];57(5):843–9. Available from: https://pubmed.ncbi.nlm.nih.gov/19524354/.
17. Ouzaid I, Panthier F, Hermieu JF, Xylinas E. Contemporary surgical and technical aspects of transurethral resection of bladder tumor [Internet]. Vol. 8, Translational Andrology and Urology. AME Publishing Company; 2019 [cited 2021 Jan 2]. p. 21–4. Available from: /pmc/articles/PMC6414345/?report=abstract.
18. Cui Y, Chen H, Liu L, Chen J, Qi L, Zu X. Comparing the efficiency and safety of bipolar and monopolar transurethral resection for non-muscle invasive bladder tumors: a systematic review and meta-analysis. J Laparoendosc Adv Surg Tech [Internet]. 2016 Mar 1 [cited 2021 Jan 2];26(3):196–202. Available from: https://pubmed.ncbi.nlm.nih.gov/26799841/
19. Zhao C, Tang K, Yang H, Xia D, Chen Z. Bipolar versus monopolar transurethral resection of nonmuscle-invasive bladder cancer: a meta-analysis [Internet]. Vol. 30, Journal of Endourology. Mary Ann Liebert Inc.; 2016 [cited 2021 Jan 2]. p. 5–12. Available from: https://pubmed.ncbi.nlm.nih.gov/26413779/.
20. V8–07: En bloc bladder tumor resection: back to oncologic basics | AUA University [Internet]. [cited 2021 Jan 7]. Available from: https://auau.auanet.org/content/v8-07-en-bloc-bladder-tumor-resection-back-oncologic-basics.
21. Kramer MW, Rassweiler JJ, Klein J, Martov A, Baykov N, Lusuardi L, et al. En bloc resection of urothelium carcinoma of the bladder (EBRUC): a European multicenter study to compare safety, efficacy, and outcome of laser and electrical en bloc transurethral resection of bladder tumor. World J Urol [Internet]. 2015 Dec 1 [cited 2021 Jan 2];33(12):1937–43. Available from: https://pubmed.ncbi.nlm.nih.gov/25910478/.
22. Chang SS, Boorjian SA, Chou R, Clark PE, Daneshmand S, Konety BR, et al. Diagnosis and treatment of non-muscle invasive bladder cancer: AUA/SUO guideline. J Urol. 2016;196:1021.
23. Miladi M, Peyromaure M, Zerbib M, Saïghi D, Debré B. The value of a second transurethral resection in evaluating patients with bladder tumours. In: European Urology [Internet]. Elsevier; 2003 [cited 2021 Jan 2]. p. 241–5. Available from: https://pubmed.ncbi.nlm.nih.gov/12600426/.

24. Herr HW. The value of a second transurethral resection in evaluating patients with bladder tumors. J Urol [Internet]. 1999 [cited 2021 Jan 2];162(1):74–6. Available from: https://pubmed.ncbi.nlm.nih.gov/10379743/.
25. HERR HW. Restaging transurethral resection of high risk superficial bladder cancer improves the initial response to bacillus calmette-guerin therapy. J Urol [Internet]. 2005 Dec [cited 2021 Jan 31];174(6):2134–7. Available from: http://www.jurology.com/doi/10.1097/01.ju.0000181799.81119.fc.
26. See WA. Can restaging transurethral resection of T1 bladder cancer select patients for immediate cystectomy? In: Herr HW, Donat SM, Dalbagni G, editors. Urologic Oncology: Seminars and Original Investigations, vol. 25. New York: Department of Urology, Memorial Sloan-Kettering Cancer Center; Elsevier; 2007. p. 276.
27. Fujimoto N, Harada S, Terado M, Sato H, MATSUMOTO T. Multiple biopsies of normal-looking urothelium in patients with superficial bladder cancer: Are they necessary? Int J Urol [Internet]. 2003 Dec 1 [cited 2021 Jan 2];10(12):631–5. Available from: https://doi.org/10.1046/j.1442-2042.2003.00724.x
28. Tran K, Severn M. Blue light cystoscopy in patients with suspected non-muscle invasive bladder carcinoma: a review of clinical utility. 2017 [cited 2021 Jan 2];1–15. Available from: https://pubmed.ncbi.nlm.nih.gov/28825777/.
29. Jocham D, Witjes F, Wagner S, Zeylemaker B, Van Moorselaar J, Grimm MO, et al. Improved detection and treatment of bladder cancer using hexaminolevulinate imaging: a prospective, phase III multicenter study. J Urol. 2005;174(3):862–6.
30. Filbeck T, Pichlmeier U, Knuechel R, Wieland WF, Rößler W. Senkung des rezidivrisikos oberflächlicher harnblasenkarzinome mittels 5-aminolävulinsäure-induzierter fluoreszenzdiagnostik: Resultate einer 5-jahres-studie. Urol - Ausgabe A [Internet]. 2003 Oct 25 [cited 2021 Jan 2];42(10):1366–73. Available from: https://link-springer-com.eresources.mssm.edu/article/10.1007/s00120-003-0355-y.
31. Xiong Y, Li J, Ma S, Ge J, Zhou L, Li D, et al. A meta-analysis of narrow band imaging for the diagnosis and therapeutic outcome of non-muscle invasive bladder cancer. PLoS One. 2017;12:e0170819.
32. Naito S, Algaba F, Babjuk M, Bryan RT, Sun YH, Valiquette L, et al. The Clinical Research Office of the Endourological Society (CROES) Multicentre Randomised Trial of Narrow Band Imaging–Assisted Transurethral Resection of Bladder Tumour (TURBT) versus conventional white light imaging–assisted turbt in primary non–muscle-invasive bladder cancer patients: trial protocol and 1-year results. Eur Urol. 2016;70(3):506–15.
33. Tschirdewahn S, Harke NN, Hirner L, Stagge E, Hadaschik B, Eisenhardt A. Narrow-band imaging assisted cystoscopy in the follow-up of patients with transitional cell carcinoma of the bladder: a randomized study in comparison with white light cystoscopy. World J Urol [Internet]. 2020 Jun 1 [cited 2021 Jan 2];38(6):1509–15. Available from: https://pubmed.ncbi.nlm.nih.gov/31471739/.
34. Pruthi RS, Baldwin N, Bhalani V, Wallen EM. Conservative Management of Low Risk Superficial Bladder Tumors. J Urol [Internet]. 2008 Jan [cited 2021 Jan 2];179(1):87–90. Available from: http://www.jurology.com/doi/10.1016/j.juro.2007.08.171.
35. Schrag D, Hsieh LJ, Rabbani F, Bach PB, Herr H, Begg CB. Adherence to surveillance among patients with superficial bladder cancer. JNCI J Natl Cancer Inst [Internet]. 2003 Apr 16 [cited 2021 Jan 3];95(8):588–97. Available from: https://academic.oup.com/jnci/article-lookup/doi/10.1093/jnci/95.8.588.
36. Mori K, Miura N, Babjuk M, Karakiewicz PI, Mostafaei H, Laukhtina E, et al. Low compliance to guidelines in nonmuscle-invasive bladder carcinoma: a systematic review. Vol. 38, Urologic oncology: seminars and original investigations. Elsevier Inc.; 2020. p. 774–82.
37. van Osch FHM, Nekeman D, Aaronson NK, Billingham LJ, James ND, Cheng KK, et al. Patients choose certainty over burden in bladder cancer surveillance. World J Urol [Internet]. 2019 Dec 1 [cited 2021 Jan 3];37(12):2747–53. Available from: https://pubmed.ncbi.nlm.nih.gov/30903352/.

38. Brown FM. Urine cytology: is it still the gold standard for screening? Urol Clin North Am [Internet]. 2000 [cited 2021 Jan 3];27(1):25–37. Available from: https://pubmed.ncbi.nlm.nih.gov/10696242/.
39. Giordano A, Soria F. Role and efficacy of current biomarkers in bladder cancer. AME Med J [Internet]. 2020 Mar 25 [cited 2021 Jan 3];5(0):6–6. Available from: http://amj.amegroups.com/article/view/5394/html
40. Lotan Y, Osullivan P, Raman JD, Shariat SF, Kavalieris L, Frampton C, et al. Clinical comparison of noninvasive urine tests for ruling out recurrent urothelial carcinoma. Urol Oncol Semin Orig Investig. 2017;35(8):531.e15–22.
41. Wright JL, Hotaling J, Porter MP. Predictors of upper tract urothelial cell carcinoma after primary bladder cancer: a population based analysis. JURO [Internet] 2009 [cited 2021 Jan 3];181:1035–9. Available from: www.jurology.com.
42. Göğüş Ç, Baltaci S, Şahinli S, Türkölmez K, Bedük Y, Göüs O. Value of selective upper tract cytology for recognition of upper tract tumors after treatment of superficial bladder cancer. Int J Urol [Internet]. 2003 May 1 [cited 2021 Jan 3];10(5):243–6. Available from: https://pubmed.ncbi.nlm.nih.gov/12694462/
43. Donin NM, Lenis AT, Holden S, Drakaki A, Pantuck A, Belldegrun A, et al. Immunotherapy for the treatment of urothelial carcinoma. J Urol [Internet]. 2017 Jan 1 [cited 2021 Jan 10];197(1):14–22. Available from: http://www.jurology.com/doi/10.1016/j.juro.2016.02.3005.
44. Old LJ, Clarke DA, Benacerraf B. Effect of bacillus calmette-guérin infection on transplanted tumours in the mouse. Nature [Internet]. 1959 [cited 2021 Jan 10];184(4682):291–2. Available from: https://www.nature.com/articles/184291a0.
45. Morales A, Eidinger D, Bruce AW. Intracavitary bacillus Calmette Guerin in the treatment of superficial bladder tumors. J Urol. 1976;116(2):180–2.
46. Babjuk M, Burger M, Compérat EM, Gontero P, Mostafid AH, Palou J, et al. European Association of Urology guidelines on non-muscle-invasive bladder cancer (TaT1 and carcinoma in situ) – 2019 update. Eur Urol. 2019;76:369.
47. Rouprêt M, Neuzillet Y, Masson-Lecomte A, Colin P, Compérat E, Dubosq F, et al. CCAFU french national guidelines 2016-2018 on bladder cancer. Prog Urol. 2016;1(27):S67–91.
48. Gandhi NM, Morales A, Lamm DL. Bacillus Calmette-Guérin immunotherapy for genitourinary cancer [Internet]. Vol. 112, BJU International. BJU Int; 2013 [cited 2021 Jan 10]. p. 288–97. Available from: https://pubmed.ncbi.nlm.nih.gov/23517232/.
49. Redelman-Sidi G, Glickman MS, Bochner BH. The mechanism of action of BCG therapy for bladder cancer-A current perspective [Internet]. Vol. 11, Nature Reviews Urology. Nature Publishing Group; 2014 [cited 2021 Jan 10]. p. 153–62. Available from: https://pubmed.ncbi.nlm.nih.gov/24492433/.
50. Lamm DL, Van der Meijden APM, Morales A, Brosman SA, Catalona WJ, Herr HW, et al. Incidence and treatment of complications of bacillus Calmette-Guerin intravesical therapy in superficial bladder cancer. J Urol [Internet]. 1992; [cited 2021 Jan 10];147(3 I):596–600. Available from: https://pubmed.ncbi.nlm.nih.gov/1538436/
51. Lamm DL, Dehaven JI, Riggs DR. Keyhole limpet hemocyanin immunotherapy of bladder cancer: Laboratory and clinical studies. In: European Urology [Internet]. S. Karger AG; 2000 [cited 2021 Jan 16]. p. 41–4. Available from: https://pubmed.ncbi.nlm.nih.gov/10828686/.
52. Lamm DL, Blumenstein BA, Crissman JD, Montie JE, Gottesman JE, Lowe BA, et al. Maintenance bacillus Calmette-Guerin immunotherapy for recurrent ta, T1 and carcinoma in situ transitional cell carcinoma of the bladder: a randomized southwest oncology group study. J Urol. 2000;163(4):1124–9.
53. Lamm DL. Efficacy and safety of bacille Calmette-Guérin immunotherapy in superficial bladder cancer. In: Clinical infectious diseases [Internet]. Clin Infect Dis; 2000 [cited 2021 Jan 10]. Available from: https://pubmed.ncbi.nlm.nih.gov/11010830/.
54. Rischmann P, Desgrandchamps F, Malavaud B, Chopin DK. BCG intravesical instillations: recommendations for side-effects management. Eur Urol [Internet]. 2000 [cited 2021 Jan 16];37(Suppl. 1):33–6. Available from: https://www.karger.com/Article/FullText/52381.

55. Sylvester RJ, Brausi MA, Kirkels WJ, Hoeltl W, Calais Da Silva F, Powell PH, et al. Long-term efficacy results of EORTC Genito-urinary group randomized phase 3 study 30911 comparing Intravesical instillations of Epirubicin, bacillus Calmette-Guérin, and bacillus Calmette-Guérin plus isoniazid in patients with intermediate- and high-risk stage ta T1 urothelial carcinoma of the bladder. Eur Urol. 2010;57(5):766–73.
56. Fernandez-Gomez J, Solsona E, Unda M, Martinez-Piñeiro L, Gonzalez M, Hernandez R, et al. Prognostic factors in patients with non-muscle-invasive bladder cancer treated with bacillus Calmette-Guérin: multivariate analysis of data from four randomized CUETO trials. Eur Urol. 2008;53(5):992–1002.
57. Fda, Cder, Mccrayk. BCG-unresponsive nonmuscle invasive bladder cancer: developing drugs and biologics for treatment guidance for industry [Internet]. 2018 [cited 2021 Jan 10]. Available from: https://www.fda.gov/Drugs/GuidanceComplianceRegulatoryInformation/Guidances/default.htmand/ or https://www.fda.gov/BiologicsBloodVaccines/GuidanceComplianceRegulatoryInformation/Guidances/default.htm.
58. Novara G, Catto JWF, Wilson T, Annerstedt M, Chan K, Murphy DG, et al. Systematic review and cumulative analysis of perioperative outcomes and complications after robot-assisted radical cystectomy. Eur Urol. 2015;67:376–401.
59. Porter MP, Penson DF. Health related quality of life after radical cystectomy and urinary diversion for bladder cancer: a systematic review and critical analysis of the literature. J Urol [Internet] 2005 [cited 2021 Jan 10]; Available from: https://www.auajournals.org/doi/abs/10.1097/01.ju.0000149080.82697.65.
60. Abrams PH, Choa RG, CGC G, Ashken MH, Green NA. A controlled trial of single dose Intravesical adriamycin in superficial bladder Tumours. Br J Urol. 1981;53:585.
61. Pan JS, Slocum HK, Rustum YM, Greco WR, Gaeta JF, Huben RP. Inhibition of implantation of murine bladder tumor by thiotepa in cauterized bladder. J Urol. 1989;142:1589.
62. Brocks CP, Büttner H, Böhle A. Inhibition of tumor implantation by intravesical gemcitabine in a murine model of superficial bladder cancer. J Urol. 2005;174:1115–18.
63. Pode D, Alon Y, Horowitz AT, Vlodavsky I, Biran S. The mechanism of human bladder tumor implantation in an in vitro model. J Urol. 1986;136(2):482–86.
64. Flaig TW, Spiess PE, Agarwal N, Bangs R, Boorjian SA, Buyyounouski MK, et al. NCCN guidelines insights: bladder cancer, Version 52018, J Natl Compr Cancer Netw. 2018.
65. Messing EM, Tangen CM, Lerner SP, Sahasrabudhe DM, Koppie TM, Wood DP, et al. Effect of intravesical instillation of gemcitabine vs saline immediately following resection of suspected low-grade non-muscle-invasive bladder cancer on tumor recurrence SWOG S0337 randomized clinical trial. JAMA J Am Med Assoc. 2018;319(18):1880–88.
66. Kang M, Jeong CW, Kwak C, Kim HH, Ku JH. Single, immediate postoperative instillation of chemotherapy in non-muscle invasive bladder cancer: a systematic review and network meta-analysis of randomized clinical trials using different drugs. Oncotarget. 2016;7(29):45479–88.
67. Naya Y, Mikami K, Takaha N, Inoue Y, Fujihara A, Kanazawa M, et al. Randomized study of intravesical pirarubicin chemotherapy with low and intermediate-risk nonmuscle-invasive bladder cancer in Japan: comparison of a single immediate postoperative intravesical instillation with short-term adjuvant intravesical instillation. Med (United States). 2018;97(42):12740.
68. Sylvester RJ, Oosterlinck W, Holmang S, Sydes MR, Birtle A, Gudjonsson S, et al. Systematic review and individual patient data meta-analysis of randomized trials comparing a single immediate instillation of chemotherapy after transurethral resection with transurethral resection alone in patients with stage pTa-pT1 urothelial carcinoma. Eur Urol. 2016;69(2):231–44.
69. Perlis N, Zlotta AR, Beyene J, Finelli A, Fleshner NE, Kulkarni GS. Immediate post- transurethral resection of bladder tumor intravesical chemotherapy prevents non-muscle- invasive bladder cancer recurrences: an updated meta-analysis on 2548 patients and quality-of-evidence review. Eur Urol. 2013;64(3):421–30.
70. Oddens JR, Van Der Meijden APM, Sylvester R. One immediate postoperative instillation of chemotherapy in low risk ta, T1 bladder cancer patients. Is it always safe? Eur Urol. 2004;46(3):336–38.

71. Tolley DA, Parmar MKB, Grigor KM, Lallemand G, Beynon LL, Fellows SJ, et al. The effect of intravesical mitomycin C on recurrence of newly diagnosed superficial bladder cancer: a further report with 7 years of followup. J Urol. 1996;155(4):1233–38.
72. Liu B, Wang Z, Chen B, Yu J, Zhang P, Ding Q, et al. Randomized study of single instillation of epirubicin for superficial bladder carcinoma: long-term clinical outcomes. Cancer Investig. 2006;24(2):60–63.
73. Türkeri L, Tanidir Y, Çal Ç, Özen H, Şahin H. Comparison of the efficacy of single or double intravesical epirubicin instillation in the early postoperative period to prevent recurrences in non-muscle-invasive urothelial carcinoma of the bladder: prospective, randomized multicenter study. Urol Int. 2010;85(3):261–65.
74. Sylvester RJ, Oosterlinck W, Van Der Meijden APM. A single immediate postoperative instillation of chemotherapy decreases the risk of recurrence in patients with stage ta T1 bladder cancer: a meta-analysis of published results of randomized clinical trials. J Urol. 2004;30(4):353–54.
75. Bouffioux C, Kurth KH, Bono A, Oosterlinck W, Kruger CB, De Pauw M, et al. Original articles: bladder cancer: intravesical adjuvant chemotherapy for superficial transitional cell bladder carcinoma: results of 2 European Organization for Research and Treatment of cancer randomized trials with mitomycin C and doxorubicin comparing. J Urol. 1995;153(3 pt 2):934–41.
76. Chou R, Buckley D, Fu R, Gore JL, Gustafson K, Griffin JC, et al. Emerging approaches to diagnosis and treatment of non–muscle-invasive bladder cancer. Comp Eff Rev. 2015;15(16).
77. Böhle A, Bock PR. Intravesical bacille Calmette-Guérin versus mitomycin C in superficial bladder cancer: formal meta-analysis of comparative studies on tumor progression. Urology. 2004;173(3):730–31.
78. Chou R, Selph S, Buckley DI, Fu R, Griffin JC, Grusing S, et al. Intravesical therapy for the treatment of nonmuscle invasive bladder cancer: a systematic review and meta-analysis. J Urol. 2017;197(5):1189–199.
79. Malmström PU, Sylvester RJ, Crawford DE, Friedrich M, Krege S, Rintala E, et al. An individual patient data meta-analysis of the long-term outcome of randomised studies comparing intravesical mitomycin C versus bacillus Calmette-Guérin for non-muscle-invasive bladder cancer. Eur Urol. 2009;56(2):247–56.
80. Zargar H, Aning J, Ischia J, So A, Black P. Optimizing intravesical mitomycin C therapy in non-muscle-invasive bladder cancer. Nat Rev Urol. 2014;11(4):220–30.
81. Au JLS, Badalament RA, Wientjes MG, Young DC, Warner JA, Venema PL, et al. Methods to improve efficacy of intravesical mitomycin C: results of a randomized phase III trial. J Natl Cancer Inst. 2001;93(8):597–604.
82. Guillaume Wientjes M, Badalament RA, Au JLS. Use of pharmacologic data and computer simulations to design an efficacy trial of intravesical mitomycin C therapy for superficial bladder cancer. Cancer Chemother Pharmacol. 1993;32:255–62.
83. Au JL-S, Badalament RA, Wientjes MG, Young DC, Warner JA, Venema PL, et al. Methods to improve efficacy of Intravesical Mitomycin C: results of a randomized phase III trial. JNCI J Natl Cancer Inst [Internet] 2001 Apr 18 [cited 2021 Jan 31];93(8):597–604. Available from: https://academic.oup.com/jnci/article-lookup/doi/10.1093/jnci/93.8.597.
84. Friedrich MG, Pichlmeier U, Schwaibold H, Conrad S, Huland H. Long-term Intravesical adjuvant chemotherapy further reduces recurrence rate compared with short-term Intravesical chemotherapy and short-term therapy with bacillus Calmette-Guérin (BCG) in patients with non-muscle-invasive bladder carcinoma. Eur Urol. 2007;52(4):1123–29.
85. Sylvester RJ, Oosterlinck W, Witjes JA. The schedule and duration of intravesical chemotherapy in patients with non-muscle-invasive bladder cancer: a systematic review of the published results of randomized clinical trials. Eur Urol. 2008;53(4):709–19.
86. Onrust SV, Wiseman LR, Goa KL. Epirubicin. A review of its intravesical use in superficial bladder cancer. Drugs and Aging. 1999;15(4):307–33.
87. Van Der Meijden APM, Brausi M, Zambon V, Kirkels W, De Balincourt C, Sylvester R, et al. Intravesical instillation of epirubicin, bacillus Calmette-Guerin and bacillus Calmette-

Guerin plus isoniazid for intermediate and high risk TA, T1 papillary carcinoma of the bladder: a European Organization for Research and Treatment of cancer Genito-Uri. J Urol. 2001;166(2):476–81.
88. Hendricksen K, Kiemeney LA, Caris C, Janzing R, Witjes W, Witjes JA. Comparison of three schedules of adjuvant intravesical epirubicin in patients with non-muscle invasive bladder cancer Eur Urol Suppl. 2008;53(5):984–91.
89. Elsawy AA, El-Assmy AM, Bazeed MA, Ali-El-Dein B. The value of immediate postoperative intravesical epirubicin instillation as an adjunct to standard adjuvant treatment in intermediate and high-risk non–muscle-invasive bladder cancer: a preliminary results of randomized controlled trial. Urol Oncol Semin Orig Investig. 2019;37(3):179.
90. Sylvester RJ, Brausi MA, Kirkels WJ, Hoeltl W, Calais Da Silva F, Powell PH, et al. Long-term efficacy results of EORTC Genito-urinary group randomized phase 3 study 30911 comparing Intravesical instillations of Epirubicin, bacillus Calmette-Guérin, and bacillus Calmette-Guérin plus isoniazid in patients with intermediate- and high-risk . Eur Urol. 2010;57(5):766–73.
91. Dinney CPN, Greenberg RE, Steinberg GD. Intravesical valrubicin in patients with bladder carcinoma in situ and contraindication to or failure after bacillus Calmette-Guérin. Urol Oncol Semin Orig Investig. 2013;31(8):1635–42.
92. Witjes JA, Van Der Heijden AG, Vriesema JLJ, Peters GJ, Laan A, Schalken JA. Intravesical gemcitabine: a phase 1 and pharmacokinetic study. Eur Urol. 2004;45(2):182–6.
93. Di Lorenzo G, Perdonà S, Damiano R, Faiella A, Cantiello F, Pignata S, et al. Gemcitabine versus bacille Calmette-Guérin after initial bacille Calmette-Guérin failure in non-muscle- invasive bladder cancer: a multicenter prospective randomized trial. Cancer. 2010;116(8):1893–1900.
94. Addeo R, Caraglia M, Bellini S, Abbruzzese A, Vincenzi B, Montella L, et al. Randomized phase III trial on gemcitabine versus mytomicin in recurrent superficial bladder cancer: evaluation of efficacy and tolerance. J Clin Oncol. 2010;28(4):543–8.
95. Skinner EC, Goldman B, Sakr WA, Petrylak DP, Lenz HJ, Lee CT, et al. SWOG S0353: phase II trial of intravesical gemcitabine in patients with nonmuscle invasive bladder cancer and recurrence after 2 prior courses of intravesical bacillus calmette-guérin. J Urol. 2013;190(4):1200–04.
96. Jones G, Cleves A, Wilt TJ, Mason M, Kynaston HG, Shelley M. Intravesical gemcitabine for non-muscle invasive bladder cancer. Cochrane Database Syst Rev. 2012 Jan 18.
97. Verweij J, Clavel M, Chevalier B. Paclitaxel (Taxol™) and docetaxel (Taxotere™): not simply two of a kind. Ann Oncol. 1994;5(6):495–505.
98. Rangel C, Niell H, Miller A, Cox C. Taxol and taxotere in bladder cancer: in vitro activity and urine stability. Cancer Chemother Pharmacol. 1994;33(6):460–64.
99. Laudano MA, Barlow LJ, Murphy AM, Petrylak DP, Desai M, Benson MC, et al. Long-term clinical outcomes of a phase I trial of Intravesical docetaxel in the Management of non- muscle- invasive bladder cancer refractory to standard intravesical therapy. Urology. 2010;75(1):134–7.
100. Barlow LJ, McKiernan JM, Benson MC. Long-term survival outcomes with intravesical docetaxel for recurrent nonmuscle invasive bladder cancer after previous bacillus Calmette-Guérin therapy. J Urol. 2013;189(3):834–39.
101. Barlow L, McKiernan J, Sawczuk I, Benson M. A single-institution experience with induction and maintenance intravesical docetaxel in the management of non-muscle-invasive bladder cancer refractory to bacille Calmette-Guérin therapy. BJU Int. 2009;104(8):1098–102.
102. Sekine H, Fukui I, Yamada T, Ohwada F, Yokokawa M, Ohshima H. Intravesical mitomycin C and doxorubicin sequential therapy for carcinoma in situ of the bladder: a longer followup result. J Urol. 1994;151(1):27–30.
103. Marttila T, Järvinen R, Liukkonen T, Rintala E, Boström P, Seppänen M, et al. Intravesical bacillus Calmette-Guérin versus combination of Epirubicin and interferon-α2a in reducing recurrence of non–muscle-invasive bladder carcinoma: FinnBladder-6 study. Eur Urol. 2016:70(2):341–47.

104. Lightfoot AJ, Breyer BN, Rosevear HM, Erickson BA, Konety BR, O'Donnell MA. Multi-institutional analysis of sequential intravesical gemcitabine and mitomycin C chemotherapy for non-muscle invasive bladder cancer. Urol Oncol Semin Orig Investig. 2014;32(1) 35.e15–19.
105. Steinberg RL, Thomas LJ, O'Donnell MA, Nepple KG. Sequential intravesical gemcitabine and docetaxel for the salvage treatment of non-muscle invasive bladder cancer. Bl Cancer. 2015;1(1):65–72.
106. Decastro GJ, Sui W, Pak JS, Lee SM, Holder D, Kates MM, et al. A phase i trial of intravesical cabazitaxel, gemcitabine and cisplatin for the treatment of nonmuscle invasive bacillus calmette-guérin unresponsive or recurrent/relapsing urothelial carcinoma of the bladder. J Urol. 2020;204(2):247–53.
107. Powles T, Eder JP, Fine GD, Braiteh FS, Loriot Y, Cruz C, et al. MPDL3280A (anti-PD-L1) treatment leads to clinical activity in metastatic bladder cancer. Nature [Internet]. 2014 Nov 27 [cited 2021 Jan 10];515(7528):558–62. Available from: https://www.nature.com/articles/nature13904.
108. Balar AV, Kamat AM, Kulkarni GS, Uchio EM, Boormans JL, Bajorin DF, et al. Pembrolizumab (pembro) for the treatment of patients with bacillus Calmette-Guérin (BCG) unresponsive, high-risk (HR) non–muscle-invasive bladder cancer (NMIBC): over two years follow-up of KEYNOTE-057. J Clin Oncol. 2020;38(15_suppl):5041.
109. Black PC, Tangen C, Singh P, McConkey DJ, Lucia S, Lowrance WT, et al. Phase II trial of atezolizumab in BCG-unresponsive non-muscle invasive bladder cancer: SWOG S1605 (NCT #02844816). J Clin Oncol. 2020;38(15_suppl):5022.
110. Yamashita M, Rosser CJ, Zhou JH, Zhang XQ, Connor RJ, Engler H, et al. Syn3 provides high levels of intravesical adenoviral-mediated gene transfer for gene therapy of genetically altered urothelium and superficial bladder cancer. Cancer Gene Ther [Internet]. 2002 [cited 2021 Jan 10];9(8):687–91. Available from: https://pubmed.ncbi.nlm.nih.gov/12136430/.
111. Benedict WF, Tao Z, Kim CS, Zhang X, Zhou JH, Adam L, et al. Intravesical Ad-IFNα causes marked regression of human bladder cancer growing orthotopically in nude mice and overcomes resistance to IFN-α protein. Mol Ther [Internet]. 2004 Sep [cited 2021 Jan 10];10(3):525–32. Available from: https://pubmed.ncbi.nlm.nih.gov/15336652/.
112. Tao Z, Connor RJ, Ashoori F, Dinney CPN, Munsell M, Philopena JA, et al. Efficacy of a single intravesical treatment with Ad-IFN/Syn 3 is dependent on dose and urine IFN concentration obtained: Implications for clinical investigation. Cancer Gene Ther [Internet]. 2006 Feb [cited 2021 Jan 10];13(2):125–30. Available from: https://pubmed.ncbi.nlm.nih.gov/16082384/.
113. Shore ND, Boorjian SA, Canter DJ, Ogan K, Karsh LI, Downs TM, et al. Intravesical rAd–IFNa/Syn3 for patients with high-grade, bacillus calmette-guerin–refractory or relapsed non–muscle-invasive bladder cancer: A phase II randomized study. J Clin Oncol [Internet]. 2017 Oct 20 [cited 2021 Jan 10];35(30):3410–6. Available from: https://ascopubs.org/doi/10.1200/JCO.2017.72.3064.
114. Boorjian SA, Alemozaffar M, Konety BR, Shore ND, Gomella LG, Kamat AM, et al. Intravesical nadofaragene firadenovec gene therapy for BCG-unresponsive non-muscle-invasive bladder cancer: a single-arm, open-label, repeat-dose clinical trial. Lancet Oncol [Internet]. 2020 Nov 1 [cited 2021 Jan 10];22(1):107–17. Available from: www.thelancet.com/oncology.
115. Rosenberg SA. IL-2: The First Effective Immunotherapy for Human Cancer. J Immunol [Internet]. 2014 Jun 15 [cited 2021 Jan 10];192(12):5451–8. Available from: https://pubmed.ncbi.nlm.nih.gov/24907378/.
116. Lee S, Margolin K. Cytokines in Cancer Immunotherapy. Cancers (Basel) [Internet]. 2011 Oct 13 [cited 2021 Jan 10];3(4):3856–93. Available from: http://www.mdpi.com/2072-6694/3/4/3856.
117. Sonpavde G, Rosser CJ, Pan C, Parikh RA, Nix J, Gingrich JR, et al. Phase I trial of ALT-801, a first-in-class T-cell receptor (TCR)-interleukin (IL)-2 fusion molecule, plus gemcitabine (G) for bacillus Calmette Guerin (BCG)-resistant non-muscle-invasive bladder cancer (NMIBC). J Clin Oncol. 2015;33(15_suppl):e15509.

118. Chamie K, Lee JH, Rock A, Rhode PR, Soon-Shiong P. Preliminary phase 2 clinical results of IL-15RαFc superagonist N-803 with BCG in BCG-unresponsive non-muscle invasive bladder cancer (NMIBC) patients. J Clin Oncol. 2019;37(15_suppl):4561.
119. Rosser CJ, Nix J, Ferguson L, Hernandez L, Wong HC. Phase Ib trial of ALT-803, an IL-15 superagonist, plus BCG for the treatment of BCG-naïve patients with non-muscle-invasive bladder cancer. J Clin Oncol. 2018;36(6_suppl):510.
120. Vicinium Treatment for Subjects With Non-muscle Invasive Bladder Cancer Previously Treated With BCG – Full Text View – ClinicalTrials.gov [Internet]. [cited 2021 Jan 10]. Available from: https://clinicaltrials.gov/ct2/show/NCT02449239.
121. Kowalski M, Guindon J, Brazas L, Moore C, Entwistle J, Cizeau J, et al. A phase II study of oportuzumab monatox: An immunotoxin therapy for patients with noninvasive urothelial carcinoma in situ previously treated with bacillus Calmette-Guérin. J Urol [Internet]. 2012 Nov [cited 2021 Jan 10];188(5):1712–8. Available from: https://pubmed.ncbi.nlm.nih.gov/22998907/
122. Rentsch CA, Bosshard P, Mayor G, Rieken M, Püschel H, Wirth G, et al. Results of the phase I open label clinical trial SAKK 06/14 assessing safety of intravesical instillation of VPM1002BC, a recombinant mycobacterium bacillus Calmette Guérin (BCG), in patients with non-muscle invasive bladder cancer and previous failure of conventional BCG therapy. Oncoimmunology [Internet]. 2020;Jan 1 [cited 2021 Jan 10];9(1). Available from: /pmc/articles/PMC7185202/?report=abstract
123. IBCN 2020: Efficacy, Safety and Tolerability of the rBCG VPM1002BC in Patients with High-Grade NMIBC Recurrence after BCG Induction with or without BCG Maintenance Therapy – SAKK 06/14 [Internet]. [cited 2021 Jan 10]. Available from: https://www.urotoday.com/conference-highlights/ibcn-2020/125268-ibcn-2020-results-of-a-phase-i-ii-single-arm-clinical-trial-assessing-efficacy-safety-and-tolerability-of-the-recombinant-bacillus-calmette-guerin-vpm1002bc-in-patients-with-non-muscle-invasive-bladder-cancer-recurrence-after-bcg-induction-with-or-without-bcg-maintenance-therapy-sakk-06-14.html.
124. Paroni R, Salonia A, Lev A, Da Pozzo LF, Cighetti G, Montorsi F, et al. Effect of local hyperthermia of the bladder on mitomycin C pharmacokinetics during intravesical chemotherapy for the treatment of superficial transitional cell carcinoma. Br J Clin Pharmacol Suppl. 2001.
125. Colombo R, Lev A, Da Pozzo LF, Freschi M, Gallus G, Rigatti P. Original articles: bladder cancer: a new approach using local combined microwave hyperthermia and chemotherapy in superficial transitional bladder carcinoma treatment. J Urol. 1995.
126. Colombo R, Da Pozzo LF, Salonia A, Rigatti P, Leib Z, Baniel J, et al. Multicentric study comparing intravesical chemotherapy alone and with local microwave hyperthermia for prophylaxis of recurrence of superficial transitional cell carcinoma. J Clin Oncol. 2003.
127. Colombo R, Salonia A, Leib Z, Pavone-Macaluso M, Engelstein D. Long-term outcomes of a randomized controlled trial comparing thermochemotherapy with mitomycin-C alone as adjuvant treatment for non-muscle-invasive bladder cancer (NMIBC). BJU Int. 2011;107(6):912–18.
128. Alfred Witjes J, Hendricksen K, Gofrit O, Risi O, Nativ O. Intravesical hyperthermia and mitomycin-C for carcinoma in situ of the urinary bladder: experience of the European Synergo® working party. World J Urol. 2009;27(3):319–24.
129. Van Der Heijden AG, Kiemeney LA, Gofrit ON, Nativ O, Sidi A, Leib Z, et al. Preliminary European results of local microwave hyperthermia and chemotherapy treatment in intermediate or high risk superficial transitional cell carcinoma of the bladder. Eur Urol. 2004;46(1):65–71.
130. Di Stasi SM, Giannantoni A, Massoud R, Dolci S, Navarra P, Vespasiani G, et al. Electromotive versus passive diffusion of mitomycin C into human bladder wall: concentration-depth profiles studies. Cancer Res. 1999;59(19):4912–18.
131. Colombo R, Brausi M, Da Pozzo LF, Salonia A, Montorsi F, Scattoni V, et al. Thermochemotherapy and electromotive drug administration of mitomycin C in superficial bladder cancer eradication: a pilot study on marker lesion. Eur Urol. 2001;39(1):95–100.
132. Di Stasi SM, Giannantoni A, Stephen RL, Capelli G, Navarra P, Massoud R, et al. Intravesical electromotive mitomycin C versus passive transport mitomycin C for high risk superficial bladder cancer: a prospective randomized study. J Urol. 2003;170(3):777–82.

133. Di Stasi SM, Giannantoni A, Giurioli A, Valenti M, Zampa G, Storti L, et al. Sequential BCG and electromotive mitomycin versus BCG alone for high-risk superficial bladder cancer: a randomised controlled trial. Lancet Oncol. 2006;7(1):43–51.
134. Gan C, Amery S, Chatterton K, Khan MS, Thomas K, O'Brien T. Sequential bacillus Calmette-Guérin/electromotive drug administration of mitomycin C as the standard intravesical regimen in high risk nonmuscle invasive bladder cancer: 2-year outcomes. J Urol. 2016;195(6):1697–1703.
135. Di Stasi SM, Valenti M, Verri C, Liberati E, Giurioli A, Leprini G, et al. Electromotive instillation of mitomycin immediately before transurethral resection for patients with primary urothelial non-muscle invasive bladder cancer: a randomised controlled trial. Lancet Oncol. 2011;12(9):871–9.
136. Railkar R, Agarwal PK. Photodynamic therapy in the treatment of bladder cancer: past challenges and current innovations. Eur Uro Focus. 2018;4(4):509–11.
137. Berg K, Selbo PK, Weyergang A, Dietze A, Prasmickaite L, Bonsted A, et al. Porphyrin-related photosensitizers for cancer imaging and therapeutic applications. J Microsc. 2005;218(2):133–47.
138. Bachor R, Reich E, Rück A, Hautmann R. Aminolevulinic acid for photodynamic therapy of bladder carcinoma cells. Urol Res. 1996;24(5):285–9.
139. Waidelich R, Stepp H, Baumgartner R, Weninger E, Hofstetter A, Kriegmair M. Clinical experience with 5-aminolevulinic acid and photodynamic therapy for refractory superficial bladder cancer. J Urol. 2001;165(6 Pt 1):1904–07.
140. Berger AP, Steiner H, Stenzl A, Akkad T, Bartsch G, Holtl L. Photodynamic therapy with intravesical instillation of 5-aminolevulinic acid for patients with recurrent superficial bladder cancer: a single-center study. Urology. 2003;61:338.
141. Filonenko EV, Kaprin AD, Alekseev BYA, Apolikhin OI, Slovokhodov EK, Ivanova-Radkevich VI, et al. 5-Aminolevulinic acid in intraoperative photodynamic therapy of bladder cancer (results of multicenter trial). Photodiagn Photodyn Ther. 2016;16:106.
142. Lee JY, Diaz RR, Cho KS, Lim MS, Chung JS, Kim WT, et al. Efficacy and safety of photodynamic therapy for recurrent, high grade nonmuscle invasive bladder cancer refractory or intolerant to bacille calmette-Guérin immunotherapy. J Urol. 2013;190:1192.
143. Bianco FJ, Justa D, Grignon DJ, Sakr WA, Pontes JE, Wood DP. Management of clinical T1 bladder transitional cell carcinoma by radical cystectomy. Urol Oncol Semin Orig Investig [Internet]. 2004 Jul [cited 2021 Jan 4];22(4):290–4. Available from: https://pubmed.ncbi.nlm.nih.gov/15283885/.
144. Stein JP. Indications for early cystectomy [Internet]. Vol. 62, Urology. Elsevier Inc.; 2003 [cited 2021 Jan 4]. p. 591–5. Available from: http://www.goldjournal.net/article/S0090429503005843/fulltext.
145. Mohamed NE, Shah QN, Kata HE, Sfakianos J, Given B. Dealing with the unthinkable: bladder and colorectal cancer patients' and informal caregivers' unmet needs and challenges in life after ostomies. Semin Oncol Nurs [Internet] 2021 Jan 7 [cited 2021 Jan 10];151111. Available from: https://linkinghub.elsevier.com/retrieve/pii/S0749208120301261.
146. Stein JP, Lieskovsky G, Cote R, Groshen S, Feng AC, Boyd S, et al. Radical cystectomy in the treatment of invasive bladder cancer: Long-term results in 1,054 patients. J Clin Oncol [Internet]. 2001 Feb 1 [cited 2021 Jan 10];19(3):666–75. Available from: https://pubmed.ncbi.nlm.nih.gov/11157016/.

Chapter 17
Neoadjuvant and Adjuvant Therapy for Muscle-Invasive Bladder Cancer

Brendan J. Guercio and Gopa Iyer

Introduction

In contrast to non-muscle-invasive bladder cancer, which has an excellent prognosis with local therapy alone, muscle-invasive bladder cancer (MIBC) is often a systemic disease at diagnosis due to clinically occult micrometastases [1, 2]. As a result, MIBC managed with surgical resection alone, specifically radical cystectomy plus pelvic lymph node dissection, results in recurrence at distant sites in up to 50% of patients [3, 4]. Maximizing chance of cure at time of radical cystectomy is key given the dismal prognosis of bladder cancer that recurs with distant metastases, which remains incurable in a majority of cases [2]. Addition of perioperative systemic therapy to surgical resection can reduce risk of recurrence and improve overall survival [5]. Herein, we will aim to summarize key evidence regarding standard perioperative systemic treatments for MIBC, as well as promising novel perioperative regimens that are currently under investigation.

Neoadjuvant Chemotherapy (NACT)

Historically, the investigation of NACT prior to radical cystectomy for MIBC began with neoadjuvant cisplatin monotherapy based on the efficacy of cisplatin observed in the metastatic setting [6]. This was followed by trials of NACT combinations [7–11] such as CMV (cisplatin, methotrexate, vinblastine), wherein the phase 3 trial

B. J. Guercio · G. Iyer (✉)
Department of Medicine, Memorial Sloan Kettering Cancer Center, New York, NY, USA
e-mail: guerciob@mskcc.org; iyerg@mskcc.org

K. L. Stratton, A. K. Morgans (eds.), *Urologic Oncology*,
https://doi.org/10.1007/978-3-030-89891-5_17

BA06 30894 showed a 16% reduction in the risk of death with three cycles of CMV versus no neoadjuvant therapy as well as an absolute improvement in 10-year survival by 6% [12, 13]. Eventually, MVAC (methotrexate, vinblastine, doxorubicin, and cisplatin) was established as a standard neoadjuvant regimen for MIBC based on the findings of SWOG-8710, a phase 3 trial demonstrating a median survival of 77 months after surgery among patients who received neoadjuvant MVAC versus 46 months among patients treated with surgery alone ($p = 0.06$ by two-sided log-rank test) and a corresponding hazard ratio (HR) for risk of death in the upfront cystectomy group of 1.33 compared to the MVAC-treated arm (95% confidence interval [CI] 1.00–1.76). In SWOG-8710, patients treated with MVAC experienced a superior pathologic complete response (pCR) rate of 38% versus 15% among patients treated with surgery alone [14]. A retrospective analysis of SWOG-8710 demonstrated a significant correlation between pathologic response at cystectomy and long-term survival, wherein patients with residual disease (>ypT0) had a HR for overall survival of 2.51 compared to patients with a complete pathologic response, defined as ypT0 (95% CI 1.47–4.27, $p = 0.0008$) [15]. Residual muscle-invasive disease (≥ypT2) appeared particularly prognostic, with a HR for overall survival of 2.24 compared to patients without muscle-invasive disease (95% CI 1.34–3.76, $p = 0.0022$) [15]. The association between pathologic response and long-term patient survival was ultimately confirmed in a meta-analysis, establishing pathologic response at cystectomy as an important surrogate endpoint for survival in MIBC [16]. MVAC was also determined superior to the competing CISCA regimen (cisplatin, cyclophosphamide, doxorubicin) [17].

In 2005, a meta-analysis including 3005 patients from 11 clinical trials demonstrated a 5% absolute increase in 5-year overall survival and a 14% decrease in the risk of death among patients with MIBC who received cisplatin-based NACT prior to local therapy compared to patients who received local therapy alone [5]. This corresponded to a 22% improvement in disease-free survival (HR 0.78, 95% CI 0.71–0.86, $p < 0.0001$ [5]. The improvement in overall survival is comparable to that seen in other tumor types in which perioperative chemotherapy is considered an established standard of care [18, 19].

As a result, cisplatin-based NACT is the current standard of care for cisplatin-eligible patients with MIBC [5, 20–22]. However, many patients do not benefit from NACT [14, 23], and inability to predict benefit and concerns about toxicity have led to low uptake of NACT in community practice. For example, an analysis of the American College of Surgeons and American Cancer Society National Cancer Data Base (NCDB), which included patients treated at both community and academic centers, showed that use of NACT for localized MIBC in 2010 was only 20.9% [24]. As a result, some clinicians have proposed clinical criteria such as presence of hydroureteronephrosis and lymphovascular invasion to refine selection of patients for NACT [25]; however, use of such criteria is not a universally accepted standard for clinical practice [26].

NACT traditionally refers to three to four cycles of cisplatin-based chemotherapy in patients with T2–T4aN0M0 disease followed by assessment for cystectomy.

In patients with disease that has spread to lymph nodes or soft tissue sites, consolidative surgical resection can be considered if a major radiographic response is achieved following six cycles of cisplatin-based chemotherapy [27–29]. Indeed, an NCDB data analysis of patients with bladder cancer involving regional lymph nodes demonstrated that treatment with perioperative chemotherapy plus surgery was associated with superior outcomes compared to either chemotherapy or surgery alone [30]. However, all patients with N1–3 and/or M1 disease should receive six cycles of chemotherapy if able prior to consolidative surgery, given a lack of compelling evidence to support a smaller number of cycles in this clinical context [31]. If uncertainty regarding lymph node involvement exists, lymph nodes 1–2 cm in diameter can be further evaluated by FDG-PET/CT with or without image-guided biopsy [32]. Notably, two phase 2 trials of neoadjuvant dose-dense MVAC (ddMVAC) allowed patients with clinical N1 disease, providing support for consideration of NACT plus cystectomy for patients with muscle-invasive disease and clinical involvement of a single regional lymph node in the true pelvis [33, 34]. Indeed one trial included 17 patients with cN1 disease and found 14 (82%) were pN0 at time of surgery, though these patients did not have biopsies before therapy to confirm nodal involvement [33].

Neoadjuvant Cisplatin-Based Chemotherapy Does Not Impact Feasibility of Curative Surgery

Multiple trials have demonstrated that NACT does not adversely impact the feasibility of radical cystectomy [7, 14, 35]. For instance, in the phase 3 trial SWOG-8710, 307 patients were randomized 1:1 to MVAC followed by cystectomy versus cystectomy alone, and radical cystectomy was ultimately completed in 82% of patients in the MVAC arm and 81% of patients treated with cystectomy alone [14].

Selection of Patients Appropriate for Cisplatin-Based Chemotherapy

Cisplatin-based chemotherapy carries risk of significant and lasting toxicity in patients with pre-existing comorbidities such as renal dysfunction and neuropathy. A consensus set of criteria for cisplatin eligibility based on a survey of the literature and genitourinary oncologists suggested that cisplatin be precluded if one or more of the following characteristics are present: (1) Eastern Cooperative Oncology Group performance status ≥2; (2) creatinine clearance <60 ml/min; (3) grade ≥2 hearing loss; (4) grade ≥2 neuropathy; or (5) New York Heart Association heart failure ≥ Class III [36].

Non-MVAC Options for NACT

Gemcitabine Plus Cisplatin

Gemcitabine plus cisplatin (GC) supplanted MVAC as the standard of care for metastatic urothelial carcinoma based on a large randomized trial showing GC to have similar efficacy and reduced toxicity compared to MVAC [37, 38]. Though neoadjuvant GC and MVAC for MIBC have never been compared head-to-head in a randomized trial, retrospective analyses have suggested these regimens have similar efficacy in the neoadjuvant setting as well [39, 40]. For example, in a retrospective study of 935 patients who received NACT for MIBC, GC-treated patients ($n = 602$) had <ypT2N0 disease at time of radical cystectomy in 44.8% of cases, compared to 43.7% among patients treated with MVAC ($n = 183$) [40]. pCR rates were also similar, occurring in 23.9% and 24.5% of patients treated with GC and MVAC, respectively [40]. Despite the absence of level I evidence comparing GC to MVAC, the GC regimen was ultimately endorsed by the National Comprehensive Cancer Network (NCCN) as a standard of care for neoadjuvant treatment of MIBC [26].

In order to increase the number of patients eligible for cisplatin-based therapy, one small study treated patients with MIBC with split-dose cisplatin 35 mg/m^2 plus gemcitabine 1000 mg/m^2 on days 1 and 8 of every 21-day cycle for a maximum of four cycles for patients with a calculated glomerular filtration rate $\geq$40 ml/min [41]. The regimen was well tolerated, with no clinically significant decline in kidney function. The study's small sample size and failure to report pathological response rates preclude firm estimates of the regimen's efficacy. Subsequent small retrospective studies of neoadjuvant split-dose cisplatin for MIBC have suggested lower rates of pCR compared to standard-dose cisplatin [42, 43], though one of these studies suggested comparable long-term survival [43].

Study of other cisplatin-based neoadjuvant regimens for MIBC is ongoing, including the combination of albumin-bound paclitaxel plus cisplatin (NCT04060459).

Dose-dense regimens The development of granulocyte growth factor support made feasible dose-dense regimens, allowing delivery of a greater total dose of chemotherapy over a given unit of time [44]. Dose-dense MVAC was first compared to MVAC in a phase 3 trial in metastatic bladder cancer by the European Organization for Research and Treatment of Cancer (EORTC) [44]. The trial randomized 263 patients to either 2-week cycles of ddMVAC plus granulocyte-stimulating factor (G-CSF) or 4-week cycles of traditional MVAC. The dose-dense regimen was found to be associated with reduced toxicity and greater clinical efficacy compared to MVAC, with a HR for mortality of 0.76 and a 5-year survival rate for ddMVAC of 21.8% versus 13.5% for MVAC [45].

This led to two single-arm trials that subsequently investigated ddMVAC with G-CSF for MIBC in the neoadjuvant setting [33, 46]. While one study treated 39 patients with 4 cycles of ddMVAC [33], the other treated 40 patients with 3 cycles

[46]. Downstaging to non-muscle-invasive disease (<ypT2N0) at time of surgical resection was observed in 49% and 53% of cases, respectively, with pCR rates of 26% and 38% [33, 46]. The dose-dense schedule also allowed a shorter time delay between chemotherapy initiation and surgical resection. While median time to surgery with non-dose-dense therapy is 16–19 weeks [14, 39], median time to surgery in the three-cycle ddMVAC trial was only 9.7 weeks [46]. However, the trials suffered features that limited generalizability of their findings [47]. For example, both trials included patients with node-positive disease, a patient population not eligible for standard NACT regimens.

In a comparative effectiveness analysis of neoadjuvant GC versus MVAC across 28 institutions adjusted using propensity scores, no statistically significant difference in pCR rate or survival was identified between 146 patients treated with GC and 66 patients treated with MVAC, 77% of which received ddMVAC [48].

Results of the randomized neoadjuvant trial SWOG S1314 presented in 2019 also suggested roughly equivalent efficacy between ddMVAC and standard GC with regard to pathologic response. The phase 2 study randomized patients with MIBC to four cycles of GC every 21 days versus four cycles of ddMVAC every 14 days [49]. With a sample size of 167 patients, the trial reported ypT0 rates for ddMVAC and GC of 32% and 35% and downstaging to non-muscle-invasive disease in 55% and 49% of patients, respectively. Survival outcomes have not been reported. Notably, SWOG S1314's primary objective was to assess the prognostic and predictive value of the COXEN score, a gene expression profile, and not to compare the efficacy of these two regimens.

In opposition to these findings stand the results of an interim analysis from the GETUG/AFU V05 VESPER trial, a phase 3 study which randomized 494 patients with MIBC to 4 cycles of perioperative GC every 3 weeks or 6 cycles of perioperative ddMVAC every 2 weeks [50, 51]. The trial enrolled patients with cT2–4 N0M0 disease for neoadjuvant treatment, while patients with pT3–4 or node-positive M0 disease at cystectomy were eligible for adjuvant therapy [51]. Of the 219 patients treated with neoadjuvant GC, 36% were ypT0N0 at time of surgery, compared to 42% of the 218 patients treated with neoadjuvant ddMVAC, with a $p = 0.02$. Downstaging to non-muscle-invasive disease at time of surgery was seen in 49% of patients treated with GC and 63% of patients treated with ddMVAC ($p = 0.007$). Finally, 77% of patients treated with ddMVAC had organ-confined disease at time of resection (<ypT3N0) compared to 63% treated with GC ($p = 0.002$). Sixty percent of patients received six cycles in the ddMVAC arm, while 84% received four cycles in the GC arm. Toxicity was reportedly manageable, with more grade 3 asthenia and GI side effects with ddMVAC. In the trial as a whole, grade 3 or higher toxicities occurred in 50% and 54% of patients treated with ddMVAC and GC, respectively. During chemotherapy, three deaths occurred in the ddMVAC arm and one in the GC arm. Progression-free and overall survival data are anticipated for 2021. Ultimately, reporting of survival outcomes from VESPER will be needed to determine whether six cycles of neoadjuvant ddMVAC is indeed superior in clinical efficacy to four cycles of standard neoadjuvant GC. In MIBC, chemotherapy with neoadjuvant intent is typically limited to three to four cycles in the interest of

avoiding overtreatment, while six cycles of chemotherapy is reserved for patients with metastatic disease. The discrepancy in cycle number between treatment arms in GETUG/AFU V05 complicates comparisons of efficacy between GC and ddM-VAC within this study.

Dose-dense GC (ddGC) has also been investigated as neoadjuvant therapy for MIBC. In a single-arm, phase 2 trial that treated patients with cT2–4a, N0–1, M0 MIBC with three cycles of 14-day ddGC before cystectomy, vascular toxicities, such as stroke and venous thromboembolism, caused the study to close early following enrollment of 31 patients, short of the 44-patient goal [34]. Of the 31 patients who were evaluable, 10 (32%, 95% CI 16–49%) at cystectomy were ypT0N0, while an additional 13% (95% CI 1–25%) had downstaging to non-muscle-invasive disease [34].

A subsequent trial of ddGC enrolled 49 patients but excluded patients with any history of cardiovascular events [52]. The trial also used different dosing, prescribing a total of six cycles prior to radical cystectomy with 2500 mg/m^2 of gemcitabine based on the metastatic phase 3 trial HE 16/03 [53], in contrast to 1200 mg/m^2 used in the first trial, and split-dose cisplatin 35 mg/m^2 on day 1 and 2 instead of 70 mg/m^2 on day 1. Sixty-seven percent of patients completed all six cycles of ddGC. Of 46 evaluable patients, 57% (95% CI, 42–70%) achieved downstaging to non-muscle-invasive disease, while 15% achieved ypT0 (95% CI, 8–28%) [52]. With a median follow-up for living patients of 25.6 months, median recurrence-free and overall survival were not reached. Unlike the prior trial of neoadjuvant ddGC, vascular toxicity in this trial was comparable to toxicities observed in prior neoadjuvant trials of standard GC, perhaps due to the splitting of cisplatin over days 1 and 2 and the upfront exclusion of patients who had experienced cardiovascular events or angina or stroke within the prior 6 months [52]. Therefore, the ddGC regimen as studied in this latter study may be reasonable for selected patients.

Non-Cisplatin-Based NACT

While cisplatin-based NACT is the current standard of care for MIBC, up to 50% of patients with MIBC are ineligible for cisplatin-containing regimens due to comorbidities such as renal dysfunction and neuropathy (see consensus criteria for cisplatin eligibility detailed earlier in this chapter) [36]. This has resulted in an urgent unmet need for alternative perioperative regimens for cisplatin-ineligible patients. However, there is currently no level I evidence to support the use of non-cisplatin-based NACT for MIBC. While carboplatin-based regimens have not been compared directly to cisplatin-based regimens in any randomized neoadjuvant trials, carboplatin-based regimens have been determined inferior to cisplatin-based regimens in the metastatic setting [54–56]. Single-arm, phase 2 trials of neoadjuvant carboplatin in combination with paclitaxel and gemcitabine [57, 58] or with nab-paclitaxel and gemcitabine [59] have resulted in greater hematologic toxicity and lower pathological response rates compared to those historically observed with cisplatin-based regimens. As a result, current guidelines recommend against the use of carboplatin-based chemotherapy for neoadjuvant purposes [20].

Pathologic Response to NACT Is a Predictor of Patient Survival

pCR at cystectomy (ypT0N0) following neoadjuvant cisplatin-based chemotherapy is a strong predictor of patient survival. For instance, a retrospective analysis of SWOG-8710 demonstrated that among 115 patients who had MVAC followed by radical cystectomy with negative margins, patients with ypT0N0 disease at cystectomy had a median overall survival of 13.6 years, compared to 10.6 years among patients with non-muscle-invasive disease at cystectomy and 3.7 years among patients with residual muscle-invasive disease [15]. The prognostic value of a complete pathologic response after NACT was further supported by findings from a meta-analysis of 13 trials with 886 patients treated with NACT followed by radical cystectomy, which showed pCR to be associated with a relative risk for mortality of 0.45 (95% CI 0.36–0.56, $p < 0.00001$) compared to residual disease [16].

Downstaging to non-muscle-invasive disease (<ypT2N0) with NACT is also associated with superior survival. For instance, in a retrospective study of 147 patients with MIBC, patients with <ypT2N0 disease after neoadjuvant MVAC experienced a 5-year overall survival of 75%, compared to only 20% among patients with ypT2 or greater disease at cystectomy [60]. The prognostic importance of residual muscle-invasive disease after NACT was confirmed in subsequent studies [15, 61], including a large retrospective analysis of 935 patients with MIBC treated with three or more cycles of NACT before radical cystectomy which demonstrated non-muscle-invasive disease at cystectomy to confer a HR for overall survival of 0.25 (95% CI 0.16–0.40, $p < 0.001$) compared to patients with residual muscle-invasive disease [40]. As a consequence, use of <ypT2N0 disease at cystectomy has been proposed as an intermediate endpoint to accelerate the investigation of novel neoadjuvant regimens for MIBC [62, 63].

Adjuvant Chemotherapy

Survival benefits observed with NACT have also led to the investigation of adjuvant chemotherapy for patients with MIBC. In theory, adjuvant therapy could offer equivalent control of micrometastatic disease to NACT while also offering certain advantages. For example, an adjuvant paradigm allows pathologic confirmation of disease extent at radical cystectomy prior to initiation of systemic therapy, thereby refining patient selection for chemotherapy to prevent over- and undertreatment [31]. Such pathologic evaluation at radical cystectomy could allow some patients with MIBC to avoid systemic therapy, given that 6–15% of patients with MIBC achieve a pCR with transurethral resection of bladder tumor (TURBT) alone and experience low probability of disease recurrence without chemotherapy [3, 14, 64, 65].

In practice, patients who undergo radical cystectomy often fail to proceed to adjuvant chemotherapy even when indicated due to the significant morbidity of the surgical procedure in conjunction with the frailty conferred by advanced age for most patients diagnosed with bladder cancer (median age 73 years) [66]. For example, a retrospective study of 1142 patients who underwent radical cystectomy showed grade 2–5 complications that could have delayed effective adjuvant chemotherapy in 30% of cases [67].

Accordingly, trials of adjuvant therapy for MIBC have been plagued by poor accrual [68–71]. The largest and most recent trial of adjuvant therapy for MIBC was EORTC 30994, in which 284 patients with pT3–4 and/or node-positive disease were randomized to adjuvant GC, MVAC, or ddMVAC, or the same regimens deferred until recurrence [71]. At a median follow-up duration of 7 years, the median overall survival in the immediate treatment group was 6.74 years (95% CI 3.85–not reached) versus 4.60 years (95% CI 2.15–6.25) in the deferred treatment group. Though the difference in median overall survival favored adjuvant therapy, the difference was not statistically significant ($p = 0.13$) [71].

Given the failure of multiple trials to achieve target accrual in the adjuvant space, Galsky et al. performed an analysis of the NCDB to examine associations of adjuvant chemotherapy with clinical outcome among patients treated between 2003 and 2006 with pT3–4 and/or node-positive bladder cancer [72]. Of the 5653 patients included in the study, 23% had received adjuvant chemotherapy. The investigators used propensity scores to control for pertinent covariates such as age and pathological tumor stage. Patients who received adjuvant chemotherapy experienced longer overall survival compared to patients who did not, with a HR of 0.70 (95% CI 0.64–0.76). Sensitivity analyses demonstrated that adjuvant chemotherapy's benefit persisted when factors not captured in the NCDB, such as performance status, were accounted for. However, the study did suffer notable limitations, including its retrospective nature and the NCDB's lack of clearly defined data on adjuvant chemotherapy regimens, disease recurrence, and timing of salvage chemotherapy [72]. The conclusions of the NCDB analysis were further supported by the results of a systematic review and meta-analysis of 945 patients enrolled in 9 randomized clinical trials of adjuvant therapy for MIBC [73]. The analysis showed a pooled HR of 0.77 (95% CI 0.59–0.99) for overall survival, with a p-value of 0.049. For the seven trials reporting disease-free survival, the pooled HR was 0.66 (95% CI 0.45–0.91, $p = 0.014$), a benefit which appeared to be of greater statistical significance among patients with node-positive disease ($p = 0.010$).

Nonetheless, given the absence of definitive data from phase 3 trials demonstrating a survival benefit from adjuvant chemotherapy and the challenges associated with administration of chemotherapy after radical cystectomy, NACT is recommended over adjuvant chemotherapy for MIBC [31]. In the absence of NACT prior to cystectomy, NCCN guidelines recommend consideration of adjuvant cisplatin-based chemotherapy for patients with pT3–4 disease, positive nodes, or positive margins at time of radical cystectomy [26].

Investigation of the optimal regimen for adjuvant chemotherapy is ongoing. GETUG/AFU V05 VESPER is an ongoing neoadjuvant and adjuvant phase 3 trial which randomized patients in its adjuvant arms with pT3/4 or node-positive M0 disease to four cycles of GC versus six cycles of ddMVAC [51]. Preliminary reports from an interim analysis reported that 57 patients were enrolled in the adjuvant arms [50]. In the adjuvant arms, 40% of patients received six cycles in the ddMVAC arm and 60% of patients received four cycles in the GC arm. While preliminary safety results pooled across the trial's neoadjuvant and adjuvant arms have been reported as reviewed earlier in this chapter, efficacy results for the adjuvant arms are not yet known.

Adjuvant Chemotherapy After NACT

Notably, implementation of adjuvant chemotherapy for patients who have already received NACT is not considered standard practice [26], even in cases where patients after NACT have pathologic predictors of poor prognosis at cystectomy, such as residual muscle-invasive or node-positive disease [15]. Data to support use of adjuvant chemotherapy in such settings is limited to lower-level evidence: in a retrospective analysis of 37 patients with pathologically node-positive disease after NACT, of whom 11 received adjuvant therapy of various regimens, adjuvant chemotherapy was associated with an improvement in recurrence-free survival, though there was no statistically significant difference in overall or disease-specific survival [74]. Potential confounders included the fact that patients who received adjuvant chemotherapy tended to be younger and had better performance status.

Biomarkers of Response to Cisplatin-Based Chemotherapy

Given the considerable toxicity inherent to cisplatin-based chemotherapy and the lack of benefit from NACT experienced by many patients with MIBC, extensive efforts have been made to identify biomarkers that can predict benefit and improve patient selection for neoadjuvant therapy (Table 17.1). For instance, a phase 3 trial by Stadler et al. investigated the potential for p53 status, assessed by immunohistochemistry, to predict benefit from cisplatin-based adjuvant chemotherapy [69]. Ultimately, the study failed to demonstrate any predictive value of p53, though the study was limited by a high patient refusal rate, lower than expected event rate, and failures to receive the assigned therapy [69]. In addition, the study's method of p53 status, by immunohistochemistry, could not detect genomic alterations resulting in lack of p53 expression.

Table 17.1 Biomarkers under investigation to guide perioperative systemic therapy for urothelial cancer

Biomarker	Key studies	Method of assessment
Biomarkers for chemotherapy		
Alterations in DDR genes	Van Allen et al. [75] Plimack et al. [76] Miron et al. [77] Liu et al. [78] Iyer et al. [52] Li et al. [79] Teo et al. [80] Geynisman et al. [81]	NGS
Intrinsic molecular subtypes	Choi et al. [82] McConkey et al. [83]	RNA seq
COXEN gene expression score	Kothari et al. [84] Flaig et al. [49]	RNA seq
Cell-free DNA	Christensen et al. [85] Patel et al. [86]	NGS
Biomarkers for immunotherapy		
PD-L1	Necchi et al. [87] Powles et al. [88] van Dijk et al. [89] Gao et al. [90]	IHC
TMB	Necchi et al. [87] Powles et al. [88] van Dijk et al. [89] Gao et al. [90]	NGS
TGF-ß expression signature	Mariathasan et al. [91] Powles et al. [88] van Dijk et al. [89]	RNA seq
Eight-gene cytotoxic T cell transcriptional signature (tGE8)	Mariathasan et al. [91] Powles et al. [88] van Dijk et al. [89] Gao et al. [90]	RNA seq
IFN-gamma signaling signature	Grande et al. [92] Necchi et al. [87] van Dijk et al. [89] Gao et al. [90]	RNA seq
Alterations in DDR genes	Teo et al. [93] Necchi et al. [87] Powles et al. [88] van Dijk et al. [89] Gao et al. [90]	NGS
Tertiary lymphoid structures	van Dijk et al. [89] Gao et al. [90]	Multiplex immunofluorescence
Intrinsic molecular subtypes	Powles et al. [88]	RNA seq

Abbreviations: *DDR* DNA damage response and repair, *IFN* interferon, *IHC* immunohistochemistry, *NGS* next-generation sequencing, *PD-L1* programmed death ligand-1, *RNA seq* RNA sequencing, *TGF* transforming growth factor, *TMB* tumor mutational burden

Intrinsic molecular subtypes of urothelial cancer have also been identified through transcriptomic profiling and are under investigation as potential predictors of chemosensitivity [82, 94–97]. Similar to breast cancer, luminal and basal-type tumors have been identified in MIBC [82, 94–96]. An unbiased clustering analysis of transcriptomic data from 412 MIBCs in the urothelial TCGA revealed 5 distinct expression subtypes, including luminal-papillary, luminal-infiltrated, luminal, basal-squamous, and neuronal [98]. These subtypes were congruent with the four subtypes identified in a prior analysis of TCGA in 2014 [96] and also confirmed the overarching luminal and basal subtypes identified in previous transcriptomic analyses of bladder cancer [82, 94–96]. Compared to basal type tumors, luminal tumors appear to have less aggressive natural histories but are also less sensitive to chemotherapy [82, 95]. In a retrospective study of patients who received cisplatin-based NACT, MIBCs with a p53-like luminal subtype (corresponding to TCGA cluster II) appeared to be chemoresistant with lower chance of downstaging to non-muscle-invasive disease at time of cystectomy [82]. A transcriptomic analysis comparing pre-treatment TURBT specimens from 343 patients with MIBC to 476 cases that did not receive NACT also showed luminal tumors to have the best overall survival regardless of NACT and basal tumors to derive the greatest survival benefit from NACT compared to surgery alone [99]. A phase 2 trial of neoadjuvant ddMVAC and bevacizumab demonstrated that patients with basal type tumors experienced a higher rate of overall survival at 5 years of 91% compared to luminal (73%) and p53-like tumors (36%) [83]. Validation of the intrinsic molecular subtypes as predictors of cisplatin or chemotherapy sensitivity or resistance will be required in larger, prospective cohorts prior to implementation in clinical practice.

Another potential predictive biomarker of interest is the COXEN (Co-eXpression ExtrapolatioN) score, a dichotomized gene expression model which accurately predicted sensitivity to cisplatin-based therapy in a cohort of 15 patients with MIBC or metastatic bladder cancer [84]. The COXEN score's ability to predict pathologic response was then tested in the phase 2 trial SWOG S1314 (NCT02177695), which randomized 237 patients with MIBC to receive either neoadjuvant ddMVAC or gemcitabine and cisplatin [49]. Preliminary results indicated that the COXEN score was not a statistically significant predictor of pathologic response in the trial's individual arms, though the COXEN gemcitabine-cisplatin score did predict for pathologic downstaging when arms were pooled [49]. No interaction between COXEN score and chemotherapy regimen as a predictor of pathologic response was detected [49]. Additional analyses focusing on genomic predictors of response are anticipated from S1314 specimens.

Additional biomarkers for prediction of response to neoadjuvant cisplatin-based chemotherapy are deleterious alterations within genes involved in DNA damage response and repair (DDR). The identification of DDR gene alterations as a biomarker of chemosensitivity began with a retrospective study of whole exome sequencing in patients with MIBC that identified an association between chemosensitivity and somatic mutations of *ERCC2* [75], a nucleotide excision repair gene that is mutated in 10–18% of bladder cancers [100]. The association between *ERCC2* alteration and chemosensitivity was subsequently validated [78], and mutations within the helicase domain were found to be particularly indicative of cisplatin sensitivity [79]. Defects in other DDR genes were also identified as predictors of response to cisplatin-based therapy [52, 76, 80]. In a study of patients on clinical trials of neoadjuvant cisplatin-based therapy, Plimack et al. demonstrated that alterations in *ATM*, *RB1*, and *FANCC* predicted pathologic response with 87% sensitivity and 100% specificity, as well as longer overall survival [76, 77]. Subsequently, a multicenter phase 2 trial of neoadjuvant ddGC for MIBC showed the presence of deleterious DDR gene alterations to have a positive predictive value for pathologic downstaging to non-muscle-invasive disease of 89% [52]. Furthermore, no patients with deleterious DDR gene alterations had disease recurrence at a median follow-up of 2 years. The capacity for DDR gene alterations to predict sensitivity to platinum-based chemotherapy may also extend to the metastatic setting, based on an analysis by Teo et al. demonstrating that the presence of deleterious alterations in various DDR genes in metastatic urothelial carcinoma was associated with longer progression-free and overall survival on platinum-based therapy, with an overall survival of 23.7 months in DDR mutant patients versus 13 months among DDR wild-type patients [93]. Finally, DDR gene alterations in urothelial cancer may also predict clinical benefit from immune checkpoint blockade, presumably due to an increase in tumor neoantigens due to deficient DNA repair resulting in greater immunogenicity [93]. As discussed later in this chapter, immune checkpoint blockade in addition to or in substitution of NACT is now under intense investigation, as is whether DDR gene alterations may help identify patients with MIBC that are most likely to benefit from neoadjuvant immune checkpoint blockade [87–90].

Finally, cell-free DNA in plasma and urine is a promising potential biomarker to guide perioperative therapy for MIBC. For instance, a study of 17 patients with MIBC receiving NACT found that detection of tumor-derived cell-free DNA in blood or urine just prior to the second cycle of NACT predicted disease recurrence with a sensitivity of 83% (95% CI 36–100%) and specificity of 100% (95% CI 42–100%) [86]. In another study of 68 patients with MIBC treated with NACT before cystectomy, analysis of circulating tumor DNA (cell-free DNA in plasma) accurately identified patients with metastatic relapse after cystectomy with a sensitivity of 100% and specificity of 98% with a median lead time over traditional imaging methods of 96 days [85]. Though available data on cell-free DNA in the context of MIBC remains limited, these promising results suggest that larger prospective studies of cell-free DNA sequencing could lead to significant improvements in the perioperative management of MIBC.

Risks of Clinical Understaging in MIBC

Given the potential for biomarkers to predict response to cisplatin-based therapy, trials are currently underway to test whether biomarker-driven strategies may allow for selection of patients who may be spared radical cystectomy after achieving a complete clinical response to NACT. This includes the phase 2 trial Alliance

A031701, wherein patients who have MIBC harboring a deleterious DDR gene alteration and achieve downstaging to noninvasive disease or a complete clinical response after cisplatin-based NACT may opt for bladder preservation (NCT03609216). The RETAIN trial is also investigating bladder sparing for MIBC patients with alterations of *ATM*, *RB1*, *FANCC*, or *ERCC2* and no clinical evidence of disease following neoadjuvant accelerated MVAC (NCT02710734) [81]. If determined safe and effective, such biomarker-driven approaches could significantly improve patient quality of life by avoiding the morbidity of definitive local therapy in a subset of patients with MIBC.

However, pending results of such studies, it is crucial to emphasize that all patients with MIBC who are able should proceed to definitive local therapy following completion of NACT, even if a complete clinical response is documented [101]. Multiple studies have identified frequent understaging by TURBT (pre- and post-NACT) and imaging when compared to pathologic staging at radical cystectomy [25, 57, 102–105]. For instance, a 77-patient phase 2 trial of NACT followed by TURBT before immediate cystectomy versus cystoscopic surveillance for patients with a clinical complete response found that, among patients with a clinical complete response who underwent immediate cystectomy ($n = 10$), 60% had persistent cancer upon surgical pathologic evaluation [57]. The substantial risk of clinical understaging has since been confirmed in multiple later studies [25, 57, 103–105]. While outside the scope of this chapter, bladder preservation through use of definitive chemoradiation in lieu of radical cystectomy may be offered to carefully selected patients with localized MIBC [106, 107].

Immune Checkpoint Blockade as Neoadjuvant Therapy

Though cisplatin-based NACT improves survival of patients with MIBC, up to 50% of patients with MIBC are ineligible for cisplatin due to comorbidities such as kidney dysfunction and neuropathy [36], resulting in an urgent unmet need for alternative neoadjuvant options. Investigation of immune checkpoint blockade as an alternative neoadjuvant strategy offers a promising opportunity to improve care for cisplatin-ineligible patients with MIBC.

Neoadjuvant Anti-programmed Death-1(PD-1)/Programmed Death Ligand-1 (PD-L1) Monotherapy

Two single-arm, phase 2 trials of anti-PD-1/PD-L1 monotherapy have been published to date. PURE-01 was a 114-patient trial of neoadjuvant pembrolizumab and enrolled patients with T2–4aN0M0 disease regardless of cisplatin eligibility [87, 108]. In contrast, ABACUS was a trial of neoadjuvant atezolizumab for 95 patients with T2–4aN0M0 disease who were cisplatin-ineligible [88]. Pathologic response rates for both trials were promising, with 31% of patients in ABACUS achieving ypT0/Tis and 42% achieving ypT0 in PURE-01. PURE-01 also recently reported results specifically for bladder cancers with >50% variant histology (n = 30), a patient population often excluded from clinical trials, and demonstrated ypT0 in 37% of patients (95% CI 28–46%) at cystectomy [108]. Toxicity profiles in both trials were manageable, with grade 3 or higher adverse events in 11% or less of patients in both trials [87, 88, 108].

Several unresolved controversies exist regarding the results of PURE-01 and ABACUS. PURE-01's relatively high pCR rate may not be generalizable given an exceptionally high frequency of PD-L1 positivity in 70% of pre-treatment tumors included in the trial [87]. Moreover, while PURE-01 reported a statistically significant association between PD-L1 CPS ≥ 10% and ypT0 at cystectomy ($p = 0.011$), ABACUS found no statistically significant association [87, 88]. Notably, comparison of PD-L1 expression between these trials is hampered by differences in PD-L1 assessment methodology. While PURE-01 defined PD-L1 positivity as a combined positive score (percentage of PD-L1-positive immune cells plus PD-L1-positive tumor cells) of 10% or higher based on the Dako 22C3 pharmDx assay [87], in ABACUS, tumors were considered PD-L1 positive if 5% or more of immune cells stained positive for PD-L1 using the Ventana SP142 assay [88]. With regard to tumor mutational burden (TMB), PURE-01 reported a significant nonlinear association between complete pathologic response and elevated TMB, while ABACUS did not [87, 88]. Future studies are clearly necessary to define the predictive capacity of PD-L1 positivity, TMB, and several other biomarkers for neoadjuvant checkpoint blockade. Additional ongoing trials are summarized in Table 17.2.

Combined Blockade of Cytotoxic T-Lymphocyte Antigen 4 (CTLA-4) and PD-1/PD-L1 in the Neoadjuvant Setting

The ABACUS trial indicated that neoadjuvant anti-PD-1/PD-L1 monotherapy may be less effective in the context of bulky disease as well as in tumors without evidence of pre-existing T cell immunity, as denoted by low levels of intraepithelial CD8+ T cells and an eight-gene cytotoxic T cell transcriptional signature, tGE8 [88]. This finding motivated investigation of combination immunotherapy as a means to increase treatment responses in higher-risk patients and tumors without pre-existing T cell immunity [89, 90].

Three phase 2 trials recently reported results after investigating the addition of anti-CTLA-4 to PD-1/PD-L1 blockade for bladder cancer in the neoadjuvant setting [89, 90, 92]. The single-arm NABUCCO trial enrolled 24 patients with stage III urothelial cancer and administered two doses of ipilimumab (anti-CTLA-4) and two doses of nivolumab (anti-PD-1) over the course of 3 total treatment days followed by surgical resection [89]. Approximately half of the patients in the NABUCCO trial were ineligible for cisplatin, while the remainder had refused standard

Table 17.2 Ongoing trials evaluating neoadjuvant immune checkpoint blockade therapy for muscle-invasive bladder cancer

Therapy	Phase	Stage eligibility	Cisplatin-eligible patients (Yes/No)	Trial identifier	Status
Anti-PD-1/PD-L1 monotherapy					
Pembrolizumab (PANDORE)	2	T2–4N0 or Nx	No	NCT03212651	Active, not recruiting
Atezolizumab	2	T2–4N0M0	No	NCT03577132	Not yet recruiting
Atezolizumab	2	T < 2, T2–4N0M0	No	NCT02451423	Recruiting
Atezolizumab (ABACUS)	2	T2–4aN0M0	No	NCT02662309	Results reported [88]; active, not recruiting
Chemotherapy-free combination regimens					
Pembrolizumab + epacadostat (PECULIAR)	2	T2–3bN0M0	Yes	NCT03832673	Not yet recruiting
Nivolumab ± urelumab	2	T2–4aN0M0	No	NCT02845323	Recruiting
Nivolumab ± lirilumab (PrE0807)	1	T2–4aN0–1 M0	No	NCT03532451	Active, not recruiting
Durvalumab ± oleclumab (BLASST-2)	1	T2–4aN0M0	No	NCT03773666	Partial results reported [109]; recruiting
Durvalumab ± olaparib		T2–4aN0M0 or T1–4aN1M0	No	NCT04579133	Not yet recruiting
Atezolizumab + cabozantinib (ABATE)	2	T2–4aN0/xM0	No	NCT04289779	Recruiting
Pembrolizumab + entinostat	2	T2–4aN0M0	No	NCT03978624	Recruiting
Nivolumab + CG0070	2	T2–4aN0–1 M0	No	NCT04610671	Recruiting
Retifanlimab ± epacadostat vs epacadostat alone (Optimus)	2	T2–3bN0M0	No	NCT04586244	Recruiting
Nivolumab + ipilimumab (NABUCCO)	1	T3–4N0 or N+	No	NCT03387761	Results reported [89]; recruiting
Nivolumab ± ipilimumab (CA209-9DJ)	2	T2–4aN0M0	No	NCT03520491	Recruiting
Durvalumab + tremelimumab (DUTRENEO)	2	T2–4N0 or N1	Yes/no	NCT03472274	Preliminary results [92]; recruiting

(continued)

Table 17.2 (continued)

Therapy	Phase	Stage eligibility	Cisplatin-eligible patients (Yes/No)	Trial identifier	Status
Durvalumab + tremelimumab	1	T2–4aN0M0	No	NCT02812420	Results reported [90]; active, not recruiting
Balstilimab + zalifrelimab + gemcitabine/cisplatin	2	T2–4N0–1 M0	Yes	NCT04430036	Recruiting
Durvalumab + radiation (RADIANT)	2	T2–4aN0M0	No	NCT04543110	Not yet recruiting
Neoadjuvant and adjuvant pembrolizumab ± enfortumab vedotin (KEYNOTE-905/ EV-303)	3	T2–4aN0M0	No	NCT03924895	Recruiting
Neoadjuvant and adjuvant nivolumab ± bempegaldesleukin	3	T2–4aN0M0	No	NCT04209114	Recruiting
Chemoimmunotherapy combinations					
Nivolumab + gemcitabine/cisplatin (BLASST-1)	2	T2–4aN0M0	Yes	NCT03294304	Results reported [110]; active, not recruiting
Nivolumab + aMVAC, with selective bladder preservation (RETAIN-2)	2	T2–3N0M0	Yes	NCT04506554	Not yet recruiting
Avelumab (AURA) ± chemotherapy	2	T2–4N0 or N+	Yes/no	NCT03674424	Recruiting
Pembrolizumab + gemcitabine/cisplatin	2	T2–4N0 or Nx	Yes	NCT02690558	Active, not recruiting
Pembrolizumab + aMVAC	2	T2–4aN0–1 M0	Yes	NCT04383743	Recruiting
Atezolizumab + gemcitabine/cisplatin	1/2	T2–4aN0/XM0	Yes	NCT02989584	Active, not recruiting
Nivolumab + gemcitabine/cisplatin with selective bladder sparing	2	T2–4aN0M0	Yes	NCT03558087	Recruiting
Gemcitabine/cisplatin + toripalimab	2	T2–4aN0M0	Yes	NCT04099589	Recruiting
Durvalumab + tremelimumab + ddMVAC (NEMIO)	1/2	T2–4aN0–1 M0	Yes	NCT03549715	Recruiting

Table 17.2 (continued)

Therapy	Phase	Stage eligibility	Cisplatin-eligible patients (Yes/No)	Trial identifier	Status
Atezolizumab + BCG + gemcitabine/cisplatin	2	T2–4aN0–1 M0	Yes	NCT04630730	Not yet recruiting
Gemcitabine/cisplatin ± neoadjuvant and adjuvant nivolumab ± neoadjuvant linrodostat (ENERGIZE)	3	T2–4aN0M0	Yes	NCT03661320	Recruiting
Gemcitabine/cisplatin ± neoadjuvant and adjuvant pembrolizumab (KEYNOTE-866)	3	T2–4aN0M0	Yes	NCT03924856	Recruiting
Gemcitabine/cisplatin ± neoadjuvant and adjuvant durvalumab (NIAGARA)	3	T2–4aN0M0	Yes	NCT03732677	Recruiting

Abbreviations: *aMVAC* accelerated methotrexate, vinblastine, doxorubicin, and cisplatin, *BCG* bacillus Calmette-Guérin, *ddMVAC* dose-dense methotrexate, vinblastine, doxorubicin, and cisplatin; *PD-1/PD-L1* programmed death-1/programmed death ligand-1

cisplatin-based therapy. Twenty-three patients (96%, 95% CI, 79–100%) underwent surgery within 12 weeks of initiating study therapy, meeting the trial's primary endpoint of feasibility. The study also reported a pCR rate (ypT0N0) of 46% (95% CI, 26–67%), and 58% (95% CI, 37–77%) of patients had no invasive disease remaining at time of resection (defined as pCR or pTisN0/pTaN0) [89]. At a median postoperative follow-up of 8.3 months, two patients developed recurrent disease and one patient in the trial had died, attributed to progression of disease. While grade 3–4 immune-related adverse events occurred in 55% of patients, 14% of these were considered clinically insignificant laboratory abnormalities [89].

A separate single-arm study of durvalumab (anti-PD-L1) plus tremelimumab (anti-CTLA-4) included 28 patients with high-risk, muscle-invasive urothelial cancer, defined by clinical T3/T4 disease, variant histology, lymphovascular invasion, hydronephrosis, and/or high-grade upper tract disease [90]. Ninety percent of patients were cisplatin-ineligible; the remainder had refused cisplatin-based chemotherapy. In the intention-to-treat analysis, the trial reported a pCR rate of 31.7%, which included patients with ypT0N0 or residual ypTisN0 at surgery. Downstaging in the intent-to-treat analysis to non-muscle-invasive disease occurred in 50% of patients. Overall survival at 1 year was 88.8%, with a relapse-free survival of 82.8% [90]. Notably, only six patients (21%) experienced grade 3 or higher immune-related adverse events, of which four were asymptomatic laboratory abnormalities.

The multicenter phase 2 DUTRENEO trial also reported results of neoadjuvant durvalumab plus tremelimumab versus chemotherapy for muscle-invasive urothelial bladder cancer (cT2–4a, N ≤ 1, M0) [92]. In this study, cisplatin-eligible patients were prospectively selected using a tumor pro-inflammatory interferon-gamma signature; patients with "hot" tumors were randomized to durvalumab 1500 mg plus tremelimumab 75 mg every 4 weeks for three cycles versus standard gemcitabine/cisplatin or ddMVAC, while patients with "cold" tumors were given standard cisplatin-based chemotherapy only. Sixty-one patients were recruited. Among patients with hot tumors, 23 received durvalumab plus tremelimumab with 8 (34.8%) achieving a pCR; 22 received standard chemotherapy, of which 8 (36.4%) achieved a pCR (odds ratio 0.923). Among patients with cold tumors, 16 received cisplatin-based chemotherapy, with 11 (68.8%) achieving pCR. Twenty-two percent of patients who received durvalumab/tremelimumab experienced grade 4 toxicities, in comparison to 36.4% of hot patients and 62.5% of cold patients who received chemotherapy [92]. The authors concluded that durvalumab plus tremelimumab appeared to be active and safe in patients with MIBC, though the interferon-gamma signature failed to select patients more likely to benefit from immunotherapy versus chemotherapy.

Overall, these findings suggest that combination anti-CTLA-4 plus anti-PD-1/PD-L1 blockade may hold promise as neoadjuvant therapy for locoregionally advanced cancers of the urothelial tract. While the aforementioned findings suggest that neoadjuvant ipilimumab plus nivolumab may have greater efficacy than durvalumab plus tremelimumab, both trials were small and cross-trial comparisons are of course fraught with caveats. The two trials of combination neoadjuvant immune checkpoint blockade featured notable differences in their respective patient populations. For example, while 42% of patients in the NABUCCO study had clinical lymph node involvement at baseline, all patients enrolled in the single-arm trial of durvalumab and tremelimumab were node-negative. There was also significant variability in cisplatin eligibility and tumor baseline characteristics. For example, only half of patients in the NABUCCO study were cisplatin-ineligible, and 63% were PD-L1 positive [89]. Differences in activity and toxicity could also be related to differences in dosing of the anti-CTLA-4 agents, given evidence of such dose dependency in melanoma [111]. Notably, these trials showed increased rates of immunotherapy-related adverse events compared to trials of anti-PD-1/PD-L1 monotherapy [88, 108], consistent with prior data from patients with metastatic urothelial cancer [112].

Neoadjuvant Combinations of Immune Checkpoint Blockade with Targeted Agents

The phase 2 trial, BLASST-2, recently reported preliminary results from the first ten-patient cohort enrolled on its single-arm study of neoadjuvant durvalumab 750 mg every 2 weeks for three cycles prior to radical cystectomy [109]. All ten patients completed three cycles of durvalumab, and there were no dose-limiting toxicities. Eight patients underwent radical cystectomy with at least 12 weeks of post-op follow-up at time of reporting. Pathologic downstaging to non-muscle-invasive disease at time of surgery was seen in 25% (2 of 8) patients with ypT0 in 12.5% (n = 1) of patients. Results of the second ten-patient cohort, which will receive durvalumab with the addition of the CD73 inhibitor oleclumab, are yet to be reported (NCT03773666).

The phase 2 NEODURVARIB trial of combination durvalumab plus olaparib prior to surgery enrolled 29 patients with cT2–4a MIBC [113]. Presented at ESMO 2020, two patients required early withdrawal due to disease progression and sepsis, but 89.7% of patients successfully underwent cystectomy, and the combination of durvalumab and olaparib prior to surgery was well tolerated with grade 3 toxicity in only 3.4% of patients. In the 26 patients who underwent cystectomy, the pCR rate was 50% [113]. The full results of the trial are yet to be published.

Addition of Neoadjuvant Immune Checkpoint Blockade to Chemotherapy

Addition of immune checkpoint blockade to chemotherapy is also under investigation in the neoadjuvant setting. The phase 2 BLASST-1 trial enrolled 41 patients with MIBC (cT2–4a, N ≤ 1, M0) and treated them with cisplatin 70 mg/m^2 on day1, gemcitabine 1000 mg/m^2 on days 1 and 8, and nivolumab 360 mg on day 8 of a 21-day cycle for 4 cycles, followed by radical cystectomy within 8 weeks [110]. In the intent-to-treat analysis, a pathologic response, defined as ≤ypT1N0 at surgery, was achieved in 65.8% of patients (n = 27), including patients with N1 disease at baseline. Most adverse events were attributed to gemcitabine and cisplatin, with grade 3 to 4 adverse events occurring in 20% of patients overall. Immune-related adverse events occurred in only three patients. No delay to cystectomy or unexpected surgical complications were observed [110].

The phase 1b/2 trial HCRN GU14-188 enrolled both cisplatin-eligible and cisplatin-ineligible patients with cT2–4aN0M0 disease [114, 115]. In the cisplatin-eligible arm, 43 patients were enrolled and treated with standard cisplatin 70 mg/m^2 on day 1 plus gemcitabine 1000 mg/m^2 on days 1 and 8 of a 21-day cycle for 4 cycles, with addition of pembrolizumab 200 mg starting on cycle 1 day 8 and given every 3 weeks for 5 doses, prior to radical cystectomy. Only patients who underwent surgery and received at least one dose of pembrolizumab were included in the efficacy analysis (36 patients of a total 43 enrolled). ypT0N0 was achieved in 44.4% of patients, while ≤pT1N0 was achieved in 61.1%. Pathologic downstaging did not correlate with PD-L1 score and occurred even in patients with cT3/4 disease. Grades 3 to 4 adverse events did occur in a number of patients, including cytopenias in 57% of patients, one grade 3 myocardial infarction, one grade 4 hyponatremia, and ten other grade 3 adverse events. Median time to surgery from the final dose of protocol therapy was 5.3 weeks. Of four patients that did not undergo cystectomy, three refused and one did not proceed due to grade 4 thrombocytopenic purpura, though all four patients were alive without recurrence at a median follow-up of 32 months. At a median follow-up of 34.2 months, the estimated 36-month recurrence-free, overall, and disease-specific survival rates were 63%, 82%, and 87%, respectively [114]. In the cisplatin-ineligible arm, 37 patients were enrolled and treated with gemcitabine 1000 mg/m^2 on days 1, 8, and 15 of a 28-day cycle for 3 cycles, with pembrolizumab 200 mg every 3 weeks starting on day 8 of cycle 1 and continued for five doses [116]. ypT0N0 was achieved in 45.2% of patients, and 51.6% of patients had downstaging to non-muscle-invasive disease. At a median follow-up of 10.8 months, the estimated 12-month recurrence-free, overall, and disease-specific survival was 74.9%, 93.8%, and 100%. Treatment-related adverse events appeared manageable and included grade 3 to 4 neutropenia in 24% of patients, anemia in 13%, and thrombocytopenia in 5%. There were grade 3 non-hematologic adverse events in 36% of patients, two of which prevented radical cystectomy. The authors noted that pathologic downstaging in this cisplatin-ineligible cohort using a cisplatin-free regimen was comparable to standard of care cisplatin-based chemotherapy [116].

Phase 3 Trials of Neoadjuvant Immune Checkpoint Blockade

Multiple phase 3 trials investigating neoadjuvant immune checkpoint blockade are currently underway. Several are employing anti-PD-1/PD-L1 inhibitors in combination with cisplatin-based chemotherapy for cisplatin-eligible patients, including ENERGIZE, a trial of neoadjuvant gemcitabine/cisplatin alone or in combination with nivolumab (neoadjuvant and adjuvant) with or without linrodostat, a selective oral IDO1 inhibitor (NCT03661320) [117]; KEYNOTE-866, a trial of neoadjuvant gemcitabine/cisplatin plus perioperative pembrolizumab (neoadjuvant and adjuvant) versus placebo (NCT03924856) [118]; and the NIAGARA trial, investigating neoadjuvant durvalumab in combination with gemcitabine/cisplatin followed by adjuvant durvalumab versus neoadjuvant gemcitabine/cisplatin alone (NCT03732677) [119]. Trials for cisplatin-ineligible patients include NCT04209114, a study of neoadjuvant and adjuvant nivolumab plus bempegaldesleukin (Bempeg/NKTR-214, a CD122-preferential IL2 pathway agonist) versus nivolumab alone versus standard of care surgery alone, and MK-3475-905/KEYNOTE-905/EV-303, a trial of perioperative pembrolizumab (both neoadjuvant and adjuvant) plus cystectomy or perioperative pembrolizumab plus enfortumab vedotin (both neoadjuvant and adjuvant) (NCT03924895). The results of these studies may transform the standard of care for preoperative management of MIBC, and their findings are eagerly awaited.

Immune Checkpoint Blockade in the Adjuvant Setting

Evaluation of immune checkpoint blockade as adjuvant therapy for MIBC is an active area of investigation. In contrast to trials of adjuvant chemotherapy, where adequate accrual has been hindered by time to recovery from cystectomy and toxicities related to cisplatin-based chemotherapy [68–71], the favorable toxicity profiles of anti-PD-1/PD-L1 agents have made accrual to adjuvant trials more feasible [120, 121].

In the phase 3 adjuvant atezolizumab trial IMvigor010, patients with (1) ypT2-4a or pN+ disease following NACT or (2) pT3-4a or pN+ if no NACT, patients were randomized to atezolizumab 1200 mg every 3 weeks for 16 cycles or observation. The trial failed to demonstrate a statistically significant improvement in disease-free survival (stratified HR 0.89, 95% CI 0.74–1.08, $p = 0.24$) or overall survival (stratified HR 0.85, 95% CI 0.66–1.09, $p = 0.20$) [120]. This also appeared true regardless of PD-L1 status, with patients categorized as IC2/3 (PD-L1 expressing immune cells by Ventana SP142 assay ≥5%) experiencing a stratified HR of 1.01 (95% CI 0.75–1.35) and patients categorized as IC0/1 (PD-L1 < 5%) with a stratified HR of 0.81 (95% CI 0.63–1.05). The authors noted that a higher percentage of patients discontinued therapy due to adverse events compared to studies in the metastatic setting.

In contrast, CheckMate-274, a phase 3, placebo-controlled trial of nivolumab following surgery in patients with high-risk, muscle-invasive urothelial carcinoma, has met its primary endpoint for improving disease-free survival according to a recent industry press release [121, 122]. This endpoint was met in all randomized patients as well as in patients with PD-L1 expression on 1% or more of tumor cells. Patients included in the study may or may not have previously received NACT. Presentation and publication of the study's full findings are eagerly awaited.

Results of Alliance A031501/AMBASSADOR, a phase 3 trial of adjuvant pembrolizumab for localized MIBC and locoregionally advanced urothelial cancer, are also expected in the near future (NCT03244384) [123]. A randomized controlled phase 2 trial of adjuvant durvalumab versus surveillance for MIBC (NCT03768570) is also ongoing. As noted above, a number of studies are also investigating adjuvant immune checkpoint blockade in conjunction with neoadjuvant immune checkpoint blockade and other neoadjuvant therapies (ENERGIZE, NCT03661320; KEYNOTE-866, NCT03924856; NIAGARA, NCT03732677; AMBASSADOR, NCT03924895).

Non-immunotherapy Investigational Treatments in the Perioperative Space

While studies in the perioperative space are extensively exploring checkpoint blockade, trials exploring other non-chemotherapy agents have been reported or are underway. A phase 2 trial of neoadjuvant erlotinib enrolled 20 patients with clinical T2 MIBC and reported a ypT0 rate of 25%, with 35% of patients downstaged to non-muscle-invasive disease and 75% with organ-confined disease [124]. Notably, all patients that achieved ypT0 or ypTis/T1 experienced a rash during treatment. At a median follow-up of 24.8 months, 50% of patients remained alive without evidence of disease recurrence.

Another neoadjuvant single-arm, phase 2 trial for MIBC investigated the combination of gemcitabine and cisplatin with the tyrosine kinase inhibitor sunitinib [125]. Of 18 patients enrolled, 15 were evaluable for efficacy endpoints. Only one patient achieved ypT0N0 at cystectomy, while five (33%) experienced downstaging to non-muscle-invasive disease, suggesting little additional activity with sunitinib. Notably, the regimen caused neutropenia requiring G-CSF support, and more than half of patients experience grade 3 or 4 adverse events.

NEO-BLADE, a phase 2 randomized placebo-controlled trial of neoadjuvant nintedanib, an oral small molecule multi-targeted kinase inhibitor of VEGFR-2, FGFR-1, and PDGFR, versus placebo with GC in locally advanced MIBC failed to demonstrate a statistically significant improvement in pCR [126]. However, patients who received nintedanib experienced a 12-month PFS rate of 89.0% compared to 74.1% in the placebo arm (HR 0.48, 95% CI 0.24–0.98, $p = 0.038$). Moreover, OS at 12 and 24 months was 96% and 89% in the nintedanib group compared to 83% and 69% in the placebo arm (HR 0.39, 95% CI 0.168–0.902, $p = 0.022$). The etiology of the improved survival in the absence of an improvement in pathologic response rate in the nintedanib arm remains unclear, and these results require confirmation in additional trials.

Ongoing perioperative trials of non-chemotherapy, non-immune checkpoint blockade regimens also include PROOF 302, a randomized double-blind, placebo-controlled trial of the FGFR inhibitor infigratinib as adjuvant therapy for invasive urothelial carcinoma with susceptible alterations of *FGFR3* (NCT04197986) [127], and a single-arm phase 1 trial investigating use of the anti-CD38 monoclonal antibody, daratumumab, prior to radical cystectomy for cisplatin-ineligible patients with MIBC (NCT03473730).

Finally, an additional area of investigation in the perioperative space is the implementation of novel drug delivery systems to boost efficacy while simultaneously limiting toxicity. In 2017, results were reported for a phase 1b trial of the novel gemcitabine-releasing intravesical system TAR-200 [128]. Among ten patients with MIBC who received treatment with TAR-200 prior to radical cystectomy, there were no treatment-related serious adverse events or discontinuations and no treatment-related cytopenias. Indeed, while pharmacokinetic analyses confirmed measurable levels of gemcitabine in urine, no gemcitabine was detected in plasma. Four of the ten patients treated had no residual muscle-invasive disease at time of cystectomy. Given these early signs of efficacy and noteworthy tolerability, this drug delivery system may warrant further investigation in the neoadjuvant space, perhaps in combination with other agents such as immune checkpoint blockade for patients that are less likely to tolerate systemic chemotherapy.

Conclusions

Level I evidence derived from multiple prospective clinical trials and a meta-analysis supports the clinically meaningful survival advantage conferred by neoadjuvant cisplatin-based chemotherapy for patients with MIBC [5]. While adjuvant chemotherapy offers potential advantages over neoadjuvant therapy, such as treatment selection based on complete histopathologic staging, trials of adjuvant chemotherapy for MIBC have been plagued by poor accrual, and therefore NACT remains preferred over adjuvant therapy whenever feasible [68–71]. Given the current inability to predict which patients will or will not benefit from neoadjuvant cisplatin-based chemotherapy, numerous biomarkers remain under investigation as potential predictors of chemosensitivity, including but not limited to alterations of DDR genes [49, 52]. Studies employing such biomarkers with intent to safely select patients for bladder sparing after NACT are also underway [81].

Following the FDA approval of several checkpoint inhibitors in metastatic UC, immunotherapy is being explored extensively in combination with NACT [110, 114]. Moreover, given the favorable toxicity profile of this treatment modality compared to chemotherapy, single-agent checkpoint blockade is being investigated in the cisplatin-ineligible patient population and as adjuvant therapy following upfront cystectomy, with at least one adjuvant study of nivolumab meeting its primary endpoint [88–90, 92, 108, 109, 113, 120, 122].

Additionally, trials of novel targeted agents, including FGFR inhibitors and multi-targeted kinase inhibitors, are another area of active investigation in the perioperative management of patients with MIBC, and the widespread adoption of next-generation sequencing will allow for genetic selection of patients in real time who are most likely to benefit from these treatments [124–127]. Additionally, novel platforms such as cell-free DNA are expected to risk stratify patients for treatment based upon the presence of radiographically undetectable minimal residual disease [85].

Clearly, the approach to MIBC is rapidly evolving. The influx of novel therapies and biomarker-based platforms will hopefully lead to an individualized approach, including both operative and organ-sparing approaches, to the management of patients with muscle-invasive disease.

References

1. AJCC Cancer Staging Manual 8th edn. Amin MB, Edge S, Greene F, Byrd DR, Brookland RK, Washington MK, et al., editors: Springer; 2016.
2. American Cancer Society. Cancer Facts and Figures. Cancer.org. 2020. Available from: https://www.cancer.org/content/dam/cancer-org/research/cancer-facts-and-statistics/annual-cancer-facts-and-figures/2020/cancer-facts-and-figures-2020.pdf.
3. Stein JP, Lieskovsky G, Cote R, Groshen S, Feng AC, Boyd S, et al. Radical cystectomy in the treatment of invasive bladder cancer: long-term results in 1,054 patients. J Clin Oncol. 2001;19(3):666–75.
4. Yafi FA, Aprikian AG, Chin JL, Fradet Y, Izawa J, Estey E, et al. Contemporary outcomes of 2287 patients with bladder cancer who were treated with radical cystectomy: a Canadian multicentre experience. BJU Int. 2011;108(4):539–45.
5. Advanced Bladder Cancer Meta-analysis C. Neoadjuvant chemotherapy in invasive bladder cancer: update of a systematic review and meta-analysis of individual patient data advanced bladder cancer (ABC) meta-analysis collaboration. Eur Urol. 2005;48(2):202–5; discussion 5–6.

6. Martinez-Piñeiro JA, Gonzalez Martin M, Arocena F, Flores N, Roncero CR, Portillo JA, et al. Neoadjuvant cisplatin chemotherapy before radical cystectomy in invasive transitional cell carcinoma of the bladder: a prospective randomized phase III study. J Urol. 1995;153(3 Pt 2):964–73.
7. Malmstrom PU, Rintala E, Wahlqvist R, Hellstrom P, Hellsten S, Hannisdal E. Five-year followup of a prospective trial of radical cystectomy and neoadjuvant chemotherapy: Nordic Cystectomy Trial I. The Nordic Cooperative Bladder Cancer Study Group. J Urol. 1996;155(6):1903–6.
8. Shipley WU, Winter KA, Kaufman DS, Lee WR, Heney NM, Tester WR, et al. Phase III trial of neoadjuvant chemotherapy in patients with invasive bladder cancer treated with selective bladder preservation by combined radiation therapy and chemotherapy: initial results of Radiation Therapy Oncology Group 89-03. J Clin Oncol. 1998;16(11):3576–83.
9. Sengelov L, von der Maase H, Lundbeck F, Barlebo H, Colstrup H, Engelholm SA, et al. Neoadjuvant chemotherapy with cisplatin and methotrexate in patients with muscle-invasive bladder tumours. Acta Oncol. 2002;41(5):447–56.
10. Sherif A, Holmberg L, Rintala E, Mestad O, Nilsson J, Nilsson S, et al. Neoadjuvant cisplatinum based combination chemotherapy in patients with invasive bladder cancer: a combined analysis of two Nordic studies. Eur Urol. 2004;45(3):297–303.
11. Bassi P, Pappagallo GL, Sperandio P. Neoadjuvant M-VAC chemotherapy of invasive bladder cancer: results of a multicenter phase III trial. J Urol. 1999;161:264A.
12. International Collaboration of T, Medical Research Council Advanced Bladder Cancer Working P, European Organisation for R, Treatment of Cancer Genito-Urinary Tract Cancer G, Australian Bladder Cancer Study G, National Cancer Institute of Canada Clinical Trials G, et al. International phase III trial assessing neoadjuvant cisplatin, methotrexate, and vinblastine chemotherapy for muscle-invasive bladder cancer: long-term results of the BA06 30894 trial. J Clin Oncol. 2011;29(16):2171–7.
13. Neoadjuvant cisplatin, methotrexate, and vinblastine chemotherapy for muscle-invasive bladder cancer: a randomised controlled trial. International collaboration of trialists. Lancet. 1999;354(9178):533–40.
14. Grossman HB, Natale RB, Tangen CM, Speights VO, Vogelzang NJ, Trump DL, et al. Neoadjuvant chemotherapy plus cystectomy compared with cystectomy alone for locally advanced bladder cancer. N Engl J Med. 2003;349(9):859–66.
15. Sonpavde G, Goldman BH, Speights VO, Lerner SP, Wood DP, Vogelzang NJ, et al. Quality of pathologic response and surgery correlate with survival for patients with completely resected bladder cancer after neoadjuvant chemotherapy. Cancer. 2009;115(18):4104–9.
16. Petrelli F, Coinu A, Cabiddu M, Ghilardi M, Vavassori I, Barni S. Correlation of pathologic complete response with survival after neoadjuvant chemotherapy in bladder cancer treated with cystectomy: a meta-analysis. Eur Urol. 2014;65(2):350–7.
17. Logothetis CJ, Dexeus FH, Finn L, Sella A, Amato RJ, Ayala AG, et al. A prospective randomized trial comparing MVAC and CISCA chemotherapy for patients with metastatic urothelial tumors. J Clin Oncol. 1990;8(6):1050–5.
18. Polychemotherapy for early breast cancer: an overview of the randomised trials. Early Breast Cancer Trialists' Collaborative Group. Lancet. 1998;352(9132):930–42.
19. Gill S, Loprinzi CL, Sargent DJ, Thome SD, Alberts SR, Haller DG, et al. Pooled analysis of fluorouracil-based adjuvant therapy for stage II and III colon cancer: who benefits and by how much? J Clin Oncol. 2004;22(10):1797–806.
20. Milowsky MI, Rumble RB, Booth CM, Gilligan T, Eapen LJ, Hauke RJ, et al. Guideline on muscle-invasive and metastatic bladder cancer (European Association of Urology guideline): American Society of Clinical Oncology clinical practice guideline endorsement. J Clin Oncol. 2016;34(16):1945–52.
21. Witjes JA, Bruins HM, Cathomas R, Compérat E, Cowan NC, Gakis G, et al. Muscle-invasive and metastatic bladder cancer. EAU Guidelines [Internet]. 2020. Available from: http://uroweb.org/guidelines/compilations-of-all-guidelines/.

22. Spiess PE, Agarwal N, Bangs R, Boorjian SA, Buyyounouski MK, Clark PE, et al. Bladder cancer, version 5.2017, NCCN clinical practice guidelines in oncology. J Natl Compr Canc Netw. 2017;15(10):1240–67.
23. Galsky MD, Hahn NM, Rosenberg J, Sonpavde G, Hutson T, Oh WK, et al. A consensus definition of patients with metastatic urothelial carcinoma who are unfit for cisplatin-based chemotherapy. Lancet Oncol. 2011;12(3):211–4.
24. Reardon ZD, Patel SG, Zaid HB, Stimson CJ, Resnick MJ, Keegan KA, et al. Trends in the use of perioperative chemotherapy for localized and locally advanced muscle-invasive bladder cancer: a sign of changing tides. Eur Urol. 2015;67(1):165–70.
25. Culp SH, Dickstein RJ, Grossman HB, Pretzsch SM, Porten S, Daneshmand S, et al. Refining patient selection for neoadjuvant chemotherapy before radical cystectomy. J Urol. 2014;191(1):40–7.
26. Flaig TW, Spiess PE, Agarwal NA, Bangs R, Boorjian SA, Buyyounouski MK, et al. NCCN Clinical Practice Guidelines in Oncology (NCCN Guidelines): Bladder cancer v6.2020. Available from: https://www.nccn.org/professionals/physician_gls/pdf/bladder.pdf.
27. Dodd PM, McCaffrey JA, Herr H, Mazumdar M, Bacik J, Higgins G, et al. Outcome of postchemotherapy surgery after treatment with methotrexate, vinblastine, doxorubicin, and cisplatin in patients with unresectable or metastatic transitional cell carcinoma. J Clin Oncol. 1999;17(8):2546–52.
28. Herr HW, Donat SM, Bajorin DF. Post-chemotherapy surgery in patients with unresectable or regionally metastatic bladder cancer. J Urol. 2001;165(3):811–4.
29. Ho PL, Willis DL, Patil J, Xiao L, Williams SB, Melquist JJ, et al. Outcome of patients with clinically node-positive bladder cancer undergoing consolidative surgery after preoperative chemotherapy: The M.D. Anderson Cancer Center Experience. Urol Oncol. 2016;34(2):59 e1–8.
30. Galsky MD, Stensland K, Sfakianos JP, Mehrazin R, Diefenbach M, Mohamed N, et al. Comparative effectiveness of treatment strategies for bladder cancer with clinical evidence of regional lymph node involvement. J Clin Oncol. 2016;34(22):2627–35.
31. Funt SA, Rosenberg JE. Systemic, perioperative management of muscle-invasive bladder cancer and future horizons. Nat Rev Clin Oncol. 2017;14(4):221–34.
32. Apolo AB, Riches J, Schoder H, Akin O, Trout A, Milowsky MI, et al. Clinical value of fluorine-18 2-fluoro-2-deoxy-D-glucose positron emission tomography/computed tomography in bladder cancer. J Clin Oncol. 2010;28(25):3973–8.
33. Choueiri TK, Jacobus S, Bellmunt J, Qu A, Appleman LJ, Tretter C, et al. Neoadjuvant dose-dense methotrexate, vinblastine, doxorubicin, and cisplatin with pegfilgrastim support in muscle-invasive urothelial cancer: pathologic, radiologic, and biomarker correlates. J Clin Oncol. 2014;32(18):1889–94.
34. Anari F, O'Neill J, Choi W, Chen DYT, Haseebuddin M, Kutikov A, et al. Neoadjuvant dose-dense gemcitabine and cisplatin in muscle-invasive bladder cancer: results of a phase 2 trial. Eur Urol Oncol. 2018;1(1):54–60.
35. Sherif A, Rintala E, Mestad O, Nilsson J, Holmberg L, Nilsson S, et al. Neoadjuvant cisplatin-methotrexate chemotherapy for invasive bladder cancer -- Nordic cystectomy trial 2. Scand J Urol Nephrol. 2002;36(6):419–25.
36. Galsky MD, Hahn NM, Rosenberg J, Sonpavde G, Hutson T, Oh WK, et al. Treatment of patients with metastatic urothelial cancer "unfit" for Cisplatin-based chemotherapy. J Clin Oncol. 2011;29(17):2432–8.
37. von der Maase H, Hansen SW, Roberts JT, Dogliotti L, Oliver T, Moore MJ, et al. Gemcitabine and cisplatin versus methotrexate, vinblastine, doxorubicin, and cisplatin in advanced or metastatic bladder cancer: results of a large, randomized, multinational, multicenter, phase III study. J Clin Oncol. 2000;18(17):3068–77.
38. von der Maase H, Sengelov L, Roberts JT, Ricci S, Dogliotti L, Oliver T, et al. Long-term survival results of a randomized trial comparing gemcitabine plus cisplatin, with methotrexate, vinblastine, doxorubicin, plus cisplatin in patients with bladder cancer. J Clin Oncol. 2005;23(21):4602–8.

39. Dash A, Pettus JA, Herr HW, Bochner BH, Dalbagni G, Donat SM, et al. A role for neoadjuvant gemcitabine plus cisplatin in muscle-invasive urothelial carcinoma of the bladder: a retrospective experience. Cancer. 2008;113(9):2471–7.
40. Zargar H, Espiritu PN, Fairey AS, Mertens LS, Dinney CP, Mir MC, et al. Multicenter assessment of neoadjuvant chemotherapy for muscle-invasive bladder cancer. Eur Urol. 2015;67(2):241–9.
41. Hussain SA, Palmer DH, Lloyd B, Collins SI, Barton D, Ansari J, et al. A study of split-dose cisplatin-based neo-adjuvant chemotherapy in muscle-invasive bladder cancer. Oncol Lett. 2012;3(4):855–9.
42. Osterman CK, Babu DS, Geynisman DM, Lewis B, Somer RA, Balar AV, et al. Efficacy of split schedule versus conventional schedule neoadjuvant cisplatin-based chemotherapy for muscle-invasive bladder cancer. Oncologist. 2019;24(5):688–90.
43. Sellers LE, Harper A, Linch MD, Davda R, Miller R, Payne H, et al. Split dose gemcitabine/cisplatin (GC) in urothelial carcinoma of the bladder: review of toxicity and response. J Clin Oncol. 2016;34(15_suppl):e16018-e.
44. Sternberg CN, de Mulder PH, Schornagel JH, Theodore C, Fossa SD, van Oosterom AT, et al. Randomized phase III trial of high-dose-intensity methotrexate, vinblastine, doxorubicin, and cisplatin (MVAC) chemotherapy and recombinant human granulocyte colony-stimulating factor versus classic MVAC in advanced urothelial tract tumors: European Organization for Research and Treatment of Cancer Protocol no. 30924. J Clin Oncol. 2001;19(10):2638–46.
45. Sternberg CN, de Mulder P, Schornagel JH, Theodore C, Fossa SD, van Oosterom AT, et al. Seven year update of an EORTC phase III trial of high-dose intensity M-VAC chemotherapy and G-CSF versus classic M-VAC in advanced urothelial tract tumours. Eur J Cancer. 2006;42(1):50–4.
46. Plimack ER, Hoffman-Censits JH, Viterbo R, Trabulsi EJ, Ross EA, Greenberg RE, et al. Accelerated methotrexate, vinblastine, doxorubicin, and cisplatin is safe, effective, and efficient neoadjuvant treatment for muscle-invasive bladder cancer: results of a multicenter phase II study with molecular correlates of response and toxicity. J Clin Oncol. 2014;32(18):1895–901.
47. Pouessel D, Gauthier H, Serrate C, Pfister C, Culine S. Dose-dense methotrexate, vinblastine, doxorubicin, and cisplatin neoadjuvant chemotherapy in bladder cancer: ready for prime time? J Clin Oncol. 2014;32(36):4168–9.
48. Galsky MD, Pal SK, Chowdhury S, Harshman LC, Crabb SJ, Wong YN, et al. Comparative effectiveness of gemcitabine plus cisplatin versus methotrexate, vinblastine, doxorubicin, plus cisplatin as neoadjuvant therapy for muscle-invasive bladder cancer. Cancer. 2015;121(15):2586–93.
49. Flaig TW, Tangen CM, Daneshmand S, Alva AS, Lerner SP, Lucia MS, et al. SWOG S1314: a randomized phase II study of co-expression extrapolation (COXEN) with neoadjuvant chemotherapy for localized, muscle-invasive bladder cancer. J Clin Oncol. 2019;37(15_suppl):4506.
50. Culine S, Gravis G, Flechon A, Soulie M, Guy L, Laguerre B, et al. Randomized phase III trial of dose-dense methotrexate, vinblastine, doxorubicin, and cisplatin (dd-MVAC) or gemcitabine and cisplatin (GC) as perioperative chemotherapy for muscle invasive urothelial bladder cancer (MIUBC): preliminary results of the GETUG/AFU V05 VESPER trial on toxicity and pathological responses. J Clin Oncol. 2020;38(6_suppl):437.
51. Pfister C, Gravis G, Pignot G, Flechon A, Soulie M, Chevreau C, et al. Randomized phase III study of gemcitabine and cisplatin (GC) versus dose dense methotrexate, vinblastine, doxorubicin and cisplatin (DD-MVAC) in the perioperative setting for patients with locally advanced transitional cell cancer of the bladder: the French GETUG/AFU V05 VESPER trial. J Clin Oncol. 2018;36(6_suppl):TPS530-TPS.
52. Iyer G, Balar AV, Milowsky MI, Bochner BH, Dalbagni G, Donat SM, et al. Multicenter prospective phase II trial of neoadjuvant dose-dense gemcitabine plus cisplatin in patients with muscle-invasive bladder cancer. J Clin Oncol. 2018;36(19):1949–56.

53. Bamias A, Dafni U, Karadimou A, Timotheadou E, Aravantinos G, Psyrri A, et al. Prospective, open-label, randomized, phase III study of two dose-dense regimens MVAC versus gemcitabine/cisplatin in patients with inoperable, metastatic or relapsed urothelial cancer: a Hellenic Cooperative Oncology Group study (HE 16/03). Ann Oncol. 2013;24(4):1011–7.
54. Bellmunt J, Ribas A, Eres N, Albanell J, Almanza C, Bermejo B, et al. Carboplatin-based versus cisplatin-based chemotherapy in the treatment of surgically incurable advanced bladder carcinoma. Cancer. 1997;80(10):1966–72.
55. Dogliotti L, Carteni G, Siena S, Bertetto O, Martoni A, Bono A, et al. Gemcitabine plus cisplatin versus gemcitabine plus carboplatin as first-line chemotherapy in advanced transitional cell carcinoma of the urothelium: results of a randomized phase 2 trial. Eur Urol. 2007;52(1):134–41.
56. Petrioli R, Frediani B, Manganelli A, Barbanti G, De Capua B, De Lauretis A, et al. Comparison between a cisplatin-containing regimen and a carboplatin-containing regimen for recurrent or metastatic bladder cancer patients. A randomized phase II study. Cancer. 1996;77(2):344–51.
57. deVere White RW, Lara PN Jr, Goldman B, Tangen CM, Smith DC, Wood DP Jr, et al. A sequential treatment approach to myoinvasive urothelial cancer: a phase II Southwest Oncology Group trial (S0219). J Urol. 2009;181(6):2476–80; discussion 80-1.
58. Smith DC, Mackler NJ, Dunn RL, Hussain M, Wood D, Lee CT, et al. Phase II trial of paclitaxel, carboplatin and gemcitabine in patients with locally advanced carcinoma of the bladder. J Urol. 2008;180(6):2384–8; discussion 8.
59. Grivas PD, Hussain M, Hafez K, Daignault-Newton S, Wood D, Lee CT, et al. A phase II trial of neoadjuvant nab-paclitaxel, carboplatin, and gemcitabine (ACaG) in patients with locally advanced carcinoma of the bladder. Urology. 2013;82(1):111–7.
60. Splinter TA, Scher HI, Denis L, Bukowski R, Simon S, Klimberg I, et al. The prognostic value of the pathological response to combination chemotherapy before cystectomy in patients with invasive bladder cancer. European Organization for Research on Treatment of Cancer--Genitourinary Group. J Urol. 1992;147(3):606–8.
61. Iyer G, Tully CM, Zabor EC, Bochner BH, Dalbagni G, Herr HW, et al. Neoadjuvant gemcitabine-cisplatin plus radical cystectomy-pelvic lymph node dissection for muscle-invasive bladder cancer: a 12-year experience. Clin Genitourin Cancer. 2020;18(5):387–94.
62. Chism DD, Woods ME, Milowsky MI. Neoadjuvant paradigm for accelerated drug development: an ideal model in bladder cancer. Oncologist. 2013;18(8):933–40.
63. Funt SA, Chapman PB. The role of neoadjuvant trials in drug development for solid tumors. Clin Cancer Res. 2016;22(10):2323–8.
64. Pagano F, Bassi P, Galetti TP, Meneghini A, Milani C, Artibani W, et al. Results of contemporary radical cystectomy for invasive bladder cancer: a clinicopathological study with an emphasis on the inadequacy of the tumor, nodes and metastases classification. J Urol. 1991;145(1):45–50.
65. Dalbagni G, Genega E, Hashibe M, Zhang ZF, Russo P, Herr H, et al. Cystectomy for bladder cancer: a contemporary series. J Urol. 2001;165(4):1111–6.
66. Cancer Stat Facts: bladder cancer. NIH NCI: surveillance, epidemiology, and end results program. Available from: https://seer.cancer.gov/statfacts/html/urinb.html.
67. Donat SM, Shabsigh A, Savage C, Cronin AM, Bochner BH, Dalbagni G, et al. Potential impact of postoperative early complications on the timing of adjuvant chemotherapy in patients undergoing radical cystectomy: a high-volume tertiary cancer center experience. Eur Urol. 2009;55(1):177–85.
68. Paz-Ares LG, Solsona E, Esteban E, Saez A, Gonzalez-Larriba J, Anton A, et al. Randomized phase III trial comparing adjuvant paclitaxel/gemcitabine/cisplatin (PGC) to observation in patients with resected invasive bladder cancer: results of the Spanish Oncology Genitourinary Group (SOGUG) 99/01 study. J Clin Oncol. 2010;28(18_suppl):LBA4518-LBA.

69. Stadler WM, Lerner SP, Groshen S, Stein JP, Shi SR, Raghavan D, et al. Phase III study of molecularly targeted adjuvant therapy in locally advanced urothelial cancer of the bladder based on p53 status. J Clin Oncol. 2011;29(25):3443–9.
70. Cognetti F, Ruggeri EM, Felici A, Gallucci M, Muto G, Pollera CF, et al. Adjuvant chemotherapy with cisplatin and gemcitabine versus chemotherapy at relapse in patients with muscle-invasive bladder cancer submitted to radical cystectomy: an Italian, multicenter, randomized phase III trial. Ann Oncol. 2012;23(3):695–700.
71. Sternberg CN, Skoneczna I, Kerst JM, Albers P, Fossa SD, Agerbaek M, et al. Immediate versus deferred chemotherapy after radical cystectomy in patients with pT3-pT4 or N+ M0 urothelial carcinoma of the bladder (EORTC 30994): an intergroup, open-label, randomised phase 3 trial. Lancet Oncol. 2015;16(1):76–86.
72. Galsky MD, Stensland KD, Moshier E, Sfakianos JP, McBride RB, Tsao CK, et al. Effectiveness of adjuvant chemotherapy for locally advanced bladder cancer. J Clin Oncol. 2016;34(8):825–32.
73. Leow JJ, Martin-Doyle W, Rajagopal PS, Patel CG, Anderson EM, Rothman AT, et al. Adjuvant chemotherapy for invasive bladder cancer: a 2013 updated systematic review and meta-analysis of randomized trials. Eur Urol. 2014;66(1):42–54.
74. Kassouf W, Agarwal PK, Grossman HB, Leibovici D, Munsell MF, Siefker-Radtke A, et al. Outcome of patients with bladder cancer with pN+ disease after preoperative chemotherapy and radical cystectomy. Urology. 2009;73(1):147–52.
75. Van Allen EM, Mouw KW, Kim P, Iyer G, Wagle N, Al-Ahmadie H, et al. Somatic ERCC2 mutations correlate with cisplatin sensitivity in muscle-invasive urothelial carcinoma. Cancer Discov. 2014;4(10):1140–53.
76. Plimack ER, Dunbrack RL, Brennan TA, Andrake MD, Zhou Y, Serebriiskii IG, et al. Defects in DNA repair genes predict response to neoadjuvant cisplatin-based chemotherapy in muscle-invasive bladder cancer. Eur Urol. 2015;68(6):959–67.
77. Miron B, Hoffman-Censits JH, Anari F, O'Neill J, Geynisman DM, Zibelman MR, et al. Defects in DNA repair genes confer improved Long-term survival after cisplatin-based neoadjuvant chemotherapy for muscle-invasive bladder cancer. Eur Urol Oncol. 2020;3(4):544–7.
78. Liu D, Plimack ER, Hoffman-Censits J, Garraway LA, Bellmunt J, Van Allen E, et al. Clinical validation of chemotherapy response biomarker ERCC2 in muscle-invasive urothelial bladder carcinoma. JAMA Oncol. 2016;2(8):1094–6.
79. Li Q, Damish AW, Frazier Z, Liu D, Reznichenko E, Kamburov A, et al. ERCC2 helicase domain mutations confer nucleotide excision repair deficiency and drive cisplatin sensitivity in muscle-invasive bladder cancer. Clin Cancer Res. 2019;25(3):977–88.
80. Teo MY, Bambury RM, Zabor EC, Jordan E, Al-Ahmadie H, Boyd ME, et al. DNA damage response and repair gene alterations are associated with improved survival in patients with platinum-treated advanced urothelial carcinoma. Clin Cancer Res. 2017;23(14):3610–8.
81. Geynisman DM, Abbosh P, Zibelman MR, Feldman R, McConkey DJ, Hahn NM, et al. A phase II trial of risk-adapted treatment for muscle invasive bladder cancer after neoadjuvant accelerated MVAC. J Clin Oncol. 2018;36(6_suppl):TPS537-TPS.
82. Choi W, Porten S, Kim S, Willis D, Plimack ER, Hoffman-Censits J, et al. Identification of distinct basal and luminal subtypes of muscle-invasive bladder cancer with different sensitivities to frontline chemotherapy. Cancer Cell. 2014;25(2):152–65.
83. McConkey DJ, Choi W, Shen Y, Lee IL, Porten S, Matin SF, et al. A prognostic gene expression signature in the molecular classification of chemotherapy-naive urothelial cancer is predictive of clinical outcomes from neoadjuvant chemotherapy: a phase 2 trial of dose-dense methotrexate, vinblastine, doxorubicin, and cisplatin with bevacizumab in urothelial cancer. Eur Urol. 2016;69(5):855–62.
84. Kothari S, Gustafson D, Killian K, Costello J, Edelman DC, Walling J, et al. COXEN prediction of antineoplastic drug sensitivity in bladder cancer patients. J Clin Oncol. 2016;34(2_suppl):365.

85. Christensen E, Birkenkamp-Demtroder K, Sethi H, Shchegrova S, Salari R, Nordentoft I, et al. Early detection of metastatic relapse and monitoring of therapeutic efficacy by ultra-deep sequencing of plasma cell-free DNA in patients with urothelial bladder carcinoma. J Clin Oncol. 2019;37(18):1547–57.
86. Patel KM, van der Vos KE, Smith CG, Mouliere F, Tsui D, Morris J, et al. Association of plasma and urinary mutant DNA with clinical outcomes in muscle invasive bladder cancer. Sci Rep. 2017;7(1):5554.
87. Necchi A, Anichini A, Raggi D, Briganti A, Massa S, Luciano R, et al. Pembrolizumab as neoadjuvant therapy before radical cystectomy in patients with muscle-invasive urothelial bladder carcinoma (PURE-01): an open-label, single-arm, phase II study. J Clin Oncol. 2018:JCO1801148.
88. Powles T, Kockx M, Rodriguez-Vida A, Duran I, Crabb SJ, Van Der Heijden MS, et al. Clinical efficacy and biomarker analysis of neoadjuvant atezolizumab in operable urothelial carcinoma in the ABACUS trial. Nat Med. 2019;25(11):1706–14.
89. van Dijk N, Gil-Jimenez A, Silina K, Hendricksen K, Smit LA, de Feijter JM, et al. Preoperative ipilimumab plus nivolumab in locoregionally advanced urothelial cancer: the NABUCCO trial. Nat Med. 2020;26:1839-1844.
90. Gao J, Navai N, Alhalabi O, Siefker-Radtke A, Campbell MT, Tidwell RS, et al. Neoadjuvant PD-L1 plus CTLA-4 blockade in patients with cisplatin-ineligible operable high-risk urothelial carcinoma. Nat Med. 2020;26:1845-1851.
91. Mariathasan S, Turley SJ, Nickles D, Castiglioni A, Yuen K, Wang Y, et al. TGFbeta attenuates tumour response to PD-L1 blockade by contributing to exclusion of T cells. Nature. 2018;554(7693):544–8.
92. Grande E, Guerrero F, Puente J, Galante I, Duran I, Dominguez M, et al. DUTRENEO trial: a randomized phase II trial of DUrvalumab and TREmelimumab versus chemotherapy as a NEOadjuvant approach to muscle-invasive urothelial bladder cancer (MIBC) patients (pts) prospectively selected by an interferon (INF)-gamma immune signature. J Clin Oncol. 2020;38(15_suppl):5012.
93. Teo MY, Seier K, Ostrovnaya I, Regazzi AM, Kania BE, Moran MM, et al. Alterations in DNA damage response and repair genes as potential marker of clinical benefit from PD-1/PD-L1 blockade in advanced urothelial cancers. J Clin Oncol. 2018;36(17):1685–94.
94. Sjodahl G, Lauss M, Lovgren K, Chebil G, Gudjonsson S, Veerla S, et al. A molecular taxonomy for urothelial carcinoma. Clin Cancer Res. 2012;18(12):3377–86.
95. Damrauer JS, Hoadley KA, Chism DD, Fan C, Tiganelli CJ, Wobker SE, et al. Intrinsic subtypes of high-grade bladder cancer reflect the hallmarks of breast cancer biology. Proc Natl Acad Sci U S A. 2014;111(8):3110–5.
96. Cancer Genome Atlas Research N. Comprehensive molecular characterization of urothelial bladder carcinoma. Nature. 2014;507(7492):315–22.
97. Lindgren D, Frigyesi A, Gudjonsson S, Sjodahl G, Hallden C, Chebil G, et al. Combined gene expression and genomic profiling define two intrinsic molecular subtypes of urothelial carcinoma and gene signatures for molecular grading and outcome. Cancer Res. 2010;70(9):3463–72.
98. Robertson AG, Kim J, Al-Ahmadie H, Bellmunt J, Guo G, Cherniack AD, et al. Comprehensive molecular characterization of muscle-invasive bladder cancer. Cell. 2017;171(3):540–56 e25.
99. Seiler R, Ashab HAD, Erho N, van Rhijn BWG, Winters B, Douglas J, et al. Impact of molecular subtypes in muscle-invasive bladder cancer on predicting response and survival after neoadjuvant chemotherapy. Eur Urol. 2017;72(4):544–54.
100. Abbosh PH, Plimack ER. Molecular and clinical insights into the role and significance of mutated DNA repair genes in bladder cancer. Bladder Cancer. 2018;4(1):9–18.
101. Apolo AB, Grossman HB, Bajorin D, Steinberg G, Kamat AM. Practical use of perioperative chemotherapy for muscle-invasive bladder cancer: summary of session at the Society of Urologic Oncology annual meeting. Urol Oncol. 2012;30(6):772–80.

102. Scher HI, Yagoda A, Herr HW, Sternberg CN, Bosl G, Morse MJ, et al. Neoadjuvant M-VAC (methotrexate, vinblastine, doxorubicin and cisplatin) effect on the primary bladder lesion. J Urol. 1988;139(3):470–4.
103. Millikan R, Dinney C, Swanson D, Sweeney P, Ro JY, Smith TL, et al. Integrated therapy for locally advanced bladder cancer: final report of a randomized trial of cystectomy plus adjuvant M-VAC versus cystectomy with both preoperative and postoperative M-VAC. J Clin Oncol. 2001;19(20):4005–13.
104. Canter D, Long C, Kutikov A, Plimack E, Saad I, Oblaczynski M, et al. Clinicopathological outcomes after radical cystectomy for clinical T2 urothelial carcinoma: further evidence to support the use of neoadjuvant chemotherapy. BJU Int. 2011;107(1):58–62.
105. Meijer RP, Nieuwenhuijzen JA, Meinhardt W, Bex A, van der Poel HG, van Rhijn BW, et al. Response to induction chemotherapy and surgery in non-organ confined bladder cancer: a single institution experience. Eur J Surg Oncol. 2013;39(4):365–71.
106. Weiss C, Rodel C. Urological cancer: Chemoradiation superior in muscle-invasive bladder cancer. Nat Rev Clin Oncol. 2012;9(7):374–5.
107. Wettstein MS, Rooprai JK, Pazhepurackel C, Wallis CJD, Klaassen Z, Uleryk EM, et al. Systematic review and meta-analysis on trimodal therapy versus radical cystectomy for muscle-invasive bladder cancer: does the current quality of evidence justify definitive conclusions? PLoS One. 2019;14(4):e0216255.
108. Necchi A, Raggi D, Gallina A, Madison R, Colecchia M, Luciano R, et al. Updated results of PURE-01 with preliminary activity of neoadjuvant pembrolizumab in patients with muscle-invasive bladder carcinoma with variant histologies. Eur Urol. 2020;77(4):439–46.
109. Wei XX, McGregor BA, Lee RJ, Gao X, Kilbridge KL, Preston MA, et al. Durvalumab as neoadjuvant therapy for muscle-invasive bladder cancer: preliminary results from the Bladder Cancer Signal Seeking Trial (BLASST)-2. J Clin Oncol. 2020;38(6_suppl):507.
110. Gupta S, Sonpavde G, Weight CJ, McGregor BA, Gupta S, Maughan BL, et al. Results from BLASST-1 (Bladder Cancer Signal Seeking Trial) of nivolumab, gemcitabine, and cisplatin in muscle invasive bladder cancer (MIBC) undergoing cystectomy. J Clin Oncol. 2020;38(6_suppl):439.
111. Ascierto PA, Del Vecchio M, Robert C, Mackiewicz A, Chiarion-Sileni V, Arance A, et al. Ipilimumab 10 mg/kg versus ipilimumab 3 mg/kg in patients with unresectable or metastatic melanoma: a randomised, double-blind, multicentre, phase 3 trial. Lancet Oncol. 2017;18(5):611–22.
112. Antonia SJ, Lopez-Martin JA, Bendell J, Ott PA, Taylor M, Eder JP, et al. Nivolumab alone and nivolumab plus ipilimumab in recurrent small-cell lung cancer (CheckMate 032): a multicentre, open-label, phase 1/2 trial. Lancet Oncol. 2016;17(7):883–95.
113. Rodriguez-Moreno JF, de Velasco G, Alvarez-Fernandez C, Collado R, Fernandez-Rodriguez R, Vazquez Estevez S, et al. Impact of the combination of durvalumab (MEDI4736) plus olaparib (AZD2281) administered prior to surgery in the molecular profile of resectable urothelial bladder cancer. NEODURVARIB trial. Ann Oncol. 2020;31(suppl_4):S589.
114. Hoimes CJ, Adra N, Fleming MT, Kaimakliotis HZ, Picus J, Smith ZL, et al. Phase Ib/II neoadjuvant (N-) pembrolizumab (P) and chemotherapy for locally advanced urothelial cancer (laUC): final results from the cisplatin (C)- eligible cohort of HCRN GU14-188. J Clin Oncol. 2020;38(15_suppl):5047.
115. Hoimes CJ, Abouassaly R, Saltzman JN, Fleming MT, Hoffman-Censits JH, Byrd T, et al. HCRN GU14-188: neoadjuvant pembrolizumab (P) and gemcitabine (G) with or without cisplatin (C) in muscle invasive urothelial cancer (MIUC). J Clin Oncol. 2016;34(15_suppl):TPS4578-TPS.
116. Kaimakliotis HZ, Adra N, Kelly WK, Trabulsi EJ, Lauer RC, Picus J, et al. Phase II neoadjuvant (N-) gemcitabine (G) and pembrolizumab (P) for locally advanced urothelial cancer (laUC): interim results from the cisplatin (C)-ineligible cohort of GU14-188. J Clin Oncol. 2020;38(15_suppl):5019.
117. Sonpavde G, Necchi A, Gupta S, Steinberg GD, Gschwend JE, Heijden MSVD, et al. A phase 3 randomized study of neoadjuvant chemotherapy (NAC) alone or in combination

with nivolumab (NIVO) ± BMS-986205 in cisplatin-eligible muscle invasive bladder cancer (MIBC). J Clin Oncol. 2019;37(15_suppl):TPS4587-TPS.
118. Siefker-Radtke AO, Steinberg GD, Bedke J, Nishiyama H, Fang X, Kataria R, et al. Phase III study of perioperative pembrolizumab (pembro) plus neoadjuvant chemotherapy (chemo) versus placebo plus neoadjuvant chemo in cisplatin-eligible patients (pts) with muscle-invasive bladder cancer (MIBC): KEYNOTE-866. J Clin Oncol. 2020;38(6_suppl):TPS599-TPS.
119. Powles T, Meeks JJ, Galsky MD, Heijden MSVD, Nishiyama H, Al-Ahmadie H, et al. A phase III, randomized, open label, multicenter, global study of efficacy and safety of durvalumab in combination with gemcitabine+cisplatin (G+C) for neoadjuvant treatment followed by durvalumab alone for adjuvant treatment in muscle-invasive bladder cancer (MIBC) (NIAGARA). J Clin Oncol. 2019;37(15_suppl):TPS4592-TPS.
120. Hussain MHA, Powles T, Albers P, Castellano D, Daneshmand S, Gschwend J, et al. IMvigor010: primary analysis from a phase III randomized study of adjuvant atezolizumab (atezo) versus observation (obs) in high-risk muscle-invasive urothelial carcinoma (MIUC). J Clin Oncol. 2020;38(15_suppl):5000.
121. Bajorin DF, Galsky MD, Gschwend JE, Tomita Y, Azrilevich A, Witjes F. A phase III, randomized, double-blind, multicenter study of adjuvant nivolumab vs placebo in patients (pts) with high-risk invasive urothelial carcinoma (UC; CheckMate 274). Ann Oncol. 2017;28(suppl_5):v295-v329.
122. Bristol Myers Squibb. Opdivo (nivolumab) significantly improves disease free-survival vs. placebo as adjuvant therapy for patients with high-risk, muscle-invasive urothelial carcinoma in phase 3 CheckMate -274 Trial 2020 [updated September 24, 2020]. Available from: https://news.bms.com/news/corporate-financial/2020/Opdivo-nivolumab-Significantly-Improves-Disease-Free-Survival-vs.-Placebo-as-Adjuvant-Therapy-for-Patients-with-High-Risk-Muscle-Invasive-Urothelial-Carcinoma-in-Phase-3-CheckMate%2D%2D274-Trial/default.aspx.
123. Apolo AB, Rosenberg JE, Kim WY, Chen RC, Sonpavde G, Srinivas S, et al. Alliance A031501: phase III randomized adjuvant study of MK-3475 (pembrolizumab) in muscle-invasive and locally advanced urothelial carcinoma (MIBC) (AMBASSADOR) versus observation. J Clin Oncol. 2019;37(7_suppl):TPS504-TPS.
124. Pruthi RS, Nielsen M, Heathcote S, Wallen EM, Rathmell WK, Godley P, et al. A phase II trial of neoadjuvant erlotinib in patients with muscle-invasive bladder cancer undergoing radical cystectomy: clinical and pathological results. BJU Int. 2010;106(3):349–54.
125. Balar AV, Iyer G, Apolo AB, Regazzi AM, Garcia-Grossman IR, Pendse D, et al. Phase II trial of neoadjuvant gemcitabine (G) and cisplatin (C) with sunitinib in patients (pts) with muscle-invasive bladder cancer (MIBC). J Clin Oncol. 2012;30(15_suppl):4581.
126. Hussain SA, Lester JF, Jackson R, Gornall M, Elliott A, Crabb SJ, et al. Phase II randomized placebo-controlled neoadjuvant trial of nintedanib or placebo with gemcitabine and cisplatin in locally advanced muscle invasive bladder cancer (NEO-BLADE). J Clin Oncol. 2020;38(6_suppl):438.
127. Daneshmand S, Grivas P, Sridhar SS, Gupta S, Bellmunt J, Sonpavde G, et al. PROOF 302: a randomized, double-blind, placebo-controlled, phase III trial of infigratinib as adjuvant therapy in patients with invasive urothelial carcinoma harboring susceptible FGFR3 alterations. J Clin Oncol. 2020;38(15_suppl):TPS5095-TPS.
128. Daneshmand S, Pohar KS, Steinberg GD, Aron M, Cutie C. Effect of GemRIS (gemcitabine-releasing intravesical system, TAR-200) on antitumor activity in muscle-invasive bladder cancer (MIBC). J Clin Oncol. 2017;35(15_suppl):e16000-e.

Chapter 18
Bladder-Sparing Approaches to Treatment of Muscle-Invasive Bladder Cancer

Amishi Bajaj and Sean Sachdev

Background

Bladder cancer is the tenth most common cancer worldwide, with an incidence steadily increasing over time, especially in developed nations [1]. Muscle-invasive bladder cancer (MIBC) is defined as bladder cancer that has invaded at least to the depth of the muscularis propria of the bladder wall, characterized as pathologic T2 by the most recent edition of American Joint Commission on Cancer (AJCC) TNM staging [2]. MIBC comprises about 30% of bladder malignancies and encompasses histologies including urothelial (formerly known as transitional cell) carcinoma – which is the most common histology in the United States, accounting for 90% of diagnoses – as well as squamous cell carcinoma (accounting for most of the remaining 10%), adenocarcinoma, and neuroendocrine carcinoma [1]. Development of urothelial carcinoma is strongly linked to tobacco usage and environmental exposure in the developed world [3], whereas squamous cell carcinoma is frequently diagnosed in regions of Africa and the Middle East and manifests in the setting of chronic irritation, such as that secondary to the protozoan infection schistosomiasis [4].

The most common presentation of MIBC is painless gross hematuria, which is often assessed by urine cytology, computed tomography (CT), or magnetic resonance (MR) urography for complete imaging of the genitourinary tract and, ultimately, cystoscopy [5]. At the time of cystoscopy, which allows for direct visualization of the bladder lumen, transurethral resection of bladder tumor

A. Bajaj · S. Sachdev (✉)
Department of Radiation Oncology, Robert H. Lurie Comprehensive Cancer Center, Northwestern University, Feinberg School of Medicine, Chicago, IL, USA
e-mail: sean.sachdev@nm.org

K. L. Stratton, A. K. Morgans (eds.), *Urologic Oncology*,
https://doi.org/10.1007/978-3-030-89891-5_18

Table 18.1 AJCC 8th edition TNM classification staging for bladder cancer

T	Tx: Primary tumor cannot be assessed T0: No evidence of primary tumor Ta: Non-invasive papillary carcinoma Tis: Carcinoma in situ T1: Tumor invades sub-epithelial connective tissue T2: Tumor invades muscularis propria pT2a: Tumor invades superficial layer (inner half) pT2b: Tumor invades deep layer (outer half) T3: Tumor invades perivesical tissue pT3a: Microscopic invasion pT3b: Macroscopic invasion T4: Tumor invasion into adjacent pelvic organs T4a: Prostate, uterus, vagina T4b: Pelvic wall or abdominal wall
N	Nx: Lymph nodes cannot be assessed N0: No lymph node metastasis N1: Single lymph node metastasis in the true pelvis (hypogastric, obturator, external iliac, or presacral) N2: Multiple regional lymph node metastases in the true pelvis (hypogastric, obturator, external iliac, or presacral) N3: Lymph node metastasis to the common iliac lymph nodes
M	M0: No distant metastasis M1: Distant metastasis

(TURBT) is commonly performed for both pathologic confirmation and tumor debulking. If muscular invasion is noted in the pathologic specimen (i.e., confirming pT2 disease), patients are additionally recommended to receive imaging to assess for metastases [6]. Table 18.1 describes AJCC 8th edition TNM classification staging for bladder cancer. For patients with muscle-invasive disease, definitive management is oft considered a subject of controversy; while surgical resection has been historically regarded as the most standard approach, bladder-sparing treatments are being increasingly utilized as an alternative, effective approach for select patients. Each of these treatment options will be addressed, with emphasis on and comparisons with bladder preservation.

Historical Approaches to MIBC

Radical Cystectomy

MIBC has historically been treated with radical cystectomy (RC), a surgery involving resection of the bladder, adjacent fat, distal ureters, and peritoneum with a pelvic lymph node dissection [7]. For men, the prostate and seminal vesicles are additionally removed; for women, the anterior vaginal wall, uterus, fallopian tubes, and ovaries are additionally removed. The standard pelvic lymph node dissection involves removal of the obturator nodes, external and internal iliac nodes, and the most inferiorly situated common iliac nodes [7]. An ongoing phase III randomized clinical trial (RCT) comparing standard pelvic lymphadenectomy to an extended lymphadenectomy for patients with pT2-T4a disease (SWOG S1011) is aiming to compare the disease-free survival (DFS) rates between these two surgical approaches [8], although results from the recently published LEA AUO AB 25/02 trial out of Europe suggest no reduction in the rate of locoregional recurrence (LRR) with extended pelvic lymph node dissection [9].

Following resection of the bladder, a urinary diversion is performed; both non-continent and continent options for urinary diversion are available. An ileal conduit is a non-continent diversion comprised of small bowel: a channel is created with the ureters attached to it, and it exits through the skin overlying the abdomen by a stoma emptying into a receptacle for urine collection [10]. An ileal conduit is the most commonly utilized type of urinary diversion following RC [10]. Two types of continent diversions include an Indiana pouch, which is a portion of ileum that is constructed to act as a urinary reservoir that allows for the patient to intermittently self-catheterize, and an orthotopic "neobladder," which is a urinary pouch created from small or large bowel (ileum, ileo colon, or sigmoid colon) and then anastomosed to the distal urethra [11]. The benefits/drawbacks of one diversion versus another and/or picking the optimal approach for a patient are beyond the scope of this chapter.

Large, retrospective, single-institution series out of the University of Southern California (USC) and Memorial Sloan Kettering Cancer Center (MSKCC) published in the early 2000s highlight outcomes after RC [12]. The USC experience reported on 633 patients with pT2-T4a disease managed with RC with a 5-year actuarial overall survival (OS) rate of 48% at a 5-year median follow-up and 32% at a 10-year median follow-up [7]. The MSKCC group studied 184 patients with pT2-T4 disease and found a 5-year OS rate of 36% and 27% at 10 years [13]. Later, the Southwest Oncology Group (SWOG), Eastern Cooperative Oncology Group (ECOG), and Cancer and Leukemia Group B (CALGB) published results of a trial investigating the implementation of neoadjuvant chemotherapy (NAC) with three cycles of methotrexate, vinblastine, doxorubicin, and cisplatin (MVAC) in patients with cT2-T4a disease receiving RC (SWOG 8710) and found improved OS with addition of NAC [14], with a 5-year OS of 50% and a 10-year OS of 34% [12]. Data from the Advanced Bladder Cancer (ABC) meta-analysis collaboration analyzed over 3000 patients from 11 trials and reported a 5% absolute improvement in OS at 5 years with the addition of platinum-based combination chemotherapy [15]. Accompanying data additionally suggests that up to 30% of patients are unable to complete planned adjuvant systemic therapy due to perioperative morbidity [16], thereby solidifying the role for NAC as standard of care.

Postoperative Radiotherapy

For patients felt to be at high risk of LRR following RC, postoperative radiotherapy (PORT) following RC may additionally be considered [17, 18]. Patients receiving PORT may include patients with higher T stage (pT3-T4), positive surgical margins, and involved lymph nodes identified during surgical dissection [19]. To date, only a single study by the National Cancer Institute of Egypt has assessed administration of PORT following RC. Patients enrolled included 236 patients with pT3-T4 disease, and radiotherapy (RT) was administered either using a conventional fractionation scheme (daily RT to a total dose of 50 Gy over 5 weeks) or in a thrice daily fashion (at 1.25 Gy per fraction with 3 hours between fractions, to a total dose of 37.5 Gy given over the course of 12 days) [17]. While the study found improved local control (87–93% vs. 50%) and DFS (44–49% vs. 25%) for patients receiving PORT compared to RC only, 68% of the study population had squamous cell carcinoma secondary to bilharzia (schistosomiasis), and it remained unclear if findings of this study apply to non-squamous cell histologies as well.

As patients with extensive disease identified on pathology were often receiving adjuvant chemotherapy as well, a subsequent study was undertaken to assess PORT with chemotherapy. A phase II trial compared adjuvant chemotherapy to adjuvant chemotherapy with sandwiched RT in patients age 70 or younger with ≥pT3b disease, grade 3 disease, or positive nodes following RC with negative margins [18]. Patients received either four cycles of adjuvant gemcitabine and cisplatin chemotherapy (n = 45) or two cycles of gemcitabine and cisplatin chemotherapy before and after RT (n = 75), with RT consisting of 45 Gy in 1.5 Gy twice daily (BID) fractions using three-dimensional conformal radiotherapy (3DCRT) [18]. The investigators found a significant improvement in LRR-free survival with the addition of PORT at 2-year follow-up (96% vs. 69%, $p < 0.01$) with trends toward improvement in DFS (68% vs. 56%, $p = 0.07$) and OS (71% vs. 60%, $p = 0.11$) [18]. While the majority of patients enrolled on the trial had unfavorable disease characteristics, again, only 53% of patients had urothelial carcinoma, with a significant number of patients having squamous cell carcinoma due to the relatively higher incidence of schistosomiasis in Egypt.

Given the excellent outcomes demonstrated with the addition of PORT by Egyptian trials with uncertainty as to whether these results would be the same for patients with urothelial carcinoma, a randomized phase II trial was developed to assess pelvic recurrence-free survival with the addition of postoperative adjuvant intensity-modulated radiotherapy (IMRT) following RC for patients with pT3-T4 urothelial carcinoma (NRG GU-001) [20]. Unfortunately, the trial was closed 2 years after opening due to poor accrual. Consequently, there remains no existing prospective data regarding outcomes with PORT in the era of more novel treatment approaches with IMRT and image-guided radiotherapy (IGRT), both of which would improve efforts to minimize dose to pelvic organs at risk (OARs) such as the bowel and rectum. In a survey of 277 radiation oncologists in the United States of America regarding management of patients with node-negative MIBC, nearly half of surveyed radiation oncologists had used PORT for indications including gross residual disease, positive margins, pathological node involvement, pT3-T4 disease, lymphovascular invasion, and high-grade disease, with use of PORT significantly associated with using IMRT on multivariable regression [21]. Data from population-based analyses has suggested improvement in OS with PORT for patients with pT4, pathological node positivity, and positive surgical margins [22].

Surgical Morbidity

As with all oncologic treatment, the survival outcomes from RC must be viewed within the greater context of treatment-related morbidity and mortality, among other factors impacting operative candidates. While the mortality rate associated with RC is estimated to be 1–3% [23–25], the postoperative complication rate may be as high as 60% or greater [26, 27]. A series of over a thousand patients from a prospective complications database analyzed at a large, tertiary academic center found that 64% of patients experienced ≥1 complication, and of those, 83% of complications were graded 2–5, with 26% of patients requiring re-admission [26]. Even with efforts to decrease surgical morbidity by transitioning to laparoscopic and robot-assisted techniques (rather than an open cystectomy approach), data from a large systematic review demonstrated a 59% 90-day complication rate with 15% of complications being classified as high grade [27]. In addition to expected operative complications such as a urinary tract infection or wound infection leading to urosepsis, wound dehiscence, hemorrhage, rectal injury, and postoperative ileus leading to small bowel obstruction, the mean in-hospital stay of 9 days for all diversion types [27] carries the additional risk of venous thromboembolism – with potential to extend to pulmonary embolism – as well as hospital-acquired infection. For patients subsequently receiving PORT, treatment-related morbidity is even greater; a single-institution experience of 78 patients treated with a single dose of pre-operative RT and PORT reported a 37% bowel obstruction rate for patients receiving PORT as compared to 8% of patients who did not receive PORT [28].

An additional consideration of great importance for patients receiving surgical management – unrelated to patient characteristics such as age, performance status, and comorbidities – is the impact of treatment facility type and case volume on oncologic outcomes and morbidity. For patients receiving RC, high hospital volume and surgical expertise have been associated with improved overall survival, with the combined effect of both being shown to decrease the risk of long-term mortality by 20% [29]. By contrast, population-based analyses on patients with MIBC receiving bladder preservation have suggested no such benefit, indicating that all types of centers may more readily offer this approach [30]. While reasonable outcomes have been demonstrated with RC, with RT classically reserved as an option for only those refusing RC or deemed inoperable, a great interest has emerged in bladder preservation options that may allow for patients to maintain a functional bladder, thereby improving quality of life.

Introduction to Bladder Preservation

Selective bladder preservation (SBP) first emerged in the 1980s with the performance of single-institution retrospective cohort studies demonstrating reasonable oncologic outcomes for patients who had been administered neoadjuvant RT with or without chemotherapy followed by cystoscopic response assessment [31]. Patients who demonstrated a complete pathologic response to neoadjuvant treatment were then designated as eligible for a bladder preservation approach and received further/completion radiotherapy, whereas those with an incomplete response on interim evaluation proceeded to RC [31]. With the rise of this new treatment paradigm came the ultimate question for appropriate patient selection: Which patients would be the best candidates for consideration of this type of treatment, as opposed to proceeding with RC upfront?

Selection Criteria

Strict selection criteria have been proposed in determining which medically operable patients are best suited for bladder preservation and include the following [32]:

- cT2-T3a disease
- Patients with unifocal disease (no definitive cutoff for size, but often ≤5–6 cm)
- Patients without extensive carcinoma in situ
- Patients who have received maximal, visibly complete TURBT
- Patients without tumor-associated hydronephrosis

Additional considerations when assessing candidacy for SBP include favorable baseline bladder function, with the idea that the bladder should only be preserved if pre-treatment capacity and voiding ability are intact, as well as adequate renal function to allow for administration of concurrent radiosensitizing platinum-based chemotherapy (cisplatin alone or as part of a combination). The rationale underlying these selection criteria will be addressed in detail in the discussion of trimodality therapy.

Selective Bladder Preservation vs. Radical Cystectomy

A number of challenges have arisen in efforts to establish SBP as an alternative treatment paradigm for patients deemed eligible for consideration based on the aforementioned selection criteria. In the absence of prospective, randomized data directly comparing SBP to RC in the management of MIBC, a multitude of factors come into play in making the final determination as to which treatment the patient will receive. Depending on the practice environment in which the patient is being evaluated, patients may be subjected to referral bias, as patients would require referral to a clinician familiar with the modality to have a discussion about SBP [33]. An additional determination that is often made at the time of surgical consultation is the patient's operability, which carries inherent selection bias that confounds any comparisons between SBP and RC, as patients who are medically frail or less likely to perform well postoperatively are more likely to be offered SBP over RC than those with minimal comorbidity and excellent performance status [34].

Yet another factor that must be taken into consideration is the difference between clinical and pathologic staging; clinical staging does not necessarily possess high accuracy for the detection of advanced disease, as historical data suggest up to 76% of patients with MIBC may have a discrepancy between clinical T stage at TURBT and final pathologic T stage at RC [35, 36]. While these data do not reflect recent advances in modern imaging techniques, with a trend toward increasing utilization of multi-parametric MRI [37, 38], they highlight that pitfalls exist in staging information available for patients receiving SBP.

While there are currently no prospective, randomized data directly comparing outcomes from SBP to RC, data from high-quality retrospective series have suggested similar survival outcomes to RC for patients receiving bladder-sparing trimodality therapy (TMT). A study of 112 patients with MIBC evaluated at a multidisciplinary clinic (in which both RC and SBP were presented as treatment options) at Princess Margaret Cancer Center utilized propensity score matching for retrospective survival analyses and reported a 5-year disease-specific survival (DSS) rate of 73.2% for patients receiving RC vs. 76.6% for patients receiving TMT, with a salvage cystectomy rate of 10.7% for patients failing TMT [39]. Accompanying these data are those from population-based analyses; a National Cancer Database (NCDB) analysis using propensity score matching for patients with cT2-3N0M0 urothelial carcinoma treated definitively with either RC or TMT found no significant difference in OS (4 year OS of 42.6% for RC vs. 39.1% for TMT, $p = 0.15$) with report of a time-varying hazard ratio [40]. Meta-analysis data reviewing 19 studies on 12,380 patients has additionally found no significant difference in OS, DSS, or progression-free survival when comparing SBP to RC [41].

The United Kingdom (UK) Medical Research Council (MRC) developed a multi-center feasibility pilot study addressing Selective bladder Preservation Against Radical Excision (SPARE), which attempted to randomize patients with cT2-3N0M0 urothelial carcinoma status post three cycles of NAC to RC or SBP [42]. Patients were randomized to the study intervention prior to a cystoscopy following NAC with plan for a fourth cycle of NAC followed by radiotherapy or RC for patients with ≤T1 residual tumor (whereas all non-responders would immediately proceed with RC following the third cycle of NAC) [42]. Unfortunately, the trial was closed due to poor accrual, leaving the need for a phase III trial assessing for non-inferiority between the two approaches.

Bladder Preservation Treatment Paradigms

While conventional treatment for SBP generally involves a multimodality approach incorporating maximal surgical resection and RT administered concurrently with radiosensitizing systemic therapy, bladder-sparing unimodality treatment approaches may be employed for certain patients. These will be addressed briefly in turn prior to discussion regarding multimodality treatment options.

Surgical Monotherapy

Transurethral Resection of Bladder Tumor

Following maximal TURBT, the clinical complete response (CR) rate for patients with cT2-T3 disease (solitary lesions, no CIS) based on repeat cystoscopic assessment (performed 3 weeks following initial TURBT) has been found to range from 10% to 20% based on small series performed in the 1980s [43, 44]. A retrospective cohort study out of MSKCC comparing 99 patients receiving TURBT as definitive therapy (of which 57% of patients had a preserved bladder) to 52 patients receiving RC found a non-significant 10-year DSS (76% for TURBT vs. 71% for RC, $p = 0.30$) [45]. Of note, most patients were found to have cT0 disease on repeat cystoscopy, and these patients had significantly better survival than the patients with residual T1 disease on restaging TURBT ($p = 0.003$) [45]. Among patients with residual tumors, 69%demonstrated relapsed disease within the bladder, of which only 53% of patients were successfully salvaged with RC [45]. These results indicate that, while some patients with no residual disease on restaging TURBT demonstrate favorable outcomes with maximal TURBT alone as definitive treatment, many patients will have relapsed disease within the bladder (of which not all cases can be salvaged), thereby making TURBT alone a suboptimal choice for definitive treatment. Small series performed from 1950 to 1970 comparing TURBT alone to RC have demonstrated consistently inferior survival rates for TURBT as monotherapy, with an estimated 5-year OS of approximately 30% [46, 47].

Partial Cystectomy

For certain patients, partial cystectomy may be a viable treatment option for those pursuing surgical management while seeking bladder preservation. Patients under consideration for this approach must be very carefully selected: the ideal would have a solitary lesion of small size, without evidence of CIS, situated in a portion of the bladder amenable to complete excision with a widely negative margin (of at least 1 cm but preferably 2 cm) [48]. Prior to partial cystectomy, the bladder would need to be adequately sampled by random biopsy (including the prostatic urethra) with no evidence of tumor involvement elsewhere in the bladder [49]. Importantly, the remaining portion of the bladder following partial cystectomy would still need to have adequate capacity to allow maintenance of normal voiding [48, 49]. For this reason, patients would not be considered optimal candidates for partial cystectomy if they had tumors involving the bladder neck, ureteral orifices, or trigone (areas in which ureteral re-implantation would be required to achieve an adequate margin) [50]. Patients would therefore also be viewed as suboptimal candidates for this approach if they had history of a recurrent bladder tumor. A handful of single-institution retrospective series, each with a relatively small cohort, has suggested a 5-year OS rate of approximately 70% with a bladder preservation rate of 65% for well-selected patients receiving partial cystectomy [51–53]. Alas, given the relatively strict selection criteria, less than 10% of patients with MIBC receive partial cystectomy [54], and even for those patients, ~25% may still require salvage RC following recurrence [55].

Radiotherapy Monotherapy

External Beam Radiotherapy

External beam radiotherapy (EBRT) alone has been utilized for patients with cT2-T4 disease; while frequently reserved for patients with significant comorbidities precluding surgery or administration of systemic therapy in the United States, this treatment option was explored in the definitive setting in Europe from 1970 to 1990 with multiple published experiences. The earliest and largest of these was a study out of Edinburgh, Scotland, reporting on 963 patients with muscle-invasive urothelial carcinoma receiving RT alone, which found a 5-year OS across all T stages of 30.3%, with worse survival associated with age 80 or greater, cT4 disease, ulcerated lesions, grade 3 disease, and size ≥7 cm [56]. These patients were treated with 4, 6, or 9 MV photon irradiation using a small field measuring 10 × 10 cm including the whole bladder in the target volume to a dose of 55 Gy in 20 fractions, and severe RT-related complications were seen in about 15% of patients [56, 57]. Another large, retrospective study out of Glasgow, Scotland, reported on 709 patients receiving radical RT, including administered doses up to 60–64 Gy in 30 fractions; treatment was designed using a four-field technique for the first 4 weeks of treatment followed by a bladder boost for the last 2 weeks [58]. Patients in this study additionally received pelvic nodal irradiation, with doses of 40.42.5 Gy [58]. The crude 5-year OS rate was reported to be 24.7%, with 5-year OS of 86.9% for T1 tumors, 49.1% for T2 tumors, 27.7% for T3 tumors, and 1.8% for T4 tumors; of interest, patients with urothelial carcinoma demonstrated improved survival compared to those with squamous cell carcinoma, and pelvic nodal irradiation did not confer an OS benefit [58]. Similar studies were undertaken in the United States; a series by Pollack et al. analyzed 135 patients treated with an average dose of 6588 ± 475 cGy with an average fractional dose of 207 ± 18 cGy and found a 5-year OS rate of 26%, consistent with the survival outcomes from other studies [59]. Across studies, 5-year local control was estimated to be 30–50%, with prognostic factors including T stage, tumor size, tumor histology, extent of resection by TURBT, and presence of hydronephrosis/CIS [56–59].

Subsequently, RT monotherapy in the modern treatment setting has been compared to the RT plus concurrent chemotherapy in both retrospective cohort studies and prospective, randomized trials like BC2001 [60, 61]. While these data will be addressed in greater detail with discussion of TMT, given their results favoring concurrent chemotherapy administration for improved survival outcomes, RT alone has fallen out of favor for treatment in the definitive setting for patients able to receive systemic therapy. For patients who are not able to receive systemic therapy due to comorbidities, contraindications, or patient preference, reasonable outcomes may be achieved with radical RT with the understanding that (1) recurrent disease will require treatment with salvage cystectomy and (2) not all pelvic recurrences may necessarily be able to undergo successful salvage treatment.

Brachytherapy

Use of brachytherapy for radical RT was initially reported on in the 1940s and was largely utilized in Europe at its peak popularity [62–65]. The earliest reports of utilization of brachytherapy included use of permanent radon seeds, with later series reporting on use of interstitial iridum-192 [62, 63, 65]. This practice largely fell out of favor due to treatment-related toxicity, including urinary leakage in the acute/sub-acute setting and late side effects of stenosis, stricture, or fistula formation. Though EBRT was therefore often the preferred radiotherapeutic technique for patients receiving unimodality treatment with RT, brachytherapy was later studied in the 1990s as a boost treatment in combination with EBRT +/– TURBT or partial cystectomy [66]. Small retrospective series have indicated excellent outcomes for well-selected patients, with estimated 5-year local control of 70%, 5-year OS ranging from 60% to 70%, and a 5-year bladder preservation rate of 90–95% [67, 68]. When administered with low-dose preoperative EBRT of 10–11 Gy (administered in 2–3 fractions, such as 3 fractions of 3.5 Gy) for prevention of iatrogenic scar formation, brachytherapy doses range from 30 to 50 Gy [66–68].

Combined Modality Treatment

Partial Cystectomy/TURBT and Chemotherapy

To improve outcomes with TURBT and partial cystectomy, clinicians additionally have considered the use of adjuvant chemotherapy, as has been done for patients receiving RC. The addition of chemotherapy was studied in both the neoadjuvant and adjuvant settings. A series out of Italy of 104 patients with cT2-4N0M0 urothelial carcinoma who had received three cycles of neoadjuvant methotrexate, vinblastine, doxorubicin, and cisplatin (MVAC) found that 60% of patients who received TURBT following NAC were alive at median follow-up of 4.5 years, with 44% of patients maintaining a functional bladder [69]. A similarly sized sample population was reported on by MSKCC, with 111 patients receiving 4 cycles of neoadjuvant MVAC, of which 26 (23.4%) were selected for partial cystectomy based on favorable response on repeat cystoscopy; though 12 patients (46%) developed bladder recurrences, patients with no residual tumor (pT0) or non-invasive residual disease (pTis) were found to have a 5-year OS of 87% [70]. Patients included in these studies were those with unifocal, solitary tumors measuring ≤5 cm with a significant response noted following NAC [70, 71]. These results encourage the use of NAC when possible if pursuing TURBT or partial cystectomy for bladder preservation, although a significant number of patients will require salvage treatment for recurrences, which account for about half of the patient population receiving this treatment.

For patients receiving chemotherapy administered in the adjuvant setting, this paradigm has also demonstrated improvements in local control compared to TURBT alone. A small retrospective analysis of 50 patients with cT2-4 disease (of which 36 patients had T3 disease) treated with TURBT followed by 2–6 cycles of cisplatin/methotrexate found a 76% post-treatment CR rate with 5-year local control of 60% [72]. Further, a phase II nonrandomized trial comparing patients receiving RC ($n = 71$) to those receiving TURBT with three cycles of adjuvant platinum-based chemotherapy ($n = 75$) found no significant difference in 5-year and 10-year cancer-specific survival ($p = 0.54$), which was reported as 64.5% and 59.8%, respectively, for patients receiving bladder preservation [73]. For the patients receiving TURBT and adjuvant chemotherapy with clinical response, 40 patients (53%) achieved an initial CR, although 56% ultimately developed recurrence or progression and 45% received salvage RC [73].

Trimodality Therapy

Treatment Overview

TMT for SBP consists of maximal safe TURBT with examination under anesthesia followed by concurrent chemoradiotherapy. TURBT allows for tumor debulking, which is especially useful for management of a relatively radioresistant tumor histology, allowing further local therapy to be delivered with adjuvant RT to ideally address residual macroscopic or microscopic disease. Chemotherapy is administered concurrently with RT to both (1) enhance radiosensitivity for the purpose of increasing fractional cell kill (local function) and (2) address any sites housing micrometastatic disease (systemic function). The most commonly utilized chemotherapy regimens for TMT include [61, 74, 75]:

- Cisplatin 35 mg/m^2, weekly up to 6 weeks
- Cisplatin-based regimens with 5-FU (fluorouracil 400 mg/m^2 on days 1–3 and 8–10 with cisplatin 15 mg/m^2 on days 1,2, 8, and 9) or paclitaxel (paclitaxel 50 mg/m^2 on days 1 and 8 and cisplatin 15 mg/m^2 on days 1, 2, 8, and 9)
- 5-FU/mitomycin-C (500 mg/m^2 5-FU days 1–5 and 16–20 with mitomycin-C 12 mg/m^2 on day 1)
- Gemcitabine 27 mg/m^2, twice weekly up to 6 weeks

A considerable amount of variation exists in radiotherapeutic management with regard to both target volume and dose: some clinicians treat a partial bladder vs. the full bladder; some pursue nodal irradiation, while others target the bladder only; some clinicians attempt to plan a focal boost to the bladder tumor; and some clinicians administer treatment using a hypofractionated regimen (55 Gy in 20 fractions), while others treat using a conventional fractionation scheme up to 64–64.8 Gy in 1.8–2 Gy daily fractions. These treatment-related considerations will be addressed in detail with discussion of radiation techniques.

Visibly completed TURBT has been strongly advocated for in patient selection based on evidence suggesting that maximal TURBT is associated with higher rates of CR, lower rate of salvage RC, and improved OS [76, 77]. A retrospective analysis of 415 patients treated at the University of Erlangen found that early tumor stage and complete TURBT were the most important factors in predicting for CR and survival [76]. However, while maximal TURBT has historically been regarded as a strict selection criterion, there is a growing body of evidence to suggest that similar outcomes may still be achieved with incomplete TURBT [38, 78]. In a retrospective series out of MGH, while the salvage RC rate was higher for patients with incomplete TURBT vs. visibly complete TURBT (42% vs. 22%, $p < 0.001$), a CR was still achieved in 57% of patients with incomplete TURBT [78]. This idea is additionally represented by a portion of the patients enrolled in the BC2001 trial, of whom greater than a third received biopsy only or an incomplete TURBT [61]. More recently, research efforts have even been directed toward the possibility of forgoing TURBT due to concern for iatrogenic tumor spread, such as with initiation of the BladderPath study out of the United Kingdom: BladderPath is a phase II/III trial randomizing patients with possible MIBC to TURBT or multiparametric MRI for clinical staging [38].

Another essential factor for appropriate patient selection is the patient's T stage, as higher T stage is associated with less likelihood of CR following TMT. Results from the MGH experience have demonstrated that the clinical CR rate for cT2 tumors was about 80% as compared to 64% for cT3-T4 disease, suggesting that patients with cT2-T3a disease have the greatest likelihood of optimal outcomes with SBP [78]. However, patients with cT4a disease were included in the vast majority of large, retrospective series exploring SBP as well as BC2001. With regard to in situ disease, early data published in the early 1990s found that extensive CIS was associated with much higher risk of LRR (40% vs. 6%, $p = 0.075$) and that absence of CIS was a significant predictor for clinical CR ($p = 0.03$); these data guided the general recommendation encouraging absence of CIS for TMT [79]. Similarly, data from the pioneering experiences at MGH have suggested that tumor-related hydronephrosis is associated with worse OS and DSS, and these results were corroborated by findings of a lesser likelihood to achieve CR for patients with tumor-related hydronephrosis in RTOG 8903 [78, 80].

Given the relatively higher incidence of urothelial carcinoma compared to other forms of MIBC, such as squamous cell carcinoma or adenocarcinoma, it is unclear if patients with non-urothelial carcinoma histologies have differences in outcomes following SBP. While prospective studies investigating patients treated with SBP such as BC2001 have limited inclusion criteria to those with urothelial carcinoma, retrospective data comparing outcomes between patients with non-urothelial carcinoma (22%, $n = 66$) and urothelial carcinoma (78%, $n = 237$) found no significant difference in CR rate (82–83%, $p = 0.9$), 10–year DSS (64–67%, $p = 0.39$), or 10-year OS (42%, $p = 0.21$) [81].

Outcomes and Literature Review

SBP was first developed following pioneering single-institution experiences by the University of Erlangen, University of Paris, and Massachusetts General Hospital (MGH) [82–84]. The University of Paris experience represents one of the earliest efforts at bladder preservation, as clinicians there initially studied concurrent chemoradiotherapy as a preoperative regimen prior to RC. After finding that 18 consecutive patients demonstrated 100% pathologic CR upon analysis of the final cystectomy specimen, it was determined that concurrent chemoradiotherapy may be utilized toward SBP [49]. The French experience reported on a cohort of 54 patients with operable cT2-T4 MIBC, all of whom were managed with concurrent chemoradiotherapy with cisplatin/5-FU and BID RT administered in a split course fashion as both induction (24 Gy) and consolidation (with an additional 20 Gy) following TURBT [82]. Re-staging cystoscopy and TURBT were performed 4–6 weeks following completion of induction chemoradiation, and consolidation treatment was administered only to those with CR; any patients with residual disease after induction received RC. At post-induction cystoscopy, 40 patients (74%) were found to have a CR; at mean follow-up of 27 +/− 12 months, three patients receiving SBP with initial CR developed recurrent disease in the pelvis, and the overall 3-year DFS rate was reported to be 62% with no significant survival difference noted between patients receiving SBP and those ultimately receiving RC [82].

The University of Erlangen initiated prospective study of SBP in the early 1980s, initially by assessing patients receiving TURBT followed by EBRT alone to 50–56 Gy in 2 Gy daily fractions; following treatment of over 100 consecutive patients in this manner, radiosensitizing platinum monotherapy (cisplatin or carboplatin) was added for treating patients thereafter [76]. A German group reported on outcomes for 415 patients, of which 79% had cT2-T4 disease, 30.3% were treated with RT alone following TURBT, and 69.6% received concurrent chemoradiotherapy following TURBT; they found a CR rate of 72% and reported that the local control following CR without muscle-invasive recurrence was 64% at 10 years [76]. The 10-year DSS was 42% for their cohort, and the bladder preservation rate was 80% [76]. Administration of radiosensitizing chemotherapy concurrently with RT was found to improve both CR rate and survival, and patients who required salvage RC due to disease persistence or recurrence still maintained a 10-year DSS of 45%, comparable to the 10-year DSS for the cohort at large [76]. Of note, patients in this German study received the entire course of concurrent chemoradiotherapy without mid-evaluation cystoscopy to evaluate response; re-staging was performed 6–8 weeks following completion of all definitive treatment. Further, the patients routed to salvage RC were only those with poorly differentiated, superficial tumors, or persistent/residual invasive disease, and patients with well-differentiated, superficial disease remaining (e.g., CIS) were allowed to continue with SBP while receiving endoscopic treatment with TURBT/intravesical therapy [76].

At a similar time in the mid-1990s, pioneers at MGH reported on an initial experience with 53 patients with cT2-4N0M0 MIBC treated consecutively with TURBT and adjuvant concurrent chemoradiotherapy to a dose of 40 Gy (using a daily fractionation scheme) with concurrent cisplatin followed by cystoscopic evaluation and further treatment to 64.8 Gy for patients with a CR or those deemed unsuitable for RC [85]. The study found an initial CR rate of 53% with 89% of patients having a functioning bladder, and the 4-year DFS was found to be 45% for the entire cohort [85]. MGH has subsequently reported on patients treated over 20 years with long-term follow-up; in their cohort of 348 patients with cT2-T4aN0M0 MIBC, all of whom were treated with maximal TURBT and concurrent chemoradiotherapy to 64–65 Gy with cisplatin (with patients receiving response assessment following 40 Gy and some patients receiving additional chemotherapy administered adjuvantly or neoadjuvantly), their findings were as follows at nearly 8-year median follow-up [78]:

- Initial CR rate: 72%
- Cystectomy rate: 29% (native bladder preservation: 71%)
  - 12% – invasive tumor recurrence noted on post-treatment surveillance
  - 17% – incomplete response noted following concurrent chemoradiotherapy
- 5-year OS, 52%; 10-year OS, 35%
- 5-year DSS, 64%; 10-year DSS, 59%
- 10-year rates of recurrence (for patients with initial CR):
  - Non-invasive: 29%
  - Invasive: 16%
  - Pelvic: 11%
  - Distant: 32%

The two most important factors predicting for OS and DSS were clinical T stage and initial CR following induction therapy [78]. NAC was not found to be associated with OS on multivariable regression analysis, and no patients required RC due to toxicity secondary to treatment from SBP [78].

Following promising results from the aforementioned single institution experiences, data obtained from cooperative group experiences undertaken by the Radiation Therapy Oncology Group (RTOG) confirmed such outcomes. These trials are briefly summarized in Table 18.2 [49]. The first published RTOG trial was RTOG 8512, which was a phase II study analyzing 42 patients with cT2-T4N0-2M0 disease receiving 40 Gy to the pelvis with 2 cycles of concurrent cisplatin followed by an additional 24 Gy with another cycle of cisplatin in the event of CR (whereas patients with residual tumor following 40 Gy and 2 cycles of cisplatin received RC) [86]. The study found an initial CR of 66%, and 42% of patients were alive with an intact bladder at 5 years [86]. This study was followed by RTOG 8802, which sought to investigate outcomes with the addition of MCV chemotherapy following TURBT but prior to concurrent chemoradiotherapy [87]. Of 91 patients studied, the 4-year risk of LRR was found to be 43%, which was similar to the reported 4-year rate of surviving with an intact bladder of 44% [87]. This was then followed by RTOG 8903, which was a phase III trial aiming to compare concurrent cisplatin

Table 18.2 Summary of Radiation Therapy Oncology Group (RTOG) trials investigating outcomes for patients receiving radiotherapy for muscle-invasive bladder cancer [49]

RTOG Trial #	Phase	Neoadj. Chemo	Concurrent Chemotherapy	Radiation Dose (Gy)	Adjuvant Chemo	*n*	CR rate	5-year OS
85-12	II	--	Cisplatin	40.0 + 24.0	--	42	66%	52%
88-02	II	MCV x 2	Cisplatin	39.6 + 25.2	--	91	75%	62%
89-03	III	MCV x 2 vs. none	Cisplatin	39.6 + 25.2	--	123	61% 55%	49% 48%
95-06	I/II	--	Cisplatin/5-FU	24.0 + 20.0[a]	--	34	67%	--
97-06	I/II	--	Cisplatin	40.8 + 24.0[a]	MCV x 3	46	74%	--
99-06	I/II	--	Cisplatin/paclitaxel	40.3 + 24.0[a]	Cisplatin/ gemcitabine x 4	80	81%	56%
02-33	II	--	Cisplatin/ paclitaxel or cisplatin/5-FU	40.3 + 24.0[a]	Cisplatin, paclitaxel, and gemcitabine x 4	93	72% 62%	71% 75%
07-12	II	--	Cisplatin/5-FU or gemcitabine	40.0 + 24.0[a] (QD or BID)	Cisplatin/ gemcitabine x 4	66	88% 78%	--

[a]Asterisk indicates BID radiotherapy delivery

with RT (standard arm) to the standard arm plus the addition of neoadjuvant MCV chemotherapy; however, this study was closed early due to high rate of severe leukopenia witnessed in patients receiving MCV [80]. Based on the 123 patients analyzed, neoadjuvant MCV was not found to be associated with CR rate, OS, or freedom from distant metastases; based on these findings, later RTOG did not incorporate NAC [80].

Subsequent RTOG trials explored utilization of BID RT, as was done by clinicians at the University of Paris (and, separately, by investigators in Egypt using PORT) with concurrent chemotherapy administration. RTOG 9506 reported on 34 patients with cT2-T4N0M0 MIBC without hydronephrosis receiving TURBT followed by induction chemoradiotherapy to 24 Gy administered BID at 3 Gy per fractions with concurrent cisplatin/5-FU; following cystoscopy and re-biopsy 4 weeks later, patients with CR received consolidation chemoradiotherapy with BID RT to the bladder to 20 Gy (for a cumulative dose of 44 Gy) [88]. While the study reported a 3-year OS of 83% with 66% of patients maintaining an intact bladder, the grades 3–4 hematologic toxicity rate of 21% declared this regimen as relatively toxic in spite of encouraging oncologic outcomes [88]. The RTOG turned to investigation of adjuvant chemotherapy with its next trial, RTOG 9706, which analyzed 52 patients with cT2-T4aN0M0 MIBC patients who received induction chemoradiotherapy (administered BID with 1.8 Gy to the pelvis in the morning followed by a 1.6 Gy boost to the tumor 4–6 hours later) with concurrent cisplatin, cystoscopic evaluation 3–4 weeks following induction, consolidation chemoradiation in the event of CR (given in 1.5 Gy BID fractions to a total dose of 45.6 Gy to the pelvis/bladder and 64.8 Gy to the tumor), and, finally, three cycles of adjuvant MCV [89]. The authors found that 74% of patients achieved CR, with only 11% of patients experiencing grades 3–4 hematologic toxicity (unlike the nearly double rate noted in RTOG 9506); however, only 45% of patients were able to receive the full three cycles of adjuvant MCV, and of the patients who received the full three cycles, 41% developed grades 3–4 hematologic toxicity [89]. Consequently, this treatment regimen was also felt to be very toxic, although the logic underlying condensing the induction phase into a shorter time frame with BID RT was sound. The subsequently performed RTOG 9906 trial also assessed BID RT but added paclitaxel to induction cisplatin and utilized an adjuvant chemotherapy regimen consisting of gemcitabine/cisplatin [90].

The RTOG trials performed most recently have continued to evaluate different variations of systemic therapy administration. RTOG 0233 was a phase II study reporting on a group of 93 patients randomized to receive cisplatin/paclitaxel or cisplatin/5-FU administered concurrently with induction RT to 40.3 Gy following TURBT, with patients then receiving consolidation chemoradiation to 64.3 Gy with the same chemotherapy given during induction in the event of downstaging to T0, Tcis, or Ta disease [74]. Patients then went on to receive adjuvant chemotherapy with gemcitabine (1000 mg/m^2), paclitaxel (50 mg/m^2), and cisplatin (35 mg/m^2) all administered on days 1 and 8. Results showed comparable rates of 5-year OS between the two arms (paclitaxel, 71%; 5-FU, 75%) with 5-year bladder-intact survival rates of 67–71% [74]. However, the study reported marked rates of toxicity, with 16 patients (35%) treated with paclitaxel and 19 (44%) treated with 5-FU developing late grades 3–4 toxicity (of which 11% and 6%, respectively, were attributed to RT) [74].

Following completion of RTOG 0233, a pooled analysis of RTOG 8802, 9506, 9706, 9906, and 0233 was published in 2014 and reported on 468 patients across the 5 studies, with clinical T stage of T2 in 61%, T3 in 35%, and T4a in 4% of patients. With median follow-up of 4.3 years among all patients and 7.8 years among survivors, the study found [91]:

- CR rate: 69%
- 5-year OS, 57%; 10-year OS, 36%
- 5-year DSS, 71%; 10-year DSS, 65%
- 10-year estimate of muscle-invasive LRR: 14%
- 10-year estimate of non-muscle invasive LRR: 36%
- 10-year estimate of distant metastasis: 35%

Most recently, RTOG 0712 reported on SBP using either cisplatin/5-FU with BID RT or gemcitabine with once daily RT following TURBT as part of induction to 40 Gy as well as consolidation to 64 Gy for those patients achieving CR on interim cystoscopic assessment; this was then followed by adjuvant cisplatin/gemcitabine [75]. Twice weekly gemcitabine emerged as an attractive systemic therapy option following completion of a phase I trial by the University of Michigan establishing good response, survival, and bladder preservation rates of this regimen, with a maximum tolerated dose of 27 mg/m^2 [92]. While not statistically powered to make a comparison between cisplatin/5-FU with BID RT and gemcitabine with once daily RT, RTOG 0712 demonstrated rates of freedom from distant metastasis exceeding 75% in both arms (cisplatin/5-FU with BID RT, 78%; gemcitabine with daily RT, 84%) with post-induction CR rates of 88% for cisplatin/5-FU with BID RT and 78% for gemcitabine with daily RT. [75] These results have encouraged further utilization of gemcitabine with daily RT as an alternative to the prior platinum-based RTOG regimens with BID RT, especially for patients with renal function precluding use of agents like cisplatin.

The largest prospective, randomized study performed in patients with MIBC is BC2001; this trial was performed in the United Kingdom and reported on 360 patients with MIBC randomized to receive either RT alone (n = 178) or RT with concurrent 5-FU/mitomycin-C (n = 182) [61]. In addition, patients were randomized to receive whole bladder radiotherapy or treatment of a partial bladder volume using a partial 2-by-2 factorial design, with permission of 2 RT schedules: (1) a conventionally fractionated schedule to 64 Gy in 32 fractions over the course of 6.5 weeks or (2) a hypofractionated approach of 55 Gy in 20 fractions over the course of 4 weeks. BC2001 found a significant improvement in 2-year locoregional DFS with the addition of concurrent chemotherapy (67% vs. 54%, p = 0.03) with trends toward improved 5-year OS (48% vs. 35%, p = 0.16; though the study was underpowered to show a difference in survival), reduced 2-year cystectomy rate (11.4% vs. 16.8%, p = 0.07), and higher grades 3–4 acute treatment-related toxicity (36% vs. 28%, p = 0.07) [61]. An exploratory analysis demonstrated a 2-year relapse rate of 18% for patients receiving concurrent chemoradiotherapy vs. 32% for patients receiving RT alone ($p = 0.01$) [61]. Subgroup analysis indicated no significant differences based on patients receiving whole-bladder RT ($n = 63$) vs. "modified volume" RT ($n = 58$) vs. elective whole-bladder RT ($n = 239$) ($p = 0.66$) or 64 Gy in 32 fractions ($n = 217$) vs. 55 Gy in 20 fractions ($n = 142$) ($p = 0.59$) [61, 93]. Two important distinctions in this study come to light when comparing patients treated on BC2001 to those treated on RTOG protocols: (1) patients were not required to receive maximal TURBT for enrollment (over a third of patients had biopsy only or incomplete TURBT); (2) no interim cystoscopic assessment or re-biopsy was performed following an induction treatment phase; treatment proceeded continuously, and first post-treatment cystoscopy was performed 6 months following completion of definitive therapy [61]. This trial validated numerous facets of modern-day treatment: use of the 5-FU/mitomycin-C regimen for radiosensitization, use of hypofractionated RT, and continuous treatment without a mid-treatment break.

Evolving Considerations

There has been great evolution of numerous considerations over time when considering the treatment paradigm for MIBC; these are depicted in Fig. 18.1 and include utilization of NAC, alterations in fractionation for RT delivery, hypoxia modification, use of molecular stratification in treatment selection, use of immunotherapy, and response evaluation. Each of these will be briefly addressed in turn.

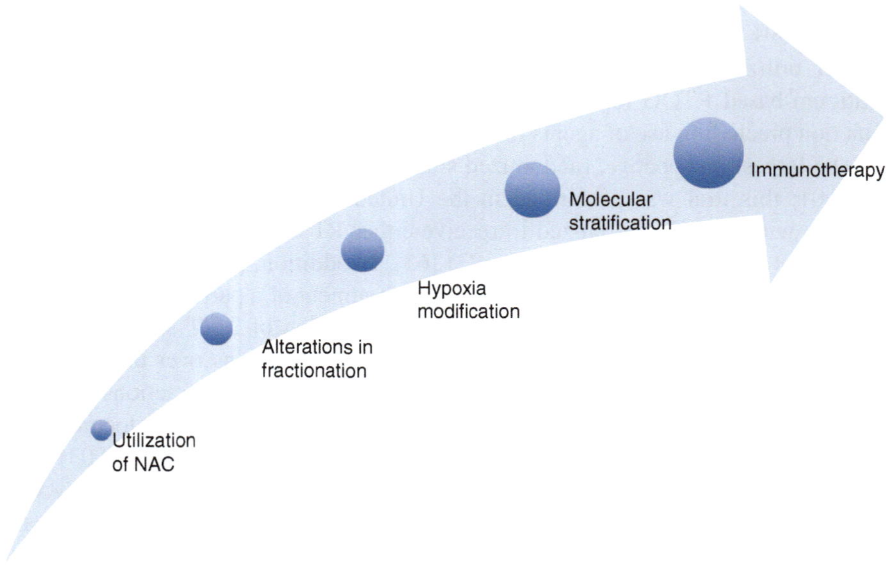

Fig. 18.1 Timeline depicting evolution of treatment considerations over time

Neoadjuvant Chemotherapy

From the initial conception of SBP using TMT in the early 1980s, NAC emerged as a treatment of interest due to the potential for tumor downstaging at the time of TURBT and the opportunity for early assessment of response to systemic therapy (with the caveat that administration of NAC would postpone initiation of definitive local treatment). While many of the largest phase III studies aimed at assessing the role of NAC prior to definitive local therapy have been performed on patients receiving RC (e.g., the Nordic 1 Cooperative Bladder Cancer Study Group, Spanish CUETO, Italian GUONE, and SWOG 8710/Intergroup 0080 trials) [14, 94–96], there are some prospective, randomized data assessing the role of NAC for patients receiving radical EBRT. A pooled analysis by the West Midlands Urological Research Group and the Australian Bladder Cancer Study Group compiled data from two pilot studies comparing radical RT to radical RT with induction cisplatin; with a total of 255 patients analyzed, no significant difference in OS was noted [97]. The MRC-EORTC published results of a large trial studying 485 patients undergoing either RC or EBRT monotherapy and randomly assigned to receive neoadjuvant MVAC (n = 491) or no NAC (n = 485); while results demonstrated that NAC was associated with higher rates of pathological CR, the 10% absolute improvement in OS at 3 years required to establish NAC as standard of care was not found [98].

With regard to NAC prior to administration of concurrent chemoradiotherapy, RTOG 8903 assessed the addition of neoadjuvant MCV to the standard of concurrent cisplatin with RT and found no impact on CR rate, freedom from distant metastasis, or OS but noted significant hematologic toxicity that led to only a 67% protocol completion rate for patients receiving MCV [80]. The outcomes for patients treated on BC2001 who received NAC were recently published: 117 patients of the initial cohort of 360 (33%) received platinum-based NAC prior to receiving RT +/− concurrent 5-FU/mitomycin-C, and no differences in local control or OS were noted between the two arms among this subgroup of patients receiving NAC [99]. However, patients receiving NAC and concurrent chemoradiotherapy were noted to have a 33% rate of grades 3–4 toxicity as compared to 22% for patients receiving NAC followed by RT alone [99]. Based on findings suggesting no significant benefit in oncologic outcomes and elevated rates of grades 3–4 toxicity, NAC has not continued to evolve as a paradigm-shifting treatment consideration.

Variations in Fractionation

Another unique aspect of TMT for MIBC has been the implementation of multiple fractionation schemes in delivering RT. Accelerated RT with BID fractionation was studied in the early TMT experience out of the University of Paris and subsequently implemented in multiple RTOG trials, including RTOG 9506, RTOG 9706, RTOG 9906, RTOG 0233, and RTOG 0712 [75, 82, 91]. Using accelerated fractionation for these studies – all of which entailed mid-treatment response assessment with cystoscopy to evaluate for CR prior to consolidation chemoradiation or cystectomy – carried the advantage of decreasing time to definitive local treatment. Unlike hyperfractionation, which utilizes a lower dose per fraction in combination with an increased number of daily fractions to ultimately yield a higher cumulative dose, accelerated fractionation yields a similar total dose to conventional fractionation (e.g., 64 Gy) with a shorter treatment package time.

There is limited existing data comparing accelerated fractionation and conventional fractionation. A prospective, randomized trial out of the Royal Marsden Hospital randomized 229 patients with cT2-T3N0-1M0 urothelial carcinoma treated from 1988 to 1998 to one of two EBRT monotherapy regimens: (1) an accelerated fractionation regimen of 60.8 Gy in 32 fractions over 26 days ($n = 129$) or (2) a conventional fractionation regimen of 64 Gy in 32 fractions over 45 days ($n = 100$) [100]. The accelerated fractionation RT was delivered using BID RT (first fraction, 1.8 Gy; second fraction, 2.0 Gy) with 6 hours between fractions and a 1-week treatment gap following the first 12 fractions. The primary endpoint was local control, and the trial was powered to detect a 20% difference. While no significant difference was noted between the two arms in terms of local control, OS, or DFS, a significantly higher rate of grades 2–3 bowel toxicity was noted in the accelerated fractionation arm when compared to the conventional fraction arm (44% vs. 26%, $p = 0.001$) [100]. While not directly comparing these two fractionation schemes in the setting of systemic therapy administration, these results indicate a greater likelihood of toxicity from accelerated fractionation without a well-established oncologic benefit.

With regard to hyperfractionation, a prospective, randomized trial conducted in Sweden randomized 168 patients with cT2-T4N0M0 MIBC to a hyperfractionated regimen of thrice daily RT (1 Gy per fraction, three times per day) to a total dose of 84 Gy or a conventional fractionation regimen of 64 Gy in 32 fractions administered once daily [101]. Both treatments were administered over the course of 8 weeks with a 2-week "rest period" in the middle of treatment. At 10-year follow up, the authors found improved rates of local control and OS for patients receiving hyperfractionation [101]. Similarly, meta-analysis data comparing hyperfractionation to conventional fractionation for bladder cancer (2 trials, 345 patients) has suggested improved OS with hyperfractionation [102]. However, findings of these data may largely be explained by the higher dose achieved with hyperfractionated RT; data from the Netherlands have underscored that dose escalation leads to improved local control, with logistic modeling calculations predicting that an increase in total dose by 10 Gy is associated with 3-year improved local control by an odds ratio of 1.44 [103].

Hypofractionation has also been utilized for SBP in the management of MIBC, especially following results of the BC2001 study, which incorporated a partial 2-by-2 factorial design in which patients could be treated with either conventional fractionation or a hypofractionated regimen of 55 Gy in 20 fractions [61]. Long-term outcomes from BC2001 never demonstrated a significant difference between conventional fractionation RT and hypofractionated RT for any trial endpoint;

however, until recently, there was no high-quality data for direct comparison [93]. A recently published, individual patient data meta-analysis of BC2001 and BCON (a phase III trial assessing use of hypoxia-modifying agents, discussed in detail in the next section) analyzed 782 patients between the two trials and aimed to establish non-inferiority of 55 Gy in 20 fractions as compared to 64 Gy in 32 fractions with regard to both locoregional control and late toxicity [104]. While the meta-analysis found comparable toxicity profiles between the two fractionation regimens (2-year late rectal toxicity, 3–6%; 2-year late bladder toxicity, 24–25%), at 10-year median follow-up, it was found that patients receiving 55 Gy in 20 fractions had a lower risk of LRR at 3 years than those treated with conventional fractionation (adjusted HR: 0.71, 95% CI: 0.52–0.96) when controlling for pre-specified prognostic factors for local control including age, sex, tumor stage, use of NAC, and extent of resection at TURBT.

Hypoxia Modification

Following data published in the late 1990s regarding modification of hypoxia-induced radioresistance using entities such as high oxygen-content gas breathing, hemoglobin oxygen affinity modifiers, and nicotinamide suggesting improvement in local control for bladder tumors [105], hypoxia modification became an area of active exploration in the 2000s, especially in the United Kingdom. Hypoxia-modifying agents such as carbogen, a mixture of carbon dioxide and oxygen, and nicotinamide, an oxidoreductase coenzyme, were investigated in phase II trials in combination with radical RT to a dose of 52.5 Gy [106]. Following demonstration of good outcomes with carbogen and nicotinamide (CON) for hypoxia modification, a phase III randomized trial (BCON) comparing RT alone to RT with CON was undertaken in patients with locally advanced bladder cancer [107]. BCON randomized 333 patients (to either RT +/− CON) while permitting fractionation schedules of either 64 Gy in 32 fractions or 55 Gy in 20 fractions. The study found no significant difference between RT and RT with CON for its primary endpoint of cystoscopic control at 6 months (76% for RT alone vs. 81% for RT with CON, $p = 0.30$) [107]; however, at 10-year follow-up, RT with CON was associated with significantly improved recurrence-free survival (27% vs. 20%, $p = 0.04$) with a trend toward improved OS (32% vs. 24%, $p = 0.07$; initially significant at 3-year follow-up) [108]. Further analysis of hypoxia modification has demonstrated that tumor necrosis on pathologic specimen obtained by TURBT predicts for better survival outcomes [109]. Researchers have additionally developed a 24-gene signature predicting for benefit from CON (HR: 0.47, 95% CI: 0.26–0.86; $p = 0.015$) with both prognostic ($p = 0.017$) and predictive ($p = 0.058$) significance [110]. While currently utilized predominantly in the United Kingdom, hypoxia modification remains an active area of interest and further study.

Molecular Stratification

Adding further nuance and complexity to the management of MIBC is the idea that molecular stratification of patients' tumors may both predict for treatment response and guide optimal management [31]. MIBC carries a heterogeneous mutational profile and is considered one of the most highly mutated cancers along with non-small cell lung cancer and squamous cell carcinoma of the head and neck; consequently, efforts to associate molecular subtypes of MIBC with patients' baseline characteristics and treatment response are underway [111]. With regard to systemic therapy administration, tumors with mutations in genes associated with DNA damage repair (*ERCC2*, *ERBB2*, *ATM*, and *RB1*) have been shown to demonstrate greater sensitivity to cisplatin [112, 113]. Similarly, increased *BCL2* expression has been found to be associated with poorer outcomes for patients receiving concurrent chemoradiotherapy and serves as a marker for patients who may benefit from NAC [114]. For predicting response to RT, existing data has demonstrated that patients with tumors highly expressing *MRE11* demonstrate better response to radical RT than those with tumors demonstrating low expression [115]. With significant heterogeneity at the molecular level, investigators at centers worldwide set out to create an international consensus on MIBC molecular subtypes and relate these classes to clinical behavior and treatment response; the authors used 1750 MIBC transcriptomic profiles from 16 published datasets as well as two additional cohorts to develop the following 6 classes [116]:

1. Luminal papillary (LumP)
2. Luminal non-specific (LumNS)
3. Luminal unstable (LumU)
4. Stroma-rich
5. Basal/squamous (Ba/Sq)
6. Neuroendocrine-like (NE-like)

The six molecular classes represented (as follows, percentage of the samples) LumP, 24%; LumNS, 8%; LumU, 15%; stroma-rich, 15%; Ba/Sq, 35%; and NE-like, 3% [116]. mRNA data were utilized to assess for associations with molecular gene signatures for bladder cancer pathways and tumor microenvironment infiltration. The consensus molecular classes were found to be associated with certain genomic alterations: LumP tumors were found to be predominantly associated with mutations in *FGFR3* and *KDM6A* as well as deletions of *CDKN2A*, whereas LumNS was largely associated with mutations in *ELF3* and alterations in *PPARG* (which were also noted in LumU tumors) [116]. Targeted sequencing data revealed that 58% and 20% of Ba/Sq tumors were associated with *TP53* and *RB1*, respectively, and 49% of Ba/Sq tumors were associated with genomic deletions of 3p14.2 [116].

Of greatest interest to clinicians was description of the association of the six molecular classes with clinical characteristics, OS, and response to treatment. These are briefly summarized in Figure 18.2 [116]. With regard to sociodemographic characteristics, patients with LumP and LumU tumors were found to be more likely to have cT2 ($p = 0.009$) or cT3-T4 ($p < 0.001$) disease compared to other molecular

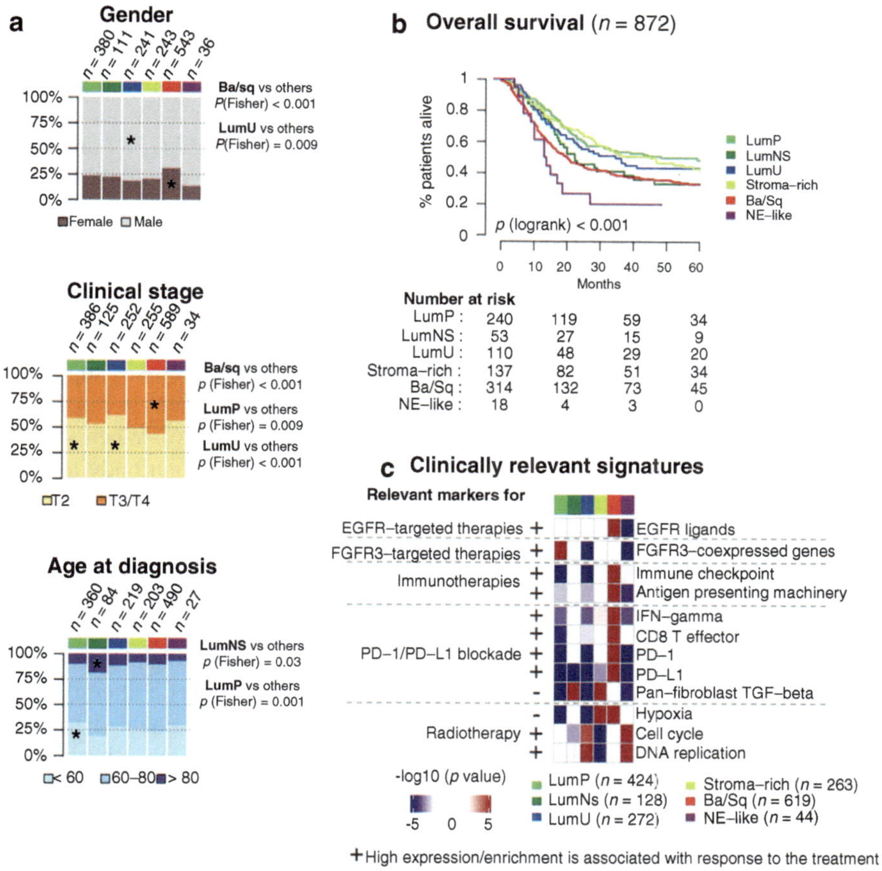

Fig. 18.2 Association of six molecular classes with clinical characteristics, survival, and response to treatment

classes. Patients with age < 60 were more likely to have LumP tumors ($p = 0.001$), whereas patients age > 80 were more likely to have LumNS tumors ($p = 0.03$). Ba/Sq tumors were far more likely to be found among females ($p < 0.001$) and those with higher clinical stage ($p < 0.001$) [116]. The association of the six molecular classes with overall survival was analyzed using a multivariable Cox regression model accounting for patients' age and clinical T, N, and M staging as covariates with the LumP class serving as a reference for comparison. While patients with LumU (HR: 1.49, 95% CI: 0.93–2.39), LumNS (HR: 1.07, 95% CI: 0.63–1.82), and stroma-rich (HR: 0.98, 95% CI: 0.65–1.49) tumors demonstrated similar OS to patients with LumP tumors, patients with Ba/Sq (HR: 1.83, 95% CI: 1.30–2.58, $p < 0.001$) and NE-like (HR: 2.34, 95% CI: 1.09–5.05, $p < 0.03$) tumors were associated with significantly worse prognosis [116].

In terms of response to different types of therapy, both LumU and NE-like tumors were felt to be associated with greater response to RT based on demonstrating significantly elevated cell cycle activity and low hypoxia signals when compared to the other classes [116]. Given that the *FGFR3* signature was both strongly and specifically activated for patients with LumP tumors, therapies targeting *FGFR3* are being investigated. Ba/Sq tumors were found to demonstrate high levels of EGFR and EGFR ligand as well as immune checkpoint markers and genes involved in the mechanisms underlying antigen presentation, all of which would suggest response to immunotherapy; however, none of the molecular classes demonstrated a profile clearly suggesting better or worse response to anti-PD1/PDL1 therapy [116]. While class-based analysis of patients receiving NAC demonstrated no significant association of consensus class with outcome, comparison of the survival curves suggested that patients with LumNS or Ba/Sq tumors may derive greater benefit from patients with NAC, whereas patients with stroma-rich tumors may not [116]. When specifically analyzing patients treated with the anti-PDL1 monoclonal antibody atezolizumab [117], patients were more likely to respond to atezolizumab if they had LumNS ($p = 0.05$), LumU ($p = 0.0044$), or NE-like ($p = 0.012$) tumors [116].

While still an area of growing investigation with need for prospective validation, association of molecular classes with treatment response has the potential to provide considerable guidance in both determination of appropriate therapy of existing options and design of clinical trials ahead. There are multiple ongoing phase II clinical trials aimed at evaluating different treatments based on genetic alterations in DNA damage response; an ongoing phase II trial looking at Risk Enabled Therapy After Initiating Chemotherapy for Bladder Cancer (RETAIN BLADDER; NCT02710734) endeavors to utilize genomic profiles (obtained from sequencing patients' TURBT specimens while they are receiving cisplatin-based NAC) as well as response to post-chemotherapy TURBT findings to risk-stratify patients [118]. The ALLIANCE trial A03171 (NCT 03609216) is an open phase II trial evaluating for potential bladder preservation in patients receiving dose-dense cisplatin/gemcitabine and has primary and secondary endpoints assessing outcomes based on presence or absence of known genetic alterations [118]. Yet another trial is assessing cisplatin/gemcitabine but with the addition of nivolumab (NCT03558087) for patients with MIBC undergoing SBP [118].

Immunotherapy

Immune checkpoint inhibition (ICI) has been established as a crucial aspect of treatment for non-bladder malignancies and is an area of ongoing investigation for treating MIBC as well. As discussed previously with utilization of molecular stratification, a role for ICI is emerging based on enhanced treatment response in certain tumor types over others. As treatment using ICI has thus far been largely explored in the locally advanced and metastatic settings, treatment paradigms incorporating ICI for patients with MIBC receiving SBP are not yet well established. There are multiple ongoing trials assessing use of ICI for patients receiving SBP followed by RT alone or concurrent chemoradiation. For patients receiving RT alone following TURBT, there are two ongoing phase II trials assessing use of RT with concurrent ICI: NCT03747419 and IMMUNOPRESERVE [119]. NCT03747419 is assessing use of the anti-PDL1 monoclonal antibody avelumab for patients ineligible to receive cisplatin. IMMUNOPRESERVE (Durvalumab Plus Tremelimumab with Concurrent Radiotherapy for Localized Muscle Invasive Bladder Cancer Treated with a Selective Bladder Preservation Approach; NCT 03702179) is a phase II trial sponsored by the Spanish Oncology Genito-Urinary Group (SOGUG) studying joint inhibition of PD1 and CTLA4 concurrently with RT (administered as 46 Gy to the pelvis with 64–66 Gy to the bladder) with the primary endpoint of pathological response at post-treatment biopsy [120].

For patients receiving concurrent chemoradiotherapy +/− ICI following TURBT, there are two phase II trials (NCT03617913 and NCT02621151) and two phase III trials (NCT03775265 [INTACT, NRG/SWOG S1806] and NCT04241185 [KEYNOTE 992]) currently open [119, 121]. NCT03617913 aims to study the CR rate with the addition of avelumab to concurrent chemoradiotherapy using either cisplatin or 5-FU/mitomycin-C, and NCT02621151 is a study investigating lead-in pembrolizumab, maximal TURBT, and adjuvant concurrent chemoradiotherapy with gemcitabine and pembrolizumab using hypofractionated RT of 52 Gy in 20 fractions [119].

NCT03775265 (INTACT, NRG/SWOG S1806) is a phase III RCT randomizing patients with MIBC status post TURBT to concurrent chemoradiotherapy with or without atezolizumab [122, 123]. Patients on S1806 are allowed to receive single-agent cisplatin, single-agent gemcitabine, or 5-FU/mitomycin-C for systemic therapy; patients randomized to the experimental arm additionally receive concurrent and adjuvant atezolizumab 1200 mg every 3 weeks for nine cycles [123]. With regard to RT administration, enrolled patients may be treated with 3DCRT or IMRT, and treatment of pelvic lymph nodes is optional; however, all patients must receive conventionally fractionated treatment to 64–64.8 Gy, as hypofractionation is not permitted on this trial [123]. For the volume to be irradiated, clinicians have the option of treating the small pelvis to 40–50 Gy (or 41.4–50.4 Gy, if treating at 1.8 Gy/fraction) followed by sequential boost(s) to either the (1) bladder tumor alone, (2) the whole bladder alone, or (3) the whole bladder with a secondary sequential boost to the bladder tumor [123]. For patients not receiving nodal RT, the treatment step involving irradiating the small pelvis would be omitted. In addition to having a primary endpoint of bladder-intact event free survival, S1806 has translational objectives of testing that nuclear *MRE11*, impaired DNA damage response genes, or tumor subtyping are prognostic [123].

NCT04241185 (KEYNOTE-992) is a phase III global, multicenter, double-blinded, placebo-controlled RCT randomizing patients with MIBC status post maximal TURBT to concurrent chemoradiotherapy with or without pembrolizumab for SBP [121]. Similar to SWOG S1806, the trial is allowing for cisplatin monotherapy, 5-FU/mitomycin-C, or gemcitabine monotherapy; however, the trial accepts both conventional fractionation (whole bladder +/− pelvic node) and hypofractionation (whole bladder only) [121]. Patients randomized to the experimental arm receive concurrent and adjuvant pembrolizumab for up to nine doses, and those on the control arm will receive a placebo. Similarly, tissue will undergo biomarker analysis. The study aims to assess the primary endpoint of bladder-intact free survival with secondary endpoints of safety, time to occurrence of NMIBC, OS, and metastasis-free survival [121].

Response Evaluation

One of the most pertinent considerations in the evolution of SBP treatment paradigms is that of mid-treatment response evaluation. Among the pioneering single institution experiences establishing use of TMT for SBP, the University of Erlangen appeared distinct from the University of Paris and MGH in that concurrent chemoradiotherapy was completed continuously without a treatment break for response evaluation. The RTOG approach has involved a treatment break following the induction phase of treatment for early response assessment (following delivery of approximately 40–42 Gy) with repeat cystoscopy and tumor site biopsy. Patients complete consolidation chemoradiation only if a complete response or superficial residual disease is noted, whereas the remaining patients are encouraged to pursue cystectomy in the event of residual/persistent disease. One merit of a mid-treatment response assessment includes early identification of non-responders with the hope that, by avoiding treatment that is not working, they may maintain excellent outcomes following receipt of RC. Further, as full-dose RT has not yet been administered at the mid-treatment point, the surgical morbidity associated with operating on previously irradiated tissue could be less/better. On the other hand, it is arguable that patients may unnecessarily be deemed "non-responders" who receive RC before the treatment has taken effect (and would otherwise have demonstrated a clinical CR following completion of planned concurrent chemoradiotherapy). Critics of a treatment break for response assessment also point to the potential for accelerated tumor clonogen repopulation with prolonging treatment package time, with data demonstrating a trend toward inferior local control with longer treatment package time [124, 125].

In contrast to the RTOG approach, patients treated on phase III trials such as BC2001 and BCON did not receive a mid-treatment break for response assessment and demonstrated comparable outcomes; in these patients, the first opportunity for repeat cystoscopy is often at 3 months post-treatment. In the absence of prospective data directly comparing outcomes for patients receiving mid-treatment cystoscopy and tumor site re-biopsy vs. those receiving continuous concurrent chemoradiotherapy following TURBT, there is no clear answer as to which approach is better. However, on the basis of several existing studies demonstrating excellent outcomes for patients treated without treatment break for response assessment, in addition to ongoing RCTs (e.g., SWOG S1806) enrolling patients treated continuously without a treatment break, it is now considered common practice to forego a mid-treatment response assessment.

Post-Treatment Follow-Up

It is essential that patients treated with SBP return for regular cancer surveillance, which is comprised of a thorough history and physical examination, cystoscopy +/− biopsy of tumor site, and urine cytology. This is completed at regular intervals; based on the National Comprehensive Cancer Network (NCCN) guidelines utilized in the United States, MIBC patients treated with SBP should undergo cystoscopy every 3 months for the first 2 years following completion of definitive intent treatment with the following additional testing to be completed every 3–6 months: CT/MR abdomen/pelvis (A/P), chest imaging (e.g., CT chest), renal function testing, complete blood count, comprehensive metabolic panel, and liver function tests [126]. Every 6–12 months, patients should additionally receive urine cytology [126].

Once the first 2 years have passed, for years 3–4, patients may undergo cystoscopy every 6 months and receive CT/MR A/P and CT chest annually, with laboratory evaluation and urine cytology to be performed only as clinically indicated [126]. At year 5, patients may receive cystoscopy annually and should continue to receive CT/MR A/P and CT chest annually. From 5 to 10 years patients are out from treatment, patients are allowed to receive cystoscopy annually with imaging and blood tests only as clinically indicated, and finally, if >10 years out from treatment, patients may elect to discontinue surveillance if they have remained disease-free in that time [126].

Management of Recurrent Disease

Locoregional Recurrence

Continuous surveillance is important for management of potential locoregional or distant recurrences. Cystoscopy with biopsy of the tumor site allows for detection of a local recurrence within the bladder, which may manifest as a superficial, non-muscle-invasive recurrence (which may then be managed with transurethral resection or intravesical therapy) or a muscle-invasive recurrence that would then require salvage cystectomy with pelvic lymphadenectomy. Regularly spaced, frequent cystoscopy allows for early detection and implementation of salvage treatment. As discussed previously with review of outcomes, patients receiving salvage treatment with RC have the potential to maintain similar survival outcomes if the local recurrence is detected and acted upon early. While most LRRs manifest within the first 2 years following completion of definitive therapy, late can recurrences even up to 5 years following treatment [127].

If patients are suspected to have recurrent disease outside the bladder that has remained contained within the pelvis, in addition to evaluation with CT/MR A/P, they may receive a positron emission tomography (PET)-CT for further assessment, which may help aid in identifying nodal involvement. Unfortunately, given the great likelihood of metastatic disease outside of the pelvis in the event of nodal involvement at the time of relapse, the rate of isolated pelvic relapse is small and estimated to range from 5% to 7% [128]. Management of nodal disease in the setting of a tumor identified within the bladder would be addressed with salvage RC with extended PLND with the option of adjuvant PORT depending on postoperative findings. Isolated nodal relapse is an uncommon scenario: management would begin with multidisciplinary input among clinicians with expertise in management of complex urologic cases. Local therapy options could include surgery (depending on multiple determining factors including size, location, local symptoms, and patient candidacy) or RT. Stereotactic body radiotherapy (SBRT) is a consideration for managing patients with oligometastatic disease, with prescribed doses up to 24–32 Gy administered up to 4–5 fractions depending on the dose constraints of adjacent OARs [129]. Strong consideration would additionally be given to administration of systemic therapy to address sites of subclinical disease not visualized on imaging at the time of diagnosis of recurrence. Patients with pelvic recurrences have a poor prognosis; even with efforts at effective salvage treatment, reported median survival ranges from 4 to 8 months [127].

Distant Recurrence

Management of metastatic disease in MIBC is quite complex; as such, extensive discussions regarding the myriad of systemic therapy options available for management in this scenario comprise a separate chapter. For patients with metastatic disease, goals of care should be identified early, and appropriate palliation should be provided when needed to sites of disease yielding local symptoms (e.g., lungs, bone) to promote improved quality of life. Distant recurrence accounts for 30–40% of relapses – with the most common sites being the lungs, liver, and bone – and carries a very poor prognosis [78, 130].

Node-Positive Disease

SBP for patients with clinically involved nodes at the time of diagnosis is an understudied area of clinical practice with no existing randomized data to guide management, as studies evaluating SBP have largely limited enrollment to patients with clinical N0 disease. While RTOG 8802 included a handful of patients with clinically involved nodes, the small size of the patient population limits meaningful interpretation [31, 87]. An ongoing ECOG/NRG study (NCT04216290, EA8185/INSPIRE) is a phase II trial randomizing patients with stage III urothelial carcinoma (any cT, cN1-2, cM0) status post three cycles or more of NAC to concurrent chemoradiotherapy with or without durvalumab, with the primary endpoint being clinical CR

[131]. Patients noting no clinical benefit at post-treatment re-staging 8 weeks following completion of treatment are planned to receive salvage RC, and planned stratifications include extent of TURBT (presence of residual disease vs. no residual disease), size of lymph nodes (1–2 cm vs. >2 cm), chemotherapy administered (cisplatin vs. non-cisplatin regimen), whether NAC was administered pre- or post-randomization, and response to pre-randomization NAC [131]. Performance of this trial marks an important step toward establishing concurrent chemoradiotherapy as a primary treatment option for management of clinically node positive MIBC, as data from population-based analyses suggest that nearly 80% of patients with node-positive nonmetastatic are managed with chemotherapy alone as opposed to SBP [132].

Quality of Life Considerations

Health-related quality of life (HRQOL) embodies a multitude of domains including physical (incorporating urinary and sexual function), social, emotional, and psychological well-being, with a diagnosis of MIBC in itself having been shown to significantly impact physical and social function based on population-based analyses on registry patients from the Surveillance, Epidemiology, and End Results (SEER) Program [133]. An important consideration for patients electing to undergo SBP is the impact on HRQOL that undergoing RC would impart. In addition to impact on urinary and sexual function, the associated urinary diversion significantly impacts daily life and body image [134]. While often not initially suspected as a HRQOL culprit, sexual dysfunction secondary to RC is one of the most significant detriments to quality of life. Along with physical changes/altered anatomy accounting for organic etiologies underlying sexual dysfunction (e.g., up to 80% of men may develop erectile dysfunction), negative psychosocial influences such as the stigma associated with urinary diversion may strain intimacy and lead to impaired sexual expression or satisfaction [135]. Existing data also suggests that urinary function and bowel habits are consistently compromised in patients undergoing RC with urinary diversion. The first validated bladder cancer-specific instrument studying HRQOL was the Bladder Cancer Index (BCI), developed in 2007; a pilot study ($n = 315$) using the BCI found that patients who had received RC scored lower than patients maintaining their native bladder in both function and bother scores across all domains (sexual, urinary, bowel) [136]. Of great interest with potential surprise, patients who had received an orthotopic neobladder demonstrated significantly lower urinary function scores as compared to patients who had received incontinent diversions [136]. The impact of RC with urinary diversion on HRQOL should be strongly considered when determining a treatment course for patients eligible for SBP which may allow them to circumvent issues related to compromised urinary, bowel, and sexual functioning.

Retrospective data reporting on HRQOL for patients receiving SBP demonstrates better outcomes for patients receiving TMT as compared to RC. A cross-sectional bi-institutional study in the United States analyzing 226 patients with MIBC eligible for RC who were disease-free for 2 years or longer administered six validated HRQOL instruments and found that TMT was associated with better HRQOL by nearly 10 points out of 100 compared to patients receiving RC ($p = 0.001$) with greater physical, social, emotional, and cognitive functioning ($p < 0.04$) [137]. As compared to RC, patients receiving TMT reported better bowel function by 4.5 points ($p = 0.02$), fewer bowel symptoms by 3–7 points ($p < 0.05$), better sexual function by 9–32 points ($p < 0.02$), and better body image by 15 points ($p < 0.001$) [137]. A cross-sectional questionnaire study performed in Sweden comparing treatment-related side effects from pelvic EBRT monotherapy ($n = 58$) to RC ($n = 251$) and population controls ($n = 310$) found that 74% of irradiated patients reported normal urinary function, and there was no statistically significant difference in distress secondary to gastrointestinal symptoms between EBRT monotherapy and RC (32% vs. 24%) [138]. A similarly high rate of preserved urinary function was reported by MGH, with 75% of patients from their retrospective cohort study demonstrating normal bladder function by urodynamic study [139]. With regard to sexual function, data from MGH suggests that the majority of male patients maintained erectile function with only 8% of male patients expressing dissatisfaction, and separate data reporting on female patients has found that over 70% of women receiving SBP maintained pre-treatment levels of sexual satisfaction [139, 140]. Overall, data from a pooled analysis of multiple RTOG studies (RTOG 8903, 9506, 9706, and 9906) has shown a late grade 3 genitourinary toxicity rate of 5.7% and late grade 3 gastrointestinal toxicity rate of 1.9% among patients retaining their native bladder, with no grades 4–5 toxicities, indicating relatively favorable late term toxicity outcomes for those receiving EBRT with concurrent chemotherapy [141].

Radiation Techniques

Simulation

CT simulation is best performed with the patient having been instructed to present to the radiation oncology clinic with an empty bladder and rectum; treating the patient with a maximally empty bladder allows for greater reproducibility by evading the perils of daily inconsistency in bladder filling. Once the patient has completely voided and made efforts to minimize rectal distension, the patient is then simulated in the supine position using a custom-made device such as a Vac-Lok (Civco, Kalona, Iowa, USA) for immobilization of the pelvis. A CT scan typically without contrast is performed from L1 through mid-femur. Depending on institutional practice, considerations may be made for using IV contrast to aid in identification of vasculature (particularly for clinicians who utilize pelvic nodal irradiation); however, it is critical that renal function be assessed prior to administration of IV contrast due to concern for contrast-induced nephropathy in patients with high risk of compromised renal function secondary to their disease. In lieu of contrast administration to aid in visualization at the time of simulation, any diagnostic imaging obtained as part of pre-treatment workup may be coregistered to guide planning. For clinicians planning on administering a bladder tumor boost, certain institutions have utilized liquid, radio-opaque markers such as lipiodol to aid in identification [142]. Based on institutional practice, some clinicians may opt to treat the patient using an adaptive RT technique with a "plan-of-the-day"; such a practice may involve simulating the patient with a maximally empty bladder, a comfortably/reproducibly full bladder, and the bladder in an intermediary state [143]. At the authors' institution, patients are simulated and treated with a maximally empty bladder and rectum for every day of treatment, and neither IV/oral contrast nor fiducial markers are utilized for treatment.

Target Volume

There is great variability in practice across the world with regard to target volume delineation, and the optimal RT target volume in TMT for SBP is considered an area of controversy. This is reflected in the protocol of ongoing phase III RCT SWOG S1806, which allows for patients to be treated with or without nodal irradiation as well as treatment of the whole bladder with or without a tumor boost or omission of a whole bladder field and treatment of the tumor only [123]. The patient's target volumes may then be defined and delineated as follows, as described per protocol of SWOG S1806 [123]:

- Gross tumor volume (GTV): Macroscopic visible tumor on imaging/cystoscopy
- Clinical target volume (CTV): Comprised of multiple entities, as stated below
  - CTV_bladder tumor: Defined by diagnostic imaging/site of TURBT (as per findings documented in operative report as well as multidisciplinary discussion with urologic surgeon at time of treatment planning)
  - CTV_prostate: Target volume encompassing prostate and prostatic urethra in male patients
  - CTV_whole bladder: Target volume encompassing the entire bladder, including the CTV_bladder tumor
  - CTV_nodal: Target volume encompassing the pelvic nodes below the common iliac bifurcation, including the presacral nodes, external iliac nodes, internal iliac nodes, and obturator nodes. These nodal regions are anatomically defined as follows:
    - Pre-sacral nodes: This lymphatic area extends from the superior aspect of S1 to the superior aspect of S3 and includes the 1 cm thickness anterior to the sacrum

- External iliac nodes: This lymph node group is contoured inferiorly up to the superior aspect of the femoral heads and is delineated by creating a 7 mm circumferential expansion around the external iliac vessels.
- Internal iliac nodes: This lymph node group is contoured inferiorly until no longer visualized or until exiting the pelvis via the greater sciatic notch and is delineated by creating a 7 mm circumferential expansion around the internal iliac vessels.
- Obturator nodes: This lymphatic area is contoured superiorly where the iliac vessel contours stop and extends inferiorly to the superior aspect of the symphysis pubis; it encompasses the 1 cm width of tissue situated medially to the obturator internus muscles from the anterior to posterior borders of the ilium.
- All nodal target volumes must be trimmed so that they do not extend outside the pelvis or into adjacent OARs such as the rectum, bowel, or bone.

- Planning target volume (PTV): Comprised of symmetric expansions of CTV to account for inter-fraction variability from internal organ motion or daily set-up. The following are recent trial-utilized values; optimal PTV expansions could be determined based on institutional preferences or analyses determining set-up/positional error.
  - PTV_bladder tumor: 5 mm to 1 cm expansion if using IMRT; 1.0–1.5 cm expansion if using 3DCRT with margin to be determined based on image-guided radiotherapy (IGRT) options available at treating institution.
  - PTV_whole bladder: 5 mm to 1 cm expansion if using IMRT; 1.0–1.5 cm expansion if using 3DCRT (except in the region of the bladder tumor, with margin of 2 cm permissible) with margin to be determined based on image-guided radiotherapy (IGRT) options available at treating institution.
  - PTV_prostate: 5 mm expansion of CTV_prostate for male patients.
  - PTV_nodal: 5 mm expansion of CTV_nodal.
  - Anisotropic expansions may be utilized to achieve dose constraints to adjacent OARs.

A treatment plan for a patient treated with 41.4 Gy to the pelvis and nodes followed by a sequential bladder boost to 64.8 Gy is portrayed in Fig. 18.3. Acceptable planning metrics ideally yield coverage $V100 \geq 95\%$ with a hotspot no greater than 110%. The OARs to delineate include the bilateral femoral heads, rectum, and small bowel, with corresponding dose constraints to be listed in the following section on dosing.

There is no clear consensus regarding treatment of pelvic nodal regions, other than that pelvic nodal irradiation can be administered using conventional fractionation, whereas hypofractionated treatments typically target the whole (or partial) bladder only. Randomized data from a trial performed in Pakistan comparing patients receiving RT to the whole pelvis ($n = 120$) to those receiving treatment to bladder only ($n = 110$) found, at 5-year median follow-up, no significant difference in DFS (47.1% vs. 46.9%, $p = 0.5$), bladder preservation rate (58.9% vs. 57.1%, $p = 0.8$), or OS (52.9% vs. 51%, $p = 0.8$) [144].

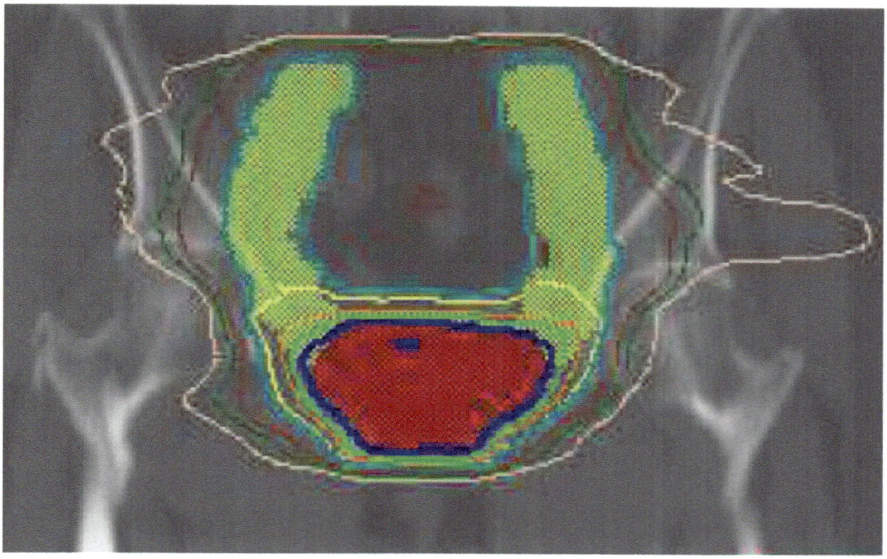

Fig. 18.3 A treatment plan for a patient treated with definitive concurrent chemoradiotherapy using IMRT for muscle-invasive bladder cancer. A prescription of 41.4 Gy was used for PTV_pelvis and nodes (lime green volume encompassed by teal isodose line) and was followed by a sequential boost of 23.4 Gy to the PTV_bladder for a cumulative dose of 64.8 Gy (red volume encompassed by dark blue isodose line). The low dose spread from IMRT is additionally depicted (pearl, 20.0 Gy; dark green, 25.0 Gy; brown, 30.0 Gy; teal, 41.4 Gy; yellow, 45.0 Gy; orange, 54.0 Gy; green, 60.0 Gy)

Therefore, the following are all accepted treatment volumes for irradiating MIBC:

- Whole pelvis irradiation encompassing bladder and lymph nodes (e.g., to 41.4 Gy), followed by cone down to whole bladder (e.g., to 55.8 Gy), followed by boost to tumor site (e.g., to 64.8 Gy)
- Whole pelvis irradiation encompassing bladder and lymph nodes (e.g., to 41.4 Gy), followed by cone down to whole bladder (e.g., to 64.8 Gy)
- Treatment of either whole bladder or tumor site only, with or without a boost
  - This is the most common method of treatment delivery in Europe, where the PTV often incorporates the CTV with a 1.5 cm expansion. In BC2001, the PTV1 consisted of the outer bladder wall with a 1.5 cm expansion, and the PTV2 consisted of the tumor site with a 1.5 cm expansion [61].

Dose

Multiple dosing schemes have been utilized in TMT for SBP. Conventionally fractionated RT is administered in 1.8–2.0 Gy per fraction once daily. Daily, conventionally fractionated RT delivers a cumulative dose of 64–64.8 Gy to either (1) the whole bladder or (2) the tumor site only (with a margin), depending on planned treatment delivery method. For patients who are receiving pelvic nodal irradiation, dose delivered to this area typically ranges from 41.4 to 50.4 Gy when administering treatment at 1.8 Gy per fraction or 40 to 50 Gy when treating with 2 Gy daily fractions. If utilizing an accelerated fractionation approach, such as in the RTOG trials (e.g., RTOG 0712), treatment may be administered in 1.5 Gy fractions twice daily (separated by at least 6 hours) [75]. For patients receiving hypofractionated RT, treatment is administered at 2.75 Gy per fraction to a cumulative dose of 55 Gy to either (1) the whole bladder or (2) the tumor site with a margin (partial bladder).

Dose Constraints (Conventional Fractionation) [75, 123]

Rectum: $V30 \leq 50\%$, $V55 \leq 10\%$
Femoral heads: Max 45 Gy
Small bowel: $V50 \leq 15$ cc, $V45 \leq 100$ cc, $V30 \leq 150$ cc

Fields

While 3DCRT has historically been utilized for management of MIBC, with wide margins (1.5 cm as per BC2001 or 2 cm as per RTOG approach) to account for organ motion and variations in set-up prior to advances in IGRT, IMRT is being increasingly utilized with the aid of cone beam CT (CBCT) for daily image guidance. IMRT carries multiple benefits, including the potential for use of simultaneous integrated boost (SIB) technique to the primary tumor site and shorter treatment delivery times with the ability to minimize dose to adjacent OARs by optimizing beam angles/dose entry, thereby providing more conformal treatment [145]. However, 3DCRT still remains frequently utilized. For patients receiving treatment with 3DCRT incorporating pelvic nodal irradiation, treatment has historically encompassed a "small pelvis" that may be treated using a four-field technique (AP/PA and opposed laterals) with the following field borders [75]:

- Superior border: Mid-sacroiliac joint
- Inferior border: Bottom of the obturator foramen
- Lateral borders: 1.5 cm margin on the pelvic brim for AP/PA fields or 2 cm beyond the CTV for the lateral fields

In designing the AP/PA fields, care must be taken to block the femoral heads. In designing the lateral fields, the rectum and small bowel should be blocked.

RTOG Approach

To summarize an example of radiotherapeutic management, the RTOG approach will be utilized as an example. Following a diagnosis of MIBC with decision to pursue SBT with TMT, a patient receives maximal TURBT and is then initiated on induction treatment of concurrent chemoradiotherapy to a dose of 40–45 Gy administered over 20–25 fractions. In the first phase of RT, the whole bladder is treated with a 2 cm margin, and the initial treatment volume incorporates the prostatic urethra in men (or the proximal 2 cm of the urethra in women) as well as the pelvic lymphatics (which may be treated using the previously described "small pelvis" technique if using 3DCRT). Following induction therapy, a repeat cystoscopy with biopsy of the primary tumor site is performed after a 2–3-week treatment break. Patients with residual disease noted on pathology are then referred for RC, whereas patients with CR (or good response with only superficial disease remaining) then proceed with the consolidation phase of treatment. In the consolidation phase of treatment, patients receive the remainder of the prescription dose, which is administered as a cone treatment down to the whole bladder (an additional 10–14 Gy) followed by a final boost to the tumor alone with a 2 cm margin (an additional 10 Gy).

Summary of Treatment Recommendations

For patients considered eligible for SBP who are receiving TMT, we recommend maximal TURBT with adjuvant concurrent chemoradiotherapy. Patients are considered optimal candidates if they present with cT2-T3aN0M0 disease with unifocal disease and without CIS or tumor-associated hydronephrosis, although consideration for bladder sparing is on a case-by-case basis. Options for concurrent systemic therapy include cisplatin monotherapy, gemcitabine monotherapy, 5-FU/mitomycin-C, or a cisplatin-based regimen with 5-FU or paclitaxel. RT regimens vary based on institutional practice but include conventionally fractionated RT of 64.8 Gy in 36 fractions to the bladder +/− pelvic nodes or hypofractionated RT of 55 Gy in 20 fractions to the whole bladder only. It is the authors' practice to perform conventionally fractionated radiotherapy, delivering 41.4 Gy in 23 fractions to the PTV encompassing the whole bladder and pelvic nodes followed by a 23.4 Gy in 13 fraction boost to the whole bladder PTV for a cumulative dose of 64.8 Gy given over 36 fractions. Consideration may additionally be given to concurrent and adjuvant immunotherapy with patient enrollment on a clinical trial.

Conclusion

SBP is an emerging treatment paradigm for definitive management of MIBC with great promise. The most effective regimen investigated to date incorporates TMT with maximal TURBT followed by RT administered with concurrent radiosensitizing chemotherapy. While currently limited to patients deemed eligible for candidacy based on strict selection criteria, future treatment directions include broadening eligibility and assessing outcomes for patients with MIBC who do not necessarily meet these criteria. Studies on HRQOL suggest comparatively higher quality of life associated with bladder sparing versus RC; while there are no prospective, randomized data to directly compare these two treatments, a steadily increasing body of literature suggests no significant difference in oncologic outcomes, which makes bladder sparing treatment very compelling. In addition to continued assessment of systemic therapy options, ICI is additionally under investigation with ongoing RCTs, and recently designed RCTs are now incorporating molecular subtyping with the ultimate goal of having these be prospectively validated. The results of ongoing RCTs prospectively investigating conventional fractionation vs. hypofractionation and pelvic nodal irradiation vs. treatment of bladder only are eagerly awaited. Further study will additionally be needed to elucidate a better understanding of optimal management for patients with node-positive disease as we approach an era of improved systemic therapy now incorporating ICI.

References

1. Saginala K, Barsouk A, Aluru JS, Rawla P, Padala SA, Barsouk A. Epidemiology of bladder cancer. Med Sci (Basel, Switzerland). 2020;8(1):15. https://doi.org/10.3390/medsci8010015.
2. Magers MJ, Lopez-Beltran A, Montironi R, Williamson SR, Kaimakliotis HZ, Cheng L. Staging of bladder cancer. Histopathology. 2019;74(1):112–34. https://doi.org/10.1111/his.13734.
3. Bray F, Ferlay J, Soerjomataram I, Siegel RL, Torre LA, Jemal A. Global cancer statistics 2018: GLOBOCAN estimates of incidence and mortality worldwide for 36 cancers in 185 countries. CA Cancer J Clin. 2018;68(6):394–424. https://doi.org/10.3322/caac.21492.
4. Mostafa MH, Sheweita SA, O'Connor PJ. Relationship between schistosomiasis and bladder cancer. Clin Microbiol Rev. 1999;12(1):97–111.
5. Zhu C-Z, Ting H-N, Ng K-H, Ong T-A. A review on the accuracy of bladder cancer detection methods. J Cancer. 2019;10(17):4038–44. https://doi.org/10.7150/jca.28989.
6. Galgano SJ, Porter KK, Burgan C, Rais-Bahrami S. The role of imaging in bladder cancer diagnosis and staging. Diagnostics (Basel, Switzerland). 2020;10(9). https://doi.org/10.3390/diagnostics10090703.
7. Stein JP, Lieskovsky G, Cote R, et al. Radical cystectomy in the treatment of invasive bladder cancer: long-term results in 1,054 patients. J Clin Oncol Off J Am Soc Clin Oncol. 2001;19(3):666–75. https://doi.org/10.1200/JCO.2001.19.3.666.
8. Muilwijk T, Akand M, Gevaert T, Joniau S. No survival difference between super extended and standard lymph node dissection at radical cystectomy: what can we learn from the first prospective randomized phase III trial? Transl Androl Urol. 2019;8(Suppl 1):S112–5. https://doi.org/10.21037/tau.2018.12.09.
9. Gschwend JE, Heck MM, Lehmann J, et al. Extended versus limited lymph node dissection in bladder cancer patients undergoing radical cystectomy: survival results from a prospective, randomized trial. Eur Urol. 2019;75(4):604–11. https://doi.org/10.1016/j.eururo.2018.09.047.
10. Siddiqui KM, Izawa JI. Ileal conduit: standard urinary diversion for elderly patients undergoing radical cystectomy. World J Urol. 2016;34(1):19–24. https://doi.org/10.1007/s00345-015-1706-1.
11. Monn MF, Kaimakliotis HZ, Cary KC, et al. Short-term morbidity and mortality of Indiana pouch, ileal conduit, and neobladder urinary diversion following radical cystectomy. Urol Oncol. 2014;32(8):1151–7. https://doi.org/10.1016/j.urolonc.2014.04.009.
12. Lukka H. In favour of bladder preservation using combined modality treatment. Can Urol Assoc J = J l'Association des Urol du Canada. 2009;3(5):412–5. https://doi.org/10.5489/cuaj.1157.

13. Dalbagni G, Genega E, Hashibe M, et al. Cystectomy for bladder cancer: a contemporary series. J Urol. 2001;165(4):1111–6.
14. Grossman HB, Natale RB, Tangen CM, et al. Neoadjuvant chemotherapy plus cystectomy compared with cystectomy alone for locally advanced bladder cancer. N Engl J Med. 2003;349(9):859–66. https://doi.org/10.1056/NEJMoa022148.
15. Neoadjuvant chemotherapy in invasive bladder cancer: update of a systematic review and meta-analysis of individual patient data advanced bladder cancer (ABC) meta-analysis collaboration. Eur Urol. 2005;48(2):202–6. https://doi.org/10.1016/j.eururo.2005.04.006.
16. Eisenberg MS, Thompson RH, Frank I, et al. Long-term renal function outcomes after radical cystectomy. J Urol. 2014;191(3):619–25. https://doi.org/10.1016/j.juro.2013.09.011.
17. Zaghloul MS, Awwad HK, Akoush HH, Omar S, Soliman O, el Attar I. Postoperative radiotherapy of carcinoma in bilharzial bladder: improved disease free survival through improving local control. Int J Radiat Oncol Biol Phys. 1992;23(3):511–7. https://doi.org/10.1016/0360-3016(92)90005-3.
18. Zaghloul MS, Christodouleas JP, Smith A, et al. Adjuvant sandwich chemotherapy plus radiotherapy vs adjuvant chemotherapy alone for locally advanced bladder cancer after radical cystectomy: a randomized phase 2 trial. JAMA Surg. 2018;153(1):e174591. https://doi.org/10.1001/jamasurg.2017.4591.
19. Christodouleas JP, Hwang W-T, Baumann BC. Adjuvant radiation for locally advanced bladder cancer? A question worth asking. Int J Radiat Oncol Biol Phys. 2016;94(5):1040–2. https://doi.org/10.1016/j.ijrobp.2016.01.015.
20. Baumann BC, Bosch WR, Bahl A, et al. Development and validation of consensus contouring guidelines for adjuvant radiation therapy for bladder cancer after radical cystectomy. Int J Radiat Oncol Biol Phys. 2016;96(1):78–86. https://doi.org/10.1016/j.ijrobp.2016.04.032.
21. Solanki AA, Martin B, Korpics M, Small C, Harkenrider MM, Mitin T. Adjuvant radiotherapy use by US radiation oncologists after radical cystectomy for muscle-invasive bladder cancer. Clin Oncol (R Coll Radiol). 2017;29(7):429–35. https://doi.org/10.1016/j.clon.2017.02.005.
22. Fischer-Valuck BW, Michalski JM, Mitra N, et al. Effectiveness of postoperative radiotherapy after radical cystectomy for locally advanced bladder cancer. Cancer Med. 2019;8(8):3698–709. https://doi.org/10.1002/cam4.2102.
23. Soulié M, Straub M, Gamé X, et al. A multicenter study of the morbidity of radical cystectomy in select elderly patients with bladder cancer. J Urol. 2002;167(3):1325–8.
24. Stimson CJ, Chang SS, Barocas DA, et al. Early and late perioperative outcomes following radical cystectomy: 90-day readmissions, morbidity and mortality in a contemporary series. J Urol. 2010;184(4):1296–300. https://doi.org/10.1016/j.juro.2010.06.007.
25. Novotny V, Hakenberg OW, Wiessner D, et al. Perioperative complications of radical cystectomy in a contemporary series. Eur Urol. 2007;51(2):392–7. https://doi.org/10.1016/j.eururo.2006.06.014.
26. Donat SM, Shabsigh A, Savage C, et al. Potential impact of postoperative early complications on the timing of adjuvant chemotherapy in patients undergoing radical cystectomy: a high-volume tertiary cancer center experience. Eur Urol. 2009;55(1):177–85. https://doi.org/10.1016/j.eururo.2008.07.018.
27. Novara G, Catto JWF, Wilson T, et al. Systematic review and cumulative analysis of perioperative outcomes and complications after robot-assisted radical cystectomy. Eur Urol. 2015;67(3):376–401. https://doi.org/10.1016/j.eururo.2014.12.007.
28. Reisinger SA, Mohiuddin M, Mulholland SG. Combined pre- and postoperative adjuvant radiation therapy for bladder cancer--a ten year experience. Int J Radiat Oncol Biol Phys. 1992;24(3):463–8. https://doi.org/10.1016/0360-3016(92)91060-z.
29. Santos F, Zakaria AS, Kassouf W, Tanguay S, Aprikian A. High hospital and surgeon volume and its impact on overall survival after radical cystectomy among patients with bladder cancer in Quebec. World J Urol. 2015;33(9):1323–30. https://doi.org/10.1007/s00345-014-1457-4.
30. Bajaj A, Martin B, Bhasin R, et al. The impact of academic facility type and case volume on survival in patients undergoing curative radiation therapy for muscle-invasive blad-

der cancer. Int J Radiat Oncol Biol Phys. 2018;100(4):851–7. https://doi.org/10.1016/j.ijrobp.2017.11.040.
31. Mirza A, Choudhury A. Bladder preservation for muscle invasive bladder cancer. Bladder cancer (Amsterdam, Netherlands). 2016;2(2):151–63. https://doi.org/10.3233/BLC-150025.
32. Hamad J, McCloskey H, Milowsky MI, Royce T, Smith A. Bladder preservation in muscle-invasive bladder cancer: a comprehensive review. Int Braz J Urol. 2020;46(2):169–84. https://doi.org/10.1590/S1677-5538.IBJU.2020.99.01.
33. Winquist E, Booth CM. Trimodality therapy for muscle-invasive bladder cancer: concurrent chemotherapy is not enough. J Clin Oncol. 2020;38(24):2709–11. https://doi.org/10.1200/JCO.19.02959.
34. Ritch CR, Balise R, Prakash NS, et al. Propensity matched comparative analysis of survival following chemoradiation or radical cystectomy for muscle-invasive bladder cancer. BJU Int. 2018;121(5):745–51. https://doi.org/10.1111/bju.14109.
35. Hollenbeck BK, Miller DC, Dunn RL, Montie JE, Wei JT. The effects of stage divergence on survival after radical cystectomy for urothelial cancer. Urol Oncol. 2005;23(2):77–81. https://doi.org/10.1016/j.urolonc.2004.08.012.
36. van Dijk PR, Ploeg M, Aben KKH, et al. Downstaging of TURBT-based muscle-invasive bladder cancer by radical cystectomy predicts better survival. ISRN Urol. 2011;2011:458930. https://doi.org/10.5402/2011/458930.
37. Marchioni M, Primiceri G, Delli Pizzi A, et al. Could bladder multiparametric MRI be introduced in routine clinical practice? Role of the new VI-RADS score: results from a prospective study. Clin Genitourin Cancer. 2020;18(5):409–415.e1. https://doi.org/10.1016/j.clgc.2020.03.002.
38. James ND, Pirrie S, Liu W, et al. Replacing TURBT with mpMRI for staging MIBC: pilot data from the BladderPath study. J Clin Oncol. 2020;38(6_suppl):446. https://doi.org/10.1200/JCO.2020.38.6_suppl.446.
39. Kulkarni GS, Hermanns T, Wei Y, et al. Propensity score analysis of radical cystectomy versus bladder-sparing trimodal therapy in the setting of a multidisciplinary bladder cancer clinic. J Clin Oncol Off J Am Soc Clin Oncol. 2017;35(20):2299–305. https://doi.org/10.1200/JCO.2016.69.2327.
40. Zhong J, Switchenko J, Jegadeesh NK, et al. Comparison of outcomes in patients with muscle-invasive bladder cancer treated with radical cystectomy versus bladder preservation. Am J Clin Oncol. 2019;42(1):36–41. https://doi.org/10.1097/COC.0000000000000471.
41. Vashistha V, Wang H, Mazzone A, et al. Radical cystectomy compared to combined modality treatment for muscle-invasive bladder cancer: a systematic review and meta-analysis. Int J Radiat Oncol Biol Phys. 2017;97(5):1002–20. https://doi.org/10.1016/j.ijrobp.2016.11.056.
42. Huddart RA, Birtle A, Maynard L, et al. Clinical and patient-reported outcomes of SPARE - a randomised feasibility study of selective bladder preservation versus radical cystectomy. BJU Int. 2017;120(5):639–50. https://doi.org/10.1111/bju.13900.
43. Herr HW. Conservative management of muscle-infiltrating bladder cancer: prospective experience. J Urol. 1987;138(5):1162–3. https://doi.org/10.1016/S0022-5347(17)43535-X.
44. Henry K, Miller J, Mori M, Loening S, Fallon B. Comparison of transurethral resection to radical therapies for stage B bladder tumors. J Urol. 1988;140(5):964–7. https://doi.org/10.1016/s0022-5347(17)41899-4.
45. Herr HW. Transurethral resection of muscle-invasive bladder cancer: 10-year outcome. J Clin Oncol. 2001;19(1):89–93. https://doi.org/10.1200/JCO.2001.19.1.89.
46. Barnes RW, Dick AL, Hadley HL, Johnston OL. Survival following transurethral resection of bladder carcinoma. Cancer Res. 1977;37(8 Pt 2):2895–7.
47. Milner WA. The role of conservative surgery in the treatment of bladder tumours. Br J Urol. 1954;26(4):375–86. https://doi.org/10.1111/j.1464-410x.1954.tb04920.x.
48. Nerli RB, Reddy M, Koura AC, Prabha V, Ravish IR, Amarkhed S. Cystoscopy-assisted laparoscopic partial cystectomy. J Endourol. 2008;22(1):83–6. https://doi.org/10.1089/end.2007.0105.

49. Park JC, Citrin DE, Agarwal PK, Apolo AB. Multimodal management of muscle-invasive bladder cancer. Curr Probl Cancer. 2014;38(3):80–108. https://doi.org/10.1016/j.currproblcancer.2014.06.001.
50. Ma B, Li H, Zhang C, et al. Lymphovascular invasion, ureteral reimplantation and prior history of urothelial carcinoma are associated with poor prognosis after partial cystectomy for muscle-invasive bladder cancer with negative pelvic lymph nodes. Eur J Surg Oncol J Eur Soc Surg Oncol Br Assoc Surg Oncol. 2013;39(10):1150–6. https://doi.org/10.1016/j.ejso.2013.04.006.
51. Kassouf W, Swanson D, Kamat AM, et al. Partial cystectomy for muscle invasive urothelial carcinoma of the bladder: a contemporary review of the M. D. Anderson Cancer Center experience. J Urol. 2006;175(6):2058–62. https://doi.org/10.1016/S0022-5347(06)00322-3.
52. Holzbeierlein JM, Lopez-Corona E, Bochner BH, et al. Partial cystectomy: a contemporary review of the Memorial Sloan-Kettering Cancer Center experience and recommendations for patient selection. J Urol. 2004;172(3):878–81. https://doi.org/10.1097/01.ju.0000135530.59860.7d.
53. Smaldone MC, Jacobs BL, Smaldone AM, Hrebinko RLJ. Long-term results of selective partial cystectomy for invasive urothelial bladder carcinoma. Urology. 2008;72(3):613–6. https://doi.org/10.1016/j.urology.2008.04.052.
54. Mistretta FA, Cyr S-J, Luzzago S, et al. Partial cystectomy with pelvic lymph node dissection for patients with nonmetastatic stage pT2-T3 urothelial carcinoma of urinary bladder: temporal trends and survival outcomes. Clin Genitourin Cancer. 2020;18(2):129–137.e3. https://doi.org/10.1016/j.clgc.2019.09.008.
55. Fahmy N, Aprikian A, Tanguay S, et al. Practice patterns and recurrence after partial cystectomy for bladder cancer. World J Urol. 2010;28(4):419–23. https://doi.org/10.1007/s00345-009-0478-x.
56. Duncan W, Quilty PM. The results of a series of 963 patients with transitional cell carcinoma of the urinary bladder primarily treated by radical megavoltage X-ray therapy. Radiother Oncol J Eur Soc Ther Radiol Oncol. 1986;7(4):299–310. https://doi.org/10.1016/s0167-8140(86)80059-7.
57. Quilty PM, Duncan W. The influence of hemoglobin level on the regression and long term local control of transitional cell carcinoma of the bladder following photon irradiation. Int J Radiat Oncol Biol Phys. 1986;12(10):1735–42. https://doi.org/10.1016/0360-3016(86)90313-5.
58. Davidson SE, Symonds RP, Snee MP, Upadhyay S, Habeshaw T, Robertson AG. Assessment of factors influencing the outcome of radiotherapy for bladder cancer. Br J Urol. 1990;66(3):288–93. https://doi.org/10.1111/j.1464-410x.1990.tb14929.x.
59. Pollack A, Zagars GK, Swanson DA. Muscle-invasive bladder cancer treated with external beam radiotherapy: prognostic factors. Int J Radiat Oncol Biol Phys. 1994;30(2):267–77. https://doi.org/10.1016/0360-3016(94)90004-3.
60. Sauer R, Birkenhake S, Kühn R, Wittekind C, Schrott KM, Martus P. Efficacy of radiochemotherapy with platin derivatives compared to radiotherapy alone in organ-sparing treatment of bladder cancer. Int J Radiat Oncol Biol Phys. 1998;40(1):121–7. https://doi.org/10.1016/s0360-3016(97)00579-8.
61. James ND, Hussain SA, Hall E, et al. Radiotherapy with or without chemotherapy in muscle-invasive bladder cancer. N Engl J Med. 2012;366(16):1477–88. https://doi.org/10.1056/NEJMoa1106106.
62. Barringer BS. Radium treatment of cancer of the bladder. Ann Surg. 1935;101(6):1425–8. https://doi.org/10.1097/00000658-193506000-00015.
63. Barringer BS. Twenty-five years of radon treatment of cancer of the bladder. JAMA. 1947;135(10):616–8.
64. Lenz M, Cahill GF. The treatment of cancer of the bladder by radium needles. Am J Roentgenol Radium Ther. 1947;58(4):486–92.
65. Wijnmaalen A, Helle PA, Koper PC, et al. Muscle invasive bladder cancer treated by transurethral resection, followed by external beam radiation and interstitial iridium-192. Int J Radiat Oncol Biol Phys. 1997;39(5):1043–52. https://doi.org/10.1016/s0360-3016(97)00375-1.

66. Rozan R, Albuisson E, Donnarieix D, et al. Interstitial iridium-192 for bladder cancer (A multicentric survey: 205 patients). Int J Radiat Oncol. 1992;24(3):469–77. https://doi.org/10.1016/0360-3016(92)91061-Q.
67. Pernot M, Hubert J, Guillemin F, et al. Combined surgery and brachytherapy in the treatment of some cancers of the bladder (partial cystectomy and interstitial iridium-192). Radiother Oncol J Eur Soc Ther Radiol Oncol. 1996;38(2):115–20. https://doi.org/10.1016/0167-8140(96)82354-1.
68. Bos MK, Marmolejo RO, Rasch CRN, Pieters BR. Bladder preservation with brachytherapy compared to cystectomy for T1-T3 muscle-invasive bladder cancer: a systematic review. J Contemp Brachytherapy. 2014;6(2):191–9. https://doi.org/10.5114/jcb.2014.43777.
69. Sternberg CN, Pansadoro V, Calabrò F, et al. Can patient selection for bladder preservation be based on response to chemotherapy? Cancer. 2003;97(7):1644–52. https://doi.org/10.1002/cncr.11232.
70. Herr HW, Scher HI. Neoadjuvant chemotherapy and partial cystectomy for invasive bladder cancer. J Clin Oncol Off J Am Soc Clin Oncol. 1994;12(5):975–80. https://doi.org/10.1200/JCO.1994.12.5.975.
71. Bazzi WM, Kopp RP, Donahue TF, et al. Partial cystectomy after neoadjuvant chemotherapy: Memorial Sloan Kettering Cancer Center contemporary experience. Int Sch Res Not. 2014;2014:702653. https://doi.org/10.1155/2014/702653.
72. Thomas R, Hall R. Radical transurethral resection and chemotherapy in. BJU Int. 1999;83(4):432–7. https://doi.org/10.1046/j.1464-410x.1999.00970.x.
73. Solsona E, Climent MA, Iborra I, et al. Bladder preservation in selected patients with muscle-invasive bladder cancer by complete transurethral resection of the bladder plus systemic chemotherapy: long-term follow-up of a phase 2 nonrandomized comparative trial with radical cystectomy. Eur Urol. 2009;55(4):911–9. https://doi.org/10.1016/j.eururo.2008.08.027.
74. Mitin T, Hunt D, Shipley WU, et al. Transurethral surgery and twice-daily radiation plus paclitaxel-cisplatin or fluorouracil-cisplatin with selective bladder preservation and adjuvant chemotherapy for patients with muscle invasive bladder cancer (RTOG 0233): a randomised multicentre phase. Lancet Oncol. 2013;14(9):863–72. https://doi.org/10.1016/S1470-2045(13)70255-9.
75. Coen JJ, Zhang P, Saylor PJ, et al. Bladder preservation with twice-a-day radiation plus fluorouracil/cisplatin or once daily radiation plus gemcitabine for muscle-invasive bladder cancer: NRG/RTOG 0712-a randomized phase II trial. J Clin Oncol Off J Am Soc Clin Oncol. 2019;37(1):44–51. https://doi.org/10.1200/JCO.18.00537.
76. Rödel C, Grabenbauer GG, Kühn R, et al. Combined-modality treatment and selective organ preservation in invasive bladder cancer: long-term results. J Clin Oncol Off J Am Soc Clin Oncol. 2002;20(14):3061–71. https://doi.org/10.1200/JCO.2002.11.027.
77. Perdonà S, Autorino R, Damiano R, et al. Bladder-sparing, combined-modality approach for muscle-invasive bladder cancer: a multi-institutional, long-term experience. Cancer. 2008;112(1):75–83. https://doi.org/10.1002/cncr.23137.
78. Efstathiou JA, Spiegel DY, Shipley WU, et al. Long-term outcomes of selective bladder preservation by combined-modality therapy for invasive bladder cancer: the MGH experience. Eur Urol. 2012;61(4):705–11. https://doi.org/10.1016/j.eururo.2011.11.010.
79. Fung CY, Shipley WU, Young RH, et al. Prognostic factors in invasive bladder carcinoma in a prospective trial of preoperative adjuvant chemotherapy and radiotherapy. J Clin Oncol Off J Am Soc Clin Oncol. 1991;9(9):1533–42. https://doi.org/10.1200/JCO.1991.9.9.1533.
80. Shipley WU, Winter KA, Kaufman DS, et al. Phase III trial of neoadjuvant chemotherapy in patients with invasive bladder cancer treated with selective bladder preservation by combined radiation therapy and chemotherapy: initial results of Radiation Therapy Oncology Group 89-03. J Clin Oncol Off J Am Soc Clin Oncol. 1998;16(11):3576–83. https://doi.org/10.1200/JCO.1998.16.11.3576.
81. Krasnow RE, Drumm M, Roberts HJ, et al. Clinical outcomes of patients with histologic variants of urothelial cancer treated with trimodality bladder-sparing therapy. Eur Urol. 2017;72(1):54–60. https://doi.org/10.1016/j.eururo.2016.12.002.

82. Housset M, Maulard C, Chretien Y, et al. Combined radiation and chemotherapy for invasive transitional-cell carcinoma of the bladder: a prospective study. J Clin Oncol Off J Am Soc Clin Oncol. 1993;11(11):2150–7. https://doi.org/10.1200/JCO.1993.11.11.2150.
83. Sauer R, Dunst J, Altendorf-Hofmann A, Fischer H, Bornhof C, Schrott KM. Radiotherapy with and without cisplatin in bladder cancer. Int J Radiat Oncol Biol Phys. 1990;19(3):687–91. https://doi.org/10.1016/0360-3016(90)90497-8.
84. Shipley WU, Prout GRJ, Einstein AB, et al. Treatment of invasive bladder cancer by cisplatin and radiation in patients unsuited for surgery. JAMA. 1987;258(7):931–5.
85. Kaufman DS, Shipley WU, Griffin PP, Heney NM, Althausen AF, Efird JT. Selective bladder preservation by combination treatment of invasive bladder cancer. N Engl J Med. 1993;329(19):1377–82. https://doi.org/10.1056/NEJM199311043291903.
86. Tester W, Porter A, Asbell S, et al. Combined modality program with possible organ preservation for invasive bladder carcinoma: results of RTOG protocol 85-12. Int J Radiat Oncol Biol Phys. 1993;25(5):783–90. https://doi.org/10.1016/0360-3016(93)90306-g.
87. Tester W, Caplan R, Heaney J, et al. Neoadjuvant combined modality program with selective organ preservation for invasive bladder cancer: results of Radiation Therapy Oncology Group phase II trial 8802. J Clin Oncol Off J Am Soc Clin Oncol. 1996;14(1):119–26. https://doi.org/10.1200/JCO.1996.14.1.119.
88. Kaufman DS, Winter KA, Shipley WU, et al. The initial results in muscle-invading bladder cancer of RTOG 95-06: phase I/II trial of transurethral surgery plus radiation therapy with concurrent cisplatin and 5-fluorouracil followed by selective bladder preservation or cystectomy depending on the initial response. Oncologist. 2000;5(6):471–6. https://doi.org/10.1634/theoncologist.5-6-471.
89. Hagan MP, Winter KA, Kaufman DS, et al. RTOG 97-06: initial report of a phase I-II trial of selective bladder conservation using TURBT, twice-daily accelerated irradiation sensitized with cisplatin, and adjuvant MCV combination chemotherapy. Int J Radiat Oncol Biol Phys. 2003;57(3):665–72. https://doi.org/10.1016/s0360-3016(03)00718-1.
90. Kaufman DS, Winter KA, Shipley WU, et al. Phase I-II RTOG study (99-06) of patients with muscle-invasive bladder cancer undergoing transurethral surgery, paclitaxel, cisplatin, and twice-daily radiotherapy followed by selective bladder preservation or radical cystectomy and adjuvant chemotherapy. Urology. 2009;73(4):833–7. https://doi.org/10.1016/j.urology.2008.09.036.
91. Mak RH, Hunt D, Shipley WU, et al. Long-term outcomes in patients with muscle-invasive bladder cancer after selective bladder-preserving combined-modality therapy: a pooled analysis of Radiation Therapy Oncology Group protocols 8802, 8903, 9506, 9706, 9906, and 0233. J Clin Oncol Off J Am Soc Clin Oncol. 2014;32(34):3801–9. https://doi.org/10.1200/JCO.2014.57.5548.
92. Oh KS, Soto DE, Smith DC, Montie JE, Lee CT, Sandler HM. Combined-modality therapy with gemcitabine and radiation therapy as a bladder preservation strategy: long-term results of a phase I trial. Int J Radiat Oncol Biol Phys. 2009;74(2):511–7. https://doi.org/10.1016/j.ijrobp.2008.08.021.
93. Hall E, Hussain SA, Porta N, et al. BC2001 long-term outcomes: a phase III randomized trial of chemoradiotherapy versus radiotherapy (RT) alone and standard RT versus reduced high-dose volume RT in muscle-invasive bladder cancer. J Clin Oncol. 2017;35(6_suppl):280. https://doi.org/10.1200/JCO.2017.35.6_suppl.280.
94. Malmström PU, Rintala E, Wahlqvist R, Hellström P, Hellsten S, Hannisdal E. Five-year followup of a prospective trial of radical cystectomy and neoadjuvant chemotherapy: Nordic Cystectomy Trial I. The Nordic Cooperative Bladder Cancer Study Group. J Urol. 1996;155(6):1903–6.
95. Martinez-Piñeiro JA, Gonzalez Martin M, Arocena F, et al. Neoadjuvant cisplatin chemotherapy before radical cystectomy in invasive transitional cell carcinoma of the bladder: a prospective randomized phase III study. J Urol. 1995;153(3 Pt 2):964–73.
96. Peyton CC, Tang D, Reich RR, et al. Downstaging and survival outcomes associated with neoadjuvant chemotherapy regimens among patients treated with cystectomy for muscle-

invasive bladder cancer. JAMA Oncol. 2018;4(11):1535–42. https://doi.org/10.1001/jamaoncol.2018.3542.
97. Wallace DM, Raghavan D, Kelly KA, et al. Neo-adjuvant (pre-emptive) cisplatin therapy in invasive transitional cell carcinoma of the bladder. Br J Urol. 1991;67(6):608–15. https://doi.org/10.1111/j.1464-410x.1991.tb15225.x.
98. Neoadjuvant cisplatin, methotrexate, and vinblastine chemotherapy for muscle-invasive bladder cancer: a randomised controlled trial. International collaboration of trialists. Lancet (London, England). 1999;354(9178):533–40.
99. Hussain SA, Porta N, Hall E, et al. Outcomes in patients with muscle-invasive bladder cancer treated with neoadjuvant chemotherapy followed by (chemo)radiotherapy in the BC2001 trial. Eur Urol. 2021;79(2):307–15. https://doi.org/10.1016/j.eururo.2020.11.036.
100. Horwich A, Dearnaley D, Huddart R, et al. A randomised trial of accelerated radiotherapy for localised invasive bladder cancer. Radiother Oncol J Eur Soc Ther Radiol Oncol. 2005;75(1):34–43. https://doi.org/10.1016/j.radonc.2004.11.003.
101. Näslund I, Nilsson B, Littbrand B. Hyperfractionated radiotherapy of bladder cancer. A ten-year follow-up of a randomized clinical trial. Acta Oncol. 1994;33(4):397–402. https://doi.org/10.3109/02841869409098435.
102. Stuschke M, Thames HD. Hyperfractionated radiotherapy of human tumors: overview of the randomized clinical trials. Int J Radiat Oncol Biol Phys. 1997;37(2):259–67. https://doi.org/10.1016/s0360-3016(96)00511-1.
103. Pos FJ, Hart G, Schneider C, Sminia P. Radical radiotherapy for invasive bladder cancer: what dose and fractionation schedule to choose? Int J Radiat Oncol Biol Phys. 2006;64(4):1168–73. https://doi.org/10.1016/j.ijrobp.2005.09.023.
104. Choudhury A, Porta N, Hall E, et al. Hypofractionated radiotherapy in locally advanced bladder cancer: an individual patient data meta-analysis of the BC2001 and BCON trials. Lancet Oncol. 2021;22(2):246–55. https://doi.org/10.1016/S1470-2045(20)30607-0.
105. Overgaard J, Horsman MR. Modification of hypoxia-induced radioresistance in tumors by the use of oxygen and sensitizers. Semin Radiat Oncol. 1996;6(1):10–21. https://doi.org/10.1053/SRAO0060010.
106. Hoskin PJ, Saunders MI, Phillips H, et al. Carbogen and nicotinamide in the treatment of bladder cancer with radical radiotherapy. Br J Cancer. 1997;76(2):260–3. https://doi.org/10.1038/bjc.1997.372.
107. Hoskin PJ, Rojas AM, Bentzen SM, Saunders MI. Radiotherapy with concurrent carbogen and nicotinamide in bladder carcinoma. J Clin Oncol Off J Am Soc Clin Oncol. 2010;28(33):4912–8. https://doi.org/10.1200/JCO.2010.28.4950.
108. Song YP, Mistry H, Choudhury A, Hoskin P. Long-term outcomes of hypoxia modification in bladder preservation: update from BCON trial. J Clin Oncol. 2019;37(7_suppl):356. https://doi.org/10.1200/JCO.2019.37.7_suppl.356.
109. Eustace A, Irlam JJ, Taylor J, et al. Necrosis predicts benefit from hypoxia-modifying therapy in patients with high risk bladder cancer enrolled in a phase III randomised trial. Radiother Oncol J Eur Soc Ther Radiol Oncol. 2013;108(1):40–7. https://doi.org/10.1016/j.radonc.2013.05.017.
110. Yang L, Taylor J, Eustace A, et al. A gene signature for selecting benefit from hypoxia modification of radiotherapy for high-risk bladder cancer patients. Clin cancer Res an Off J Am Assoc Cancer Res. 2017;23(16):4761–8. https://doi.org/10.1158/1078-0432.CCR-17-0038.
111. Matulay JT, Kamat AM. Advances in risk stratification of bladder cancer to guide personalized medicine. F1000Research. 2018;7. https://doi.org/10.12688/f1000research.14903.1.
112. Robertson AG, Kim J, Al-Ahmadie H, et al. Comprehensive molecular characterization of muscle-invasive bladder cancer. Cell. 2017;171(3):540–556.e25. https://doi.org/10.1016/j.cell.2017.09.007.
113. Choi W, Porten S, Kim S, et al. Identification of distinct basal and luminal subtypes of muscle-invasive bladder cancer with different sensitivities to frontline chemotherapy. Cancer Cell. 2014;25(2):152–65. https://doi.org/10.1016/j.ccr.2014.01.009.

114. Mitra AP. Molecular substratification of bladder cancer: moving towards individualized patient management. Ther Adv Urol. 2016;8(3):215–33. https://doi.org/10.1177/1756287216638981.
115. Choudhury A, Nelson LD, Teo MTW, et al. MRE11 expression is predictive of cause-specific survival following radical radiotherapy for muscle-invasive bladder cancer. Cancer Res. 2010;70(18):7017–26. https://doi.org/10.1158/0008-5472.CAN-10-1202.
116. Kamoun A, de Reyniès A, Allory Y, et al. A consensus molecular classification of muscle-invasive bladder cancer. Eur Urol. 2020;77(4):420–33. https://doi.org/10.1016/j.eururo.2019.09.006.
117. Balar AV, Galsky MD, Rosenberg JE, et al. Atezolizumab as first-line treatment in cisplatin-ineligible patients with locally advanced and metastatic urothelial carcinoma: a single-arm, multicentre, phase 2 trial. Lancet. 2017;389(10064):67–76. https://doi.org/10.1016/S0140-6736(16)32455-2.
118. Grivas P. DNA damage response gene alterations in urothelial cancer: ready for practice? Clin Cancer Res an Off J Am Assoc Cancer Res. 2019;25(3):907–9. https://doi.org/10.1158/1078-0432.CCR-18-2512.
119. Patel VG, Oh WK, Galsky MD. Treatment of muscle-invasive and advanced bladder cancer in 2020. CA Cancer J Clin. 2020;70(5):404–23. https://doi.org/10.3322/caac.21631.
120. Cuellar MA, Medina A, Girones R, et al. Phase II trial of durvalumab plus tremelimumab with concurrent radiotherapy as bladder-sparing therapy in patients with localized muscle invasive bladder cancer: a SOGUG study. J Clin Oncol. 2020;38(15_suppl):TPS5097-TPS5097. https://doi.org/10.1200/JCO.2020.38.15_suppl.TPS5097.
121. Balar AV, James ND, Shariat SF, et al. Phase III study of pembrolizumab (pembro) plus chemoradiotherapy (CRT) versus CRT alone for patients (pts) with muscle-invasive bladder cancer (MIBC): KEYNOTE-992. J Clin Oncol. 2020;38(15_suppl):TPS5093-TPS5093. https://doi.org/10.1200/JCO.2020.38.15_suppl.TPS5093.
122. Jiang DM, Chung P, Kulkarni GS, Sridhar SS. Trimodality therapy for muscle-invasive bladder cancer: recent advances and unanswered questions. Curr Oncol Rep. 2020;22(2):14. https://doi.org/10.1007/s11912-020-0880-5.
123. Singh P, Tangen C, Efstathiou JA, et al. INTACT: phase III randomized trial of concurrent chemoradiotherapy with or without atezolizumab in localized muscle invasive bladder cancer—SWOG/NRG1806. J Clin Oncol. 2020;38(6_suppl):TPS586-TPS586. https://doi.org/10.1200/JCO.2020.38.6_suppl.TPS586.
124. Maciejewski B, Majewski S. Dose fractionation and tumour repopulation in radiotherapy for bladder cancer. Radiother Oncol J Eur Soc Ther Radiol Oncol. 1991;21(3):163–70. https://doi.org/10.1016/0167-8140(91)90033-d.
125. Moonen L, vd Voet H, de Nijs R, Horenblas S, Hart AA, Bartelink H. Muscle-invasive bladder cancer treated with external beam radiation: influence of total dose, overall treatment time, and treatment interruption on local control. Int J Radiat Oncol Biol Phys. 1998;42(3):525–30. https://doi.org/10.1016/s0360-3016(98)00263-6.
126. Flaig TW, Spiess PE, Agarwal N, et al. Bladder cancer, version 3.2020, NCCN clinical practice guidelines in oncology. J Natl Compr Canc Netw. 2020;18(3):329–54. https://doi.org/10.6004/jnccn.2020.0011.
127. Witjes JA, Bruins M, Cathomas R, et al. European Association of Urology guidelines. 2020 Edition. In: Vol presented. European Association of Urology Guidelines Office. 2020. http://uroweb.org/guideline/bladder-cancer-muscle-invasive-and-metastatic/.
128. Kassam SN, Aziz Z, Hung LS, Sridhar SS. A case of isolated rectal recurrence of muscle invasive bladder cancer. Can Urol Assoc J = J l'Association des Urol du Canada. 2013;7(5–6):E376–80. https://doi.org/10.5489/cuaj.1223.
129. Reshko LB, Richardson MK, Spencer K, Kersh CR. Stereotactic body radiation therapy (SBRT) in pelvic lymph node oligometastases. Cancer Invest. 2020;38(10):599–607. https://doi.org/10.1080/07357907.2020.1801713.
130. Wallmeroth A, Wagner U, Moch H, Gasser TC, Sauter G, Mihatsch MJ. Patterns of metastasis in muscle-invasive bladder cancer (pT2-4): an autopsy study on 367 patients. Urol Int. 1999;62(2):69–75. https://doi.org/10.1159/000030361.

131. Joshi M, Kim S, Solanki AA, et al. EA8185: Phase II study of bladder-sparing chemoradiation (chemoRT) with durvalumab in clinical stage III, node-positive urothelial carcinoma (INSPIRE), ECOG-ACRIN/nrg collaboration. J Clin Oncol. 2021;39(6):TPS500
132. Haque W, Verma V, Butler EB, Teh BS. Chemotherapy versus chemoradiation for node-positive bladder cancer: practice patterns and outcomes from the National Cancer Data Base. Bladder Cancer (Amsterdam, Netherlands). 2017;3(4):283–91. https://doi.org/10.3233/BLC-170137.
133. Smith AB, Jaeger B, Pinheiro LC, et al. Impact of bladder cancer on health-related quality of life. BJU Int. 2018;121(4):549–57. https://doi.org/10.1111/bju.14047.
134. Shih C, Porter MP. Health-related quality of life after cystectomy and urinary diversion for bladder cancer. Meng M V, ed. Adv Urol. 2011;2011:715892. https://doi.org/10.1155/2011/715892.
135. Modh RA, Mulhall JP, Gilbert SM. Sexual dysfunction after cystectomy and urinary diversion. Nat Rev Urol. 2014;11(8):445–53. https://doi.org/10.1038/nrurol.2014.151.
136. Gilbert SM, Wood DP, Dunn RL, et al. Measuring health-related quality of life outcomes in bladder cancer patients using the Bladder Cancer Index (BCI). Cancer. 2007;109(9):1756–62. https://doi.org/10.1002/cncr.22556.
137. Mak KS, Smith AB, Eidelman A, et al. Quality of life in long-term survivors of muscle-invasive bladder cancer. Int J Radiat Oncol Biol Phys. 2016;96(5):1028–36. https://doi.org/10.1016/j.ijrobp.2016.08.023.
138. Henningsohn L, Wijkström H, Dickman PW, Bergmark K, Steineck G. Distressful symptoms after radical radiotherapy for urinary bladder cancer. Radiother Oncol J Eur Soc Ther Radiol Oncol. 2002;62(2):215–25. https://doi.org/10.1016/s0167-8140(01)00455-8.
139. Zietman AL, Sacco D, Skowronski U, et al. Organ conservation in invasive bladder cancer by transurethral resection, chemotherapy and radiation: results of a urodynamic and quality of life study on long-term survivors. J Urol. 2003;170(5):1772–6. https://doi.org/10.1097/01.ju.0000093721.23249.c3.
140. Kachnic LA, Shipley WU, Griffin PP, et al. Combined modality treatment with selective bladder conservation for invasive bladder cancer: long-term tolerance in the female patient. Cancer J Sci Am. 1996;2(2):79–84.
141. Efstathiou JA, Bae K, Shipley WU, et al. Late pelvic toxicity after bladder-sparing therapy in patients with invasive bladder cancer: RTOG 89-03, 95-06, 97-06, 99-06. J Clin Oncol Off J Am Soc Clin Oncol. 2009;27(25):4055–61. https://doi.org/10.1200/JCO.2008.19.5776.
142. Freilich JM, Spiess PE, Biagioli MC, et al. Lipiodol as a fiducial marker for image-guided radiation therapy for bladder cancer. Int Braz J Urol. 2014;40(2):190–7. https://doi.org/10.1590/S1677-5538.IBJU.2014.02.08.
143. Kibrom AZ, Knight KA. Adaptive radiation therapy for bladder cancer: a review of adaptive techniques used in clinical practice. J Med Radiat Sci. 2015;62(4):277–85. https://doi.org/10.1002/jmrs.129.
144. Tunio MA, Hashmi A, Qayyum A, Mohsin R, Zaeem A. Whole-pelvis or bladder-only chemoradiation for lymph node-negative invasive bladder cancer: single-institution experience. Int J Radiat Oncol Biol Phys. 2012;82(3):e457–62. https://doi.org/10.1016/j.ijrobp.2011.05.051.
145. Foroudi F, Wilson L, Bressel M, et al. A dosimetric comparison of 3D conformal vs intensity modulated vs volumetric arc radiation therapy for muscle invasive bladder cancer. Radiat Oncol. 2012;7:111. https://doi.org/10.1186/1748-717X-7-111.

Chapter 19
Treatment of Metastatic Bladder Cancer

Yu Fujiwara, Hirotaka Miyashita, and Matthew D. Galsky

Introduction

The treatment options for patients with locally advanced or metastatic bladder cancer (BC) have been limited for decades. The main first-line treatment has been platinum-based chemotherapy, and the role of second-line chemotherapy had been limited until the development of immune checkpoint inhibitors. Approximately 25% of patients with bladder cancer present with muscle-invasive disease, of whom half may ultimately progress to metastatic disease, while ~5% present with metastatic disease de novo [1]. The most common histology of cancer in the urinary tract is urothelial carcinoma (UC), and the bladder is the most common primary site. UC consists of approximately 90% of BC, and the evidence of treatment of BC is mainly based on the trials for UC [2]. The median overall survival (OS) of patients with metastatic BC was about 3 months prior to the development of chemotherapeutic regimens with activity in this disease, and more contemporary clinical trials report median OS of ~15 months [3, 4]. Several clinical factors have been associated with prognosis in prior studies. The Karnofsky or Eastern Cooperative Oncology Group performance status (KPS $\leq$ 80% or ECOG PS > 1) and visceral metastases (lung, liver, or bone) were found as prognostic factors among patients who received methotrexate, vinblastine, doxorubicin, and cisplatin (MVAC) or paclitaxel, gemcitabine, and cisplatin (PGC) in the first-line setting [5, 6]. In the second-line setting, a study

Y. Fujiwara · M. D. Galsky (✉)
Department of Medicine, Icahn School of Medicine at Mount Sinai, Mount Sinai Beth Israel, New York, NY, USA
e-mail: yu.fujiwara@mountsinai.org; matthew.galsky@mssm.edu

H. Miyashita
Tisch Cancer Institute, Icahn School of Medicine at Mount Sinai, New York, NY, USA
e-mail: hirotaka.miyashita@mountsinai.org

K. L. Stratton, A. K. Morgans (eds.), *Urologic Oncology*,
https://doi.org/10.1007/978-3-030-89891-5_19

evaluating vinflunine for platinum-refractory patients showed that anemia (hemoglobin <10 g/dL), liver metastases, and ECOG PS (>0) were related to poor prognosis [7]. Molecular features associated with prognosis that have been extensively validated have been more elusive though molecular subtypes of bladder cancer defined by gene expression profiling so seem to confer some prognostic information.

First-Line Treatment for Metastatic Bladder Cancer

The first-line treatment for patients with locally advanced or metastatic BC has been limited until the development of immune checkpoint blockade in the late 2010s. Currently, gemcitabine plus cisplatin (GC) and MVAC are the main options for cisplatin-eligible patients (Fig. 19.1), and carboplatin-based chemotherapy (i.e., gemcitabine plus carboplatin) has been the mainstay of treatment for patients ineligible for cisplatin. Programmed cell death protein 1 (PD-1)/programmed death-ligand 1 (PD-L1) blockade with pembrolizumab or atezolizumab is a potential option for cisplatin-ineligible patients harboring tumors with increased PD-L1

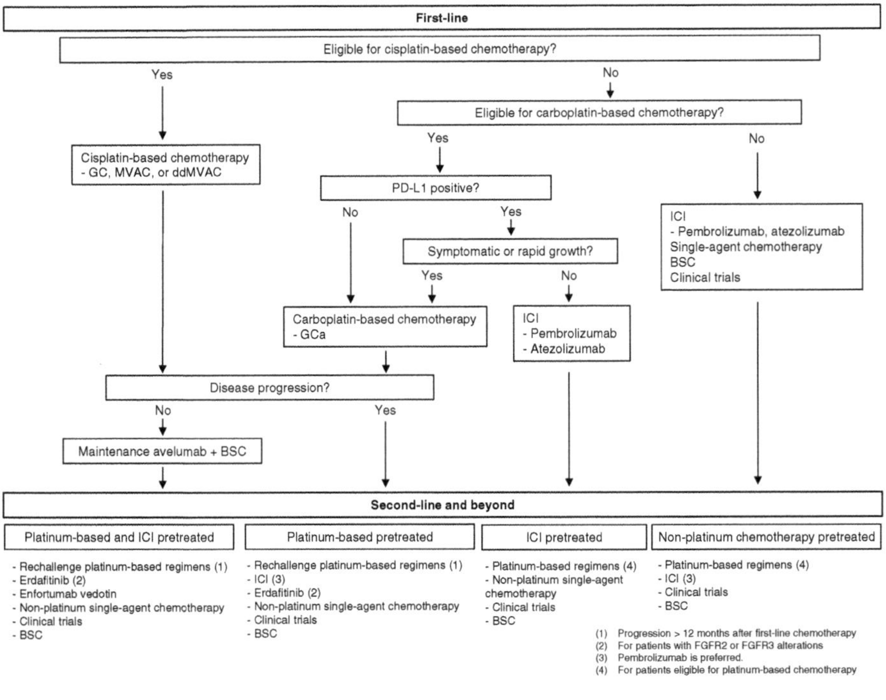

Fig. 19.1 Treatment algorithm for metastatic urothelial cancer. Abbreviation: GC gemcitabine and cisplatin, MVAC methotrexate, vinblastine, doxorubicin and cisplatin, ddMVAC dose-dense MVAC, GCa gemcitabine and carboplatin, ICI immune checkpoint inhibitor, BSC best supportive care, PD-L1 programmed death-ligand 1

expression though initial chemotherapy with switch maintenance PD-1/PD-L1 blockade has emerged as a preferred strategy. For patients that are "chemotherapy ineligible," PD-1/PD-L1 blockade remains a potential treatment option.

Treatment for Cisplatin-Eligible Patients

In the 1990s, cisplatin-based chemotherapy was shown to improve the OS in patients with advanced UC. At first, MVAC showed survival improvement when compared with cisplatin alone [8]. MVAC had toxicities such as myelosuppression and mucositis. Several platinum-based doublets with newer cytotoxic drugs, such as the combination of GC, were subsequently explored in phase 2 trials demonstrating promising activity [9]. A phase 3 trial comparing GC with MVAC showed a similar response rate and OS, albeit with less toxicity with GC, and GC became a standard first-line regimen [4, 10]. Dose-dense MVAC (ddMVAC) with granulocyte colony-stimulating factor demonstrated less toxicity and potentially better long-term survival rates compared with classical MVAC in a phase 3 trial [11]. Dose-dense GC was also compared with ddMVAC but no OS difference was observed [12]. GC was compared with paclitaxel plus GC (PGC) in a phase 3 trial (EORTC study 30987). Although subgroup analyses showed an OS improvement among patients who met all eligibility criteria and patients with primary BC, PGC had more toxicities and showed no significant survival benefit in the overall population [13]. Together, these series of single-arm and randomized studies have solidified the role of GC and ddMVAC as standard first-line options for cisplatin-eligible patients with metastatic UC (Table 19.1).

Treatment for Cisplatin-Ineligible Patients

Carboplatin-Based Chemotherapy

The risks versus benefits of cisplatin-based chemotherapy for patients with metastatic UC require individualized shared medical decisions. However, criteria for "cisplatin-ineligibility" have been harmonized for clinical trial eligibility purposes which can also offer some guidance for routine clinical care which include the following: ECOG PS >1, glomerular filtration rate (GFR) ≤ 60, grade ≥ 2 hearing loss, grade ≥ 2 peripheral neuropathy, and the New York Heart Association $\geq$ III heart failure [14]. Renal impairment, common in patients with UC based on age-associated physiologic declines in GFR, age- and smoking-related comorbidities, and potential tumor-related ureteral obstruction, is the most common reason for "cisplatin ineligibility." The development of chemotherapeutic regimens that balance safety and efficacy for this subset of patients with metastatic UC has been pursued for decades. A phase 2/3 randomized controlled trial (RCT) which compared gemcitabine plus

Table 19.1 Standard treatment regimens for locally advanced or metastatic urothelial cancer

Study	Eligibility	Number	Phase	Intervention	Treatment detail	Response rate (%)	Median PFS (months)	Median OS (months)	Reference
First-line regimens									
Loehrer 1992	NA	269	III	MVAC vs cisplatin	MVAC (methotrexate 30 mg/m^2 on days 1, 15, 22; vinblastine 3 mg/m^2 on day 2, 15, 22; doxorubicin 30 mg/m^2 on day 2; cisplatin 70 mg/m^2 on day 2, every 28 days)	39 vs 12	10.0 vs 4.3	12.5 vs 8.2	[8]
von der Maase 2000	NA	405	III	GC vs MVAC	GC (gemcitabine 1000 mg/m^2 on days 1, 8, 15; cisplatin 70 mg/m^2 on day 2, every 21 days)	49 vs 46	7.7 vs 8.3	14.0 vs 15.2	[10]
Sternberg 2006	NA	263	III	ddMVAC vs MVAC	ddMVAC (methotrexate 30 mg/m^2 on days 1; vinblastine 3 mg/m^2 on day 2; doxorubicin 30 mg/m^2 on day 2; cisplatin 70 mg/m^2 on day 2 with G-CSF on days 3–7, every 15 days)	64 vs 50	9.5 vs 8.1	15.1 vs 14.9	[11]
Bellmunt 2012	NA	626	III	PGC vs GC	PGC (paclitaxel 80 mg/m^2 on days 1, 8; gemcitabine 1000 mg/m^2 on days 1, 8, 15; cisplatin 70 mg/m^2 on day 2, every 21 days)	55.5 vs 43.6	8.3 vs 7.6	15.8 vs 12.7	[13]

De Santis 2012	With renal dysfunction	238	II/III	GCa vs M-CAVI	GCa (gemcitabine 1000 mg/m^2 on days 1, 8; carboplatin AUC 4.5 on day 1, every 21 days) M-CAVI (methotrexate 30 mg/m^2 on days 1, 15, 22; carboplatin AUC 4.5 on day 1; vinblastine 3 mg/m^2 on days 1, 15, 22, every 28 days)	41.2 vs 30.3	5.8 vs 4.2	9.3 vs 8.1	[15]
Vuky 2020	Cisplatin-ineligible	374	II	Pembrolizumab	Pembrolizumab (200 mg on day 1, every 21 days)	28.6	2.2	11.3	[19]
Balar 2017	Cisplatin-ineligible	123	II	Atezolizumab	Atezolizumab (1200 mg on day 1, every 21 days)	23.0	2.7	15.9	[17]
Powles 2020	Disease-controlled with platinum-based chemotherapy	700	III	Maintenance avelumab vs BSC	Maintenance avelumab: four to six cycles of GC or GCa following avelumab (10 mg/kg on day 1, every 14 days)	–	3.7 vs 2.0	21.4 vs 14.3	[21]
Second-line regimens (for patients with progression after platinum-based chemotherapy)									
Fradet 2019	NA	542	III	Pembrolizumab vs chemotherapy[a]	Pembrolizumab (200 mg on day 1, every 21 days) Paclitaxel (175 mg/m^2 on day 1), docetaxel (75 mg/m^2 on day 1), or vinflunine (320 mg/m^2 on day1), every 21 days	21.1 vs 11.0	2.1 vs 3.3	10.1 vs 7.3	[25]
Powles 2018	NA	931	III	Atezolizumab vs chemotherapy[b]	Atezolizumab (1200 mg on day 1, every 21 days) Paclitaxel (175 mg/m^2 on day 1), docetaxel (75 mg/m^2 on day 1), or vinflunine (320 mg/m^2 on day1), every 21 days	13.4 vs 13.4	2.1 vs 4.0	8.6 vs 8.0	[23]

(continued)

Table 19.1 (continued)

Study	Eligibility	Number	Phase	Intervention	Treatment detail	Response rate (%)	Median PFS (months)	Median OS (months)	Reference
Sharma 2017	NA	270	II	Nivolumab	Nivolumab (3 mg/kg, every 14 days)	19.6	2.0	8.74	[27]
Patel 2018	NA	249	I	Avelumab	Avelumab (10 mg/kg, every 14 days)	17.0	6.6	6.5	[29]
Powles 2017	NA[c]	191	I/II	Durvalumab	Durvalumab (10 mg/kg every 14 days)	17.8	1.5	18.2	[30]
	Later regimens								
Loriot 2019	FGFR alteration and progression after one or more chemotherapies[b]	99	II	Erdafitinib	Erdafitinib (8 mg daily, can be increased to 9 mg daily if serum phosphate level < 5.5 mg/dL on day 14)	40	5.5	13.8	[39]
Rosenberg 2019	Previously treated with platinum-based regimen and anti-PD-1/L1 therapy.	125	II	Enfortumab vedotin	Enfortumab vedotin (1.25 mg/kg on days 1, 8, 15, every 28 days)	44	5.8	11.7	[42]
Bellmunt 2009	Previously treated with platinum-based regimen	370	III	Vinflunine vs BSC	Vinflunine (320 mg/m^2 on day 1, every 21 days)	8.6 vs 0	3.0 vs 1.5	6.9 vs 4.3	[31]

Abbreviation: *NA* not available; *FGFR* fibroblast growth factor receptor; *PD-1* programmed cell death protein 1; *PD-L1* programmed death-ligand 1; *MVAC* methotrexate, vinblastine, doxorubicin, and cisplatin; *GC* gemcitabine and cisplatin; *ddMVAC* dose-dense MVAC; *PGC* paclitaxel, gemcitabine, and cisplatin; *GCa* gemcitabine and carboplatin; *M-CAVI* methotrexate, carboplatin, and vinblastine; *BSC* best supportive care; *PFS* progression-free survival; *OS* overall survival

[a]Investigators' choice from paclitaxel, docetaxel, or vinflunine

[b]The study did not specify previous exposure to PD-1/PD-L1 inhibitors as inclusion criteria

[c]The study did not selectively include patients with progression after platinum-based regimen. Nevertheless, 99.5% of patients included had received prior chemotherapy, and 95% of them had received platinum-based chemotherapy

carboplatin (GCa) with methotrexate, carboplatin, and vinblastine (M-CAVI) showed less toxicity and higher response rate in GCa than M-CAVI (overall response rate (ORR), 42% vs 30%) although no significant difference in ORR and OS was observed (EORTC study 30986) [15]. A recent phase 2 RCT evaluating the efficacy of vinflunine plus gemcitabine (VG) compared with GCa showed higher ORR in VG than GCa, but no significant difference was observed in OS and progression-free survival (PFS) [16]. Therefore, GCa has become a favored first-line regimen for cisplatin-ineligible patients with metastatic UC.

Immune Checkpoint Blockade

PD-1/PD-L1 inhibitors demonstrated early after in UC in expansion cohorts of phase I studies in solid tumors leading to the rapid initiation of larger studies. Atezolizumab, a PD-L1 inhibitor, was evaluated in the IMvigor210 phase 2 trial. In cohort 1 of this study, 119 cisplatin-ineligible chemotherapy-naïve patients with locally advanced or metastatic UC regardless of PD-L1 expression status were enrolled, and atezolizumab demonstrated an ORR of 23%, median PFS of 2.7 months, and median OS of 15.9 months [17]. Another trial (KEYNOTE-052) which evaluated the efficacy of pembrolizumab, a PD-1 inhibitor, for 370 cisplatin-ineligible patients showed an ORR of 29% with CR of 9%, median PFS of 2.2 months, and median OS of 11.3 months. Notably, ORR was 47% in patients with high PD-L1 expression (combined positive score (CPS) ≥10%) and 20% in patients with CPS <10%, respectively [18, 19]. Based on these results, atezolizumab and pembrolizumab were approved by the US Food and Drug Administration (FDA) in 2017 for cisplatin-ineligible patients regardless of the PD-L1 expression status in the first-line setting. However, the interim results of two phase 3 studies (IMvigor130 and KEYNOTE-361) which compared PD-1/PD-L1 inhibitors plus chemotherapy, PD-L1/PD-L1 inhibitor monotherapy, and chemotherapy showed poorer survival outcomes among patients with low PD-L1 expressing tumors who received PD-1/PD-L1 inhibitor monotherapy than those who received platinum-based chemotherapy. Therefore, for cisplatin-ineligible patients, the FDA prescribing label was changed to limit atezolizumab and pembrolizumab to patients with tumor harboring high levels of PD-L1 expression based on the appropriate assay for the particular PD-1/PD-L1 inhibitor. The FDA prescribing label did permit the use of these therapies for patients deemed "platinum-ineligible" (i.e., "chemotherapy-ineligible") regardless of the PD-L1 expression status. The evidence to select either carboplatin-based chemotherapy or PD-1/PD-L1 inhibitor monotherapy for cisplatin-ineligible patients is insufficient. Because of the higher response rate in carboplatin-based chemotherapy (ORR, 41.2% in EORTC Study 30986) compared with that in PD-1/PD-L1 inhibitor monotherapy (ORR, around 20% in IMvigor210 and KEYNOTE-052), patients with rapid progression or visceral crisis might be better to be treated with carboplatin-based chemotherapy. However, the incidence of grade 3 or more adverse events (AEs) is higher in chemotherapy, and patients with poor performance status or slower tumor growth may prefer PD-1/PD-L1 inhibitor monotherapy.

Maintenance Immune Checkpoint Blockade

Standard first-line platinum-based chemotherapy for metastatic UC is typically administered for up to six cycles, in the absence of prohibitive side effects or disease progression, and then discontinued due to the likelihood of cumulative side effects in the absence of additional benefit. Given the generally short duration of response upon discontinuation of chemotherapy, and the efficacy of PD-1/PD-L1 blockade as second-line treatment, initiating immune checkpoint blockade upon cessation of chemotherapy in a switch maintenance approach has been explored. In a phase 2 trial (GU14-182) which compared switch maintenance pembrolizumab with placebo subsequently after platinum-based chemotherapy, pembrolizumab demonstrated an improvement in PFS (5.4 versus 3.0 month; hazard ratio, HR 0.64 [95% confidence interval, CI, 0.41–0.98]) [20]. In parallel, the strategy to use avelumab, a PD-L1 inhibitor, as maintenance therapy was studied in a phase 3 trial (JAVELIN Bladder 100) [21]. Patients who received four to six cycles of GC/GCa without disease progression were randomly assigned to receive best supportive care with or without maintenance avelumab. Maintenance avelumab prolonged OS and PFS in the overall population (OS: 21.4 versus 14.3 months; HR 0.56 [95% CI 0.40–0.79]; PFS: 3.7 versus 2.0 months; HR 0.62 [95% CI 0.52–0.75]) and in the PD-L1-positive population. As a result, maintenance immune checkpoint blockade after initial platinum-based chemotherapy has been embraced as a standard treatment approach.

Treatment in the Second-Line and Beyond Setting

Cytotoxic chemotherapy, typically with taxanes, had been a common approach for patients with metastatic UC progressing despite first-line chemotherapy. However, ORR with this approach was relatively low and better strategies were pursued. An understanding of the tumor microenvironment and the molecular features of UC has led to the development of multiple new therapeutic classes in the second-line and beyond setting.

Immune Checkpoint Blockade

Traditionally, single-agent cytotoxic chemotherapy was the main treatment option in the second-line and beyond setting before the development of immunotherapy. The development of immune checkpoint blockade led to the expansion of therapeutic options and changed the second-line and beyond treatment scheme. Currently, five anti-PD-1/PD-L1 antibodies (pembrolizumab, atezolizumab, nivolumab, durvalumab, and avelumab) are FDA-approved in the second-line setting. Atezolizumab was first approved as it showed promising activity among patients with advanced UC progressed during or after the previous platinum-based chemotherapy in the early-phase trials [22]. Several cancer cell and tumor microenvironment features were associated with a high likelihood of response to atezolizumab, such as PD-L1 expression, tumor mutational burden, and molecular subtype, but none of these has been integrated into clinical decision-making [22]. The efficacy of atezolizumab was subsequently confirmed by the phase 3 trial (IMvigor211) that compared atezolizumab with conventional single-agent chemotherapy (paclitaxel, docetaxel, or vinflunine). Although this study did not meet its primary endpoint in patients with PD-L1 high expressing tumors, there was a suggestion of better outcomes with atezolizumab versus chemotherapy in the intent-to-treat population though this was considered exploratory given the hierarchical statistical analysis plan (i.e., improved OS needed to be demonstrated in the patients with PD-L1 high expressing tumors before hypothesis testing could formally occur in the intent-to-treat population) [23]. In contrast with atezolizumab, pembrolizumab improved the median OS (10.1 versus 7.3 months; HR 0.7 [95% CI 0.57–0.85]) in platinum-refractory patients compared with chemotherapy (paclitaxel, docetaxel, or vinflunine) in the phase 3 trial (KEYNOTE-045). Pembrolizumab also demonstrated better response rate (21% vs 11%) and less severe toxicity (17% vs 50%) [24, 25]. Pembrolizumab in patients with high PD-L1 expression (CPS $\geq$ 10) achieved similar ORR (20.3%) to the overall population, suggesting OS benefit was independent of the PD-L1 expression level. Other immune checkpoint inhibitors including nivolumab (PD-1 inhibitor), avelumab (PD-L1 inhibitor), and durvalumab (PD-L1 inhibitor) were also shown to have promising efficacy in early-phase clinical trials which resulted in FDA approval. The phase 1/2 CheckMate 032 trial evaluating nivolumab monotherapy for recurrent or platinum-ineligible patients showed 24% of ORR regardless of PD-L1 expression [26]. Another phase 2 CheckMate 275 trial assessing nivolumab monotherapy showed a similar ORR (19.6%) and median OS of 8.7 months [27]. This trial found that higher tumor mutational burden was associated with improved ORR, PFS, and OS [28]. Avelumab and durvalumab were also found to have adequate ORR (17% with avelumab and 17% with durvalumab) in early-phase clinical trials regardless of the PD-L1 expression status [29, 30].

Chemotherapy

Given the results of KEYNOTE-045 and IMvigor211 trials, single-agent chemotherapy with taxanes (or vinflunine in countries where this therapy is available) is now usually reserved for patients with contraindications to immune checkpoint inhibitors though newer therapies have further decreased the use of these therapies. In Europe, vinflunine is approved for second-line use based on the phase 3 trial result which compared vinflunine with best supportive care among 370 patients previously treated with platinum-based chemotherapy. This trial demonstrated no significant difference in OS (6.9 versus 4.6 months; HR 0.88 [95%CI 0.69–1.12]) though a trend toward better outcomes was observed [31]. Other agents such as taxanes, gemcitabine, and ifosfamide were shown in previous studies to have 10–20% response rate [32–35].

FGFR Inhibitors

Fibroblast growth factor receptor (FGFR) is known to control cell proliferation, survival, migration, and differentiation in cancer cells [36]. Alterations of FGFR lead to oncogenesis which is seen among several cancer types including UC though UC harbors among the highest frequency of somatic FGFR3 alterations [36]. Generally, alterations of FGFR3 are seen in approximately 20% of patients with advanced UC, and FGFR2 or FGFR3 is commonly involved in the luminal I subtype [36, 37]. Initially, dovitinib, a multi-targeted inhibitor of tyrosine kinases including FGFR3, was investigated for platinum-refractory patients with or without FGFR mutations. However, this phase 2 trial did not show substantial activity with dovitinib [38]. Subsequently, more potent and selective FGFR3 inhibitors were developed and demonstrated activity on UC. Erdafitinib, a pan-FGFR inhibitor, was approved by the FDA for platinum-refractory patients as erdafitinib showed efficacy in patients with FGFR mutations (FGFR3 gene mutation or FGFR2/3 gene fusions) with 42% of ORR, median PFS of 5.5 months, and median OS of 13.8 months, respectively. Of note, about 70% of patients who were previously treated with immune checkpoint blockade gained response in this trial [39]. In any grade AEs, hyperphosphatemia was seen in 77% of patients, followed by stomatitis (58%) and diarrhea (50%). Other important AEs with erdafitinib are hand-foot syndrome, nail changes (onycholysis, 18%; paronychia, 17%; nail dystrophy, 16%; nail disorder, 8%), and ocular events including dry eye and central serous retinopathy which require dry eye prophylaxis with ocular demulcents and regular ophthalmologic examinations during the first 4 months of treatment and every 3 months afterward [39]. Several studies are ongoing to evaluate other pan-FGFR inhibitors and an FGFR3-specific antibody to develop therapeutic options for patients with FGFR alterations.

Enfortumab Vedotin

Enfortumab vedotin is an antibody-drug conjugate (ADC) that is composed of an anti-nectin-4 monoclonal antibody conjugated to monomethyl auristatin E (called vedotin), a micro-tubule-disrupting agent [40]. Nectin-4 is a transmembrane protein and related to oncogenesis in cancer cells. Several solid tumors such as urothelial, breast, gastric, and lung carcinoma are known to have high expression of Nectin-4 [41]. A phase 2 trial (EV-201) demonstrated the efficacy of enfortumab vedotin in 125 patients with locally advanced or metastatic UC who had progression after platinum-based chemotherapy and immunotherapy, resulting in FDA approval in 2019. This study showed an ORR of 44%, median PFS of 5.8 months, and median OS of 11.7 months [42]. Grade ≥3 treatment-related adverse events (TRAEs) were seen in 54% of patients, and the common grade ≥3 TRAEs were neutropenia (8%), anemia (7%), and fatigue (6%). Currently, a phase 3 trial that compares enfortumab vedotin with chemotherapy (paclitaxel, docetaxel, or vinflunine) for patients previously treated with platinum-based chemotherapy and immunotherapy is ongoing (EV-301, NCT03474107). Concurrently, another phase 3 trial (EV-302, NCT04223856) will compare enfortumab vedotin plus pembrolizumab with GC/GCa in the first-line setting.

Future Perspective of Treatment

Combination Treatment with Immunotherapy

To explore the potential benefits of the combination therapy using immune checkpoint inhibitors and other agents, several phase 3 trials are ongoing both in the first-line and the later line settings. Especially, the IMvigor130 trial comparing atezolizumab, atezolizumab plus GC/GCa, and GC/GCa showed significant improvement of PFS with atezolizumab plus GC/GCa compared with GC/GCa (stratified HR 0.82 [95% CI 0.70–0.96]) but did not show OS benefit in the interim analysis (stratified HR 0.83 [95% CI 0.69–1.0]). This study is ongoing and the final OS analysis is awaited [43]. Another phase 3 study, KEYNOTE-361, compared pembrolizumab plus GC/GCa versus GC/GCa. Although there was a trend toward improvement in PFS (HR 0.78 [95% CI 0.65–0.93]) and OS (HR 0.86 [95% CI 0.72–1.02]) for patients treated with pembrolizumab plus GC/GCa, the study results did not reach statistical significance per the pre-specified statistical plan [44]. Another potential combination is the dual immune checkpoint inhibitors as the efficacy of this strategy was shown in other cancers such as renal cell carcinoma and lung cancer [45, 46]. Nivolumab plus ipilimumab (a cytotoxic T-lymphocyte antigen 4 [CTLA-4] inhibitor) was investigated in the CheckMate 032, phase 2 trial. In this study, 274 patients who showed progression on prior platinum-based chemotherapy were assigned to either nivolumab monotherapy or nivolumab plus ipilimumab which had two cohorts with different dose. Nivolumab (1 mg/kg) plus ipilimumab (3 mg/kg) provided the greatest efficacy among three cohorts in ORR (38.8%), PFS (4.9 months), and OS (15.3 months) [47]. Currently, a phase 3 trial comparing nivolumab plus ipilimumab versus platinum-based chemotherapy in the first-line setting is ongoing (CheckMate 901, NCT03036098). Dual immune checkpoint inhibitors in the first-line setting were also investigated in the DANUBE trial (NCT02516241) which compared durvalumab (PD-L1 inhibitor) versus durvalumab plus tremelimumab (CTLA-4 inhibitor) versus GC/GCa. However, this study did not meet the primary endpoint that was the OS benefit from durvalumab monotherapy compared with GC/GCa in the high PD-L1 expression group and OS benefit from durvalumab plus tremelimumab compared with GC/GCa regardless of PD-L1 expression status [48]. There is another study, the NILE trial (NCT03682068), which evaluates the efficacy of durvalumab plus GC/GCa, durvalumab plus tremelimumab with GC/GCa, and GC/GCa alone. This study is ongoing and will provide insights into the efficacy of dual immune checkpoint inhibitors with chemotherapy.

Molecular-Targeted Therapy and ADC

In addition to immunotherapy, other therapeutic agents have been explored. Angiogenesis inhibitors targeting the vascular endothelial growth factor (VEGF) pathway were investigated for advanced or metastatic BC. Ramucirumab, a monoclonal antibody that inhibits the VEGF receptor-2 (VEGFR2), was explored in a phase 3 trial (RANGE). Ramucirumab plus docetaxel was compared with docetaxel alone for platinum-refractory patients. Although PFS was significantly longer in ramucirumab plus docetaxel therapy (4.1 versus 2.8 months; HR 0.70 [95% CI 0.57–0.85]), it did not improve OS (9.4 versus 7.9 months; HR 0.89 [95% CI 0.72–1.09]) [49]. Bevacizumab, a monoclonal antibody targeting VEGF-A, plus GC was evaluated in the first-line setting in a phase 3, CALGB 90601 trial. Similarly, this combination improved PFS (HR 0.77 [95%CI 0.63–0.93]) but did not prolong OS (HR 0.87 [95% CI 0.72–1.06]) compared with GC alone [50]. Although these trials showed the potential efficacy of angiogenesis inhibitors, no agents are currently approved. The combination of angiogenesis inhibitors with PD-1/PD-L1 blockade has also been evaluated. Cabozantinib, a multi-targeted inhibitor of tyrosine kinases including VEGFR2, with nivolumab alone or with ipilimumab demonstrated a modest ORR in a phase 1 trial [51]. Lenvatinib, another multi-targeted inhibitor of tyrosine kinase including VEGFR1-3, with pembrolizumab demonstrated 25% of ORR for solid tumors in a phase 1 trial [52]. A phase 3 trial comparing lenvatinib plus pembrolizumab with pembrolizumab alone for platinum-ineligible patients in the first-line setting is ongoing (NCT03898180). Other potential options are ADCs. Sacituzumab govitecan, a Trop-2-directed antibody conjugated to a topoisomerase I inhibitor (SN-38), has been widely investigated for solid tumors and obtained approval for previously treated metastatic triple-negative breast cancer in 2020 [53]. Two cohorts of a basket phase 2 trial (NCT03547973) showed an ORR of ~30% in patients with metastatic UC who progressed after platinum-based chemotherapy and immunotherapy and in platinum-ineligible patients with immunotherapy failure [54, 55]. The cohort 3 of this study which evaluates sacituzumab govitecan plus pembrolizumab for patients after failure of platinum-based chemotherapy or immunotherapy and a phase 3 trial (NCT04527991) which compares sacituzumab govitecan with chemotherapy (docetaxel, paclitaxel, or vinflunine) after the failure of platinum-based chemotherapy and immunotherapy are ongoing. Another promising candidate of ADC is trastuzumab deruxtecan, composed of an anti-HER2 (human epidermal growth factor receptor 2) antibody linked to a cytotoxic topoisomerase I inhibitor. Approximately 30% to 50% of UC is known to express HER2 [56]. It showed clinical efficacy among HER2-positive solid tumors such as breast and gastric cancer [57–59]. A phase 2 trial for HER2 expressing tumors including BC (NCT04482309) and another trial evaluating trastuzumab deruxtecan plus nivolumab for breast cancer and UC (NCT03523572) are now conducted.

Treatment for Metastatic Non-urothelial Bladder Cancer

Since the majority of BC is UC and most clinical trials have been conducted for patients with UC, there is a lack of evidence regarding treatment options for patients with locally advanced or metastatic non-urothelial BC. There are no standardized therapeutic options for this population. Therefore, patients with non-urothelial histology are encouraged to get molecular profiling techniques including next-generation sequencing and participate in the clinical trials. If there is a lack of trials, this population can be treated with GC/GCa, ifosfamide plus paclitaxel plus cisplatin, or paclitaxel plus carboplatin plus gemcitabine based on the results of phase 2 studies in the first-line setting [60–62].

References

1. Burger M, Catto JW, Dalbagni G, Grossman HB, Herr H, Karakiewicz P, et al. Epidemiology and risk factors of urothelial bladder cancer. Eur Urol. 2013;63(2):234–41. https://doi.org/10.1016/j.eururo.2012.07.033.
2. Witjes JA, Bruins HM, Cathomas R, Compérat EM, Cowan NC, Gakis G, et al. European Association of Urology guidelines on muscle-invasive and metastatic bladder cancer: summary of the 2020 guidelines. Eur Urol. 2020; https://doi.org/10.1016/j.eururo.2020.03.055.
3. Babaian RJ, Johnson DE, Llamas L, Ayala AG. Metastases from transitional cell carcinoma of urinary bladder. Urology. 1980;16(2):142–4. https://doi.org/10.1016/0090-4295(80)90067-9.
4. von der Maase H, Sengelov L, Roberts JT, Ricci S, Dogliotti L, Oliver T, et al. Long-term survival results of a randomized trial comparing gemcitabine plus cisplatin, with methotrexate, vinblastine, doxorubicin, plus cisplatin in patients with bladder cancer. J Clin Oncol. 2005;23(21):4602–8. https://doi.org/10.1200/jco.2005.07.757.
5. Bajorin DF, Dodd PM, Mazumdar M, Fazzari M, McCaffrey JA, Scher HI, et al. Long-term survival in metastatic transitional-cell carcinoma and prognostic factors predicting outcome of therapy. J Clin Oncol. 1999;17(10):3173–81. https://doi.org/10.1200/jco.1999.17.10.3173.
6. Bellmunt J, Albanell J, Paz-Ares L, Climent MA, González-Larriba JL, Carles J, et al. Pretreatment prognostic factors for survival in patients with advanced urothelial tumors treated in a phase I/II trial with paclitaxel, cisplatin, and gemcitabine. Cancer. 2002;95(4):751–7. https://doi.org/10.1002/cncr.10762.
7. Bellmunt J, Choueiri TK, Fougeray R, Schutz FA, Salhi Y, Winquist E, et al. Prognostic factors in patients with advanced transitional cell carcinoma of the urothelial tract experiencing treatment failure with platinum-containing regimens. J Clin Oncol. 2010;28(11):1850–5. https://doi.org/10.1200/jco.2009.25.4599.
8. Loehrer PJ Sr, Einhorn LH, Elson PJ, Crawford ED, Kuebler P, Tannock I, et al. A randomized comparison of cisplatin alone or in combination with methotrexate, vinblastine, and doxorubi-

cin in patients with metastatic urothelial carcinoma: a cooperative group study. J Clin Oncol. 1992;10(7):1066–73. https://doi.org/10.1200/jco.1992.10.7.1066.
9. Kaufman D, Raghavan D, Carducci M, Levine EG, Murphy B, Aisner J, et al. Phase II trial of gemcitabine plus cisplatin in patients with metastatic urothelial cancer. J Clin Oncol. 2000;18(9):1921–7. https://doi.org/10.1200/jco.2000.18.9.1921.
10. von der Maase H, Hansen SW, Roberts JT, Dogliotti L, Oliver T, Moore MJ, et al. Gemcitabine and cisplatin versus methotrexate, vinblastine, doxorubicin, and cisplatin in advanced or metastatic bladder cancer: results of a large, randomized, multinational, multicenter, phase III study. J Clin Oncol. 2000;18(17):3068–77. https://doi.org/10.1200/jco.2000.18.17.3068.
11. Sternberg CN, de Mulder P, Schornagel JH, Theodore C, Fossa SD, van Oosterom AT, et al. Seven year update of an EORTC phase III trial of high-dose intensity M-VAC chemotherapy and G-CSF versus classic M-VAC in advanced urothelial tract tumours. Eur J Cancer. 2006;42(1):50–4. https://doi.org/10.1016/j.ejca.2005.08.032.
12. Bamias A, Dafni U, Karadimou A, Timotheadou E, Aravantinos G, Psyrri A, et al. Prospective, open-label, randomized, phase III study of two dose-dense regimens MVAC versus gemcitabine/cisplatin in patients with inoperable, metastatic or relapsed urothelial cancer: a Hellenic Cooperative Oncology Group study (HE 16/03). Ann Oncol. 2013;24(4):1011–7. https://doi.org/10.1093/annonc/mds583.
13. Bellmunt J, von der Maase H, Mead GM, Skoneczna I, De Santis M, Daugaard G, et al. Randomized phase III study comparing paclitaxel/cisplatin/gemcitabine and gemcitabine/cisplatin in patients with locally advanced or metastatic urothelial cancer without prior systemic therapy: EORTC Intergroup Study 30987. J Clin Oncol. 2012;30(10):1107–13. https://doi.org/10.1200/jco.2011.38.6979.
14. Galsky MD, Hahn NM, Rosenberg J, Sonpavde G, Hutson T, Oh WK, et al. A consensus definition of patients with metastatic urothelial carcinoma who are unfit for cisplatin-based chemotherapy. Lancet Oncol. 2011;12(3):211–4. https://doi.org/10.1016/s1470-2045(10)70275-8.
15. De Santis M, Bellmunt J, Mead G, Kerst JM, Leahy M, Maroto P, et al. Randomized phase II/III trial assessing gemcitabine/carboplatin and methotrexate/carboplatin/vinblastine in patients with advanced urothelial cancer who are unfit for cisplatin-based chemotherapy: EORTC study 30986. J Clin Oncol. 2012;30(2):191–9. https://doi.org/10.1200/jco.2011.37.3571.
16. Holmsten K, Jensen NV, Mouritsen LS, Jonsson E, Mellnert C, Agerbæk M, et al. Vinflunine/gemcitabine versus carboplatin/gemcitabine as first-line treatment in cisplatin-ineligible patients with advanced urothelial carcinoma: a randomised phase II trial (VINGEM). Eur J Cancer. 2020;127:173–82. https://doi.org/10.1016/j.ejca.2019.08.033.
17. Balar AV, Galsky MD, Rosenberg JE, Powles T, Petrylak DP, Bellmunt J, et al. Atezolizumab as first-line treatment in cisplatin-ineligible patients with locally advanced and metastatic urothelial carcinoma: a single-arm, multicentre, phase 2 trial. Lancet. 2017;389(10064):67–76. https://doi.org/10.1016/s0140-6736(16)32455-2.
18. Balar AV, Castellano D, O'Donnell PH, Grivas P, Vuky J, Powles T, et al. First-line pembrolizumab in cisplatin-ineligible patients with locally advanced and unresectable or metastatic urothelial cancer (KEYNOTE-052): a multicentre, single-arm, phase 2 study. Lancet Oncol. 2017;18(11):1483–92. https://doi.org/10.1016/s1470-2045(17)30616-2.
19. Vuky J, Balar AV, Castellano D, O'Donnell PH, Grivas P, Bellmunt J, et al. Long-term outcomes in KEYNOTE-052: phase II study investigating first-line pembrolizumab in cisplatin-ineligible patients with locally advanced or metastatic urothelial cancer. J Clin Oncol. 2020;38(23):2658–66. https://doi.org/10.1200/jco.19.01213.
20. Galsky MD, Pal SK, Mortazavi A, Milowsky MI, George S, Gupta S, et al. Randomized double-blind phase II study of maintenance pembrolizumab versus placebo after first-line chemotherapy in patients (pts) with metastatic urothelial cancer (mUC): HCRN GU14-182. J Clin Oncol. 2019;37(15_suppl):4504. https://doi.org/10.1200/JCO.2019.37.15_suppl.4504.
21. Powles T, Park SH, Voog E, Caserta C, Valderrama BP, Gurney H, et al. Avelumab maintenance therapy for advanced or metastatic urothelial carcinoma. N Engl J Med. 2020;383(13):1218–30. https://doi.org/10.1056/NEJMoa2002788.

22. Rosenberg JE, Hoffman-Censits J, Powles T, van der Heijden MS, Balar AV, Necchi A, et al. Atezolizumab in patients with locally advanced and metastatic urothelial carcinoma who have progressed following treatment with platinum-based chemotherapy: a single-arm, multicentre, phase 2 trial. Lancet. 2016;387(10031):1909–20. https://doi.org/10.1016/s0140-6736(16)00561-4.
23. Powles T, Durán I, van der Heijden MS, Loriot Y, Vogelzang NJ, De Giorgi U, et al. Atezolizumab versus chemotherapy in patients with platinum-treated locally advanced or metastatic urothelial carcinoma (IMvigor211): a multicentre, open-label, phase 3 randomised controlled trial. Lancet. 2018;391(10122):748–57. https://doi.org/10.1016/s0140-6736(17)33297-x.
24. Bellmunt J, de Wit R, Vaughn DJ, Fradet Y, Lee JL, Fong L, et al. Pembrolizumab as second-line therapy for advanced urothelial carcinoma. N Engl J Med. 2017;376(11):1015–26. https://doi.org/10.1056/NEJMoa1613683.
25. Fradet Y, Bellmunt J, Vaughn DJ, Lee JL, Fong L, Vogelzang NJ, et al. Randomized phase III KEYNOTE-045 trial of pembrolizumab versus paclitaxel, docetaxel, or vinflunine in recurrent advanced urothelial cancer: results of >2 years of follow-up. Ann Oncol. 2019;30(6):970–6. https://doi.org/10.1093/annonc/mdz127.
26. Sharma P, Callahan MK, Bono P, Kim J, Spiliopoulou P, Calvo E, et al. Nivolumab monotherapy in recurrent metastatic urothelial carcinoma (CheckMate 032): a multicentre, open-label, two-stage, multi-arm, phase 1/2 trial. Lancet Oncol. 2016;17(11):1590–8. https://doi.org/10.1016/s1470-2045(16)30496-x.
27. Sharma P, Retz M, Siefker-Radtke A, Baron A, Necchi A, Bedke J, et al. Nivolumab in metastatic urothelial carcinoma after platinum therapy (CheckMate 275): a multicentre, single-arm, phase 2 trial. Lancet Oncol. 2017;18(3):312–22. https://doi.org/10.1016/s1470-2045(17)30065-7.
28. Galsky MD, Saci A, Szabo PM, Han GC, Grossfeld G, Collette S, et al. Nivolumab in patients with advanced platinum-resistant urothelial carcinoma: efficacy, safety, and biomarker analyses with extended follow-up from CheckMate 275. Clin Cancer Res. 2020;26(19):5120–8. https://doi.org/10.1158/1078-0432.Ccr-19-4162.
29. Patel MR, Ellerton J, Infante JR, Agrawal M, Gordon M, Aljumaily R, et al. Avelumab in metastatic urothelial carcinoma after platinum failure (JAVELIN Solid Tumor): pooled results from two expansion cohorts of an open-label, phase 1 trial. Lancet Oncol. 2018;19(1):51–64. https://doi.org/10.1016/s1470-2045(17)30900-2.
30. Powles T, O'Donnell PH, Massard C, Arkenau HT, Friedlander TW, Hoimes CJ, et al. Efficacy and safety of durvalumab in locally advanced or metastatic urothelial carcinoma: updated results from a phase 1/2 open-label study. JAMA Oncol. 2017;3(9):e172411. https://doi.org/10.1001/jamaoncol.2017.2411.
31. Bellmunt J, Théodore C, Demkov T, Komyakov B, Sengelov L, Daugaard G, et al. Phase III trial of vinflunine plus best supportive care compared with best supportive care alone after a platinum-containing regimen in patients with advanced transitional cell carcinoma of the urothelial tract. J Clin Oncol. 2009;27(27):4454–61. https://doi.org/10.1200/jco.2008.20.5534.
32. Witte RS, Elson P, Bono B, Knop R, Richardson RR, Dreicer R, et al. Eastern Cooperative Oncology Group phase II trial of ifosfamide in the treatment of previously treated advanced urothelial carcinoma. J Clin Oncol. 1997;15(2):589–93. https://doi.org/10.1200/jco.1997.15.2.589.
33. Lorusso V, Pollera CF, Antimi M, Luporini G, Gridelli C, Frassineti GL, et al. A phase II study of gemcitabine in patients with transitional cell carcinoma of the urinary tract previously treated with platinum. Italian Co-operative Group on Bladder Cancer. Eur J Cancer. 1998;34(8):1208–12. https://doi.org/10.1016/s0959-8049(98)00030-6.
34. Roth BJ, Dreicer R, Einhorn LH, Neuberg D, Johnson DH, Smith JL, et al. Significant activity of paclitaxel in advanced transitional-cell carcinoma of the urothelium: a phase II trial of the Eastern Cooperative Oncology Group. J Clin Oncol. 1994;12(11):2264–70. https://doi.org/10.1200/jco.1994.12.11.2264.
35. McCaffrey JA, Hilton S, Mazumdar M, Sadan S, Kelly WK, Scher HI, et al. Phase II trial of docetaxel in patients with advanced or metastatic transitional-cell carcinoma. J Clin Oncol. 1997;15(5):1853–7. https://doi.org/10.1200/jco.1997.15.5.1853.

36. Haugsten EM, Wiedlocha A, Olsnes S, Wesche J. Roles of fibroblast growth factor receptors in carcinogenesis. Mol Cancer Res. 2010;8(11):1439–52. https://doi.org/10.1158/1541-7786.Mcr-10-0168.
37. Knowles MA, Hurst CD. Molecular biology of bladder cancer: new insights into pathogenesis and clinical diversity. Nat Rev Cancer. 2015;15(1):25–41. https://doi.org/10.1038/nrc3817.
38. Milowsky MI, Dittrich C, Durán I, Jagdev S, Millard FE, Sweeney CJ, et al. Phase 2 trial of dovitinib in patients with progressive FGFR3-mutated or FGFR3 wild-type advanced urothelial carcinoma. Eur J Cancer. 2014;50(18):3145–52. https://doi.org/10.1016/j.ejca.2014.10.013.
39. Loriot Y, Necchi A, Park SH, Garcia-Donas J, Huddart R, Burgess E, et al. Erdafitinib in locally advanced or metastatic urothelial carcinoma. N Engl J Med. 2019;381(4):338–48. https://doi.org/10.1056/NEJMoa1817323.
40. Challita-Eid PM, Satpayev D, Yang P, An Z, Morrison K, Shostak Y, et al. Enfortumab vedotin antibody-drug conjugate targeting Nectin-4 is a highly potent therapeutic agent in multiple preclinical cancer models. Cancer Res. 2016;76(10):3003–13. https://doi.org/10.1158/0008-5472.Can-15-1313.
41. Heath EI, Rosenberg JE. The biology and rationale of targeting nectin-4 in urothelial carcinoma. Nat Rev Urol. 2020. https://doi.org/10.1038/s41585-020-00394-5.
42. Rosenberg JE, O'Donnell PH, Balar AV, McGregor BA, Heath EI, Yu EY, et al. Pivotal trial of enfortumab vedotin in urothelial carcinoma after platinum and anti-programmed death 1/programmed death ligand 1 therapy. J Clin Oncol. 2019;37(29):2592–600. https://doi.org/10.1200/jco.19.01140.
43. Galsky MD, Arija JÁA, Bamias A, Davis ID, De Santis M, Kikuchi E, et al. Atezolizumab with or without chemotherapy in metastatic urothelial cancer (IMvigor130): a multicentre, randomised, placebo-controlled phase 3 trial. Lancet. 2020;395(10236):1547–57. https://doi.org/10.1016/s0140-6736(20)30230-0.
44. Alva A, Csőszi T, Ozguroglu M, Matsubara N, Geczi L, Cheng SY, et al. Pembrolizumab (P) combined with chemotherapy (C) vs C alone as first-line (1L) therapy for advanced urothelial carcinoma (UC): KEYNOTE-361. Ann Oncol. 2020;31:S1142–S215. https://doi.org/10.1016/annonc/annonc325.
45. Motzer RJ, Tannir NM, McDermott DF, Arén Frontera O, Melichar B, Choueiri TK, et al. Nivolumab plus ipilimumab versus sunitinib in advanced renal-cell carcinoma. N Engl J Med. 2018;378(14):1277–90. https://doi.org/10.1056/NEJMoa1712126.
46. Hellmann MD, Paz-Ares L, Bernabe Caro R, Zurawski B, Kim SW, Carcereny Costa E, et al. Nivolumab plus ipilimumab in advanced non-small-cell lung cancer. N Engl J Med. 2019;381(21):2020–31. https://doi.org/10.1056/NEJMoa1910231.
47. Sharma P, Siefker-Radtke A, de Braud F, Basso U, Calvo E, Bono P, et al. Nivolumab alone and with ipilimumab in previously treated metastatic urothelial carcinoma: CheckMate 032 nivolumab 1 mg/kg plus ipilimumab 3 mg/kg expansion cohort results. J Clin Oncol. 2019;37(19):1608–16. https://doi.org/10.1200/jco.19.00538.
48. Powles T, van der Heijden MS, Castellano D, Galsky MD, Loriot Y, Petrylak DP, et al. Durvalumab alone and durvalumab plus tremelimumab versus chemotherapy in previously untreated patients with unresectable, locally advanced or metastatic urothelial carcinoma (DANUBE): a randomised, open-label, multicentre, phase 3 trial. Lancet Oncol. 2020;21(12):1574–88. https://doi.org/10.1016/s1470-2045(20)30541-6.
49. Petrylak DP, de Wit R, Chi KN, Drakaki A, Sternberg CN, Nishiyama H, et al. Ramucirumab plus docetaxel versus placebo plus docetaxel in patients with locally advanced or metastatic urothelial carcinoma after platinum-based therapy (RANGE): overall survival and updated results of a randomised, double-blind, phase 3 trial. Lancet Oncol. 2020;21(1):105–20. https://doi.org/10.1016/s1470-2045(19)30668-0.
50. Rosenberg JE, Ballman KV, Halabi S, Watt C, Hahn OM, Steen PD, et al. CALGB 90601 (Alliance): randomized, double-blind, placebo-controlled phase III trial comparing gemcitabine and cisplatin with bevacizumab or placebo in patients with metastatic urothelial carcinoma. J Clin Oncol. 2019;37(15_suppl):4503. https://doi.org/10.1200/JCO.2019.37.15_suppl.4503.

51. Apolo AB, Nadal R, Girardi DM, Niglio SA, Ley L, Cordes LM, et al. Phase I study of cabozantinib and nivolumab alone or with ipilimumab for advanced or metastatic urothelial carcinoma and other genitourinary tumors. J Clin Oncol. 2020;38(31):3672–84. https://doi.org/10.1200/jco.20.01652.
52. Taylor MH, Lee CH, Makker V, Rasco D, Dutcus CE, Wu J, et al. Phase IB/II trial of lenvatinib plus pembrolizumab in patients with advanced renal cell carcinoma, endometrial cancer, and other selected advanced solid tumors. J Clin Oncol. 2020;38(11):1154–63. https://doi.org/10.1200/jco.19.01598.
53. Bardia A, Mayer IA, Vahdat LT, Tolaney SM, Isakoff SJ, Diamond JR, et al. Sacituzumab govitecan-hziy in refractory metastatic triple-negative breast cancer. N Engl J Med. 2019;380(8):741–51. https://doi.org/10.1056/NEJMoa1814213.
54. Tagawa ST, Faltas BM, Lam ET, Saylor PJ, Bardia A, Hajdenberg J, et al. Sacituzumab govitecan (IMMU-132) in patients with previously treated metastatic urothelial cancer (mUC): results from a phase I/II study. J Clin Oncol. 2019;37(7_suppl):354. https://doi.org/10.1200/JCO.2019.37.7_suppl.354.
55. Tagawa ST, Balar A, Petrylak DP, Grivas P, Agarwal N, Sternberg CN, et al. Initial results from TROPHY-U-01: a phase II open-label study of sacituzumab govitecan in patients (Pts) with metastatic urothelial cancer (mUC) after failure of platinum-based regimens (PLT) or immunotherapy. Ann Oncol. 2019;30:v890–v1. https://doi.org/10.1093/annonc/mdz394.049.
56. Mejri N, Sellami R, Lamia C, Raoudha D, Hmida NB, Sriha B, et al. Status of Her2 over expression in muscle invasive urothelial bladder carcinoma: report of 21 cases. Urol Ann. 2014;6(1):63–7. https://doi.org/10.4103/0974-7796.127033.
57. Tsurutani J, Iwata H, Krop I, Jänne PA, Doi T, Takahashi S, et al. Targeting HER2 with trastuzumab deruxtecan: a dose-expansion, phase I study in multiple advanced solid tumors. Cancer Discov. 2020;10(5):688–701. https://doi.org/10.1158/2159-8290.Cd-19-1014.
58. Modi S, Saura C, Yamashita T, Park YH, Kim SB, Tamura K, et al. Trastuzumab deruxtecan in previously treated HER2-positive breast cancer. N Engl J Med. 2020;382(7):610–21. https://doi.org/10.1056/NEJMoa1914510.
59. Shitara K, Bang YJ, Iwasa S, Sugimoto N, Ryu MH, Sakai D, et al. Trastuzumab deruxtecan in previously treated HER2-positive gastric cancer. N Engl J Med. 2020;382(25):2419–30. https://doi.org/10.1056/NEJMoa2004413.
60. Hussain M, Vaishampayan U, Du W, Redman B, Smith DC. Combination paclitaxel, carboplatin, and gemcitabine is an active treatment for advanced urothelial cancer. J Clin Oncol. 2001;19(9):2527–33. https://doi.org/10.1200/jco.2001.19.9.2527.
61. Galsky MD, Iasonos A, Mironov S, Scattergood J, Donat SM, Bochner BH, et al. Prospective trial of ifosfamide, paclitaxel, and cisplatin in patients with advanced non-transitional cell carcinoma of the urothelial tract. Urology. 2007;69(2):255–9. https://doi.org/10.1016/j.urology.2006.10.029.
62. Smith DC, Mackler NJ, Dunn RL, Hussain M, Wood D, Lee CT, et al. Phase II trial of paclitaxel, carboplatin and gemcitabine in patients with locally advanced carcinoma of the bladder. J Urol. 2008;180(6):2384–8; discussion 8. https://doi.org/10.1016/j.juro.2008.08.075.

Chapter 20
Treatment of Upper Tract Urothelial Carcinoma

Kathleen M. Olson, Kassem S. Faraj, Parminder Singh, and Mark D. Tyson

Terminology, Units, Abbreviations

AC	Adjuvant chemotherapy
CSS	Cancer-specific survival
CIS	Carcinoma in situ
CI	Confidence interval
ddMVAC	Dose-dense methotrexate, vinblastine, doxorubicin, cisplatin
GC	Gemcitabine/cisplatin
HR	Hazard ratio
LND	Lymph node dissection
MVAC	Methotrexate, vinblastine, doxorubicin, cisplatin
NAC	Neoadjuvant chemotherapy
OS	Overall survival
PFS	Progression-free survival
RNU	Radical nephroureterectomy
RFS	Recurrence-free survival
UTUC	Upper tract urothelial carcinoma
UC	Urothelial carcinoma

K. M. Olson · K. S. Faraj · M. D. Tyson (✉)
Department of Urology, Mayo Clinic Arizona, Phoenix, AZ, USA
e-mail: Olson.kathleen1@mayo.edu; Faraj.kassem@mayo.edu; Tyson.mark@mayo.edu

P. Singh
Department of Medicine/Division of Hematology and Oncology, Mayo Clinic Arizona, Phoenix, AZ, USA
e-mail: Singh.Parminder@mayo.edu

K. L. Stratton, A. K. Morgans (eds.), *Urologic Oncology*,
https://doi.org/10.1007/978-3-030-89891-5_20

Background

Epidemiology

Upper tract urothelial carcinoma (UTUC) accounts for approximately 10% of all urothelial cancers [1, 2]. Renal pelvis tumors are twice as common as ureteral tumors, and concomitant carcinoma in situ (CIS) occurs in up to 31% of cases [1]. This is usually a disease of the elderly with a mean age around 70 years [1]. Around 60% of patients present with invasive disease, including 10% with metastatic disease [1]. Histologically, pure urothelial carcinoma is most common, but variant histological subtypes are observed in up to 25% of cases, with squamous differentiation being the most common [3]. Variant histological subtypes are often associated with worse prognoses, especially the sarcomatoid, micropapillary, and small cell variants [3, 4].

Urothelial carcinoma (UC) can affect the entire urothelium and tends to be a multifocal disease. Consequently, it is not uncommon for patients to be diagnosed with synchronous or metachronous UC of the upper and lower tracts [5]. About 10% of patients with history of bladder cancer develop UTUC, whereas up to 50% of patients with UTUC subsequently develop bladder cancer [5]. Thus, depending on the patient's risk status, assessment of the entire urothelium may be needed at various intervals during the management and surveillance of patients with UC.

Risk Factors

Tobacco use, aristolochic acid (AA) intake, alcohol consumption, occupational exposures (aniline dyes), anti-inflammatory medication (phenacetin), chemotherapeutics (cyclophosphamide), and genetic disorders are all risk factors for developing UTUC.

Tobacco use increases the risk of developing UTUC by as much as six-fold, and the risk increases with cumulative smoking exposure [6]. In addition, continued smoking is associated with worse prognosis in patients with a UTUC diagnosis, and smoking cessation can mitigate these adverse outcomes [7].

Aristolochic acid is a substance found in plants that has been attributed to advanced renal disease and UTUC. It irreversibly injures the renal cortex, leading to extensive interstitial fibrosis and end-stage renal disease [8]. Its exposure can either be through environmental contamination of agricultural products by aristolochic contaminated plants or ingestion of aristolochic based herbal remedies [8, 9]. The former is the likely etiology in cases of Balkan endemic nephropathy, where exposure to the substance occurs through contamination of locally grown wheat, while the latter was identified in individuals consuming high doses of AA in a herbal mix used in weight loss clinics [8, 10]. The association with UTUC was suspected in early reports of cellular atypia in patients with aristolochic induced nephropathy and case reports of patients with aristolochic induced nephropathy who developed urothelial cell carcinoma [11, 12]. One later study reported that up to half of patients with aristolochic induced nephropathy are subsequently found to have urothelial carcinoma [13].

Alcohol consumption has also been linked to UTUC. In a case-control study, alcohol consumption was significantly higher in patients with urothelial carcinoma (OR 1.23). Strengthening the causal link, a dose-response was observed with higher consumption associated with increasing risk [14].

Exposures to other substances such as analgesics, cyclophosphamide, and arsenic have been weakly associated with increased risk of developing UTUC, but results have been inconsistent [6, 9, 15–17].

Genetic Factors

The molecular changes observed in patients with UTUC are similar to those seen in bladder cancer [18]. The most common mutations seen in sporadic UTUC include alterations in FGFR3, KMT2D, KDM6A, STAG2, cdkN2A, TP53, PIK3CA, and TSC1 [19]. Additionally, mutations in the mismatch repair process can be associated with UTUC in patients with Lynch syndrome and can be present in around 5% of patients diagnosed with UTUC [20].

Lynch Syndrome

Upper tract urothelial carcinoma is the third most common cancer in Lynch syndrome [21]. Lynch syndrome is caused by germline mutations in the mismatch repair genes MLH1, MSH2, MSH6, or PMS2. Mutations in these genes lead to microsatellite errors during replication [22]. These patients are up to 22 times more likely to develop UTUC compared to the general population [21]. The Amsterdam Criteria I and II can be used to help identify families who are likely to have Lynch syndrome [23]. According to the EAU guidelines, the diagnosis of Lynch syndrome should be suspected in patients with one or more of the following: (1) metachronous Lynch syndrome-related cancer (colorectal, endometrial, ovarian, stomach, small intestine), (2) age <65 years with UTUC, (3) first-degree relative with a Lynch-related cancer younger than 50 years of age, or (4) two first-degree relatives with Lynch syndrome-related cancer [24]. If any of the above is suspected, patients can be referred for germline testing and individual/family genetic counseling for follow-up and evaluation for other Lynch-related cancers.

Diagnosis

Evaluation for UTUC is most often prompted by presenting symptoms. Symptoms of UTUC can include microscopic hematuria, gross hematuria, flank pain, or constitutional symptoms in advanced cases [24]. The gold standard cross-sectional imaging test is a CT scan with intravenous contrast and delayed images (CT urogram), where the classic finding is a filling defect on delayed imaging (Fig. 20.1). CT urogram has high accuracy for diagnosing UTUC, with around 92% sensitivity and 95% specificity [25]. In patients who cannot undergo CT imaging, MRI with delayed imaging is also an option, though the sensitivity is lower at around 63% [26].

Another critical tool used in the diagnosis, management, and surveillance of patients with UTUC is cystoscopy. Assessing the bladder mucosa is important, as concomitant bladder cancer is present in up to 30% of patients presenting with UTUC [27]. Once the diagnosis of UTUC is suspected, pathological evaluation is important in determining management options. Pathologic specimens are obtained through either ureteroscopic biopsy or percutaneous biopsy. Ureteroscopy has the benefit of allowing direct visualization of the tumors (Fig. 20.2) and multiple techniques for obtaining tissue. These include ureteral brush biopsy, forceps biopsy, or basket biopsy [28]. Percutaneous biopsy approaches are typically performed by interventional radiology teams using ultrasound or CT-guided approaches. Though case reports exist describing possible tumor seeding after biopsy, studies have reported extremely low rates of seeding with percutaneous biopsy making this approach a good alternative when endoscopic biopsy attempts have failed [29, 30].

Urine tests can also be used in the evaluation of these patients. Urine cytology is less sensitive for UTUC than for bladder cancer; however cytology obtained from barbotaged urine can have sensitivities over 90% [31]. Fluorescence in situ hybridization (FISH) analysis is another urine-based biomarker, but the performance is suboptimal, with a sensitivity of 50% [32].

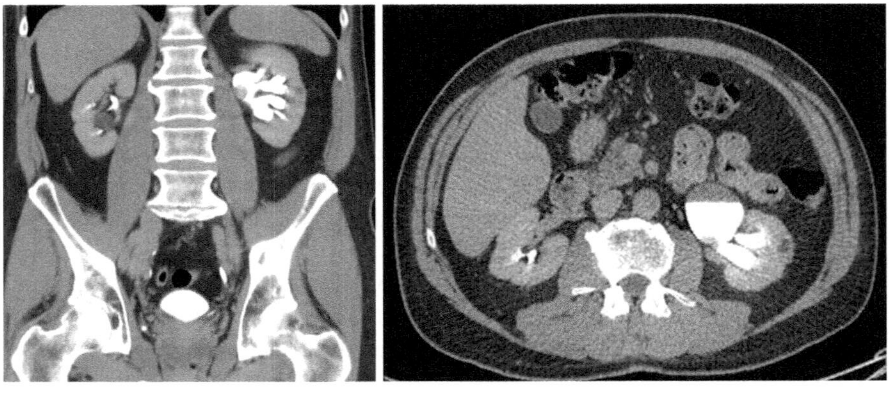

Fig. 20.1 CT images of suspected upper tract urothelial carcinoma in the left renal pelvis. Delayed images demonstrate filling defect in the renal pelvis suspicious of urothelial carcinoma

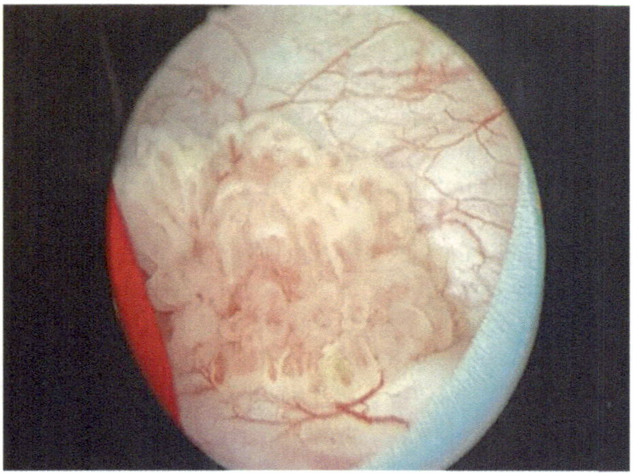

Fig. 20.2 Ureteroscopic image of papillary tumor in the renal pelvis that was confirmed to be a non-invasive low-grade urothelial carcinoma

Enhanced Imaging Modalities

In cases where the suspected area is not clearly visualized, visualization can be supplemented with enhanced imaging modalities. These enhanced imaging modalities have demonstrated efficacy in the diagnosis of patients with urothelial cancer of the bladder, though there is less data available regarding use in the upper tracts [33, 34].

While the use of enhanced ureteroscopy in the upper tracts is not typical, some data suggest it may be a useful adjunct. Kata et al. assessed the diagnostic ability of blue light ureteroscopy and found that it detected more UTUC tumors than both CT urogram and white light ureteroscopy with over 95% of tumors detected on blue light [35, 36]. Narrow-band imaging (NBI) has also been evaluated for use in the upper tracts and has been shown to improve tumor detection by 23% [37]. While these technologies have demonstrated promising results in the detection and localization of UTUC, and especially CIS, their value as it relates to oncologic outcomes will need to be verified in the setting of one or more clinical trials.

Staging

Accurate staging may be difficult, due to limitations in obtaining sufficient samples during biopsy; however there are several nomograms that can be used that can help one predict the probability of invasive or non-organ confined disease with relatively good accuracy [38–40]. Staging is done using the TNM classification for staging tumors [41]:

TX Primary tumor cannot be assessed.
T0 No evidence of primary tumor.

Ta: Non-invasive papillary carcinoma
Tis: Carcinoma in situ

T1 Tumor invades subepithelial connective tissue.
T2 Tumor invades muscularis.
T3 Tumor invades beyond muscularis into the periureteric fat (ureter).
Tumor invades beyond muscularis into the peripelvic fat or renal parenchyma (renal pelvis).
T4 Tumor invades adjacent organs or through the kidney into perinephric fat.
NX Regional lymph nodes cannot be assessed.
N0 No regional lymph node metastasis.
N1 Metastasis in a single lymph node 2 cm or less in greatest dimension.
N2 Metastasis in a single lymph node 2 cm or greater in greatest dimension or multiple lymph nodes.
M0 No distant metastasis.
M1 Distant metastasis.

Prognosis

There are several factors that have been found to be prognostic in the management of patients with UTUC. In general, prognostic factors can be grouped into three categories: pre-operative/clinical factors, surgical/pathologic factors, and molecular markers [42].

Pre-operative Factors

Certain demographic factors and overall patient health have been found to be prognostic factors for UTUC. Age has been identified as an independent predictor of worse cancer-specific survival (CSS) and overall survival (OS) in patients with UTUC in retrospective studies [38]. In addition, elderly patients have been found to present with more aggressive disease [38, 42]. With regard to ethnicity, some data has suggested poorer survival outcomes in persons of color [1]. Other patient-level factors include poor performance status [39], obesity [43], and tobacco use [7, 40, 44].

There are several disease-specific factors that affect survival as well. Ureteral tumor location and multifocal tumors have been described as factors associated with worse prognosis in retrospective studies [45, 46]. However, studies have been inconsistent with regard to the effect of tumor location on survival outcomes [43]. High tumor stage is a known factor associated with worse outcomes in patients with UTUC, but there are limitations in predicting tumor stage prior to surgery. As discussed previously, several nomograms aim to decrease this limitation by using histological and radiological factors to predict invasive disease [47, 48]. With surgical timing, delay to definitive radical nephroureterectomy (RNU) >3 months in patients with high-risk disease has been associated with more aggressive pathological features and worse recurrence-free survival (RFS) and CSS in some studies, though these results have not been consistent [49–51]. Other factors that have been associated with worse oncological outcomes include pre-operative hydronephrosis [52], higher American Society of Anesthesiologist score [53], and previous/synchronous bladder cancer [54].

Surgical/Post-operative Factors

Pathological tumor stage is an important factor for the prognosis of patients with UTUC. Based on several studies, tumor stage has been found to be a significant factor associated with oncological outcomes, with a steep reduction in survival with advanced tumor stage. For instance, examples of 5-year CSS rates for pTa/pT1, pT2, pT3, and pT4 disease are >90%, 70–80%, 50–55%, and 0–35% [45, 55–58]. Tumor grade is also an established factor associated with survival, where high-grade disease is significantly associated with worse outcomes compared to low-grade disease [58]. Lymph node involvement is an important factor associated with worse RFS and CSS [55, 56] with lymph node-positive patients demonstrating significantly worse 5-year RFS and CSS, compared to patients with no evidence of lymph node involvement (29.0% vs 73.4% and 35.3% vs. 77.3%, respectively) [58]. Lymphovascular invasion is found in approximately 20% of patients after RNU and is associated with a greater risk of mortality and recurrence [59]. Another operative outcome that has important prognostic implications is the status of the soft tissue surgical margin at the time of RNU. In a multicenter review, a positive margin was associated with worse metastasis-free survival and CSS [60]. Other factors that have been associated with worse oncological outcomes include sessile tumor growth [61], larger tumor size [62], tumor multifocality [56], and tumor necrosis [63].

Molecular Markers

The prognostic role of multiple biomarkers has been investigated in UTUC. However, the rarity of the disease limits definitive conclusions related to these biomarkers. Examples of the types of markers include cell adhesion molecules (E-Cadherin, Beta-Catenin, Parvin-Beta, CD24), markers associated with microsatellite instability, cell differentiation (Uroplakin III), angiogenesis (HIF-1 alpha), cell cycle regulation (p53), cell proliferation (Ki-67, EGFR), apoptosis (Bcl-2), vascular invasion, PD-1 pathway, and inflammatory cells (C-reactive protein, leukocytes) [42].

Management

The management of patients with localized UTUC is typically dictated by the patient's tumor risk status as well as the patient's comorbidities. Risk stratification into low- or high-risk groups can typically be determined by the tumor's histological and radiographic appearance [24]. Some studies and guidelines have suggested risk stratification as follows [24, 64]:

- High-risk
  - Hydronephrosis
  - Tumor >2 cm
  - High-grade cytology
  - Multifocal
  - Prior radical cystectomy for high-grade disease
  - Variant histology
- Low-risk
  - Unifocal
  - Tumor <2 cm
  - Low-grade cytology
  - Low-grade biopsy
  - Non-invasive on imaging

Management of localized UTUC can be split into two categories: kidney-sparing approaches and radical surgery. Low-risk patients are typically better suited for kidney-sparing techniques which include endoscopic procedures, percutaneous tumor resection, segmental ureteral resection, and intracavitary chemotherapy instillation.

Endoscopic Management

Endoscopic procedures including ureteroscopy with tumor ablation, fulguration, or resection are commonly used for both diagnostic and therapeutic purposes in patients with UTUC. Multiple studies have demonstrated the efficacy of endoscopic management, but most are limited by a retrospective and single-institutional design. In one study with a median follow-up of 54 months, 68% of patients had disease recurrence, and 19% eventually proceeded with RNU [65]. Fortunately, the vast majority of these recurrences (approximately 75%) can be retreated endoscopically using close surveillance strategies [66]. Therefore, appropriately selected patients with UTUC can be managed with endoscopic surgery, but recurrences often occur and about one-third of patients may be at risk for progression and eventually need radical nephroureterectomy.

A Special Note on Ureteroscopy

When ureteroscopy is planned as the management option in a patient with UTUC, there are a few key points to consider. The location of the tumor will dictate what kind of ureteroscope is used (i.e., flexible or semirigid). We prefer to start assessments by first placing a safety wire into the collecting system. If a small tumor is anticipated, a flexible ureteroscope can be advanced under fluoroscopic guidance over the wire to the area of disease taking care to ensure that the entire collecting system and ureter are inspected at some point during the case. The morphology and size of the tumor dictate the appropriate treatment option once the tumor is visualized. For tumors that appear papillary and on a stalk, a ureteroscopic biopsy forceps or stone basket can be used to remove the tumor. The remaining tumor burden should be ablated with holmium:YAG, neodymium:YAG, thulium laser ablation, or Bugbee fulguration. If a semirigid ureteroscope is used for a ureteral tumor, a ureteroscopic resectoscope can be used [67, 68]. This is helpful in cases with flat tumors or when the above options are not adequate for sampling. After completion of the treatment, a ureteral stent should be considered in cases of extensive manipulation, resection, or injury to the collecting system.

Percutaneous Surgery

When tumors are too large to be managed by ureteroscopy and renal preservation is desired, a percutaneous approach can be considered. Percutaneous access is obtained in standard fashion prior to the surgery or at the time of surgery by ultrasound or fluoroscopic approach. The percutaneous tract is then dilated to 30 Fr using balloon dilation system. Next, a rigid nephroscope is placed through sheath and used to identify and remove the tumor using a cold cup forceps [28]. If needed, a resectoscope can be used to resect and fulgurate the base of the tumor. Additional small tumors may occur throughout the collecting system and can be managed using a flexible nephroscope and ablative techniques. A second-look nephroscopy is often done a few days after the index surgery to ensure all tumor has been treated [28]. An 8–14 Fr nephrostomy tube or a ureteral stent can be left in place at the conclusion of the surgery at the surgeon's discretion.

Segmental Ureteral Resection

When there is a large ureteral tumor burden that cannot be addressed endoscopically and/or renal preservation is imperative, segmental ureteral resection can be considered. In terms of efficacy of this approach, a population-based study found that

5-year cancer-specific mortality rates were similar between the RNU and segmental ureteral resection and this was not conditionally changed on multivariable analysis [69]. However, not unexpectedly, there are some data to suggest that this approach is associated with higher risk of recurrence. This is clearly due, at least in part, to the risk of metachronous recurrences in urothelium which is otherwise removed with RNU. In a systematic review and meta-analysis of 4797 total patients, segmental ureterectomy was associated with a shorter 5-year RFS despite presenting with lower stages and grades [70]. Thus, segmental resection is likely associated with a greater risk of recurrence compared to radical surgery, especially in patients with high-risk features.

Intracavitary Instillation

Adjuvant Therapy

UTUC has the propensity to recur, and studies have investigated methods to reduce the risk of recurrence, with similar goals as the methods used in bladder cancer. Intravesical adjuvant instillation with either chemotherapy or BCG is effective in reducing the risk of recurrence in patients with non-muscle-invasive bladder cancer [71]. Similar concepts have been investigated in UTUC with inconsistent results. However, the data are mostly from nonrandomized retrospective comparisons which are heavily biased toward the null due to confounding by indication [58, 72, 73]. Therefore, it is unclear what the true benefit of topical therapy is in the adjuvant setting.

Primary Ablative Therapy

MitoGel

For select cases when surgical resection is not an option, topical therapy can be considered as a primary ablative option. A recently published open-label, single-arm, phase 3 trial evaluated the safety and efficacy of a mitomycin-containing reverse thermal gel as a primary chemoablative agent for low-grade tumors. Seventy-one patients received at least one dose via retrograde stent (4 mg/mL, dosed according to volume in patient's collecting system). Fifty-nine percent of these patients achieved a complete response on ureteroscopy at 3 months, and 70% showed durability at 12 months. This treatment was associated with some adverse effects including ureteral stenosis in 44% of patients [74]. Chemoablative therapy can be considered in patients with low-grade, large volume UTUC above the ureteropelvic junction where endoscopic management may be difficult and/or in those with significant comorbidities who cannot tolerate a major operation.

Radical Surgery

Radical nephroureterectomy remains the treatment of choice for many patients with UTUC. It is most often used in cases of patients with high-grade disease, independent of location, but is also used for those with low-grade tumors with high-risk features.

Low-Grade Disease

Radical nephroureterectomy is indicated as first-line treatment in patients with low-grade tumors with high-risk characteristics. These include hydronephrosis, size greater than 2 cm, multifocality, prior radical cystectomy for bladder cancer, or variant histology [75, 76]. These factors increase the risk of higher stage at time of surgery and need for more aggressive initial treatment for oncological safety. Recurrence-free survival and cancer-specific survival in patients with low-grade disease undergoing RNU are 88.3% and 89.1% at 5 years, respectively [58]. In addition, those with early recurrence despite adequate kidney sparing therapy may benefit from subsequent radical RNU. Those patients who fail initial endoscopic management and proceed to have RNU have similar 5-year OS compared to those who had immediate RNU (64% vs. 59%, respectively), and 43% had progression to, or occult, high-grade disease [72]. Additionally, RNU may be most appropriate for patients who are unable to have close follow-up [75, 76].

High-Grade Disease

The primary role of RNU is in those with localized high-grade disease. Margulis et al. showed a RFS and CSS for those with high-grade disease to be 57.2% and 63.1% at 5 years, respectively [58]. Patients found to have pT3 disease at time of RNU had a RFS of 48.0% and CSS of 54.0% at 5 years [58]. Those with pT4 had a RFS and CSS probability after RNU of 4.7% and 12.2% at 5 years, respectively [58].

Pre-operative Considerations

Preparing a patient to undergo RNU requires careful planning and patient education. Prompt surgery after diagnosis is important to avoid disease progression due to delays in treatment. We hesitate to argue for a definitive timepoint during which surgery should be performed since the predicted risk of metastatic disease increases with each day, but the general rule from the literature is that surgery should be performed within 12 weeks [50, 51, 72, 73, 77]. However, it is not likely that surgery at 11 weeks is substantially different in terms of risk than surgery at 13 weeks, and, in general, we advocate for surgery as soon as possible since delayed surgery is associated with decreased OS [73, 77].

Patients should have pre-operative evaluation with their primary care doctor for clearance and medical optimization. Patients who are actively smoking at time of diagnosis should be counseled on risks, and tobacco cessation should be encouraged. Tobacco use not only increases the risk for recurrence and mortality after RNU but is also associated with poor healing and risk of blood clot [7, 78]. Nutritional status should be optimized, diabetic sugar control evaluated, and obese patients encouraged to lose weight prior to surgery. Other important comorbidities that may contribute to anesthetic risks or post-operative recovery should be appropriately evaluated and treated prior to undergoing surgery.

Antimicrobial prophylaxis is recommended in patients undergoing renal surgery, and we typically use a single dose of a second-generation cephalosporin prior to incision. Urinalysis and culture prior to surgery and evaluation of prior positive cultures can aid in antibiotic selection. Any positive culture must be treated prior to surgery.

All patients undergoing RNU should be counseled on risk of dialysis. There is low risk of progression to dialysis in those patients with normally functioning kidneys and overall good health. However, loss of nephrons and chemotherapy may lead to chronic kidney disease (CKD) in even the healthiest of patients. Patients with GFR <60 mL/min, solitary functioning kidney, or proteinuria are referred to nephrology prior to surgery in our practice [79].

Pre-operative planning also requires evaluation of bloodwork and review of imaging. Complete blood count and basic metabolic panel should be obtained prior to surgery. A type and screen should be performed on all patients, and blood products should be prepared prior to start of surgery for certain cases. Pre-operative review of abdominal imaging is essential to identify number of ureters, arteries, and veins and prepare for any aberrant anatomy. Staging studies of the chest prior to surgery are critical as well.

Surgical Technique

Outcome Comparison for RNU Technique

Choosing a method for RNU depends on the surgeon's comfort with the approach and patient characteristics. Current techniques include open, laparoscopic, and robot-assisted techniques. Whether open or minimally invasive, adherence to basic oncologic principles is paramount to decrease recurrence rates. Strict avoidance of entry into the urinary tract during dissection and complete ureteral resection is essential. Contact between tumor and instruments should be avoided, and the specimen must be removed en bloc using a protective system such as endobag to prevent tumor spillage or seeding [80]. Removal of the entire tumor with a clear margin is essential, as a positive surgical margin is a poor prognostic factor after RNU. The 5-year CSS and metastasis-free survival in patients with positive surgical margin compared to those with negative margin were shown to be 59.1% vs. 83.3% and 51.6% vs. 79.3%, respectively [81].

With the advent of minimally invasive surgery and increasing use of robotics in surgery, several groups have compared oncologic outcome and surgical outcomes based on surgical approach. While the quality of evidence varies, the results of these studies showed that RFS, CSS, OS, and bladder specific recurrence do not significantly differ based on open, laparoscopic, or robotic approach [82–87]. Walton et al. showed comparable outcomes between open and laparoscopic RNU; however, the laparoscopic RNU group had fewer node-positive patients compared to the open RNU group (2.9% vs. 6.8%, $p = 0.041$) [83]. One limitation of these studies is possible selection bias with physicians choosing laparoscopic approach for those with expected N0 disease or smaller tumors. When looking specifically at locally advanced disease (pT3/pT4), data is conflicting [88]. Ariane et al. showed 5-year RFS and CSS in pT3/pT4 patients who had laparoscopic RNU were comparable to open RNU [85]. Conversely, one of the few randomized prospective studies showed a significant difference in metastasis-free survival and CSS between open and laparoscopic RNU [89]. A total of 80 patients were randomized to either open or laparoscopic RNU, and, in patients with high-grade or pT3 disease, significantly better oncologic outcomes were seen in the open RNU group [89]. There is less available literature on comparison of robotic RNU to other approaches, but data suggest equivalent oncologic outcomes [86, 87, 90]. However, robotic RNU is associated with higher frequency of concurrent lymph node dissection when compared to laparoscopic RNU and fewer positive surgical margins when compared to open RNU [87]. Robotic-assisted RNU may become the surgical technique of choice with increasing access to robotic systems and training in residency as it does not seem to compromise oncologic control for most patients and enables lymphadenectomy compared to laparoscopic approaches. A final concern unique to minimally invasive approaches is trocar site or peritoneal seeding from pneumoperitoneum used for visualization. A few studies have reported rare retroperitoneal and trocar site tumor deposition after laparoscopic surgery, but departures from sound oncologic surgical principles were the likely cause in these cases [91, 92].

Minimally invasive and open RNU differs slightly in terms of peri-operative factors but has similar rates of complications. Blood loss appears to be higher in open RNU and surgical time longer in minimally invasive RNU [84, 85]. Time to discharge is significantly lower in laparoscopic or robotic RNU compared to open RNU, but robotic RNU is associated with the highest in-hospital costs [86, 89]. Post-operative complication rate after RNU is about 15%, and incidence does not differ based on operative approach [85]. Complications observed include wound infections, post-operative bleeding, ileus, incisional hernia, and pneumothorax [84]. The majority of complications (8.9%) observed were Clavien I and II, and a total of 4.3% of patients had Clavien III or higher complications [85].

Bladder Cuff Resection

Approach to bladder cuff management is as varied as the approach to RNU. Oncologic surgical principles again are key to prevent tumor spillage and ensure good outcomes. Due to the vast number of approaches to bladder cuff management, the goals in this section will be to review those most frequently used. Depending on the technique planned, the ureter is typically clipped as distally as possible during the nephrectomy portion to prevent tumor spillage. In some cases, applying two clips and using electrocautery to transect the ureter between clips can be used. Cautery is thought to destroy any tumor cells at the site of transection and prevent tumor spillage. For large distal tumors that involve the ureteral orifice or protrude into the bladder, larger bladder cuff, en bloc partial, or radical cystectomy may be required to achieve an appropriate oncologic resection.

Endoscopic

There are multiple endoscopic approaches to bladder cuff management including the "pluck" technique and the intussusception technique as well as variations upon these techniques [93]. The "pluck" technique or transurethral resection of ureteral orifice should only be performed in the absence of bladder tumors and can be used for patients with proximal UTUC [94]. For all endoscopic techniques, the patient should be placed in dorsal lithotomy position. A resectoscope is inserted, and the bladder inspected to ensure intravesical absence of areas suspicious for tumor prior to initiating resection. The ureteral orifice on the ipsilateral side of disease is identified and resected aggressively with Collins knife through the intramural tunnel until fat is visualized. The patient is then repositioned for the nephrectomy portion, and once the ureter is dissected more proximally, it is able to be "plucked" as the distal dissection has already been performed. While this is not our preferred technique, operative time is reported to be the principal advantage of this technique compared to other bladder cuff techniques [95].

Another commonly described endoscopic technique is the intussusception technique. This is only indicated for tumors of the renal pelvis as it requires division of the ureter. A ureteral catheter is placed within the ureter, and, after dissection of the ureter and completion of the nephrectomy, two ties are placed around the distal ureter and the ureter is divided between. A resectoscope is then inserted and using a Collins knife, the bladder cuff incision is made. After the incision is made, the ureteral catheter is pulled into the bladder to allow for the ureter to intussuscept into the bladder and catheter, and specimens are then removed through the urethra. This approach is associated with an 18.7% failure rate for complete ureteral removal, and 15.6% of patients required a second incision for ureteral excision [96].

Open Technique

The open technique for bladder cuff resection can be used with either open or minimally invasive approaches for the nephrectomy portion of the surgery. The principal rationale for this technique in minimally invasive cohorts is that an open incision is going to be required for extraction anyhow. If a midline laparotomy or thoracoabdominal incision is not used, a second incision such as a Pfannenstiel, Gibson, or low midline incision can be used to access the bladder and ureter. After making the incision and bluntly dissecting the space of Retzius, the distal ureter is identified at the location where it crosses over the common iliac artery. Previously placed ureteral clips should be located after dissecting peritoneum off the ureter and vessels and mobilizing the ureter. The ureter is then dissected toward the intramural tunnel, ligating the superficial pedicle of the bladder to allow for better visualization and access to the intramural tunnel. If performing a completely extravesical approach, the ureter is dissected away from the detrusor muscle through the intramural tunnel until there appears to be a circumferential area of bladder mucosa surrounding the ureter. The bladder must be completely drained prior to resecting the bladder cuff. It is helpful to apply a stay stitch at one end of the planned cystotomy to prevent tissue from retracting. We have also found that placing Shallcross or other clamp across the planned bladder cuff and dividing on the bladder side of the clamp prevent tumor spillage and aid in manipulation of the tissues. Prior to division of the bladder cuff, it is important to ensure the contralateral ureteral orifice will not be resected. For a transvesical technique, the bladder is drained after dissection of distal ureter and anterior cystotomy made. The ipsilateral ureteral orifice is identified and dissected with a 1 cm bladder mucosal margin around the orifice. All cystotomies are then closed in a two-layer fashion using absorbable suture.

Laparoscopic Technique

Pure laparoscopic management of bladder cuff can be approached transvesically or via endoscopic stapler, though neither of these are our preferred technique. The transvesical technique is a minimally invasive approach that mimics the en bloc resection principles of open bladder cuff management [97]. The patient is first placed in lithotomy and bladder distended after inserting cystoscope. One to two 5 mm ports are placed into the bladder under direct visualization. The ureteral orifice is controlled by passing an endoloop around the opening. A ureteral catheter is then passed into the ureter to identify the intramural portion and ensure adequate bladder cuff excision. A Collins knife is typically used to incise the bladder cuff until adipose tissue is seen ensuring entry into the extravesical space. The orifice is then grasped with laparoscopic instrument and retracted into the bladder so the endoloop can be passed more proximally along the ureter. The ureteral catheter is then removed and endoloop tightened to prevent tumor spillage. This is a technically difficult option, and history of prior pelvic radiation or concurrent UCC of the bladder is a contraindication to this approach [98].

The laparoscopic stapling technique is used by many physicians due to the decreased operative time and avoidance of urinary tract entry. Prior to the laparoscopic portion of the case, cystoscopy is used to cauterize the ipsilateral ureteral orifice. Once the patient is repositioned and laparoscopic ports placed, the nephrectomy is performed prior to dissection of the distal ureter. The ureter is then dissected to intramural tunnel, ligating the lateral pedicle as needed. The detrusor is dissected off the ureter by applying traction to the ureter. Once dissection is completed, the ureter should be retracted as much as possible without avulsing the ureter with hopes of retracting a rim of bladder mucosa through the dissected intramural tunnel. The endovascular stapler is then placed as distally as possible. Some downsides of using this technique include incomplete pathologic evaluation of the bladder cuff and distal margin due to staples and high risk of incomplete bladder cuff and distal ureteral resection [99]. Using stapling device also poses the theoretical risk of stone encrustation of the staple line. A recent study by Tsivian et al. reported data on a variation of the laparoscopic technique in which a LigaSure device is used rather than stapler to avoid this issue [100].

Robotic Technique

Robotic RNU and bladder cuff excision have been increasing in popularity due to access to robotic equipment and increased robotic surgical training. While some studies report the transvesical technique with second cystotomy used to intravesically dissect the intramural ureter, most studies report use of an extravesical technique which is our preferred approach [101]. Patients are placed in a supine position with the arms tucked and the table flexed and rotated. This permits a side-docking approach and easy rotation of the boom when using the Da Vinci XI system. Ports can be placed in the traditional RNU template when planning on single docking (RNU and bladder cuff performed without repositioning the robot – though we do not hesitate to re-dock when exposure is suboptimal). For this technique, 8 mm ports are placed in a row after catheter insertion and bladder decompression (Fig. 20.3). The most superior port is placed about 2 fingerbreadths below the costal margin at the mid-clavicular line. As the more inferior ports are placed, each should be placed slightly more medially than the previous port to allow for bladder cuff dissection. If robotic stapler is planned to be used on the hilar structures, the larger 12 mm robotic port is often placed just left of the camera port to accommodate size of stapler. Inner cannula can be used to accommodate smaller instruments when stapler is not on the field. Assistant ports are placed along midline with 10–12 mm port just above the umbilicus and 5 mm port about 1 handbreadth superior to this. Adjustments may be needed depending upon patient size to avoid arm collisions. Other techniques have described success with assistant port placement in line with robotic trocars [102]. The single docking is beneficial in that it does not require reposition or more port placement, but this port positioning can make bladder cuff dissection more difficult, especially with the older Davinci Si models. A double docking technique, conversely, does require robotic repositioning and increased number of ports but improves bladder access and visualization. With the advent of the Da Vinci XI, the rotation of the boom is a very efficient process and can enable better triangulation in the pelvis when performing the distal ureteral dissection. For a right-sided RNU, the camera port is placed just above the level of the umbilicus with two robotic ports placed to the left of the camera about one handbreadth apart and one robotic port to the right of the camera (Fig. 20.3). These should all be placed close to the level of the umbilicus. Assistant ports are placed on the patient's right. This set up is mirrored for left-sided nephroureterectomies.

No matter the port placement, the dissection and bladder cuff management are the same. After ports are placed, the ureter is identified as it crosses the common iliac and is dissected distally, ligating the lateral pedicle to the bladder for visualization. It is helpful to use the fourth arm to retract the bladder to the contralateral side for better visualization (Fig. 20.4). Once the intramural tunnel is identified, a clip is placed as distally as possible on the ureter to prevent tumor spillage during the subsequent dissection. The ureter is then placed on traction, and the detrusor is dissected off until a rim of bladder mucosa is seen clearly around the ureter. At this point, an absorbable stitch is placed at the superior aspect of the planned bladder cuff and tied. The bladder is drained via catheter. The fourth arm can be helpful in either retracting the bladder or retracting the suture upward. Bladder cuff incision is then initiated using robotic scissors and electrocautery as needed. After opening the incision partially, it can be helpful to close the cystotomy using the previously placed suture while visualization is optimal. In addition, the contralateral ureteral orifice can be identified through the cystotomy to prevent injury. Bladder cuff excision is completed alternating between incision and closure until the ureter is completely dissected free. The cystotomy is then closed in a second layer using absorbable suture. After this, a second set of robotic ports can be placed if using the double docking technique, and the surgeon will proceed with the nephrectomy portion of the procedure.

Outcome Comparison

At present, there is no clearly superior bladder cuff technique from an oncologic perspective [93]. Data on bladder cuff recurrence vary based on the study and are likely dependent on operator skill and comfort level with the technique, disease characteristics, and length of follow-up. Current research suggests that recurrence within the bladder, which typically presents within the first 3–4 years after surgery, occurs in 21–40% of patients after RNU but is seen more frequently (30–64%) in patients with incomplete ureteral or bladder cuff excisions [103–106]. Therefore, complete resection is likely more important than the specific technique. There is

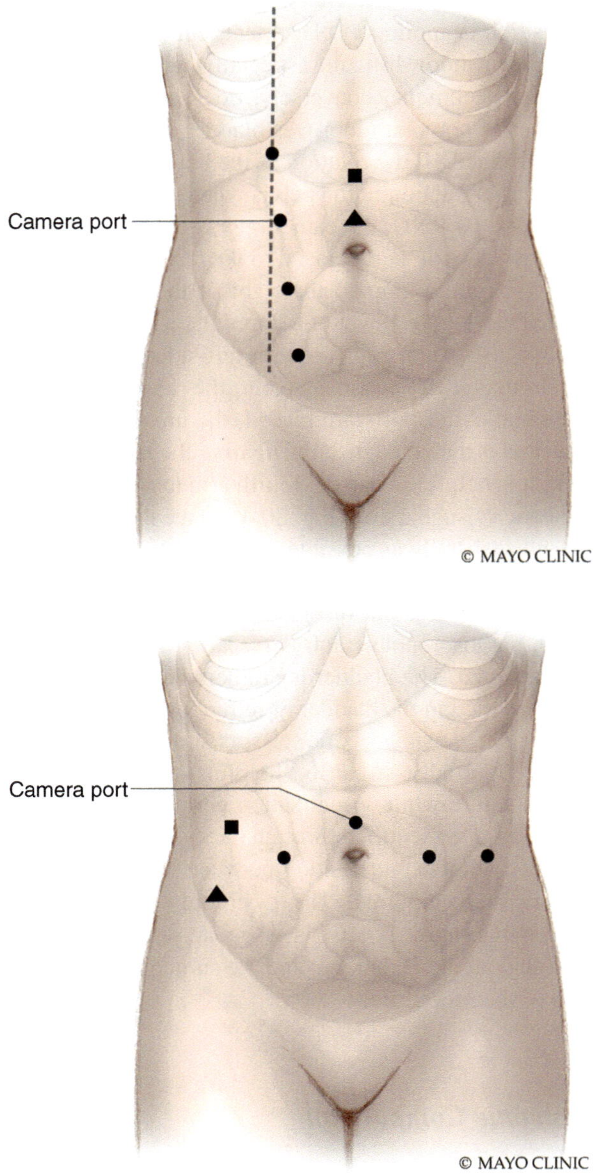

Fig. 20.3 Robotic port placement for nephroureterectomy. Dotted line indicates mid-clavicular line. Circular ports are robotic port sites, square ports are 5 mm ports, and triangular ports are 12 or 15 mm ports. The top image depicts port placement for single docking approach. Image depicts port placement for bladder cuff

some consensus, however, with multiple studies showing increased risk of bladder cuff recurrence in patients undergoing laparoscopic or endoscopic approaches [107, 108]. Endoscopic approaches, in particular, have fallen out of favor due to concerns regarding inadequate distal ureteral resection, prolonged exposure of the bladder to ureteral mucosa in the case of the intussusception technique, and seeding of the extravesical space [94, 96, 98, 105, 109, 110].

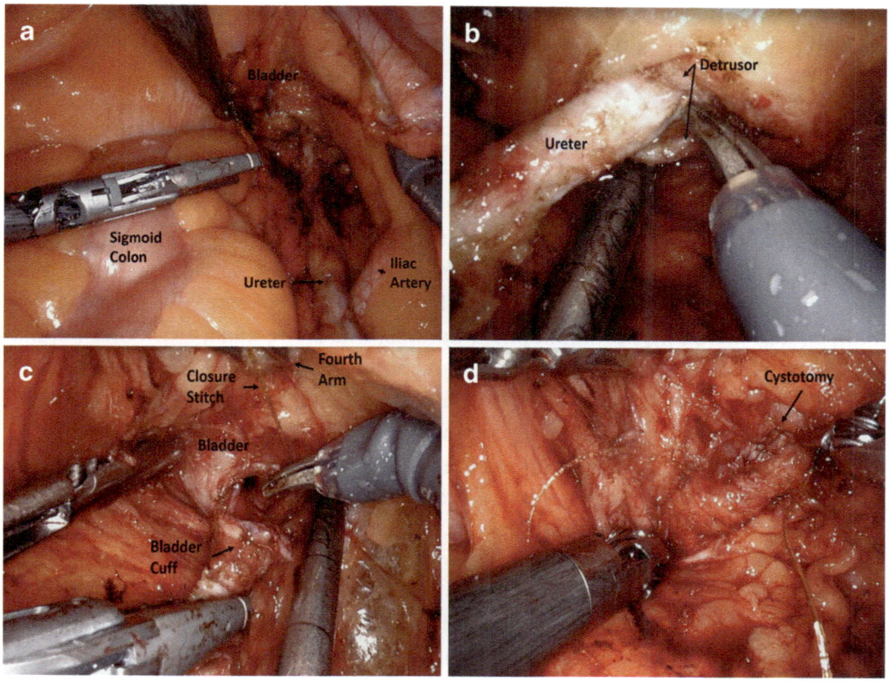

Fig. 20.4 Robotic extravesical bladder cuff technique – (**a**) initial dissection of distal ureter and landmark anatomy. (**b**) Ureter is placed on traction to facilitate dissection of detrusor off the intramural tunnel. (**c**) Prior to incising the bladder, stitch is placed at the superior extent of the cystotomy to prevent retraction of the mucosa after incision is made. The fourth arm is placed on the bladder for better visualization. (**d**) View of cystotomy after a single layer of closure

There is minimal data on the robotic bladder cuff approach with regard to bladder recurrences and oncologic outcomes. However, early studies report comparable OS and CSS as well as intravesical recurrence [86]. Looking at retroperitoneal recurrence and distant metastases, there appears to be no difference between the endoscopic and open techniques [111]. In addition, RFS and CSS do not appear to differ between open and endoscopic bladder cuff techniques [95]. Another factor to evaluate when comparing oncologic outcomes and prognosis based on distal bladder cuff management is positive margin rate [112]. A comparison of current bladder cuff literature by Phe et al. showed that the highest reported positive margin rates were for the laparoscopic stapling technique with rates as high as 25% [112]. As previously discussed, positive margins are a predictor for poor prognosis, suggesting that the laparoscopic technique is possibly inferior. Therefore, while there is no clear data to suggest a superior technique, laparoscopic stapling and endoscopic techniques should be used with caution due to higher rates of bladder recurrences and positive surgical margins. The open technique has not consistently been shown to be superior, but due to the need for extraction site incision for the kidney, this technique may provide the highest level of oncologic control with the lowest learning curve and without subjecting the patient to excess incisions, prolonged operative time, or repositioning.

Post-operative Care

Post-operative care for patients status post RNU follows typical renal surgery pathways. Patients who underwent flank incision or other open surgery approach may require a longer duration of pain control measures. Pain management should be multi-modal including acetaminophen, opioids, muscle relaxants, or other adjunct measures such as topical thermal therapy or abdominal binder. A multi-modal approach allows for decreased use of opioids and earlier mobility. In some cases, epidural or patient-controlled analgesia may be necessary.

Diet and activity should be initiated early. Clear liquids on the day of surgery with progression to solids as tolerated are the typical diet progression for patients regardless of operative approach. Patients should be encouraged to ambulate the day after surgery. Early ambulation and normal diet can lead to earlier discharge and improved recovery.

Thromboembolic and respiratory prophylaxis is essential for a successful recovery. Sequential compression devices or thromboembolic deterrent stockings (TED) are recommended post-operatively to avoid venous thromboembolic (VTE) events. Patients at higher risk for VTE should be placed on pharmacologic prophylaxis such a subcutaneous heparin in combination with mechanical prophylaxis measures. Early activity is also protective against VTE. Patients who undergo laparoscopic or open surgeries will often take shallow inspirations due to pain and may have decreased respirations secondary to opioid use. Deep breathing and use of incentive spirometer are recommended to prevent atelectasis and respiratory infection.

Catheter management is partially dependent on bladder cuff approach and concerns for urine leak post-operatively. Jackson-Pratt drain is useful when placed intraoperatively to monitor for urine leak and fluid output. It is our practice to test drain creatinine the morning of post-operative day 1. If body fluid creatinine of the drain is normal, the drain is removed, and the catheter is removed the following week. A cystogram is often performed prior to catheter removal to ensure watertight bladder cuff closure and adequate healing prior to catheter removal. Patients with normal body fluid creatinine at time of discharge may not require a cystogram prior to catheter removal. Cystogram showing extravasation from bladder cuff indicates need of a longer course of drainage with the catheter and serial cystograms prior to removal. In patients with elevated drain creatinine at the time of discharge, longer drain course and monitoring of drain output are essential. Once drain output decreases and body fluid creatinine is consistent with serum, the drain can be safely removed, and cystogram performed. Providers should have high suspicion for urine leak in those patients with failure to progress or those who present with ileus even in presence of previously normal body fluid creatinine.

Lymph Node Dissection

Curative and Diagnostic Role

Lymph node dissection (LND) should be performed at the time of RNU in high-risk tumors. Regional lymph nodes are the most common metastatic site for UTUC, and up to 30% of patients with muscle invasive UTUC will present with positive lymph nodes at the time of surgery [113, 114]. Lymph node dissection for invasive urothelial carcinoma of the bladder is routinely performed as it may provide survival and prognostic benefit [115, 116]. For UTUC, however, it is unclear as to whether lymph node dissection is curative. Conclusions on the curative role of LND in UTUC are limited due to small study population, lack of well-defined patient selection criteria, lack of standardized LND template, and retrospective nature of studies. In one prospective study using standardized LND templates based on tumor location, patients who underwent LND for renal pelvis cancers pT2 or higher had significantly greater OS and CSS compared to those who did not undergo lymphadenectomy (OS 86.1% vs. 48.0%, CSS 89.8% vs. 51.7%) [117]. No survival improvement was seen in tumors localized to the ureter [117]. A large retrospective review of >2800 patients showed that there was no survival difference in patients who had pN0 compared to pNX disease [118]. This study is limited due to lack of standardized templates, retrospective nature, and possible selection bias of physicians choosing not to perform LND on low-risk patients. Multiple studies have shown that patients with muscle-invasive disease who were pN0 had significantly improved survival compared to those who were pNX [119, 120]. In the ≥pT2 population, 5-year disease-free survival and CSS in those who underwent LND compared to those who did not were 64% vs. 37% and 67% vs. 40%, respectively [121]. Therefore, the curative benefit of LND appears to be greatest in patients with muscle-invasive disease and those with enlarged nodes on imaging.

Lymph node dissection for UTUC is an excellent prognostic tool and helps to identify patients who would benefit from adjuvant systemic therapy since positive lymph nodes and extranodal extension are predictive of decreased survival [122–124]. Patients with pathologically node-positive disease, regardless of grade, had RFS and CSS rates of 29.0% and 35.3% at 5 years, respectively [58]. Those who have not undergone neoadjuvant chemotherapy with extranodal extension have been shown to have significantly higher disease recurrence (HR 2.0, 95% CI 1.44–2.78) and significantly higher cancer-specific mortality (HR 1.97, 95% CI 1.38–2.81) compared to those with positive lymph nodes without extranodal extension [122]. Therefore, extranodal extension appears to be a more powerful predictor of recurrence and poor survival compared to the number of positive nodes alone. Lymph node density has also been thought to be a prognostic factor with those patients having a lymph node density >30% having poorer outcomes [125]. Recent studies have failed to reproduce this finding [122].

Template

One of the main issues with current lymph node dissection research is lack of a standardized template. Fajkovic et al. showed that the median number of lymph nodes removed in regional lymphadenectomy is four and that there is no prognostic value to the number of nodes removed or number of positive nodes [122]. However, other studies have shown that the number of nodes removed does matter. For instance, to achieve a 75% probability of finding one or more positive lymph node, at least eight lymph nodes must be removed [126]. However, if the appropriate template is used, fewer number of nodes may be needed in the dissection for diagnostic and curative resection.

Regional template largely depends on location of tumor. In a study by Kondo et al., sites of tumor deposition via lymphatic spread are well defined (Table 20.1) [127]. Regional template based on this lymphatic spread should include ipsilateral hilar and adjacent paraaortic or paracaval nodes, for pelvic or proximal ureteral tumors, and should include pelvic nodes, for distal ureteral tumors [120, 127–134]. Extended templates are shown in Fig. 20.5 [117]. This differs from the regional template in the following ways: (1) renal pelvis tumor LND inferior boundary at the IMA, (2) addition of retrocaval nodes for right sided renal pelvis tumors, (3) addition of retrocaval nodes for upper 2/3 ureteral mass, and (4) inferior boundary of aortic bifurcation for upper 2/3 ureteral masses.

Complications

Complications of LND are often related to uncontrolled lymphatic drainage. Comparison between patients who had lymph node dissection at time of RNU compared to RNU alone showed higher incidence of lymphorrhea, chyle fistula, and thigh numbness [117]. The incidence of all grade complications is not increased by addition of LND at time of RNU [117].

Table 20.1 Primary site of lymph node metastases based on tumor location

Tumor location within ureter	Primary landing zone: Right ureter	Primary landing zone: Left ureter
Renal pelvis	Renal hilum, paracaval, retrocaval	Renal hilum, paraaortic
Upper 2/3 ureter	Renal hilum, retrocaval, inter-aortocaval	Renal hilum, paraaortic
Lower ureter	Inferior to aortic bifurcation	Inferior to aortic bifurcation

Based on data from Kondo et al. [127]

Intravesical Therapy After Radical Nephroureterectomy

Patients with UTUC are high risk for recurrence within the bladder. Current research suggests recurrence within the bladder occurs in 21–40% of patients after RNU [103–106]. Therapies to avoid recurrence are highly sought after to avoid further surgeries, decrease risk for upper tract seeding in the contralateral solitary kidney, and prevent decreased renal function due to ureteral or bladder obstruction of the solitary kidney. Post-operative instillation of intravesical chemotherapy has been shown to decrease intravesical recurrence. Use of intravesical Mitomycin-c (40 mg in 40 mL) at the time of catheter removal after RNU leads to an 11% absolute risk reduction and 40% relative risk reduction of intravesical recurrence [106]. Instillation of piparubicin within 48 hours after RNU also leads to decreased recurrence rates [135]. A meta-analysis of five trials using intravesical chemotherapy after RNU showed similar risk reduction without serious adverse events related to intravesical therapy [136]. Only 20.5% of patients who received post-operative intravesical therapy had bladder recurrence compared to 36.7% having bladder recurrence in those who did not receive intravesical therapy [136]. Factors

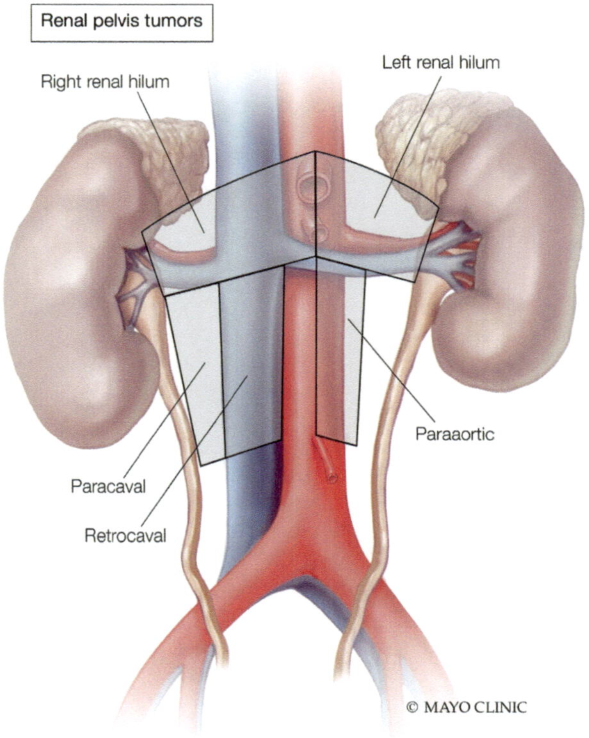

Fig. 20.5 Lymph node dissection template based on location of primary tumor

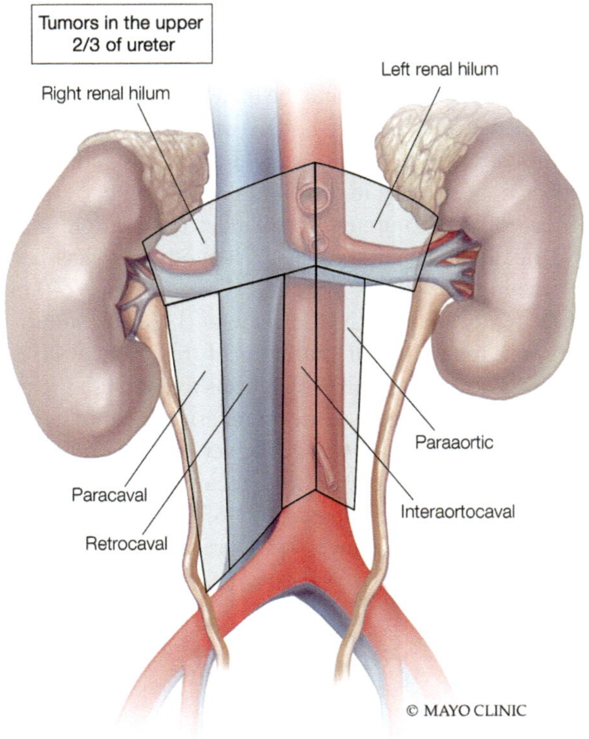

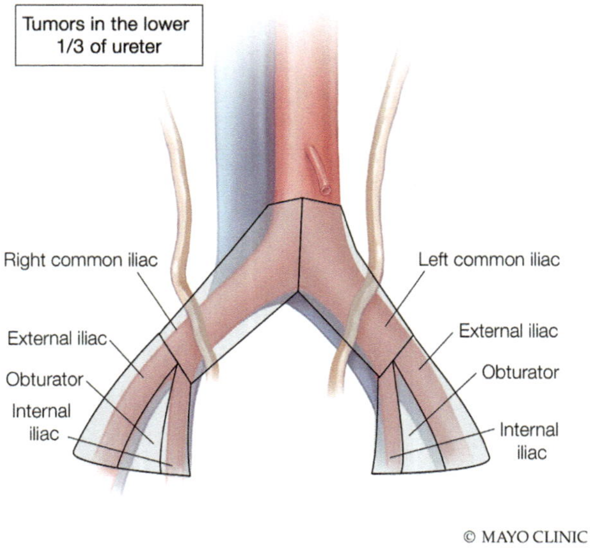

Fig. 20.5 (continued)

associated with increased risk of intravesical recurrence include advanced age, male gender, tumor within the ureter, higher tumor stage, concomitant CIS, lymph node involvement, and prior bladder cancer [107, 137]. Intravesical recurrence does not appear to affect CSS or OS in those with muscle-invasive upper tract disease. However, in those with non-muscle-invasive UTUC, bladder recurrence is associated with significantly decreased CSS and OS [138]. Current recommendation on timing of instillation is to perform the instillation within 10 days of surgery [80]. A cystogram may be performed prior to instillation, but is not necessary [106]. Therefore, while it is unclear if survival is improved with the use of intravesical therapy, use of MMC or other intravesical agents does significantly reduce bladder recurrence.

Systemic Chemotherapy

Neoadjuvant

Neoadjuvant chemotherapy (NAC) use in UTUC has been growing in popularity due to increasing studies showing beneficial effects for UC. Multiple retrospective reviews have shown favorable clinical and pathologic response to NAC. After receiving NAC, up to 80% of patients demonstrate clinical response on imaging studies [139]. Neoadjuvant chemotherapy is associated with significantly decreased incidence of advanced disease stage at time of RNU compared to those receiving RNU alone [140–143]. In a study by Matin et al., pathologic specimens were compared between subjects who were diagnosed with high-grade UTUC and underwent either RNU or NAC followed by RNU. The results showed significant difference in the incidence of pT2 and pT3 or higher-stage tumors favoring the NAC group, when compared to the RNU group (pT2, 48.8% vs. 65.4%; ≥pT3, 27.9% vs. 47.7%) [140]. A second retrospective study reported pathologic downstaging in 27% of patients with high-grade UTUC who received NAC [144]. In addition, pathologic complete response on RNU specimen has been observed in 6–15% of patients after neoadjuvant chemotherapy [140–142, 144].

Evaluation of patients with high-grade cT2-4 disease who underwent neoadjuvant chemotherapy showed that those with pathologic downstaging or pathologic complete response had improved OS [144]. In addition, a literature review by Loew et al. pooled results from six studies showing a 56% OS benefit for those receiving NAC [145]. Kubota et al. compared RFS, CSS, and OS in those patients receiving either NAC and RNU or RNU alone with locally advanced UTUC [146]. They found that NAC use is associated with significantly prolonged RFS and CSS but found no significant improvement in OS [146]. In summary, NAC appears to be effective for UTUC in patients with clinically advanced disease, high-grade disease on biopsy specimen, or other high-risk features. Further prospective trials are needed to define selection criteria demonstrating clear effect.

First-line NAC for UTUC is typically cisplatin-based, though carboplatin is frequently used in those patients who cannot tolerate cisplatin. The majority of studies showing improved oncologic outcomes combine patients receiving cisplatin (GC, MVAC, MVEC, MEP), carboplatin, and occasionally docetaxel-based chemotherapy into the NAC group [143–146]. Oncologic outcomes in these retrospective case control studies between gemcitabine/cisplatin versus gemcitabine/carboplatin have shown no difference in progression-free survival (PFS), CSS, or OS at about 40 months [143, 146]. When looking at quality of life during NAC, gemcitabine/cisplatin is associated with higher rates of gastrointestinal symptoms, decreased physical and functional quality of life, and fatigue compared to gemcitabine/carboplatin [147]. Research on this topic is limited due to infrequent use of neoadjuvant chemotherapy in an already rare disease and retrospective and observational nature of studies. We routinely recommend neoadjuvant chemotherapy in patients with high suspicion of muscle-invasive or locally advanced disease.

Adjuvant

Adjuvant chemotherapy (AC) for UTUC is more widely accepted than NAC due to larger volume of evidence and recent randomized trials showing oncologic benefit. Common chemotherapy used in the adjuvant setting is typically platinum-based though studies have included paclitaxel or other non-platinum-based regimens [145]. Multiple retrospective studies have failed to show that AC provides oncologic benefit in high-risk UTUC patients or have only shown improvement in OS and CSS in small subgroups such as those with LVI [148, 149]. One of the most recent trials, the POUT trial, is a phase 3, open-label, multi-center, randomized control trial of 255 muscle-invasive and/or lymph node-positive UTUC patients without metastases [150]. The patients were randomized to surveillance or four cycles platinum-based AC within 90 days from surgery. At 3 years, the RFS rate in the AC group was 71% compared to only 53% in the RNU alone group [150]. A total of 44% of patients within the AC group developed acute grade 3 or worse chemotherapy-related adverse events including decreased neutrophils or platelets, nausea or vomiting, and neutropenic fever [150]. A second randomized control trial published in 2019 showed improved OS, CSS, and PFS in high-risk UTUC patients who received GC after RNU compared to those who had RNU alone [151]. When looking at the combined results from AC trials in the meta-analysis by Loew et al., the pooled results for OS, CSS, and RFS for the AC group were significantly favorable at 0.77, 0.79, and 0.52, respectively [145]. Therefore, while initial studies did not show significant benefit in use of AC for UTUC, multiple recent randomized trials and retrospective trials have shown improved oncologic outcomes when using AC within the immediate post-operative period in patients with muscle-invasive disease, positive lymph nodes, or LVI [145, 150–152]. We routinely recommend patients to receive adjuvant platinum-based chemotherapy if they had not received it in neoadjuvant setting.

Surveillance

Patients with UTUC are at high risk for recurrence. This risk is present regardless of the treatment modality. It is recommended that these patients undergo cystoscopic surveillance as often as every 3 months for the first year and then at longer intervals afterward [24, 153]. In patients who have <pT2 disease who underwent renal preservation surgery, surveillance should include a combination of ureteroscopy and upper tract cross-sectional imaging with delayed phases at 3–12-month intervals. Concurrent cross-sectional chest imaging is recommended for higher-risk patient undergoing renal preservation surgery.

Metastatic UTUC

Primary Nephroureterectomy

There have been some studies that assess the role of RNU in the setting of metastatic disease, but its role is currently limited. An analysis by Moschini et al. reviewed data from an international, multicenter, multidisciplinary database and evaluated the impact of surgery on the primary tumor site on cancer-specific mortality and overall mortality in patients with metastatic urothelial cell carcinoma. There were 326 patients in the analysis of which 47 (14%) were treated with surgery of the primary site. Nineteen of these patients had a primary UTUC, while the remainder suffered from a primary bladder cancer. On multivariable analysis, surgery was associated with superior cancer-specific mortality (HR 0.59) compared to patients who only received chemotherapy [154]. This benefit was only seen in patients with a single metastatic site. Another study by Nazzani et al. reviewed data from the SEER database that included 1174 patients with metastatic UTUC, 38% of whom underwent RNU. The study found that surgery was a predictor for lower cancer-specific mortality which was confirmed on multivariable analysis and after inverse probability of treatment weighting adjustment [155]. However, retrospective studies evaluating the effect local therapy in patients with metastatic disease are highly influenced by immortal time bias, and caution should be exercised when interpreting these effect estimates. In our practice, a RNU is considered in select patients with metastatic UTUC who have demonstrated a favorable response after systematic therapy.

Metastasectomy

Data on surgical resection of metastatic disease is very limited, but some retrospective studies have shed light on this management approach. For instance, Siefker-Radtke et al. reported outcomes on 31 patients with metastatic urothelial cell carcinoma who underwent metastasectomy. Sites of metastasis included the lung, distant lymph nodes, brain, and subcutaneous tissue. All visible gross disease was resected in 97% of patients. The 5-year survival after metastasectomy was 33% suggesting that surgery may provide some survival benefit in these patients [156]. Another study by Lehmann et al. reported the German exposure of metastasectomy across 15 centers. This included 44 patients with metastatic bladder or UTUC who underwent complete resection of detectable metastasis. The 5-year OS after surgery was 28% which again suggests that there may be a survival benefit with surgery in patients with metastatic urothelial cell carcinoma [157]. There have been additional studies that have reported an oncological benefit of surgical resection in patients with metastatic UTUC after systematic therapy, where optimal patients are those who have had a favorable response and/or have limited areas of metastasis [158, 159]. We consider surgical resection of metastatic sites in highly selected motivated patients who have a favorable response to systemic therapy and have oligometastatic disease.

Systemic Therapy

First-Line Therapy

Platinum-Based Chemotherapy

Urothelial carcinoma is generally regarded as chemo-sensitive disease. Cisplatin-based combination chemotherapy is typically the first-line option in managing patients with metastatic UTUC. Data on platinum-based chemotherapy for UTUC is mostly extrapolated from studies assessing advanced urothelial cell cancer studies that involve bladder cancer. Most first-line regimens include gemcitabine/cisplatin (GC) or dose-dense methotrexate/vinblastine/doxorubicin/cisplatin (ddMVAC). MVAC was historically the first-line regimen, as this demonstrated complete remission in around 36% of patients with metastatic urothelial cell carcinoma but was associated with toxicity, with significant rates of grade 3+ myelosuppression, mucositis, sepsis, and some reports of drug-related deaths [160]. Both GC and ddMVAC have been associated with, at least similar or in the case of ddMVAC, superior, oncological outcomes compared to MVAC. In addition, these regimens are much better tolerated than standard MVAC [161, 162]. With regard to efficacy of cisplatin-based chemotherapy in metastatic UTUC, a study by Moschini et al. evaluated three EORTC studies that assessed efficacy of MVAC and/or GC in patients with advanced urothelial cell carcinoma and investigated whether tumor location affected survival in these patients. In 1039 patients, progression-free and overall survival did not differ between bladder and UTUC, suggesting that outcomes between the two disease processes are similar after treatment with cisplatin-based chemotherapy [163]. However most of the patients with UTUC may have previously undergone a RNU and may not have suitable kidney function. As a result, these patients may receive carboplatin instead of cisplatin. The two drugs are not considered equivalent in efficacy; however carboplatin is very active in this disease [164]. The overall goal of chemotherapy is to achieve disease remission or stabilization which can help improve survival of the patient. Most patients will progress and succumb to their disease after subsequent lines of therapy.

Checkpoint Inhibitors

Checkpoint inhibitors are antibodies designed to target the programmed death (PD-1) pathway and prevent tumor cells from binding PD-1/PD-L1 receptors/ligands on T cells. As a result, these immune cells can be activated and exhibit their normal functions that include stimulating cytokine release and cytotoxic activity of tumor cells [165].

There are currently five immune checkpoint inhibitors approved for advanced urothelial carcinoma including pembrolizumab, atezolizumab, nivolumab, durvalumab, and avelumab. Pembrolizumab and atezolizumab are also approved for first-line cisplatin-ineligible patients who have high expression of PD-L1 in tumor-infiltrating immune cells. Pembrolizumab was approved based on KEYNOTE-052 which was a multicenter single-arm phase 2 study that assessed first-line pembrolizumab in cisplatin-ineligible patients with metastatic urothelial cancer [166]. Three-hundred and seventy-four patients were enrolled, 59 of whom had UTUC. In the patients with UTUC, 13 (22%) achieved an objective radiological response. In the entire cohort, including advanced metastatic bladder cancer, disease control was achieved in 173 (47%) of patients, and 17 (5%) achieved a complete response. A PD-L1 expression cutoff of 10% was associated with a higher frequency of response to therapy. Sixty-two percent of patients experienced an adverse effect, with 16% experiencing a grade 3 or worse complication. Another study assessed the effects of atezolizumab, a PD-L1 inhibitor, in patients with metastatic urothelial cell carcinoma. This study similarly focused on patients with metastatic urothelial carcinoma who were previously untreated and cisplatin ineligible. In 119 patients who received therapy, the objective response rate was 23%, and complete response was 9%. In the 33 patients with UTUC, there was an objective response in 13 (39%) patients. This drug was well-tolerated overall with 35% of patients experiencing some form of adverse effect [167].

In the subsequent large phase III trials exploring checkpoint inhibitors irrespective of patients' PD-L1 expression status and after prior exposure to chemotherapy, response rates were in the range of 15–20%. The response rates were quite similar among other agents (Table 20.2).

Immunotherapy can also be used in the maintenance setting, after achieving response to chemotherapy or at the time of progression irrespective of patients' PD-L1 expression status. Avelumab is the only checkpoint inhibitor approved for maintenance therapy in patients with advanced urothelial carcinoma. The approval was based on a large phase III clinical trial randomizing 700 patients, who had received platinum-based chemotherapy and had no progression, to avelumab and

Table 20.2 Immune checkpoint inhibitors used in the metastatic urothelial carcinoma after platinum failure

Drug	Objective response rate %	Response lasting more than 6 months
Atezolizumab [168]	15%	84%
Pembrolizumab [169]	21.1%	72%
Nivolumab [170]	19.6%	77%
Durvalumab [171]	20.4%	81%
Avelumab [172]	18.2%	NA

best supportive care vs best supportive care alone. The trial met its primary end point with median overall survival in the avelumab arm 21 months vs 14 months (HR 0.69, $p = 0.001$) in the supportive care. The adverse effects were consistent with known toxicities of avelumab [173].

Immune checkpoint inhibitors provide potential to achieve a complete remission in a small group of patients and thus are integral to the treatment paradigm of patients with advanced UC despite very low response rates. First-line checkpoint inhibitors are generally used in clinical practice in patients with low volume disease. These agents may not cause immediate debulking of the cancer as observed with more traditional cytotoxic therapy [169]. For this reason, patients who are symptomatic from their disease and are suitable for chemotherapy are best served with combination chemotherapy in the beginning of the treatment and then can transition to immunotherapy after they have achieved some degree of response as a maintenance strategy. Immune checkpoint therapy brings its own set of challenges with autoimmune side effects which require an astute physician to diagnose and treat them in a timely fashion with immunosuppressive medication as they can potentially become life-threatening [174].

Second-Line Therapy

Enfortumab is a medication in a new class of therapies called antibody drug conjugates. This is a highly sophisticated pharmacologic system designed to deliver cytotoxic payloads using an antibody directed toward the specific tumor antigens. Enfortumab delivers monomethyl auristatin E (MMAE), a microtubule inhibitor that inhibits cell division, to tumors expressing nectin-4, which is overexpressed in UC cells. It is approved for patients with advanced urothelial carcinoma who had previously received platinum-based chemotherapy and an immune checkpoint inhibitor. The drug was investigated in a large phase II clinical trial in patients who were previously heavily treated. Forty-four percent patients had a response with 12% achieving complete response. The response onset was very quick and was observed across all subgroups. Estimated median PFS was 5.8 months. This is a significant improvement over traditional second-line cytotoxic therapy. Despite targeting the chemotherapy to the tumor cell, the drug has significant toxicities including fatigue, alopecia, neuropathy, rash, decreased appetite, and dysgeusia. Few patients also reported severe Steven-Johnson-like syndrome and neutropenia. However, no toxicity-related death was reported [175].

Erdafitinib is another new in class FGFR3 inhibitor which is approved for advanced urothelial carcinoma patients, harboring alterations in FGFR3, who had progressed after platinum-based chemotherapy. This is a potent oral small molecule tyrosine kinase inhibitor of FGFR1-4. The drug was evaluated in an uncontrolled single arm phase II study in patients harboring these alterations. Forty percent of the patients had confirmed response with 3% patients achieving complete response. Median PFS was 5.5 months. Treatment-related grade 3 or high side effects were observed in 46% of the patients including hyponatremia (11%), stomatitis (10%), and asthenia (7%). Other less common but significant toxicity includes hyperphosphatemia, retinal detachment, and skin toxicity [176].

Salvage or Third-Line Therapy

In patients who require additional systemic therapy following recurrence or progression after initial therapy for metastatic disease, there are several options that have been investigated. Historically, systemic chemotherapy has been administered in this setting. One option that had been commonly used in Europe was vinflunine, a microtubule inhibitor. A study by Bellmunt et al. assessed its efficacy in this setting. This was a phase 3 trial that compared vinflunine plus supportive care vs supportive care after disease progression following platinum-based therapy [177]. The study included 370 patients who were randomly assigned to the two treatment modalities. On multivariable analysis, vinflunine was associated with significantly greater survival benefit, reducing the death risk by 23%, and the median survival for this regimen was longer than in those who only received supportive care (6.9 vs 4.3 months). Other agents that have been studied include gemcitabine, pemetrexed, and taxanes, as single agents, and have demonstrated similar effects [178–180]. Combination chemotherapeutic options have also been reported in this setting and have generally achieved better response rates compared to single agents, though with the cost of increased adverse effects. Examples of combination therapy include paclitaxel/gemcitabine and paclitaxel/carboplatin [181, 182].

If patients previously responded to cisplatin-based chemotherapy, repeating a cisplatin-based regimen may be an effective option. For instance, Han et al. assessed the efficacy of standard MVAC in the setting of patients who failed first-line gemcitabine/cisplatin. The overall response rate was 30% and a complete response was achieved in 6.7% of patients. The median OS was 10.9 months. This was not without toxicities, as 63.3% of patients experienced a grade 3 neutropenia and 30% experienced a grades 3–4 thrombocytopenia [183]. Another study by Edeline et al. assessed accelerated dose MVAC in the setting of patients who failed gemcitabine-platinum therapy. There were 45 patients who were reviewed, 61% of whom experienced a response, with 10% achieving a complete response. The median OS was 14.2 months. Regarding toxicities, 69% of patients experienced a grades 3–4 adverse reaction [184]. In general, there are very few patients who would be suitable for any chemotherapy after initial lines of therapy. We always encourage patients with good performance status to explore clinical trial or offer palliative care.

References

1. Raman JD, Messer J, Sielatycki JA, Hollenbeak CS. Incidence and survival of patients with carcinoma of the ureter and renal pelvis in the USA, 1973-2005. BJU Int. 2011;107(7):1059–64.
2. Siegel RL, Miller KD, Jemal A. Cancer statistics, 2017. CA Cancer J Clin. 2017;67(1):7–30.
3. Rink M, Robinson BD, Green DA, Cha EK, Hansen J, Comploj E, et al. Impact of histological variants on clinical outcomes of patients with upper urinary tract urothelial carcinoma. J Urol. 2012;188(2):398–404.
4. Desai FS, Nongthombam J, Singh LS. Retrospective evaluation of risk factors and immunohistochemical findings for pre-neoplastic and neoplastic lesions of upper urinary tract in patients with chronic nephrolithiasis. Asian Pac J Cancer Prev. 2015;16(18):8293–8.
5. Azemar MD, Comperat E, Richard F, Cussenot O, Roupret M. Bladder recurrence after surgery for upper urinary tract urothelial cell carcinoma: frequency, risk factors, and surveillance. Urol Oncol. 2011;29(2):130–6.
6. Pommer W, Bronder E, Klimpel A, Helmert U, Greiser E, Molzahn M. Urothelial cancer at different tumour sites: role of smoking and habitual intake of analgesics and laxatives. Results of the Berlin Urothelial Cancer Study. Nephrol Dial Transplant. 1999;14(12):2892–7.
7. Rink M, Xylinas E, Margulis V, Cha EK, Ehdaie B, Raman JD, et al. Impact of smoking on oncologic outcomes of upper tract urothelial carcinoma after radical nephroureterectomy. Eur Urol. 2013;63(6):1082–90.
8. Cosyns JP. Aristolochic acid and 'Chinese herbs nephropathy' - a review of the evidence to date. Drug Saf. 2003;26(1):33–48.
9. Colin P, Koenig P, Ouzzane A, Berthon N, Villers A, Biserte J, et al. Environmental factors involved in carcinogenesis of urothelial cell carcinomas of the upper urinary tract. BJU Int. 2009;104(10):1436–40.
10. Jelakovic B, Karanovic S, Vukovic-Lela I, Miller F, Edwards KL, Nikolic J, et al. Aristolactam-DNA adducts are a biomarker of environmental exposure to aristolochic acid. Kidney Int. 2012;81(6):559–67.
11. Cosyns JP, Jadoul M, Squifflet JP, De Plaen JF, Ferluga D, van Ypersele de Strihou C. Chinese herbs nephropathy: a clue to Balkan endemic nephropathy? Kidney Int. 1994;45(6):1680–8.
12. Cosyns JP, Jadoul M, Squifflet JP, Van Cangh PJ, van Ypersele de Strihou C. Urothelial malignancy in nephropathy due to Chinese herbs. Lancet. 1994;344(8916):188.
13. Nortier JL, Martinez MM, Schmeiser HH, Arlt VM, Bieler CA, Petein M, et al. Urothelial carcinoma associated with the use of a Chinese herb (Aristolochia fangchi). N Engl J Med. 2000;342(23):1686–92.
14. Zaitsu M, Kawachi I, Takeuchi T, Kobayashi Y. Alcohol consumption and risk of upper-tract urothelial cancer. Cancer Epidemiol. 2017;48:36–40.
15. Yang MH, Chen KK, Yen CC, Wang WS, Chang YH, Huang WJ, et al. Unusually high incidence of upper urinary tract urothelial carcinoma in Taiwan. Urology. 2002;59(5):681–7.
16. Saint-Jacques N, Parker L, Brown P, Dummer TJ. Arsenic in drinking water and urinary tract cancers: a systematic review of 30 years of epidemiological evidence. Environ Health. 2014;13:44.
17. Brenner DW, Schellhammer PF. Upper tract urothelial malignancy after cyclophosphamide therapy: a case report and literature review. J Urol. 1987;137(6):1226–7.
18. Lee JY, Kim K, Sung HH, Jeon HG, Jeong BC, Seo SI, et al. Molecular characterization of urothelial carcinoma of the bladder and upper urinary tract. Transl Oncol. 2018;11(1):37–42.

19. Sfakianos JP, Cha EK, Iyer G, Scott SN, Zabor EC, Shah RH, et al. Genomic characterization of upper tract urothelial carcinoma. Eur Urol. 2015;68(6):970–7.
20. Metcalfe MJ, Petros FG, Rao P, Mork ME, Xiao L, Broaddus RR, et al. Universal point of care testing for Lynch syndrome in patients with upper tract urothelial carcinoma. J Urol. 2018;199(1):60–5.
21. Roupret M, Yates DR, Comperat E, Cussenot O. Upper urinary tract urothelial cell carcinomas and other urological malignancies involved in the hereditary nonpolyposis colorectal cancer (lynch syndrome) tumor spectrum. Eur Urol. 2008;54(6):1226–36.
22. van der Post RS, Kiemeney LA, Ligtenberg MJ, Witjes JA, Hulsbergen-van de Kaa CA, Bodmer D, et al. Risk of urothelial bladder cancer in Lynch syndrome is increased, in particular among MSH2 mutation carriers. J Med Genet. 2010;47(7):464–70.
23. Vasen HF, Mecklin JP, Khan PM, Lynch HT. The international collaborative group on hereditary non-polyposis colorectal cancer (ICG-HNPCC). Dis Colon Rectum. 1991;34(5): 424–5.
24. Roupret M, Babjuk M, Comperat E, Zigeuner R, Sylvester RJ, Burger M, et al. European Association of Urology guidelines on upper urinary tract urothelial carcinoma: 2017 update. Eur Urol. 2018;73(1):111–22.
25. Janisch F, Shariat SF, Baltzer P, Fajkovic H, Kimura S, Iwata T, et al. Diagnostic performance of multidetector computed tomographic (MDCTU) in upper tract urothelial carcinoma (UTUC): a systematic review and meta-analysis. World J Urol. 2020;38(5):1165–75.
26. Takahashi N, Glockner JF, Hartman RP, King BF, Leibovich BC, Stanley DW, et al. Gadolinium enhanced magnetic resonance urography for upper urinary tract malignancy. J Urol. 2010;183(4):1330–65.
27. Cosentino M, Palou J, Gaya JM, Breda A, Rodriguez-Faba O, Villavicencio-Mavrich H. Upper urinary tract urothelial cell carcinoma: location as a predictive factor for concomitant bladder carcinoma. World J Urol. 2013;31(1):141–5.
28. Samson P, Smith AD, Hoenig D, Okeke Z. Endoscopic management of upper urinary tract urothelial carcinoma. J Endourol. 2018;32(S1):S10–S6.
29. Joseph JP, Potretzke TA, Packiam V, Sharma V, Toussi A, Miest TS, et al. Percutaneous image-guided core needle biopsy for upper tract urothelial carcinoma. Urology. 2020;135:95–100.
30. Huang SY, Ahrar K, Gupta S, Wallace MJ, Ensor JE, Krishnamurthy S, et al. Safety and diagnostic accuracy of percutaneous biopsy in upper tract urothelial carcinoma. BJU Int. 2015;115(4):625–32.
31. Malm C, Grahn A, Jaremko G, Tribukait B, Brehmer M. Diagnostic accuracy of upper tract urothelial carcinoma: how samples are collected matters. Scand J Urol. 2017;51(2):137–45.
32. Johannes JR, Nelson E, Bibbo M, Bagley DH. Voided urine fluorescence in situ hybridization testing for upper tract urothelial carcinoma surveillance. J Urol. 2010;184(3):879–82.
33. Fradet Y, Grossman HB, Gomella L, Lerner S, Cookson M, Albala D, et al. A comparison of hexaminolevulinate fluorescence cystoscopy and white light cystoscopy for the detection of carcinoma in situ in patients with bladder cancer: a phase III, multicenter study. J Urol. 2007;178(1):68–73; discussion.
34. Mukherjee P, George AJP, Yadav BK, Jeyaseelan L, Kumar RM, Mukha RP, et al. The impact of narrow band imaging in the detection and resection of bladder tumor in transitional cell carcinoma of the bladder: a prospective, blinded, sequential intervention randomized controlled trial. Urology. 2019;128:55–61.
35. Kata SG, Aboumarzouk OM, Zreik A, Somani B, Ahmad S, Nabi G, et al. Photodynamic diagnostic ureterorenoscopy: a valuable tool in the detection of upper urinary tract tumour. Photodiagn Photodyn Ther. 2016;13:255–60.
36. Ahmad S, Aboumarzouk O, Somani B, Nabi G, Kata SG. Oral 5-aminolevulinic acid in simultaneous photodynamic diagnosis of upper and lower urinary tract transitional cell carcinoma - a prospective audit. BJU Int. 2012;110(11 Pt B):E596–600.
37. Traxer O, Geavlete B, de Medina SG, Sibony M, Al-Qahtani SM. Narrow-band imaging digital flexible ureteroscopy in detection of upper urinary tract transitional-cell carcinoma: initial experience. J Endourol. 2011;25(1):19–23.

38. Shariat SF, Godoy G, Lotan Y, Droller M, Karakiewicz PI, Raman JD, et al. Advanced patient age is associated with inferior cancer-specific survival after radical nephroureterectomy. BJU Int. 2010;105(12):1672–7.
39. Martinez-Salamanca JI, Shariat SF, Rodriguez JC, Chromecki TF, Ficarra V, Fritsche HM, et al. Prognostic role of ECOG performance status in patients with urothelial carcinoma of the upper urinary tract: an international study. BJU Int. 2012;109(8):1155–61.
40. Crivelli JJ, Xylinas E, Kluth LA, Rieken M, Rink M, Shariat SF. Effect of smoking on outcomes of urothelial carcinoma: a systematic review of the literature. Eur Urol. 2014;65(4):742–54.
41. Brierly JD, Gospodarowicz MK, Wittekind C. TNM classification of malignant tumours. Wiley-Blackwell; 2017.
42. Lughezzani G, Burger M, Margulis V, Matin SF, Novara G, Roupret M, et al. Prognostic factors in upper urinary tract urothelial carcinomas: a comprehensive review of the current literature. Eur Urol. 2012;62(1):100–14.
43. Isbarn H, Jeldres C, Shariat SF, Liberman D, Sun M, Lughezzani G, et al. Location of the primary tumor is not an independent predictor of cancer specific mortality in patients with upper urinary tract urothelial carcinoma. J Urol. 2009;182(5):2177–81.
44. Ehdaie B, Chromecki TF, Lee RK, Lotan Y, Margulis V, Karakiewicz PI, et al. Obesity adversely impacts disease specific outcomes in patients with upper tract urothelial carcinoma. J Urol. 2011;186(1):66–72.
45. Akdogan B, Dogan HS, Eskicorapci SY, Sahin A, Erkan I, Ozen H. Prognostic significance of bladder tumor history and tumor location in upper tract transitional cell carcinoma. J Urol. 2006;176(1):48–52.
46. Ouzzane A, Colin P, Xylinas E, Pignot G, Ariane MM, Saint F, et al. Ureteral and multifocal tumours have worse prognosis than renal pelvic tumours in urothelial carcinoma of the upper urinary tract treated by nephroureterectomy. Eur Urol. 2011;60(6):1258–65.
47. Chen XP, Xiong GY, Li XS, Matin SF, Garcia M, Fang D, et al. Predictive factors for worse pathological outcomes of upper tract urothelial carcinoma: experience from a nationwide high-volume centre in China. BJU Int. 2013;112(7):917–24.
48. Favaretto RL, Shariat SF, Savage C, Godoy G, Chade DC, Kaag M, et al. Combining imaging and ureteroscopy variables in a preoperative multivariable model for prediction of muscle-invasive and non-organ confined disease in patients with upper tract urothelial carcinoma. BJU Int. 2012;109(1):77–82.
49. Boorjian S, Ng C, Munver R, Palese MA, Vaughan ED Jr, Sosa RE, et al. Impact of delay to nephroureterectomy for patients undergoing ureteroscopic biopsy and laser tumor ablation of upper tract transitional cell carcinoma. Urology. 2005;66(2):283–7.
50. Sundi D, Svatek RS, Margulis V, Wood CG, Matin SF, Dinney CP, et al. Upper tract urothelial carcinoma: impact of time to surgery. Urol Oncol. 2012;30(3):266–72.
51. Waldert M, Karakiewicz PI, Raman JD, Remzi M, Isbarn H, Lotan Y, et al. A delay in radical nephroureterectomy can lead to upstaging. BJU Int. 2010;105(6):812–7.
52. Ito Y, Kikuchi E, Tanaka N, Miyajima A, Mikami S, Jinzaki M, et al. Preoperative hydronephrosis grade independently predicts worse pathological outcomes in patients undergoing nephroureterectomy for upper tract urothelial carcinoma. J Urol. 2011;185(5):1621–6.
53. Berod AA, Colin P, Yates DR, Ouzzane A, Audouin M, Adam E, et al. The role of American Society of Anesthesiologists scores in predicting urothelial carcinoma of the upper urinary tract outcome after radical nephroureterectomy: results from a national multi-institutional collaborative study. BJU Int. 2012;110(11 Pt C):E1035–40.
54. Mullerad M, Russo P, Golijanin D, Chen HN, Tsai HH, Donat SM, et al. Bladder cancer as a prognostic factor for upper tract transitional cell carcinoma. J Urol. 2004;172(6 Pt 1):2177–81.
55. Lughezzani G, Jeldres C, Isbarn H, Sun M, Shariat SF, Alasker A, et al. Nephroureterectomy and segmental ureterectomy in the treatment of invasive upper tract urothelial carcinoma: a population-based study of 2299 patients. Eur J Cancer. 2009;45(18):3291–7.
56. Novara G, De Marco V, Gottardo F, Dalpiaz O, Bouygues V, Galfano A, et al. Independent predictors of cancer-specific survival in transitional cell carcinoma of the upper urinary tract: multi-institutional dataset from 3 European centers. Cancer. 2007;110(8):1715–22.

57. Park J, Ha SH, Min GE, Song C, Hong B, Hong JH, et al. The protective role of renal parenchyma as a barrier to local tumor spread of upper tract transitional cell carcinoma and its impact on patient survival. J Urol. 2009;182(3):894–9.
58. Margulis V, Shariat SF, Matin SF, Kamat AM, Zigeuner R, Kikuchi E, et al. Outcomes of radical nephroureterectomy: a series from the Upper Tract Urothelial Carcinoma Collaboration. Cancer. 2009;115(6):1224–33.
59. Kikuchi E, Margulis V, Karakiewicz PI, Roscigno M, Mikami S, Lotan Y, et al. Lymphovascular invasion predicts clinical outcomes in patients with node-negative upper tract urothelial carcinoma. J Clin Oncol. 2009;27(4):612–8.
60. Colin P, Ouzzane A, Yates DR, Audenet F, Pignot G, Arvin-Berod A, et al. Influence of positive surgical margin status after radical nephroureterectomy on upper urinary tract urothelial carcinoma survival. Ann Surg Oncol. 2012;19(11):3613–20.
61. Langner C, Hutterer G, Chromecki T, Rehak P, Zigeuner R. Patterns of invasion and histological growth as prognostic indicators in urothelial carcinoma of the upper urinary tract. Virchows Arch. 2006;448(5):604–11.
62. Simone G, Papalia R, Loreto A, Leonardo C, Sentinelli S, Gallucci M. Independent prognostic value of tumour diameter and tumour necrosis in upper urinary tract urothelial carcinoma. BJU Int. 2009;103(8):1052–7.
63. Zigeuner R, Shariat SF, Margulis V, Karakiewicz PI, Roscigno M, Weizer A, et al. Tumour necrosis is an indicator of aggressive biology in patients with urothelial carcinoma of the upper urinary tract. Eur Urol. 2010;57(4):575–81.
64. Roupret M, Colin P, Yates DR. A new proposal to risk stratify urothelial carcinomas of the upper urinary tract (UTUCs) in a predefinitive treatment setting: low-risk versus high-risk UTUCs. Eur Urol. 2014;66(2):181–3.
65. Cutress ML, Stewart GD, Wells-Cole S, Phipps S, Thomas BG, Tolley DA. Long-term endoscopic management of upper tract urothelial carcinoma: 20-year single-centre experience. BJU Int. 2012;110(11):1608–17.
66. Krambeck AE, Thompson RH, Lohse CM, Patterson DE, Segura JW, Zincke H, et al. Endoscopic management of upper tract urothelial carcinoma in patients with a history of bladder urothelial carcinoma. J Urol. 2007;177(5):1721–6.
67. Moore K, Khastgir J, Ghei M. Endoscopic management of upper tract urothelial carcinoma. Adv Urol. 2009;2009:620604.
68. Liatsikos EN, Dinlenc CZ, Kapoor R, Smith AD. Transitional-cell carcinoma of the renal pelvis: ureteroscopic and percutaneous approach. J Endourol. 2001;15(4):377–83; discussion 97.
69. Jeldres C, Lughezzani G, Sun M, Isbarn H, Shariat SF, Budaus L, et al. Segmental ureterectomy can safely be performed in patients with transitional cell carcinoma of the ureter. J Urol. 2010;183(4):1324–9.
70. Veccia A, Antonelli A, Checcucci E, Falagario U, Carrieri G, Guruli G, et al. Segmental ureterectomy for upper tract urothelial carcinoma: a systematic review and meta-analysis of comparative studies. Clin Genitourin Cancer. 2020;18(1):E10–20.
71. Diagnosis and treatment of non-muscle invasive bladder cancer: AUA/SUO joint guideline: American Urological Association. Available from: http://www.auanet.org/guidelines/non-muscle-invasive-bladder-cancer-(aua/suo-joint-guideline-2016.
72. Gadzinski AJ, Roberts WW, Faerber GJ, Wolf JS Jr. Long-term outcomes of immediate versus delayed nephroureterectomy for upper tract urothelial carcinoma. J Endourol. 2012;26(5):566–73.
73. Lee JN, Kwon S, Choi G, Kim H, Kim T-H, Kwon TG, et al. Impact of surgical wait time on oncologic outcomes in upper urinary tract urothelial carcinoma. J Surg Oncol. 2014;110
74. Kleinmann N, Matin SF, Pierorazio PM, Gore JL, Shabsigh A, Hu B, et al. Primary chemoablation of low-grade upper tract urothelial carcinoma using UGN-101, a mitomycin-containing reverse thermal gel (OLYMPUS): an open-label, single-arm, phase 3 trial. Lancet Oncol. 2020;21(6):776–85.
75. Roupret M, Colin P, Yates D. A new proposal to risk stratify urothelial carcinomas of the upper urinary tract (UTUCs) in a predefinitive treatment setting: low-risk versus high-risk UTUCs. Eur Urol. 2013;66

76. Seisen T, Colin P, Rouprêt M. Risk-adapted strategy for the kidney-sparing management of upper tract tumours. Nat Rev Urol. 2015;12(3):155–66.
77. Xia L, Taylor BL, Pulido JE, Guzzo TJ. Impact of surgical waiting time on survival in patients with upper tract urothelial carcinoma: a national cancer database study. Urol Oncol. 2018;36(1):10.e5–10.e22.
78. Simsir A, Sarsik B, Cureklibatir I, Sen S, Gunaydin G, Cal C. Prognostic factors for upper urinary tract urothelial carcinomas: stage, grade, and smoking status. Int Urol Nephrol. 2011;43(4):1039–45.
79. Smith JA, Howards SS, Preminger GM, Hinman F. Hinman's atlas of urologic surgery. 3rd ed. Philadelphia: Elsevier/Saunders; 2012. xxix, 1151 p.
80. Roupret M, Babjuk M, Comperat E, Zigeuner R, Sylvester RJ, Burger M, et al. European Association of Urology guidelines on upper urinary tract urothelial cell carcinoma: 2015 update. Eur Urol. 2015;68(5):868–79.
81. Colin P, Ouzzane A, Yates DR, François A, Pignot G, Arvin-Berod A, et al. Influence of positive surgical margin status after radical nephroureterectomy on upper urinary tract urothelial carcinoma survival. Ann Surg Oncol. 2012;19(11):3613–20.
82. Favaretto RL, Shariat SF, Chade DC, Godoy G, Kaag M, Cronin AM, et al. Comparison between laparoscopic and open radical nephroureterectomy in a contemporary group of patients: are recurrence and disease-specific survival associated with surgical technique? Eur Urol. 2010;58(5):645–51.
83. Walton TJ, Novara G, Matsumoto K, Kassouf W, Fritsche HM, Artibani W, et al. Oncological outcomes after laparoscopic and open radical nephroureterectomy: results from an international cohort. BJU Int. 2011;108(3):406–12.
84. Ni S, Tao W, Chen Q, Liu L, Jiang H, Hu H, et al. Laparoscopic versus open nephroureterectomy for the treatment of upper urinary tract urothelial carcinoma: a systematic review and cumulative analysis of comparative studies. Eur Urol. 2012;61(6):1142–53.
85. Ariane MM, Colin P, Ouzzane A, Pignot G, Audouin M, Cornu JN, et al. Assessment of oncologic control obtained after open versus laparoscopic nephroureterectomy for upper urinary tract urothelial carcinomas (UUT-UCs): results from a large French multicenter collaborative study. Ann Surg Oncol. 2012;19(1):301–8.
86. Clements MB, Krupski TL, Culp SH. Robotic-assisted surgery for upper tract urothelial carcinoma: a comparative survival analysis. Ann Surg Oncol. 2018;25(9):2550–62.
87. Rodriguez JF, Packiam VT, Boysen WR, Johnson SC, Smith ZL, Smith ND, et al. Utilization and outcomes of nephroureterectomy for upper tract urothelial carcinoma by surgical approach. J Endourol. 2017;31(7):661–5.
88. Peyronnet B, Seisen T, Dominguez-Escrig JL, Bruins HM, Yuan CY, Lam T, et al. Oncological outcomes of laparoscopic nephroureterectomy versus open radical Nephroureterectomy for upper tract urothelial carcinoma: an European Association of Urology Guidelines Systematic Review. Eur Urol Focus. 2019;5(2):205–23.
89. Simone G, Papalia R, Guaglianone S, Ferriero M, Leonardo C, Forastiere E, et al. Laparoscopic versus open nephroureterectomy: perioperative and oncologic outcomes from a randomised prospective study. Eur Urol. 2009;56(3):520–6.
90. Aboumohamed AA, Krane LS, Hemal AK. Oncologic outcomes following robot-assisted laparoscopic nephroureterectomy with bladder cuff excision for upper tract urothelial carcinoma. J Urol. 2015;194(6):1561–6.
91. Rouprêt M, Smyth G, Irani J, Guy L, Davin JL, Saint F, et al. Oncological risk of laparoscopic surgery in urothelial carcinomas. World J Urol. 2009;27(1):81–8.
92. Ong AM, Bhayani SB, Pavlovich CP. Trocar site recurrence after laparoscopic nephroureterectomy. J Urol. 2003;170(4 Pt 1):1301.
93. Macejko AM, Pazona JF, Loeb S, Kimm S, Nadler RB. Management of distal ureter in laparoscopic nephroureterectomy--a comprehensive review of techniques. Urology. 2008;72(5):974–81.
94. Abercrombie GF, Eardley I, Payne SR, Walmsley BH, Vinnicombe J. Modified nephroureterectomy. Long-term follow-up with particular reference to subsequent bladder tumours. Br J Urol. 1988;61(3):198–200.

95. Walton TJ, Sherwood BT, Parkinson RJ, Obakponovwe O, Thomas SA, Taylor MC, et al. Comparative outcomes following endoscopic ureteral detachment and formal bladder cuff excision in open nephroureterectomy for upper urinary tract transitional cell carcinoma. J Urol. 2009;181(2):532–9.
96. Giovansili B, Peyromaure M, Saighi D, Dayma T, Zerbib M, Debre B. Stripping technique for endoscopic management of distal ureter during nephroureterectomy: experience of 32 procedures. Urology. 2004;64(3):448–52; discussion 52.
97. Gill IS, Soble JJ, Miller SD, Sung GT. A novel technique for management of the en bloc bladder cuff and distal ureter during laparoscopic nephroureterectomy. J Urol. 1999;161(2):430–4.
98. Wein AJ, Kavoussi LR, Campbell MF. Campbell-Walsh urology / editor-in-chief, Alan J. Wein ; [editors, Louis R. Kavoussi ... et al.]. 10th ed. Philadelphia: Elsevier Saunders; 2012.
99. Steinberg JR, Matin SF. Laparoscopic radical nephroureterectomy: dilemma of the distal ureter. Curr Opin Urol. 2004;14(2):61–5.
100. Tsivian A, Benjamin S, Sidi AA. A sealed laparoscopic nephroureterectomy: a new technique. Eur Urol. 2007;52(4):1015–9.
101. Nanigian DK, Smith W, Ellison LM. Robot-assisted laparoscopic nephroureterectomy. J Endourol. 2006;20(7):463–5; discussion 5–6.
102. Zargar H, Krishnan J, Autorino R, Akca O, Brandao LF, Laydner H, et al. Robotic nephroureterectomy: a simplified approach requiring no patient repositioning or robot redocking. Eur Urol. 2014;66(4):769–77.
103. Raman JD, Ng CK, Boorjian SA, Vaughan ED Jr, Sosa RE, Scherr DS. Bladder cancer after managing upper urinary tract transitional cell carcinoma: predictive factors and pathology. BJU Int. 2005;96(7):1031–5.
104. Zigeuner RE, Hutterer G, Chromecki T, Rehak P, Langner C. Bladder tumour development after urothelial carcinoma of the upper urinary tract is related to primary tumour location. BJU Int. 2006;98(6):1181–6.
105. Xylinas E, Rink M, Cha EK, Clozel T, Lee RK, Fajkovic H, et al. Impact of distal ureter management on oncologic outcomes following radical nephroureterectomy for upper tract urothelial carcinoma. Eur Urol. 2014;65(1):210–7.
106. O'Brien T, Ray E, Singh R, Coker B, Beard R. Prevention of bladder tumours after nephroureterectomy for primary upper urinary tract urothelial carcinoma: a prospective, multicentre, randomised clinical trial of a single postoperative intravesical dose of mitomycin C (the ODMIT-C trial). Eur Urol. 2011;60(4):703–10.
107. Xylinas E, Kluth L, Passoni N, Trinh QD, Rieken M, Lee RK, et al. Prediction of intravesical recurrence after radical nephroureterectomy: development of a clinical decision-making tool. Eur Urol. 2014;65(3):650–8.
108. Saika T, Nishiguchi J, Tsushima T, Nasu Y, Nagai A, Miyaji Y, et al. Comparative study of ureteral stripping versus open ureterectomy for nephroureterectomy in patients with transitional carcinoma of the renal pelvis. Urology. 2004;63(5):848–52.
109. Jones DR, Moisey CU. A cautionary tale of the modified "pluck" nephroureterectomy. Br J Urol. 1993;71(4):486.
110. Arango O, Bielsa O, Carles J, Gelabert-Mas A. Massive tumor implantation in the endoscopic resected area in modified nephroureterectomy. J Urol. 1997;157(5):1839.
111. Li WM, Shen JT, Li CC, Ke HL, Wei YC, Wu WJ, et al. Oncologic outcomes following three different approaches to the distal ureter and bladder cuff in nephroureterectomy for primary upper urinary tract urothelial carcinoma. Eur Urol. 2010;57(6):963–9.
112. Phe V, Cussenot O, Bitker MO, Roupret M. Does the surgical technique for management of the distal ureter influence the outcome after nephroureterectomy? BJU Int. 2011;108(1):130–8.
113. Zigeuner R, Pummer K. Urothelial carcinoma of the upper urinary tract: surgical approach and prognostic factors. Eur Urol. 2008;53(4):720–31.
114. Arancibia MF, Bolenz C, Michel MS, Keeley FX Jr, Alken P. The modern management of upper tract urothelial cancer: surgical treatment. BJU Int. 2007;99(5):978–81.
115. Leissner J, Hohenfellner R, Thuroff JW, Wolf HK. Lymphadenectomy in patients with transitional cell carcinoma of the urinary bladder; significance for staging and prognosis. BJU Int. 2000;85(7):817–23.

116. Herr HW, Bochner BH, Dalbagni G, Donat SM, Reuter VE, Bajorin DF. Impact of the number of lymph nodes retrieved on outcome in patients with muscle invasive bladder cancer. J Urol. 2002;167(3):1295–8.
117. Kondo T, Hara I, Takagi T, Kodama Y, Hashimoto Y, Kobayashi H, et al. Template-based lymphadenectomy in urothelial carcinoma of the renal pelvis: a prospective study. Int J Urol. 2014;21(5):453–9.
118. Lughezzani G, Jeldres C, Isbarn H, Shariat SF, Sun M, Pharand D, et al. A critical appraisal of the value of lymph node dissection at nephroureterectomy for upper tract urothelial carcinoma. Urology. 2010;75(1):118–24.
119. Roscigno M, Shariat SF, Margulis V, Karakiewicz P, Remzi M, Kikuchi E, et al. Impact of lymph node dissection on cancer specific survival in patients with upper tract urothelial carcinoma treated with radical nephroureterectomy. J Urol. 2009;181(6):2482–9.
120. Brausi MA, Gavioli M, De Luca G, Verrini G, Peracchia G, Simonini G, et al. Retroperitoneal lymph node dissection (RPLD) in conjunction with nephroureterectomy in the treatment of infiltrative transitional cell carcinoma (TCC) of the upper urinary tract: impact on survival. Eur Urol. 2007;52(5):1414–8.
121. Roscigno M, Cozzarini C, Bertini R, Scattoni V, Freschi M, Da Pozzo LF, et al. Prognostic value of lymph node dissection in patients with muscle-invasive transitional cell carcinoma of the upper urinary tract. Eur Urol. 2008;53(4):794–802.
122. Fajkovic H, Cha EK, Jeldres C, Donner G, Chromecki TF, Margulis V, et al. Prognostic value of extranodal extension and other lymph node parameters in patients with upper tract urothelial carcinoma. J Urol. 2012;187(3):845–51.
123. Roupret M, Hupertan V, Seisen T, Colin P, Xylinas E, Yates DR, et al. Prediction of cancer specific survival after radical nephroureterectomy for upper tract urothelial carcinoma: development of an optimized postoperative nomogram using decision curve analysis. J Urol. 2013;189(5):1662–9.
124. Roscigno M, Brausi M, Heidenreich A, Lotan Y, Margulis V, Shariat SF, et al. Lymphadenectomy at the time of nephroureterectomy for upper tract urothelial cancer. Eur Urol. 2011;60(4):776–83.
125. Bolenz C, Shariat SF, Fernandez MI, Margulis V, Lotan Y, Karakiewicz P, et al. Risk stratification of patients with nodal involvement in upper tract urothelial carcinoma: value of lymph-node density. BJU Int. 2009;103(3):302–6.
126. Roscigno M, Shariat SF, Freschi M, Margulis V, Karakiewizc P, Suardi N, et al. Assessment of the minimum number of lymph nodes needed to detect lymph node invasion at radical nephroureterectomy in patients with upper tract urothelial cancer. Urology. 2009;74(5):1070–4.
127. Kondo T, Nakazawa H, Ito F, Hashimoto Y, Toma H, Tanabe K. Primary site and incidence of lymph node metastases in urothelial carcinoma of upper urinary tract. Urology. 2007;69(2):265–9.
128. Skinner D. The pelvic ureter. J R Soc Med. 1978;71(7):541.
129. McCarron JP, Mills C, Vaughn ED Jr. Tumors of the renal pelvis and ureter: current concepts and management. Semin Urol. 1983;1(1):75–81.
130. Heney NM, Nocks BN, Daly JJ, Blitzer PH, Parkhurst EC. Prognostic factors in carcinoma of the ureter. J Urol. 1981;125(5):632–6.
131. Grabstald H, Whitmore WF, Melamed MR. Renal pelvic tumors. JAMA. 1971;218(6):845–54.
132. Cummings KB. Nephroureterectomy: rationale in the management of transitional cell carcinoma of the upper urinary tract. Urol Clin North Am. 1980;7(3):569–78.
133. Batata MA, Whitmore WF, Hilaris BS, Tokita N, Grabstald H. Primary carcinoma of the ureter: a prognostic study. Cancer. 1975;35(6):1626–32.
134. Batata M, Grabstald H. Upper urinary tract urothelial tumors. Urol Clin North Am. 1976;3(1):79–86.
135. Ito A, Shintaku I, Satoh M, Ioritani N, Aizawa M, Tochigi T, et al. Prospective randomized phase II trial of a single early intravesical instillation of pirarubicin (THP) in the prevention of bladder recurrence after nephroureterectomy for upper urinary tract urothelial carcinoma: the THP Monotherapy Study Group Trial. J Clin Oncol. 2013;31(11):1422–7.

136. Fang D, Li XS, Xiong GY, Yao L, He ZS, Zhou LQ. Prophylactic intravesical chemotherapy to prevent bladder tumors after nephroureterectomy for primary upper urinary tract urothelial carcinomas: a systematic review and meta-analysis. Urol Int. 2013;91(3):291–6.
137. Elalouf V, Xylinas E, Klap J, Pignot G, Delongchamps NB, Saighi D, et al. Bladder recurrence after radical nephroureterectomy: predictors and impact on oncological outcomes. Int J Urol. 2013;20(11):1078–83.
138. Yamashita S, Ito A, Mitsuzuka K, Tochigi T, Namima T, Soma F, et al. Clinical implications of intravesical recurrence after radical nephroureterectomy for upper urinary tract urothelial carcinoma. Int J Urol. 2016;23(5):378–84.
139. Meng X, Chao B, Vijay V, Silver H, Margolin EJ, Balar A, et al. High response rates to neoadjuvant chemotherapy in high-grade upper tract urothelial carcinoma. Urology. 2019;129:146–52.
140. Matin SF, Margulis V, Kamat A, Wood CG, Grossman HB, Brown GA, et al. Incidence of downstaging and complete remission after neoadjuvant chemotherapy for high-risk upper tract transitional cell carcinoma. Cancer. 2010;116(13):3127–34.
141. Liao RS, Gupta M, Schwen ZR, Patel HD, Kates M, Johnson MH, et al. Comparison of pathological stage in patients treated with and without neoadjuvant chemotherapy for high risk upper tract urothelial carcinoma. J Urol. 2018;200(1):68–73.
142. Almassi N, Gao T, Lee B, Stein RJ, Haber GP, Ornstein MC, et al. Impact of neoadjuvant chemotherapy on pathologic response in patients with upper tract urothelial carcinoma undergoing extirpative surgery. Clin Genitourin Cancer. 2018;16(6):e1237–e42.
143. Hosogoe S, Hatakeyama S, Kusaka A, Hamano I, Iwamura H, Fujita N, et al. Platinum-based neoadjuvant chemotherapy improves oncological outcomes in patients with locally advanced upper tract urothelial carcinoma. Eur Urol Focus. 2018;4(6):946–53.
144. Martini A, Daza J, Poltiyelova E, Gul Z, Heard JR, Ferket BS, et al. Pathological downstaging as a novel endpoint for the development of neoadjuvant chemotherapy for upper tract urothelial carcinoma. BJU Int. 2019;124:665–71.
145. Leow JJ, Chong YL, Chang SL, Valderrama BP, Powles T, Bellmunt J. Neoadjuvant and adjuvant chemotherapy for upper tract urothelial carcinoma: a 2020 systematic review and meta-analysis, and future perspectives on systemic therapy. Eur Urol. 2021;79(5):635–54.
146. Kubota Y, Hatakeyama S, Tanaka T, Fujita N, Iwamura H, Mikami J, et al. Oncological outcomes of neoadjuvant chemotherapy in patients with locally advanced upper tract urothelial carcinoma: a multicenter study. Oncotarget. 2017;8(60):101500–8.
147. Fukushi K, Narita T, Hatakeyama S, Yamamoto H, Soma O, Matsumoto T, et al. Quality-of-life evaluation during platinum-based neoadjuvant chemotherapies for urothelial carcinoma. Int J Clin Oncol. 2017;22(2):366–72.
148. Lee KS, Kim KH, Yoon YE, Choi KH, Yang SC, Han WK. Impact of adjuvant chemotherapy in patients with upper tract urothelial carcinoma and lymphovascular invasion after radical nephroureterectomy. Korean J Urol. 2015;56(1):41–7.
149. Hellenthal N, Shariat S, Margulis V, Karakiewicz P, Roscigno M, Bolenz C, et al. Adjuvant chemotherapy for high risk upper tract urothelial carcinoma: results from the upper tract urothelial carcinoma collaboration. J Urol. 2009;182:900–6.
150. Birtle A, Johnson M, Chester J, Jones R, Dolling D, Bryan RT, et al. Adjuvant chemotherapy in upper tract urothelial carcinoma (the POUT trial): a phase 3, open-label, randomised controlled trial. Lancet. 2020;395(10232):1268–77.
151. Luo Y, Feng BF, Wei DC, Han YL, Li MC, Zhao JH, et al. [Prospective controlled observation of effect of adjuvant chemotherapy on survival and prognosis of high-risk upper tract urothelial carcinoma patients underwent radical nephroureterectomy]. Zhonghua Yi Xue Za Zhi. 2019;99(40):3158–63.
152. Cho KS, Joung JY, Seo HK, Cho IC, Chung HS, Chung J, et al. Renal safety and efficacy of cisplatin-based chemotherapy in patients with a solitary kidney after nephroureterectomy for urothelial carcinoma of the upper urinary tract. Cancer Chemother Pharmacol. 2011;67(4):769–74.

153. Bladder cancer: national comprehensive cancer network. Available from: https://www.nccn.org/professionals/physician_gls/PDF/bladder.pdf.
154. Moschini M, Xylinas E, Zamboni S, Mattei A, Niegisch G, Yu EY, et al. Efficacy of surgery in the primary tumor site for metastatic urothelial cancer: analysis of an international, multicenter, multidisciplinary database. Eur Urol Oncol. 2020;3(1):94–101.
155. Nazzani S, Preisser F, Mazzone E, Marchioni M, Bandini M, Tian Z, et al. Survival effect of nephroureterectomy in metastatic upper urinary tract urothelial carcinoma. Clin Genitourin Cancer. 2019;17(3):e602–e11.
156. Siefker-Radtke AO, Walsh GL, Pisters LL, Shen Y, Swanson DA, Logothetis CJ, et al. Is there a role for surgery in the management of metastatic urothelial cancer? The M. D. Anderson experience. J Urol. 2004;171(1):145–8.
157. Lehmann J, Suttmann H, Albers P, Volkmer B, Gschwend JE, Fechner G, et al. Surgery for metastatic urothelial carcinoma with curative intent: the German experience (AUO AB 30/05). Eur Urol. 2009;55(6):1293–9.
158. Miller RS, Freiha FS, Reese JH, Ozen H, Torti FM. Cisplatin, methotrexate and vinblastine plus surgical restaging for patients with advanced transitional cell carcinoma of the urothelium. J Urol. 1993;150(1):65–9.
159. Dodd PM, McCaffrey JA, Herr H, Mazumdar M, Bacik J, Higgins G, et al. Outcome of postchemotherapy surgery after treatment with methotrexate, vinblastine, doxorubicin, and cisplatin in patients with unresectable or metastatic transitional cell carcinoma. J Clin Oncol. 1999;17(8):2546–52.
160. Sternberg CN, Yagoda A, Scher HI, Watson RC, Geller N, Herr HW, et al. Methotrexate, vinblastine, doxorubicin, and cisplatin for advanced transitional cell carcinoma of the urothelium. Efficacy and patterns of response and relapse. Cancer. 1989;64(12):2448–58.
161. von der Maase H, Sengelov L, Roberts JT, Ricci S, Dogliotti L, Oliver T, et al. Long-term survival results of a randomized trial comparing gemcitabine plus cisplatin, with methotrexate, vinblastine, doxorubicin, plus cisplatin in patients with bladder cancer. J Clin Oncol. 2005;23(21):4602–8.
162. von der Maase H, Hansen SW, Roberts JT, Dogliotti L, Oliver T, Moore MJ, et al. Gemcitabine and cisplatin versus methotrexate, vinblastine, doxorubicin, and cisplatin in advanced or metastatic bladder cancer: results of a large, randomized, multinational, multicenter, phase III study. J Clin Oncol. 2000;18(17):3068–77.
163. Moschini M, Shariat SF, Roupret M, De Santis M, Bellmunt J, Sternberg CN, et al. Impact of primary tumor location on survival from the European Organization for the Research and Treatment of Cancer advanced urothelial cancer studies. J Urol. 2018;199(5):1149–57.
164. Linardou H, Aravantinos G, Efstathiou E, Kalofonos C, Anagnostopoulos A, Deliveliotis C, et al. Gemcitabine and carboplatin combination as first-line treatment in elderly patients and those unfit for cisplatin-based chemotherapy with advanced bladder carcinoma: phase II study of the Hellenic Co-operative Oncology Group. Urology. 2004;64(3):479–84.
165. Ribas A. Tumor immunotherapy directed at PD-1. N Engl J Med. 2012;366(26):2517–9.
166. Balar AV, Castellano D, O'Donnell PH, Grivas P, Vuky J, Powles T, et al. First-line pembrolizumab in cisplatin-ineligible patients with locally advanced and unresectable or metastatic urothelial cancer (KEYNOTE-052): a multicentre, single-arm, phase 2 study. Lancet Oncol. 2017;18(11):1483–92.
167. Balar AV, Galsky MD, Rosenberg JE, Powles T, Petrylak DP, Bellmunt J, et al. Atezolizumab as first-line treatment in cisplatin-ineligible patients with locally advanced and metastatic urothelial carcinoma: a single-arm, multicentre, phase 2 trial. Lancet. 2017;389(10064):67–76.
168. Rosenberg JE, Hoffman-Censits J, Powles T, van der Heijden MS, Balar AV, Necchi A, et al. Atezolizumab in patients with locally advanced and metastatic urothelial carcinoma who have progressed following treatment with platinum-based chemotherapy: a single-arm, multicentre, phase 2 trial. Lancet. 2016;387(10031):1909–20.
169. Bellmunt J, de Wit R, Vaughn DJ, Fradet Y, Lee JL, Fong L, et al. Pembrolizumab as second-line therapy for advanced urothelial carcinoma. N Engl J Med. 2017;376(11):1015–26.

170. Sharma P, Retz M, Siefker-Radtke A, Baron A, Necchi A, Bedke J, et al. Nivolumab in metastatic urothelial carcinoma after platinum therapy (CheckMate 275): a multicentre, single-arm, phase 2 trial. Lancet Oncol. 2017;18(3):312–22.
171. Powles T, O'Donnell PH, Massard C, Arkenau HT, Friedlander TW, Hoimes CJ, et al. Efficacy and safety of durvalumab in locally advanced or metastatic urothelial carcinoma: updated results from a phase 1/2 open-label study. JAMA Oncol. 2017;3(9):e172411.
172. Patel MR, Ellerton J, Infante JR, Agrawal M, Gordon M, Aljumaily R, et al. Avelumab in metastatic urothelial carcinoma after platinum failure (JAVELIN Solid Tumor): pooled results from two expansion cohorts of an open-label, phase 1 trial. Lancet Oncol. 2018;19(1):51–64.
173. Powles T, Park SH, Voog E, Caserta C, Valderrama BP, Gurney H, et al. Avelumab maintenance therapy for advanced or metastatic urothelial carcinoma. N Engl J Med. 2020;383(13):1218–30.
174. Kottschade L, Brys A, Peikert T, Ryder M, Raffals L, Brewer J, et al. A multidisciplinary approach to toxicity management of modern immune checkpoint inhibitors in cancer therapy. Melanoma Res. 2016;26(5):469–80.
175. Rosenberg JE, O'Donnell PH, Balar AV, McGregor BA, Heath EI, Yu EY, et al. Pivotal trial of enfortumab vedotin in urothelial carcinoma after platinum and anti-programmed death 1/ programmed death ligand 1 therapy. J Clin Oncol. 2019;37(29):2592–600.
176. Loriot Y, Necchi A, Park SH, Garcia-Donas J, Huddart R, Burgess E, et al. Erdafitinib in locally advanced or metastatic urothelial carcinoma. N Engl J Med. 2019;381(4):338–48.
177. Bellmunt J, Theodore C, Demkov T, Komyakov B, Sengelov L, Daugaard G, et al. Phase III trial of vinflunine plus best supportive care compared with best supportive care alone after a platinum-containing regimen in patients with advanced transitional cell carcinoma of the urothelial tract. J Clin Oncol. 2009;27(27):4454–61.
178. McCaffrey JA, Hilton S, Mazumdar M, Sadan S, Kelly WK, Scher HI, et al. Phase II trial of docetaxel in patients with advanced or metastatic transitional-cell carcinoma. J Clin Oncol. 1997;15(5):1853–7.
179. Joly F, Tchen N, Chevreau C, Henry-Amar M, Priou F, Chinet-Charrot P, et al. Clinical benefit of second line weekly paclitaxel in advanced urothelial carcinoma (AUC): a GETUG phase II study. J Clin Oncol. 2004;22(14):411s-s.
180. Sweeney CJ, Roth BJ, Kabbinavar FF, Vaughn DI, Arning M, Curiel RE, et al. Phase II study of pemetrexed for second-line treatment of transitional cell cancer of the urothelium. J Clin Oncol. 2006;24(21):3451–7.
181. Kouno T, Ando M, Yonemori K, Matsumoto K, Shimizu C, Katsumata N, et al. Weekly paclitaxel and carboplatin against advanced transitional cell cancer after failure of a platinum-based regimen. Eur Urol. 2007;52(4):1115–22.
182. Otto T, Bex A, Krege S, Walz PH, Rubben H. Paclitaxel-based second-line therapy for patients with advanced chemotherapy-resistant bladder carcinoma (M1): a clinical phase II study. Cancer. 1997;80(3):465–70.
183. Han KS, Joung JY, Kim TS, Jeong IG, Seo HK, Chung J, et al. Methotrexate, vinblastine, doxorubicin and cisplatin combination regimen as salvage chemotherapy for patients with advanced or metastatic transitional cell carcinoma after failure of gemcitabine and cisplatin chemotherapy. Br J Cancer. 2008;98(1):86–90.
184. Edeline J, Loriot Y, Culine S, Massard C, Albiges L, Blesius A, et al. Accelerated MVAC chemotherapy in patients with advanced bladder cancer previously treated with a platinum-gemcitabine regimen. Eur J Cancer. 2012;48(8):1141–6.

Index

K. L. Stratton, A. K. Morgans (eds.), *Urologic Oncology*, https://doi.org/10.1007/978-3-030-89891-5

N

Batch number: 08998949

Printed by Printforce, the Netherlands